Assessing Psychological Trauma and PTSD

Assessing Psychological Trauma and PTSD

SECOND EDITION

Edited by
John P. Wilson
Terence M. Keane

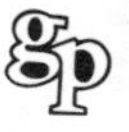

THE GUILFORD PRESS
New York London

A Division of Guilford Publications, Inc.
72 Spring Street, New York, NY 10012
www.guilford.com

Printed in the United States of America

This book is printed on acid-free paper.

Last digit is print number: 9 8 7 6 5 4 3 2 1

Library of Congress Cataloging-in-Publication Data

Assessing psychological trauma and PTSD / edited by John P. Wilson, Terence M. Keane.—2nd ed.
p. cm.
Includes bibliographical references and index.
ISBN 1-59385-035-2 (hardcover: alk. paper)
1. Post-traumatic stress disorder—Diagnosis. 2. Psychodiagnostics. 3. Neuropsychological tests. I. Wilson, John P. (John Preston) II. Keane, Terence Martin.
RC552.P67A85 2004
616.85′21—dc22

2004005746

The legacy of the 20th century is that of unparalleled scientific and cultural advancement of the human race and, at the same time, the creation of weapons of mass destruction, unprecedented world and regional wars that have claimed the lives of over 100 million people, and the specter of the annihilation of the species by nuclear holocaust.

The advent of posttraumatic stress disorder (PTSD) as a scientific–medical diagnosis in 1980 made possible the careful assessment and evaluation of the consequences of traumas, small and catastrophic, to the well-being of individuals and humankind as a whole. In many ways, the advent of PTSD as a trauma-related condition can be understood as an evolutionary development in response to the prevalence of human violence and trauma-inducing situations that dominated the 20th century.

This book is dedicated to the ameliorative, constructive processes of world peace, justice, and human rights and to the movement toward eliminating the conditions that cause trauma, PTSD, and injuries to the human spirit.

About the Editors

John P. Wilson, PhD, is Professor of Psychology at Cleveland State University, a Fulbright Scholar, and a widely recognized international expert on posttraumatic stress disorder. He is also cofounder and Past President of the International Society for Traumatic Stress Studies as well as a Diplomate and Fellow of the American Academy of Experts in Traumatic Stress and a Fellow of the American Institute of Stress. Dr. Wilson is the coeditor of *Countertransference in the Treatment of PTSD,* with Jacob D. Lindy, and *Treating Psychological Trauma and PTSD,* with Matthew J. Friedman and Jacob D. Lindy.

Terence M. Keane, PhD, is Professor and Vice Chairman of Research in Psychiatry at the Boston University School of Medicine. He is also Chief of Psychology and Director of the National Center for PTSD at the VA Boston Healthcare System. Past President of the International Society for Traumatic Stress Studies (ISTSS), Dr. Keane has published six books and over 160 articles on the assessment and treatment of posttraumatic stress disorder. His contributions to the field have been recognized by many honors, including the Robert Laufer Award for Outstanding Scientific Achievement from ISTSS, a Fulbright Scholarship, and an Outstanding Research Contribution Award and the Distinguished Service Award from the Division of Public Service Psychologists of the American Psychological Association. Dr. Keane is a Fellow of the American Psychological Association and the American Psychological Society and has lectured and conducted workshops internationally on topics related to psychological trauma.

Contributors

Deane Aikins, PhD, Department of Veterans Affairs Medical Center, National Center for PTSD, and Department of Psychiatry, Yale University School of Medicine, New Haven, Connecticut

John Briere, PhD, Department of Psychiatry and the Behavioral Sciences, Keck School of Medicine, University of Southern California, Los Angeles, California

Richard A. Bryant, PhD, School of Psychology, University of New South Wales, Sydney, Australia

Todd C. Buckley, PhD, Department of Veterans Affairs, National Center for PTSD, VA Boston Healthcare System, and Department of Psychiatry, Boston University School of Medicine, Boston, Massachusetts

Juesta M. Caddell, PhD, Research Triangle Institute, Research Triangle Park, North Carolina; Department of Psychiatry and Behavioral Sciences, Duke University Medical Center, Durham, North Carolina

Lori Ebert, PhD, Research Triangle Institute, Research Triangle Park, North Carolina

John A. Fairbank, PhD, Department of Psychiatry and Behavioral Sciences, Duke University Medical Center, Durham, North Carolina

Matthew J. Friedman, MD, PhD, Department of Veterans Affairs Medical Center, National Center for PTSD, White River Junction, Vermont; Departments of Psychiatry and Pharmacology, Dartmouth Medical School, Hanover, New Hampshire

Bonnie L. Green, PhD, Department of Psychiatry, Georgetown University Medical Center, Washington, DC

Jessica L. Hamblen, PhD, Department of Veterans Affairs Medical Center, National Center for PTSD, White River Junction, Vermont

B. Kathleen Jordan, PhD, Research Triangle Institute, Research Triangle Park, North Carolina; Department of Psychiatry and Behavioral Sciences, Duke University Medical Center, Durham, North Carolina

Danny G. Kaloupek, PhD, Department of Psychiatry, Boston University School of Medicine, and Department of Veterans Affairs, National Center for PTSD, VA Boston Healthcare System, Boston, Massachusetts

Joan Kaufman, PhD, Department of Psychiatry, Child and Adolescent Research and Education Program, Yale University School of Medicine, New Haven, Connecticut

Terence M. Keane, PhD, Department of Veterans Affairs, National Center for PTSD, VA Boston Healthcare System, and Department of Psychiatry, Boston University School of Medicine, Boston, Massachusetts

Rachel Kimerling, PhD, Palo Alto Veterans Affairs Healthcare System, National Center for PTSD, Menlo Park, California

Jeffrey A. Knight, PhD, Department of Veterans Affairs, National Center for PTSD—Behavioral Sciences Division, VA Boston Healthcare System, and Department of Psychiatry, Boston University School of Medicine, Boston, Massachusetts

John Krystal, MD, Department of Psychiatry, Yale University School of Medicine, New Haven, Connecticut

Tina Lee, MD, Palo Alto Veterans Affairs Healthcare System, National Center for PTSD, Menlo Park, California

Patti Levin, LICSW, PsyD, private practice, Cambridge, Massachusetts

Toni Luxenberg, PsyD, private practice, Brookline, Massachusetts

Charles R. Marmar, MD, Department of Psychiatry, University of California, San Francisco, and Posttraumatic Stress Disorder Program, Department of Veterans Affairs Medical Center, San Francisco, California

Nada Martinek, MPH, Department of Psychiatry, University of Queensland, Brisbane, Australia

Linda J. Metzger, PhD, Department of Psychiatry, Harvard Medical School, Boston, Massachusetts; Department of Veterans Affairs Medical Center, Manchester, New Hampshire

Thomas J. Metzler, MA, Department of Psychiatry, University of California, San Francisco, and Posttraumatic Stress Disorder Program, Department of Veterans Affairs Medical Center, San Francisco, California

Mark W. Miller, PhD, Department of Psychiatry, Boston University School of Medicine, and Department of Veterans Affairs, National Center for PTSD, VA Boston Healthcare System, Boston, Massachusetts

Thomas A. Moran, JCD, Case Western Reserve University School of Law, Cleveland, Ohio

Kathleen O. Nader, DSW, Two Suns, Cedar Park, Texas

Lisa M. Najavits, PhD, Department of Psychiatry, Harvard Medical School, Boston, Massachusetts; Trauma Research Program, McLean Hospital, Belmont, Massachusetts

Fran H. Norris, PhD, Departments of Psychiatry and Community and Family Medicine, Dartmouth Medical School, Lebanon, New Hampshire; National Center for PTSD, White River Junction, Vermont

Scott P. Orr, PhD, Department of Psychiatry, Harvard Medical School, Boston, Massachusetts; Department of Veterans Affairs Medical Center, Manchester, New Hampshire

Christian Otte, PhD, Department of Psychiatry, University of California, San Francisco, and Posttraumatic Stress Disorder Program, Department of Veterans Affairs Medical Center, San Francisco, California

Annabel Prins, PhD, Palo Alto Veterans Affairs Healthcare System, National Center for PTSD, Menlo Park, California

Beverley Raphael, MD, Centre for Mental Health, NSW Health Department, Sydney, Australia

William E. Schlenger, PhD, Research Triangle Institute, Research Triangle Park, North Carolina; Department of Psychiatry and Behavioral Sciences, Duke University Medical Center, Durham, North Carolina; Department of Psychology, North Carolina State University, Raleigh, North Carolina

Paula P. Schnurr, PhD, Department of Veterans Affairs Medical Center, National Center for PTSD, White River Junction, Vermont; Department of Psychiatry, Dartmouth Medical School, Hanover, New Hampshire

Jane Stafford, PhD, Department of Veterans Affairs, National Center for PTSD, VA Boston Healthcare System, Boston, Massachusetts

Marlene Steinberg, MD, private practice, Northampton, Massachusetts

Amy E. Street, PhD, Department of Veterans Affairs, National Center for PTSD, VA Boston Healthcare System, and Department of Psychiatry, Boston University School of Medicine, Boston, Massachusetts

Casey T. Taft, PhD, Department of Veterans Affairs, National Center for PTSD—Behavioral Sciences Division, VA Boston Healthcare System, and Department of Psychiatry, Boston University School of Medicine, Boston, Massachusetts

Daniel S. Weiss, PhD, Department of Psychiatry, University of California, San Francisco, San Francisco, California

Darrah Westrup, PhD, Palo Alto Veterans Affairs Healthcare System, National Center for PTSD, Menlo Park, California

John P. Wilson, PhD, Department of Psychology, Cleveland State University, Cleveland, Ohio

Sally Wooding, PhD, Centre for Mental Health, NSW Health Department, Sydney, Australia

Acknowledgments

This book was designed to advance our collective knowledge about the methods and procedures by which we gain insight and information about psychological trauma and its effects on human behavior. Since the publication of the first edition in 1997, the field of traumatic stress studies has seen rapid advances in all domains of scientific inquiry about posttraumatic stress disorder (PTSD) and the understanding of acute and chronic forms of traumatic stress. This volume reflects many of these advances, which range from neuroscience studies of brain functions to cross-cultural differences in trauma response.

We wish to thank the many persons who have worked behind the scenes to bring this second edition to life. At Cleveland State University, graduate assistants Stephanie Schultz and Mike Dougherty were stalwart in their daily efforts. The staffs at the National Center for PTSD in Boston and Vermont provided much research support. We give special thanks to Fred Lerner, information scientist affiliated with the PILOTS database (*www.ncptsd.org*) at the Veterans Affairs Regional and Medical Center, White River Junction, Vermont.

Finally, kudos to Kathleen D. Letizio of the Center for PTSD in Cleveland, Ohio, who oversaw the day-to-day editing and preparation of the chapters. Her unswerving dedication ensured the timely production of this second edition. Words of gratitude and thanks are insufficient to recognize her efforts and dedication, which went beyond the call of duty time and time again.

Contents

PART V. Psychosocial Development and Gender Issues

PART VI. Assessing Traumatic Injury in Litigation

Assessing Psychological Trauma and PTSD

Introduction

JOHN P. WILSON

Since the publication of the first edition of this book, the field of traumatic stress studies has continued to grow at a unprecedented rate. The scientific studies of psychological trauma proliferate, and new professional journals have emerged to accommodate this flood of information. University curricula now include courses on posttraumatic stress disorder (PTSD), crisis interventions, psychological debriefings, and stress medicine.

Today, some two decades after the classification of PTSD as a diagnostic category in DSM-III (1980) of the American Psychiatric Association (APA), we have an international database (PILOTS at *www.ncptsd.org*) that contains more than 25,000 references and annotations of peer-reviewed scientific articles. There are currently seven national centers for PTSD in the United States that conduct investigative studies in different areas of trauma research. PTSD has become a household word, and the terrorist attacks on the World Trade Center in New York City in 2001 made it patently clear that traumatic stress is a part of daily living in our times.

The second edition of *Assessing Psychological Trauma and PTSD* contains many advances in organization, complexity, and scope. In total, the new edition contains six parts, as opposed to three in the original edition, and has a new organizational structure.

Part I focuses on conceptual and diagnostic approaches to understanding trauma and PTSD. In Chapter 1, John P. Wilson presents an overview of PTSD and complex PTSD. The chapter details the psychobiological basis of understanding PTSD as a prolonged stress syndrome that comprises five interrelated sets of symptom clusters that were not present before the traumatic experience. This chapter details the logic of the diagnostic criteria for PTSD in DSM-IV-TR (2000). It also provides an analysis of complex PTSD, reflecting traumatic damage to the self-structure, personal identity, and interpersonal relationships. In Chapter 2, Richard A. Byrant examines acute stress disorder (ASD), a diagnostic category added to DSM-IV in 1994. In recent years, acute stress disorders have gained the attention of researchers and clinicians who are carefully studying the short-term effects of traumatic exposure.

Part II focuses attention on standardized psychometric measures, clinical protocols, epidemiological methods, and projective techniques of assessing trauma and PTSD. In Chapter 3, Fran H. Norris and Jessica L. Hamblen present an overview of more than 20 measures of civilian trauma and PTSD. Practitioners and researchers concerned with selecting appropriate measures of stressor exposure and PTSD will find this a good place to begin. Similarly, in Chapter 4, Daniel S. Weiss reviews the recent advances in structured clinical interview techniques for PTSD, such as the Clinician-Administered PTSD Scale (CAPS), the SCID module for PTSD, and others. This chapter is particularly useful for clinicians or researchers who wish to use a structured, standardized protocol to assess and probe posttraumatic reactions and symptom formation. In Chapter 5, Marlene Steinberg updates and expands the research and clinical use of the structural clinical interview for dissociative disorders. Because dissociative reactions are part of the diagnostic criteria for both ASD and PTSD, this chapter is especially valuable in learning how to inquire about the possible existence of dissociative processes and disorders that may coexist with acute or chronic reactions to trauma. In Chapter 6, Charles R. Marmar, Thomas J. Metzler, and Christian Otte present data on objective, self-report measures of peritraumatic dissociative experiences (i.e., those that occur concurrently with exposure to traumatic stressors). Research studies have documented the utility of the PDEQ scale to assess dissociative reactions and to predict the later onset of PTSD symptoms. The 10-item PDEQ scale is especially advantageous in research or treatment settings because it is a short scale and easy to administer. In Chapter 7, Daniel S. Weiss presents the current research findings on the Impact of Event Scale—Revised (IES-R), a 22-item scale that measures the diagnostic criteria for PTSD. The IES-R is among the most widely used instruments to assess PTSD, partly because of its reliability, construct validity, and ease of administration. This revised chapter includes new data on the statistical preparation of the IES-R that are most relevant to clinical practice and forensic settings. In Chapter 8, Toni Luxenberg and Patti Levin update research on the clinical applicability of the Rorschach test in the assessment and treatment of trauma. As a projective measure of personality assessment, the Rorschach protocol for PTSD is especially valuable in uncovering unconscious perceptual processes associated with trauma and provides a tool for in-depth evaluation of PTSD and its impact on psychological functioning. In Chapter 9, William E. Schlenger, B. Kathleen Jordan, Juesta M. Caddell, Lori Ebert, and John A. Fairbank present an updated analysis of epidemiological methods for assessing trauma and PTSD. Included in this important chapter is new information that grew out of the studies of the terrorist attacks on September 11, 2001, in New York. In Chapter 10, Terence M.

Keane, Amy E. Street, and Jane Stafford present new information on assessing military-related trauma, including a review of the range of available instruments that are specialized for use in military populations.

Part III is devoted to the assessment of the psychobiology of PSTD. In Chapter 11, Scott P. Orr, Linda J. Metzger, Mark W. Miller, and Danny G. Kaloupek present the psychophysiological methods of assessing PTSD. Similarly, in Chapter 12, Jeffrey A. Knight and Casey T. Taft review the research and advances in the neuropsychological assessment of PTSD. The neuropsychological assessment of PTSD is especially important when issues of brain injury, head trauma, toxic exposure, or other stressors have caused injury to neuropsychological functioning. Chapter 13 presents neuroimaging studies of PTSD. Using the most recent advances in brain imaging techniques (e.g., MRIs, fMRIs, PET scans, etc.) enables investigators to look inside the brain to discern both structural and functional changes produced by traumatic exposure. Joan Kaufman, Deane Aikens, and John Krystal provide a rich chapter to assist therapists, researchers, and others in understanding the nature of the brain–behavior relationship in posttraumatic conditions. In Chapter 14, Matthew J. Friedman presents for the first time a chapter dedicated to understanding pharmacological probes and assessment considerations for PTSD. This unique chapter, along with the other three in this section, illustrates that the neuropsychological knowledge of PTSD is now at the center stage of scientific inquiry.

Part IV focuses on assessing trauma, loss, and PTSD in medical settings. Chapter 15, by Todd C. Buckley, Bonnie L. Green, and Paula P. Schnurr reviews the growing research evidence concerned with trauma-related disorders in medical settings. This chapter also provides information about the link between PTSD and health-related problems (e.g., diabetes, blood pressure, endocrine functioning, etc.). In Chapter 16, Lisa M. Najavits presents the data showing the relationship between PTSD and substance abuse. This chapter is especially important to therapists, substance abuse counselors, inpatient treatment providers, and inpatient substance abuse specialty programs in which the assessment of comorbidity between PTSD and substance abuse is an important diagnostic or treatment consideration. In Chapter 17, Beverley Raphael, Nada Martinek, and Sally Wooding focus on the relationship between traumatic bereavement, loss, and PTSD. This chapter reviews the relationship and overlaps between traumatic bereavement and PTSD, with guidelines for assessing and treating complex reactions to trauma that results in loss or death.

Part V assesses trauma and PTSD in gender, cultural, and psychosocial development. In Chapter 18, Kathleen O. Nader presents a comprehensive review of psychological assessment of PTSD in children. As the chapter points out, there are special considerations when assessing psychological trauma within a developmental framework that include age, type of methodological procedure, and the nature of the traumatic stressor. Similarly, in Chapter 19,

John Briere discusses the psychological assessment of child abuse effects in adults. Briere highlights some of the difficulties that practitioners face when trying to evaluate the long-term sequelae of childhood abuse. In Chapter 20, Rachel Kimerling, Annabel Prins, Darrah Westrup, and Tina Lee review the specific issues of gender differences in response to psychological trauma. A growing set of studies has shown that males and females respond in different ways to some traumatic situations and that understanding these often subtle differences is critical to proper assessment and treatment.

Part VI is concerned solely with the forensic/clinical assessment of psychological trauma and PTSD. In Chapter 21, John P. Wilson and Thomas A. Moran present an overview of the special considerations in assessment in the context of legal issues. Guidelines are presented regarding assessment, forensic procedures, and expert witness testimony. This chapter is especially useful to attorneys, adjudicators, and administrators concerned with legal considerations involving traumatic injuries and PTSD.

PART I

Understanding and Assessing Trauma and PTSD

CHAPTER 1

PTSD and Complex PTSD

Symptoms, Syndromes, and Diagnoses

JOHN P. WILSON

Two decades have now passed since the medical–psychiatric term "post-traumatic stress disorder" (PTSD) was introduced into the third edition of the *Diagnostic and Statistical Manual of Mental Disorders* (DSM-III) of the American Psychiatric Association (1980). Since then, the proliferation of professional journals dedicated to trauma studies, reference books, and professional societies and the perfusion of interest in PTSD into mainstream areas of medicine, law, the social sciences, academic curricula, and social policymaking has become worldwide in scope (Wilson & Raphael, 1993; Wilson & Keane, 1997; Wilson, Friedman, & Lindy, 2001; Williams & Somers, 2002).

The United States, Australia, and Croatia, for example, have national centers for the study and treatment of PTSD, especially victims of war. Private hospitals have specialized inpatient units for the treatment of PTSD. International centers treat asylum seekers, refugees, and war and torture victims suffering from PTSD and its associated comorbidities (Wilson & Drozdek, in press). Access to PTSD informational materials is readily available on Internet websites (e.g., *ncptsd.org*). National media interest in PTSD intensified after the terrorist attacks on the World Trade Center towers on September 11, 2001. Prestigious newspapers, such as *The New York Times*, ran full-page articles on PTSD, its history, diagnosis, and treatment. Traumatic events of daily life or those of catastrophic proportions remind us that they are as much a part of history as the greatest scientific and cultural achievements of humankind.

Viewed historically, research conducted during the last half of the 20th century and the recognition of PTSD as an "official" psychiatric diagnosis gave birth to more vigorous and widespread scientific pursuits of knowledge about the disorder (Wilson et al., 2001). Although all of the stones of discovery have not yet been overturned, scientific inquiry progresses toward understanding the conditions and consequences that produce the human suffering, injuries, and physical and mental scars that are manifestations of traumatization.

The purpose of this chapter is to describe PTSD and complex forms of PTSD in terms of stress response syndromes, symptoms, and diagnoses. I focus on explaining PTSD in its interrelated organismic aspects and how the consequences of trauma affect the mind, body, and spirit. I discuss PTSD as a syndrome of dynamically related psychobiological processes that include the brain, the nervous and hormonal systems, psychological systems of memory, cognition, emotion, motivation, perception, and behavioral expressions of the organismic changes caused by trauma. I discuss PTSD within a holistic framework of five synergistically related symptom clusters that were not present before the traumatic event. Finally, I present a set of recommendations regarding diagnoses of PTSD and other disorders.

THE PSYCHOBIOLOGICAL DIMENSIONS OF POSTTRAUMATIC STRESS DISORDERS

Figure 1.1 presents a simplified conceptual model of PTSD as a prolonged stress response syndrome. The figure diagrams the development and function of six categories of psychological processes that constitute the structure and mechanisms of PTSD as a stress disorder. These categories represent the epigenesis of posttraumatic stress syndromes.

Traumatic Experience

Traumatic events are defined by the existence of stressors that have differential effects on organismic functioning. Traumatic stressors exist on a continuum. As defined by the current criterion A1 for PTSD in DSM-IV-TR (American Psychiatric Association, 2000), "the person experienced, witnessed, or was confronted with an event or events that involved actual or threatened death or serious injury, or a threat to the physical integrity of the self or others" (p. 467; see Table 1.1). In response to these stressors, the person's reaction involves fear and horror (emotions), helplessness (a learned behavior), or denial (cognitive alterations and ego defenses). These psychological reactions to trauma constitute criterion A2 for PTSD (see Table 1.1).

Primary Psychobiological Substrates

There are two primary interrelated substrates of PTSD as a prolonged stress response system: biological and psychological. The *biological* process refers to the neurophysiological substrates that are innate, preprogrammed capacities of the organism. The *psychological* processes involve perception, memory,

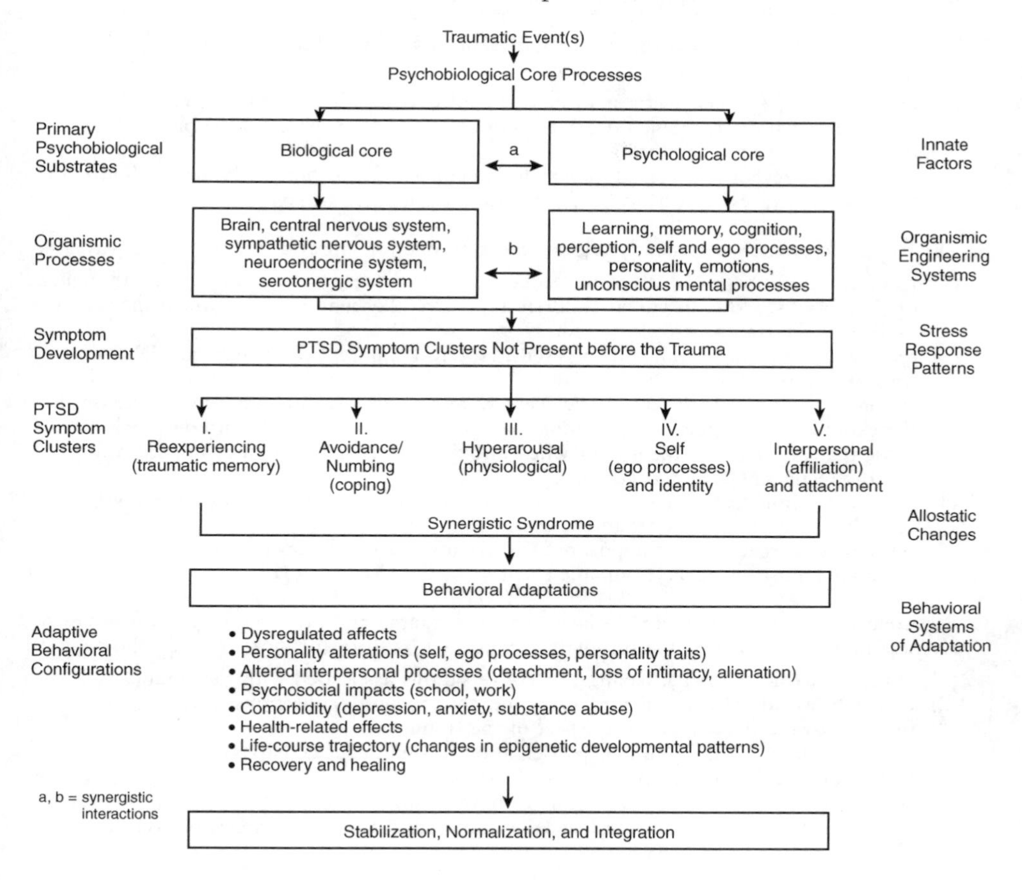

FIGURE 1.1. Psychobiological dimensions of PTSD.

cognition, learning, personality processes, and the self-structure. The two primary substrates are the organismic "soil" from which PTSD develops and forms adaptive patterns of behavior—the epigenesis of traumatic stress development.

Organismic Processes

The organismic processes in PTSD are manifestations of synergistic interactions between the biological and psychological systems in terms of adaptive responses to traumatic experiences. As organismic processes (see Figure 1.1), they reflect integrated holistic system dynamics; that is, the symptoms influence all aspects of psychological functioning. Assessing how PTSD symptom clusters "trigger" each other is important to accurate clinical assessment procedures.

TABLE 1.1. DSM-IV-TR Diagnostic Criteria for PTSD

A. The person has been exposed to a traumatic event in which both of the following were present:
   (1) the person experienced, witnessed, or was confronted with an event or events that involved actual or threatened death or serious injury, or a threat to the physical integrity of self or others
   (2) the person's response involved intense fear, helplessness, or horror. **Note:** In children, this may be expressed instead by disorganized or agitated behavior.

B. The traumatic event is persistently reexperienced in one (or more) of the following ways:
   (1) recurrent and intrusive distressing recollections of the event, including images, thoughts, or perceptions. **Note:** In young children, repetitive play may occur in which themes or aspects of the trauma are expressed.
   (2) recurrent distressing dreams of the event. **Note:** In children, there may be frightening dreams without recognizable content.
   (3) acting or feeling as if the traumatic event were recurring (includes a sense of reliving the experience, illusions, hallucinations, and dissociative flashback episodes, including those that occur on awakening or when intoxicated). **Note:** In young children, trauma-specific reenactment may occur.
   (4) intense psychological distress at exposure to internal or external cues that symbolize or resemble an aspect of the traumatic event
   (5) physiological reactivity on exposure to internal or external cues that symbolize or resemble an aspect of the traumatic event

C. Persistent avoidance of stimuli associated with the trauma and numbing of general responsiveness (not present before the trauma), as indicated by three (or more) of the following:
   (1) efforts to avoid thoughts, feelings, or conversations associated with the trauma
   (2) efforts to avoid activities, places, or people that arouse recollections of the trauma
   (3) inability to recall an important aspect of the trauma
   (4) markedly diminished interest or participation in significant activities
   (5) feeling of detachment or estrangement from others
   (6) restricted range of affect (e.g., unable to have loving feelings)
   (7) sense of a foreshortened future (e.g., does not expect to have a career, marriage, children, or a normal life span)

D. Persistent symptoms of increased arousal (not present before the trauma), as indicated by two (or more) of the following:
   (1) difficulty falling or staying asleep
   (2) irritability or outbursts of anger
   (3) difficulty concentrating
   (4) hypervigilance
   (5) exaggerated startle response

E. Duration of the disturbance (symptoms in Criteria B, C, and D) is more than 1 month.

F. The disturbance causes clinically significant distress or impairment in social, occupational, or other important areas of functioning.

Specify if:
   Acute: if duration of symptoms is less than 3 months
   Chronic: if duration of symptoms is 3 months or more

Specify if:
   With Delayed Onset: if onset of symptoms is at least 6 months after the stressor

Note. From American Psychiatric Association (2000, pp. 467–468).

Symptom Development: Five Stress-Related Clusters

PTSD symptoms develop in the aftermath of trauma (Green & Schnurr, 2000). New psychological, physiological, and behavioral patterns of reactivity develop that were not present before the trauma. The development of new symptoms may aggravate or add to preexisting psychological or psychiatric disorders. Clinically, PTSD can present with other Axis I and Axis II psychiatric disorders in many different combinations.

PTSD Symptom Clusters

The domain of PTSD symptom clusters is defined by five interrelated sets of symptoms: (1) the reexperiencing of trauma; (2) avoidance, numbing, and coping patterns; (3) hyperarousal; (4) self and ego processes; and (5) interpersonal affiliative patterns of attachment, bonding, intimacy, and love (Wilson et al., 2001). These five symptom clusters emerge from the primary substrates and are manifestations of changes in the organism's baseline functioning. In an overly simplified sense, posttraumatic adaptations constitute a new "set point" of behavioral functioning.

Adaptive Behavioral Configurations

Once PTSD symptom clusters develop from the primary psychobiological substrates, they comprise different and complex configurations of behavioral adaptation. These behavioral configurations include (1) dysregulated affects, (2) personality alterations, (3) altered interpersonal processes, and (4) a broad range of psychosocial consequences, including current health, academic, and occupational functioning (Schnurr & Green, 2004).

PTSD as a dynamic stress-response syndrome varies in severity and intensity and can develop at any point in the lifespan (e.g., childhood, adolescence, adulthood, old age; Pynoos & Nader, 1993). There are acute, chronic, and delayed-onset patterns of the disorder that may be episodic in manifestation. PTSD can be successfully treated and resolved, but it may reoccur on reactivation by new stressors, life crises, and trauma-specific stimuli or cues (TSCs) that reawaken the disorder.

PTSD AS A PSYCHOBIOLOGICAL SYNDROME

It is useful to understand PTSD as a normal, organismically based response pattern to extremely stressful life events. PTSD is a *psychobiological syndrome* that comprises an interrelated set of symptoms that cohere to form a prolonged stress reaction to trauma. As a syndrome, PTSD is synergistic in nature; the symptom clusters dynamically influence each other in behavioral manifestations.

Trauma affects all dimensions of behavioral functioning and psychological responses to physical and psychological injuries. The whole person is wounded by trauma; individuals have posttraumatic physiological reactions, emotions, perceptions, and cognitive attributions about the trauma experience that caused their injuries. Traumatic impact, such as emotional horror at witnessing a brutal unexpected death, for example, is not only emotionally overwhelming, distressing, and difficult to cope with but also triggers the release of neurohormones and activates "fight-or-flight" readiness. The traumatic event may also challenge belief systems concerned with meaning, faith, and expectancies about humanity and life itself. The effects of trauma can produce changes in worldview, beliefs about human nature, patterns of intimacy, interpersonal relationships, and conceptions of oneself and personal identity. Trauma does not occur in a vacuum or an isolated state. Its effects are multidimensional in terms of posttraumatic psychological functioning, influencing motivation, goal striving, and levels of consciousness about the self in the world.

Trauma's impact on the individual is holistic in nature, and effects on one part of the whole generate reciprocal effects on the other parts—a complex mind–body or psychobiological phenomenon. It is important to note that semantically the word "trauma" derives from Greek and Latin roots (cf. *traumatos*), in which "trauma" means injury to the body and results in a state of being wounded. Physical trauma causes injury to bodily integrity and normal biological functioning. Psychological trauma causes injury to the mind and its inherent processes and functions, including the ego, identity, and self-structure. Psychological trauma is caused by an *external* event that affects *internal* psychological phenomena at multiple levels of functioning and in conscious and unconscious modalities of awareness and behavior (Wilson et al., 2001).

Psychological and physical trauma perfuse the intricacies of psychological functioning like a stream of water cascading down a long hillside, with its shallow rocky areas, dropoff cliffs, collecting pools, and changes in the volume of flow and pressure. If one builds a dam to contain the stream, the water deepens and grows in pressure and potential to generate energy. If the dam gives way and collapses, the water may destroy everything in its path. Similarly, the "energy" of psychological trauma may dam up and burst forth in accumulated power to create deleterious effects to the well-being of the person and his or her relationships.

THE BRAIN'S COMMAND AND CONTROL CENTER OF STRESS RESPONSE

PTSD, as a psychobiological syndrome, is only one manifestation of the human stress-response system. Under conditions of stress, the organism energizes itself to cope with the need or perception to react in a situation of threat or danger that poses a challenge to well-being, coping resources, and adaptation. The evocation of the stress-response system is psychobiological in nature: (1) the person appraises, perceives, or is physically affected by a trauma; and (2) the biological response is instinctively activated to function congruently with stressor demands. The brain, as the central processing unit (CPU), mobilizes the sympathetic nervous system (SNS) to do its job of "switching on" the "fight–flight" response. The body, under brain controls, responds to action in an automatic way, commanding the cardiovascular, hormonal, muscular, nervous, and other systems to confront the trauma situation. The brain's control center activates one of the many "computer programs" hardwired into the central nervous system to release neurotransmitters that carry chemical messages to activate and energize the body's adrenergic and noradrenergic response systems, which regulate heart rate, blood vessels and nerve conduction. The adrenergic systems are part of the hypothalamic–pituitary–adrenocortical (HPA) axis, extending in a reciprocal fashion from the brain to the adrenal glands located on the kidneys, which release a neurohormone, cortisol, in response to stress. In a systematic fashion, activation of the brain and SNS by a traumatic event switches on the control apparatus in the brain, increasing arousal and readiness to respond by neurons carrying informational messages to each other. These neuronal relay systems are like neighbors telephoning one another to warn of a dangerous situation. Upon perception of threat or danger, the brain releases corticotropin-releasing factor, known as CRF, which sends chemical messages to other areas of the brain, which are awakened and "called to duty" to deal with stress and trauma.

In the HPA axis of the body, the brain releases adrenocorticotropic hormone (ACTH; *adreno* = adrenal gland; *cortico* = cortical or brain; *tropic* = zone or area), which circulates through the blood to the kidney, triggering the release of glucocorticoids (*gluco* = glucose or sugar), which in turn increase metabolic energy for muscular and nervous system response to stress and trauma. When this occurs, the system is "fired up," "primed," and "energized," with the "engine," performing at a metaphorical high speed of "revolutions per minute" (RPMs). Once activated, the stress-response systems execute their preprogrammed functions under the central control of the brain. The neurohormonal programs activate their programmed sequence until switched off and the program terminates. However, one of the unique aspects of PTSD is that the stress-response program may not switch off but continue to operate as if the threat were actively persistent and still present as an anxiety- or fear-provoking danger.

The activation of the adaptive, psychobiological stress-response system is genetically designed to meet the external demands of trauma or those posed by situations of extreme stress. Under normal conditions, the hyperarousal state activated by threat or danger will decrease and return to its baseline function. The system responds by generating more "fuel" and "power" to cope until the demands have been met and they are no longer required. At this point, the system can return to homeostatic functioning.

HOMEOSTASIS AND ALLOSTASIS: POSTTRAUMATIC CHANGES IN BASELINE FUNCTIONS

Homeostasis describes the return to baseline or normal functioning. As traditionally conceptualized, homeostasis means equilibrium, balance, or average regulatory baseline function in biological systems (Miller, 1978). However, recent studies of PTSD have shown that following traumatic stress experiences, a homeostatic condition may not be reestablished, especially with traumas that are prolonged or repetitive in nature. The different types of events that define traumatic situations may cause *prolonged hyperarousal states* in which the organism does not return to homeostasis. Rather, it continues to function *as if* the trauma were continuous and ongoing in daily life. It is as if the "computer controlled" software in the brain's CPU fails, rendering the "on" switch locked into position so that the SNS is in continuous high gear, increasing the neurohormonal responses of the engineering system that governs adrenaline, noradrenaline, glucocorticoids, and other stress hormones (e.g., serotonin, acetylcholine, etc.) to the status of an emergency, even *after* the crisis has terminated. "Allostasis" refers to the posttraumatic stress-response pattern to seek stability in functioning following a change in the homeostatic baseline.

ALLOSTASIS: STABILITY AFTER STRESS-INDUCED ORGANISMIC CHANGES IN FUNCTIONING

> At every level of living systems numerous variables are kept in steady state, within a range of stability . . . when these fail, the structure and process of the system alter markedly.
>
> —J. G. Miller (1978, p. 38)

In recent research studies, Bruce McEwen (1998) has described the nature of allostasis and allostatic load mechanisms. He notes: "the core of the body's response to challenge—is twofold, turning on an allostatic response that initiates a complex adaptive pathway, and then shutting off this response when the threat is past. . . . However, if the inactivation is inefficient, there is overexposure to other hormones. Over weeks, months, or years, exposure to increased secretions of stress hormones can result in allostatic load and its pathophysiologic consequences" (pp. 171–172). It is possible to think of *one* aspect of PTSD as an organismic syndrome of *dysregulated affective responding*. The failure of the system to shut down and adapt is also known as a process of *allostasis*, wherein the organism attempts to recalibrate its "set point" of functioning. This "set point" is not homeostatic but a recalibrated and changed baseline level of functioning. In simple terms, the organism's "engine" has a higher level of nervous system arousal after extreme stress; the system is still on "red alert" status despite a change in the external environment. *Allostasis is an attempt at stability through the changes induced by the trauma experience.* The state of traumatization reflects the state of ongoing injury or changes in system function until stabilization is achieved and normal functioning returns to baseline.

PTSD as a psychobiological state is a *dysregulated system* whose manifestations are biobehavioral, internal, and external in nature. Posttraumatic literally means "after injury," and in PTSD the prolonged stress-response patterns constitute a dynamic syndrome of symptoms and behavioral dispositions. It may include changes in personality (e.g., self, personal identity) and cognitive processing, memory, perception, motivation, and interpersonal relations. PTSD as a prolonged stress-response pattern disrupts *optimal functioning*. However, not all persons develop a full-blown diagnosable disorder; some will manifest acute reactions, acute stress disorders (ASD), and relatively high levels of stress reactions that do not meet the criteria for being considered pathological (i.e., partial PTSD).

It is important to understand that PTSD is not a unidimensional phenomenon. The psychological effects of trauma are expressed on all levels of organismic functioning: physical; psychological; social; spiritual; interpersonal; and systems of belief, ideology, values, and meaning. As a psychiatric disorder, PTSD is currently defined in diagnostic manuals as a limited set of clinical symptoms with specific sets of algorithmic criteria. To be considered an illness or psychiatric disorder, PTSD must impair areas of psychological functioning. More recently, complex PTSD has referred to a more inclusive set of symptoms, reactions, and behaviors that embrace trauma's impact to the self-structure, ego identity, and patterns of affiliation, intimacy, and attachment (Wilson et al., 2001).

THE CORE TRIAD OF PTSD SYMPTOM CLUSTERS

What are the core characteristics of PTSD as a stress disorder that distinguish its uniqueness? First, PTSD is a normal, biologically hardwired pattern of reactivity to extremely stressful situations. The stress patterns have subtypes of symptom constellations, depending on the nature of the trauma and the nature of the person. The events that are scientifically defined as traumatic are anchored at the extreme end of the stressor continuum. Generally, they are events or experiences that involve threat or danger to physical integrity and psychological well-being. Since the initial definition of PTSD in DSM-III of the American Psychiatric Association (1980), revisions have been made to the stressor criterion (A1), underscoring the need to provide conceptual clarity about the causality of the disorder. The growth of empirical research has established that the lifetime exposure to events associated with the development of PTSD are not uncommon, with 60.7% of men and 51.2% of women experiencing situations that could cause either acute or prolonged stress reactions (Kessler, Sonnega, Bromet, Hughes, & Nelson, 1995).

The lifetime prevalence of rates of PTSD varies greatly, from 1% to 30% or more for combat veterans and other trauma populations with high levels of trauma exposure. Across several studies, the highest lifetime prevalence for PTSD is associated with the sudden loss of a loved one; interpersonal assaultive violence; sexual assault (Breslau, 1998); and exposure to massive, catastrophic trauma, such as combat, torture, the atomic bomb at Hiroshima in 1945, the Nazi concentration camps, the terrorist attacks on the World Trade Center in 2001, and the 1993 bombing of the Murrah Federal Building in Oklahoma City (North & Pfefferbaum, 2002; Friedman, 2000). Once exposed to major trauma and the onset of PTSD, the individual is at a substantial risk to develop other psychiatric disorders, especially major depression, generalized anxiety disorder, and substance abuse (Breslau, 1998; McFarlane, 2001). As a conservative rule of thumb index, about 10% of women and 5% of men will develop PTSD during their lifetimes (Kessler et al., 1995). For severely traumatized persons, especially those who are not treated and/or who develop additional psychiatric problems (i.e., comorbidity) such as major depression or alcoholism, the symptoms and deleterious effects of PTSD can last a lifetime (Friedman, 2000). Moreover, until the condition stabilizes and the normal processes of stress recovery are set into motion, PTSD has the power to impair functioning, disrupt lives, and alter an individual's sense of identity, self-worth, and systems of faith, meaning, and purpose in living. What makes PTSD unique as a psychiatric disorder is that the syndrome is caused by an identifiable external force that may be an act of God, a random act of nature, or the willful malevolence of human design.

The nature and process of adaptation to trauma varies according to age, ego strength, and prior traumatization (Friedman, 2000). Posttraumatic adaptive behaviors have many configurations as psychobiological syndromes. The constellation of symptoms in PTSD is determined by several factors: (1) the pretraumatic mental health and personality characteristics of the person; (2) the nature, duration, and severity of the traumatic event; (3) the posttraumatic recovery environment and access to support, treatment, and resources to restore normal functioning; (4) the level of injury sustained to the body and the psyche, especially internal, core aspects of personality, identity, and ego processes; and (5) critical stages of epigenetic lifespan development (Erikson, 1968; Pynoos & Nader, 1993; Green, Wilson, & Lindy, 1985; Wilson et al., 2001; Wilson, 2002b; Wilson, 2003b; Breslau, 1998). These factors determine the configuration of PTSD symptoms that have subtypes and specific typologies in which the dynamics show different forms of modal expressions in behavior. For example, some persons will reexperience the trauma more frequently and intensely in flashbacks, intrusive recollections, and dreams than others. Some individuals will manifest profound numbing and extreme avoidance tendencies, and for others, their self-structure will be fragmented and dissolved by assaults on their personhood (Kalsched, 1996). Thus, depending on the depth and thoroughness of psychological assessment, PTSD symptoms will show *variable profile configurations*, with different constellations of symptoms being more pronounced than others. These variations in profile configurations are expressions of the multidimensional psychobiological nature of PTSD at any moment in time.

PTSD IS A MULTIDIMENSIONAL EPISODIC STRESS SYNDROME

Clinical assessment procedures consider the predictable fluctuations and cycles of symptom presentations (Wang, Wilson, & Mason, 1996). PTSD is not a static, unidimensional entity but a fluctuating, episodic multidimensional stress-response pattern that affects integrative psychological functioning on many levels: (1) memory, cognition, and information processing; (2) perception; (3) affect regulation; (4) motivational striving; (5) coping and ego-defensive functioning; (6) ego processes and personal identity; (7) stress tolerance capacities; (8) interpersonal relations and capacity for attachment and intimacy; and (9) life-course trajectory in the epigenesis of ego and personality development (Wilson et al., 2001). The multileveled impact of PTSD on organismic functioning produces syndrome constellations that are built on the triad of core PTSD symptoms: (1) reexperiencing, reliving, or reenacting traumatic memories; (2) avoidance tendencies, psychic numbing, and coping behaviors; and (3) psychobiological changes and physiological reactivity (hyperarousal) that was not present before the traumatic experience.

THE PSYCHOLOGICAL ARCHITECTURE OF PTSD

The core triad of PTSD symptoms are like a three-pronged support base for the larger syndrome, which sits atop its foundation. The "psychological architecture" of PTSD includes the tripod foundation and horizontal or vertical extensions that, figuratively, have different shapes to accommodate the functions of the self. The architectural principle of "form follows function" applies to understanding the structure of PTSD. *As a stress syndrome, PTSD is a psychobiologically driven organismic function of adaptation to abnormal, excessive, or extreme stressor events that tax individual coping resources.* The function of the stress-response syndrome is to meet environmental and intrapsychic challenges presented by the trauma (Kalsched, 1996). As a prolonged stress pattern, PTSD is a behavioral organization (i.e., structural form) adapted to meet allostatic loads imposed on the system. To be considered a psychiatric disorder, the symptoms must cause clinically significant impairments in functioning (i.e., DSM-IV-TR, PTSD Criterion F; see Table 1.1). The behavioral organization of PTSD constitutes its psychological structure, which can assume many complex forms as adaptive processes.

The psychological architecture of PTSD can be further analyzed to understand the relationship of structure to function. The triad of PTSD symptoms reflects the basic psychological processes of (1) memory, information, and cognitive processing; (2) coping and ego-defensive mechanisms; and (3) the mechanisms of the central nervous system associated with the capacity of either *external* or *internal* stimuli (e.g., memories of the traumatic event) to reevoke and switch on the preprogrammed neurophysiological stress response. The symptoms are synergistic processes that influence each other tridirectionally in terms of manifestations. For example, a reminder of a traumatic stressor will activate the adrenergic response system, and heart rate will increase. The person will experience increased physiological arousal and a readiness to respond to a situation or an evoking stimulus. Similarly, a sudden increase in heart rate, anxiety, or physical arousal may automatically be associated with thoughts or memories about the trauma, which, in turn, rekindle affects. In either case, external or internal activators of the trauma experience may then lead to avoidance behaviors, such as removing painful memories, avoiding things that are associated with the event, or using alcohol to alleviate emotional pain, tension, and psychic distress. In this manner, we can see that the symptom triad of (1) *reexperiencing* (traumatic memory), (2) increased *physiological reactivity*, and (3) *avoidance* behaviors are dynamically interrelated. However, before further examining their synergistic nature, I discuss each of the core triad symptom clusters separately, as well as two additional ones *not* officially listed in the current DSM-IV-TR (American Psychiatric Association, 2000) diagnostic manual. The two additional clusters include traumatic damage to the self-structure (e.g., ego identity, self-esteem) and interpersonal affiliative patterns (e.g., bonding, attachment, intimacy, and love).

DIAGNOSTIC MANUALS (DSM-IV AND ICD-10): CRITERIA, SYMPTOMS, AND ASSOCIATED FEATURES

Since the advent of PTSD as a diagnostic illness, first classified in DSM-III (American Psychiatric Association, 1980), the manual for diagnosis has undergone revisions to make the criteria congruent with clinical wisdom and scientific findings from research studies (American Psychiatric Association, 1980, 1987, 1994, 2000). Psychotherapists, clinicians, counselors, attorneys, academics, and administrative personnel routinely rely on these criteria in their work, and they utilize the official diagnostic criteria listed in either the DSM-IV or the *International Classification of Diseases* (ICD-10; World Health Organization, 1992). The criteria are set forth as a decision-making algorithm of the *minimal* number of symptoms that must be present to properly establish a positive diagnosis and to differentiate PTSD from other Axis I (major clinical disorders) or Axis II (personality disorders) psychiatric conditions. The diagnostic manuals also include sections on "associated features," which are narrative descriptions of other symptoms or behaviors that appear with the stress disorder but that may not be sufficient or necessary in themselves to constitute a prime characteristic of the syndrome for diagnostic purposes. The diagnostic criteria for each of the core triad of PTSD symptoms also share some of the same symptoms and features of other disorders, for example, depressive disorders, anxiety disorders, and specific personality disorders, such as borderline personality disorder and paranoid personality disorder.

To ensure some measure of conceptual clarity and clinical usefulness, I present a review of the current DSM-IV (American Psychiatric Association, 1994, 2000) diagnostic criteria for PTSD and then a much expanded set of criteria based on an allostatic model of PTSD by Wilson and colleagues (2001). To aid the discussion, refer to the DSM-IV-TR (American Psychiatric Association, 2000) diagnostic criteria for PTSD presented in Table 1.1.

TRAUMATIC MEMORY: REEXPERIENCING, RELIVING, AND REENACTING THE TRAUMA EXPERIENCE

How do persons reexperience traumatic events? The hallmark feature of PTSD is traumatic memory and forms of reliving, reexperiencing, or reenacting aspects of the original trauma. The memory of the trauma experience then becomes encoded in the brain and body in a variety of different ways. As a part of the syndrome, the individual reexperiences or reenacts the trauma in psychological systems: memory, perception, affect, cognition, motivation, and interpersonal social relations.

PROCESSING, STORAGE, AND RETRIEVAL OF TRAUMATIC MEMORIES

Once encoded in memory, the trauma may be behaviorally reexperienced in different ways: in frequency, in duration, in severity, in intensity, and in its influence on behaviors. *Reexperiencing phenomena involves cognitive processing, information storage, and retrieval from memory.* It can also be revivified at different levels of awareness (i.e., conscious, preconscious, and unconscious). Unconscious forms of reexperiencing are especially subtle and intricately expressed in overt reenactment manifestations in behaviors that have a psychological isomorphism with actions during the trauma (Blank, 1985b; Wilson & Zigelbaum, 1986; Wilson, 1989; Wilson et al., 2001). Unconscious reenactments of trauma parallel specific aspects of the actions that occurred during the chronology of the trauma experience (Wilson, 1989). The posttraumatic dynamics of the trauma experience can occur at different time intervals, ranging from peritraumatic reliving immediately after the onset of the trauma to days, weeks, months, or years afterward (Marmar, Weiss, & Metzler, 1997). As discovered by Freud (1910/1957), Janet (1890), Jung (1928) and other pioneering analysts, the unconscious is timeless, and therefore a traumatic memory can intrude involuntarily and unexpectedly at any point in the life cycle, especially when other life crises, traumas, or similar experiences rekindle memory and activate thoughts and affects associated with the disturbing experience—even decades after its disruptive or pathological effects have terminated. In this sense, it is meaningful to speak of traumatic experiences as timeless, having the power to resurface in conscious actions and behavioral dispositions at any point in the life cycle (Wilson et al., 2001).

DSM-IV-TR PTSD B CRITERIA: REEXPERIENCING TRAUMA—FIVE CLUSTERS WITH 16 SYMPTOM FORMS

DSM-IV-TR (American Psychiatric Association, 2000) diagnostic criteria for the core triad of PTSD symptoms includes traumatic memory, that is, the phenomenon of reexperiencing, reliving, or reenacting the traumatic event. DSM-IV-TR lists five sets of symptom clusters for the reexperiencing category, which actually contains 16 individual forms of consciously or unconsciously reliving trauma. Specifically, the diagnostic criteria indicate that the traumatic event is "persistently reexperienced" in one or more of five symptom clusters: (1) memory, (2) dreams, (3) reliving, (4) increased psychological (emotional) distress, and (5) increased physiological arousal.

Traumatic Memory

The first PTSD reexperiencing criterion, B1, involves "recurrent and intrusive distressing recollections" of the event, which include three specific subtypes, "images, thoughts, or perceptions." The B1 reexperiencing criterion concerns all aspects of traumatic memory. Note that this includes raw images, such as a visual memory of parts of the experience, perceptual processes (i.e., visual, olfactory, sensory, tactile, or kinesthetic), and organized or disorganized forms of thought (see Table 1.1).

Traumatic Dreams

The second PTSD reexperiencing criterion, (B2), involves these same traumatic memory processes in dream and sleep cycles: "recurrent distressing dreams of the [traumatic] event" or anxious dreams in children that express themes directly or indirectly in connection with the trauma. By logical inference, dreaming is a form of thought during the sleep cycle, and so dreams also contain "images, thoughts, and perceptions."

Emotional and Behavioral Forms of Reliving Trauma: Two Prongs

The third PTSD reexperiencing criterion, B3, is the most complex of the traumatic memory clusters. Its complexity is due to the two-pronged nature of this particular criterion, which states that the person reexperiences by "acting or feeling as if" the traumatic event were recurring (includes a sense of reliving the experience, illusions, hallucinations, and dissociative flashback episodes, including those that occur on awakening or when intoxicated)." Here, it is noted that the PTSD B3 criterion includes subtypes of reexperiencing the trauma that are *behavioral* (i.e., "acting as if") and *affective* ("feeling as if") with four distinct subforms involving: memory (reliving); perceptions (illusions as false sensory perceptions); hallucinations (hearing voices or seeing persons, places, or objects) that are anchored in the trauma experience; and dissociative flashback episodes. Trauma-based hallucinatory experiences are different from psychotic hallucinations precisely because the content of the hallucinations is trauma rooted and clearly identifiable as factually "real" upon careful analysis of the trauma history. Many PTSD patients have been misdiagnosed as paranoid schizophrenic, psychotic, or delusional because of their reports of trauma-based hallucinatory experiences (Blank, 1985b; Wilson, 1988).

The last of the PTSD B3 subtypes involves dissociative episodes, commonly known as "flashbacks," "zoning out," or "switching off." Dissociative psychological processes refer to an alteration in mental state—a change in the normal personality and behavior of the person and how he or she masters experience and the specific style and quality of his or her cognitive processes, especially the integrative functions of consciousness. In PTSD-related dissociation, a "dis-association" occurs upon reactivation of traumatic memory through associative learning processes. TSCs (Wilson et al., 2001) can evoke disturbing thoughts, feelings, and memories of the traumatic experience. Once activated, either consciously or unconsciously, the painful recollections and affects may be so anxiety producing and profoundly distressing to the person that he or she uses dissociative processes to protect him- or herself from the painful reliving of the trauma. It is clinically advantageous to view dissociative processes as self-protection mechanisms. The person alters his or her awareness of what he or she is feeling or reliving or fears will reoccur in the future. *Dissociation means that individuals' awareness of themselves or the environment (i.e., specific situations, places, persons, activities) alters and transforms into a* qualitatively *different state of being, which is discernible to others who are attuned to their personality functioning.* In depersonalization, for example, individuals alter awareness of themselves and feel as though they are observing their actions "outside their bodies," in a detached dream-like state of awareness. In such an altered state of consciousness, a PTSD (B3) dissociative flashback, the person may feel that he or she is in a surreal daze in which awareness of reality and the sequence of events that occurred while dissociated were reduced. The dissociative changes in conscious self-awareness and self-monitoring capacity are metaphorically similar to a dimmer switch on a light; the more it is turned down, the lower the available lighting by which to see one's environment. In dissociative flashback episodes in PTSD, the dimmer switch may alternate in brightness intensity, from total darkness to intolerable brightness. Moreover, dissociative episodes may occur when the person has lowered his or her cognitive controls through alcohol consumption or on awakening from sleep and transitioning from one state of mental activity (hypnogogic) to another (hypnopompic).

Increased Psychological and Physiological Distress

The last two (B4, B5) PTSD symptom categories of the traumatic memory cluster are psychobiological changes in response to "internal or external cues that symbolize or resemble an aspect of the traumatic event." Specifically, the B4 reexperiencing criterion concerns increased emotional reactivity upon reactivation of memories by associative learning—TSC or a stimulus of a more generalized nature, which triggers the painful emotions originally experienced at the time of the traumatic event (i.e., peritraumatic affectivity) or afterward (Marmar et al., 1997). Similarly, the B5 reexperiencing criterion reflects increased "physiological reactivity" (hyperarousal) in association with TSCs or other activating stimuli. The increased physiological reactivity (e.g., blood pressure, sweating, heart palpitations, hyperventilation, urinary urgency, flushing, etc.) indicates that the fight–flight stress response patterns have been switched on or amplified in intensity (Friedman, 1994). As part of allostasis following trauma, the body remains in a state of readiness (i.e., by degrees of hyperarousal potential). When an event, TSC, or situation signifies a potential threat or activates encoded memories of the traumatic experience, the command and control centers of the brain activate the engineering mechanisms of the adrenergic response system to execute their functions. Like soldiers scurrying to their battle stations, the neuronal messengers of the stress-response system respond to a potential red-alert status and prepare the organism to cope and adapt as necessary. As a posttraumatic stress response symptom, increased physiological reactivity "on exposure to internal or external cues that symbolize or resemble an aspect of the traumatic event" is a biobehavioral indicator of the specificity of PTSD as an integrated organismic state whose baseline functions were shifted by trauma and recalibrated at a new set point level. The new level is an index of allostatic load and recalibration of the organisms set point of responsiveness to the perception of threat, harm, or challenge to its integrity as a system (McEwen, 1998).

UNDERSTANDING AND ASSESSING THE 16 FORMS OF REEXPERIENCING TRAUMA

In summary, the reexperiencing cluster of PTSD diagnostic symptoms (criteria B1–B5) reflects the manner in which traumatic memory functions. Examination of each of the separate symptom clusters reveals a total of 16 different forms of reexperiencing a trauma in conscious or unconscious behavioral manifestations, altered states of awareness (dissociation), sensory and perceptual processes, and somatic symptoms of hyperarousal. These 16 symptoms are listed for purposes of clarity in understanding their structure and function in traumatic memory. They are important, too, as part of any clinical assessment process for PTSD diagnosis. Currently, DSM-IV-TR requires only one symptom from this entire cluster to establish the diagnosis of PTSD. Note: All symptoms are in direct or indirect reference to the traumatic event.

- B1. *Intrusive distressing recollections of trauma*—three symptoms
  1. Images (raw images, primary process thinking, visual or fragmented memories, "flicker-flashes," freeze-frame images)
  2. Thoughts (coherent, disorganized)
  3. Perceptions (sensory/perceptual processes, e.g., tactile, kinesthetic, visual, olfactory, auditory)
- B2. *Dreams associated with trauma*—3 symptoms
  4. Images (same as B1)
  5. Thoughts (same as B1)
  6. Perceptions (same as B1)
- B3. *Response predisposition: Acting or feeling "as if"*—4 x 2 modalities: modality I, "acting as if," or modality II, "feeling as if" = eight symptoms
  - 7 and 8. Reliving (revisualization or acting out prior trauma experiences)
  - 9 and 10. Illusions (perceptual, sensory, etc.)
  - 11 and 12. Trauma-rooted hallucinations (trauma-based sensory/perceptual hallucinations)
  - 13 and 14. Dissociative processes (depersonalization, derealization, amnesia, etc.)
- B4. *Increased psychological distress on exposure to trauma-related stimuli*—one symptom
  15. Anxiety, fear, sadness, terror, or other negative affects
- B5. *Increased physiological reactivity on exposure to trauma-related stimuli*—one symptom
  16. Somatic manifestations of hyperarousal states evoked by trauma-relevant cues (e.g., sweating, heart palpitations)

THE RELATIONSHIP BETWEEN REEXPERIENCING TRAUMA AND DEFENSIVE AVOIDANCE

It is important to the understanding of PTSD to note that the distress associated with reexperiencing a traumatic experience cannot be tolerated for prolonged periods of time without periods of rest, relief, and the ability to resume activities of daily living.

The wisdom of the organism is that there are many forms of coping and of warding off the pain of reliving traumatic life experiences. Traditionally, these intrapsychic and behavioral activities have been studied as coping adaptations to stress or as ego defensive processes associated with threat, anxiety, and somatic states of tension, agitation, and intolerable affects (Wilson et al., 2001). In a broader perspective, reexperiencing phenomena are reciprocal in structure to psychic mechanisms that are designed to control degrees of distress produced by the stress-response system. McEwen (1998) found that chronic activation of the stress-response system generates wear and tear on the organism, especially if the system fails to switch off after trauma or cannot do so because of repeated demands for use or because of the breakdown of the neurohormonal engineering system, when parts lose their effectiveness, fail, or just wear out from overuse. Therefore, we can view the avoidance cluster of PTSD diagnostic criteria as forms of coping with dysregulated stress-response systems. These PTSD symptoms, referred to as "avoidance and numbing behaviors," were not in the organism's repertoire prior to trauma and can be adaptive or maladaptive in nature.

DSM-IV-TR PTSD C CRITERIA: AVOIDANCE AND NUMBING OF RESPONSIVENESS NOT PRESENT BEFORE THE TRAUMA

How do persons distance and protect themselves from traumatic impact to their sense of well-being? The diagnostic C criteria of DSM-IV-TR (American Psychiatric Association, 2000) consists of seven symptoms of avoidance mechanisms and changed patterns of coping with stress that are different from pretraumatic baseline (see Table 1.1).

Trauma-Related Active and Passive Avoidance Tendencies

The PTSD C1 and C2 criteria involve efforts to avoid "thoughts, feelings, conversations . . . activities, places, or people" that are associated with the trauma. These symptoms reflect the aversive nature of reexperiencing trauma and the efforts the person undertakes to avoid being exposed to reminders that would stimulate unwanted memories and feelings associated with the trauma experience.

Loss of Memory and Inability to Recall Aspects of the Trauma Experience

The PTSD C3 avoidance criterion, "inability to recall an important aspect of the trauma," is indicative of amnesia or gaps in the chronology of the trauma experience itself. The inability to recall important aspects of the trauma may be the product of dissociated affects and memories of the most critical, salient, or overwhelming moments of trauma experience. The "loss" of memory for critical events may be caused by repression, blocking, or denial or by state-dependent learning (Wilson, 1989), in which the informational content of experience was encoded in extreme states of hyperarousal (e.g., terror of annihilation, defenselessness at the witnessing of a horrific death, or the total disavowal of the unimaginable circumstances that occurred within a relatively brief or protracted period of time). In a clinical situation, amnesia may be difficult to assess until the trauma narrative unfolds and the missing pieces of the jigsaw puzzle can be assembled into a complete form. In many cases, gaps in the chronology of the trauma story are indications of the most crucial memories that required removal from active storage in order to cope with the extraordinary intensity and powerful impact of stressors to individual well-being.

Diminished Interest in Normal Activities of Daily Living following Trauma

How does PTSD affect activities of daily living? The PTSD C4 avoidance criterion specifies "markedly diminished interest or participation in significant activities." This criterion reflects a disengagement from activities that the person enjoyed or participated in prior to the traumatic experience. The loss of interest in previously enjoyed hobbies, recreation, or daily routines is often a manifestation of depression and a desire to withdraw from others in order to "lick one's wounds." A traumatic experience may precipitate a reordering of priorities, and activities once valued may not seem enjoyable, desirable, appealing, or meaningful. Nevertheless, the salient feature of the C4 avoidance criterion is that there are readily discernible posttraumatic changes in behavior.

Social Detachments and Emotional Anesthesia (Psychic Numbing)

How do PTSD and avoidance symptoms affect social and interpersonal relations? The PTSD C5 and C6 symptoms of avoidance and psychic numbing are manifestations of changes in *interpersonal* relations and *intrapsychic* capacities to tolerate affect. The C5 avoidance criteria, "feelings of detachment or estrangement from others," is characteristic of tendencies of isolation, withdrawal, social disengagement, preference for solitary activities, and geographical distance from others in a safe or secured environment. On the other hand, the C6 avoidance criteria, "restricted range of affect," is a form of shutting down emotional responsiveness; it is emotional anesthesia, psychic closing-off, or a restricted capacity for affect tolerance. Manifestations of psychic numbing take many forms, including a loss of normal capacity to experience emotions, diminished sensuality and sexuality, a loss of spirituality, and the outward appearance of being emotionally flat, nonresponsive, vapid, unfeeling, indifferent, cold, and lacking in vitality. These emotional states can be considered as coping efforts to control the level of hyperarousal inherent in PTSD as a dysregulated stress-response syndrome. The person afflicted with PTSD over controls his or her emotional responsiveness by preemptive mechanisms to prevent feeling vulnerable to the internal distress of traumatic memory and forms of reexperiencing behavior. In a simplified way, the nonverbalized thinking is: "if I don't feel, I cannot be hurt any further than I currently am by the trauma." In its basic function, psychic numbing is a security operation, attempting to impose controls on the neurohormonal engineering systems that have failed to switch off, leaving the person feeling vulnerable to turbulent affects that persist *as if* the trauma is still occurring. In severe cases of chronic PTSD, the person may feel that to become emotionally vulnerable to the painful, unresolved aspects of trauma is tantamount to dying. Elsewhere, this phenomenon has been described as self-dissolution and deintegration, wherein the component parts of the self-structure (e.g., coherence, connection, autonomy, vitality, agency, etc.) fragment and result in a loss of ego continuity, self-sameness, and personal identity (Wilson, 2002b, 2003b; Wilson & Drozdek, in press).

Psychological Myopia: Changes in Future Orientation

The last avoidance criterion for PTSD, C7, is identified as a "sense of a foreshortened future." This symptom means that the person feels as though his or her expected course of lifespan development will be truncated, short-lived, or profoundly altered in uncertain and anxiety-provoking ways. The specter of a sense of foreshortened future may lead to an urgency to live life fully in the present and, consequently, to engage in risk-taking and acting-out behaviors. When a strong sense of foreshortened future predominates the individual's future orientation and planning, the immediacy of the present is overvalued. The result is *psychological myopia*, in which tomorrow may never exist in the eyes of the person. Such a worldview and diminished sense of future orientation may mask depression, feelings of learned helplessness, and loss of control over outcomes in daily living. In response, the individual may engage in risky, impulsive, and self-destructive patterns of behavior.

DSM-IV-TR PTSD D CRITERIA: PERSISTENT SYMPTOMS OF INCREASED AROUSAL NOT PRESENT BEFORE THE TRAUMA

How do persons manifest hyperarousal behaviors as stress-related changes in behavior? Five interrelated symptoms define DSM-IV-TR PTSD D criteria of "persistent symptoms of increased arousal" that were not present before the trauma. These symptoms reflect psychobiological changes in allostasis, hyperarousal of the adrenergic response system, and their behavioral expressions as PTSD symptoms (see Table 1.1).

Sleep Cycle Disturbances

The PTSD D1 hyperarousal criterion (difficulty falling or staying asleep) reflects sleep disturbances and includes disruptions of the early, middle, or terminal phase of the cycle. Accompanying the difficulties with sleeping are night sweats, problems returning to sleep upon early awakening, nightmares, night terrors, somnambulism, agitation, and restless activity while sleeping, which may be attended by vocalizations (e.g., gasps, screams, crying, talking, making references to the trauma experience, etc.).

Anger, Irritability, and Hostility

The PTSD D2 hyperarousal criterion, "irritability or outbursts of anger," is another manifestation of dysregulation of the stress-response system. Persons with PTSD are sometimes quick to react with irritability, hostility, anger, cynicism, confrontation, and anxious agitation at annoying circumstances. They are often restless and impatient. They have proverbial short fuses, quick tempers, and "fast draw" dispositions. Recent studies (Bremner, 2002) have shown that the basal ganglia area of the limbic system associated with anger and aggression are effected as part of the prolonged stress-response pattern. For some persons, especially those with a history of combat, aggression, or self-defense being necessary to survival, the subcortical brain structures associated with aggression appear to be in a state of kindling, a neurological ready-alert mode of functioning. On provocation, even minimal, they may be predisposed to act automatically in irritable, angry ways that, in turn, may trigger a sequence of increased aggressiveness.

Impairment in Cognitive Processing of Information

How do states of hyperarousal in PTSD influence thinking, concentration, academic performance, and other cognitive functions? The PTSD D3 criterion, difficulty concentrating, is another manifestation of hyperarousal. We can think of this symptom as part of a larger constellation of cognitive processing deficits in PTSD, which include difficulties in encoding, processing, and retrieving information. These cognitive impairments of executive function also include attention deficits (e.g., shifts in focus, drifting, inability to solve problems or follow directions, etc.). Students who have PTSD may also manifest hyperarousal in the form of irritability, anxiety, tension, agitation, inattention, "zoning out," oppositional tendencies, problems with conduct and following rules, restlessness, and discomfort associated with reexperiencing phenomena. PTSD symptoms of this type are easily misdiagnosed as hyperactive attention-deficit disorder (ADD or ADHD) because of the similarity in overt behavioral patterns. Problems of cognitive information processing in PTSD can be understood as the effect of accumulative, hyperarousal states jamming the information processing centers of the brain, impairing concentration, attention, and memory. The somatic dysregulation of affect in PTSD creates "noise," "signals," or "interference," which disrupts the normal operation of the brain's CPU for high-order cognitive processes. The dysregulated affects in PTSD are like weather storms that disrupt radio and television reception, resulting in "lost" information and poor quality reception.

Hypervigilance: Excessive Alertness to Threat and Danger and Readiness to Respond

The PTSD D4 (hypervigilance) and D5 (exaggerated startle response) criteria both reflect psychobiological changes in behavioral dispositions. These symptoms can be considered as manifestations of hyperarousal of the SNS, reflecting allostatic processes of altered thresholds of response and initial response patterns (Wilson et al., 2001). The person suffering from PTSD continues to function in a "red alert" status of readiness, behaviorally primed for another stressful event.

Hypervigilance is a behavioral disposition and a readiness to respond to stimuli, especially cues that have trauma-specific relevance to their traumatic experience (TSCs). As part of PTSD-related hypervigilance (*hyper* = excessive; *vigilance* = alert, awake, watchful), the individual is on guard and scans the environment for cues, signs, or situations that signify a threat or potential problem. Hypervigilance consists of cognitive, affective, somatic, and behavioral dimensions. In regard to perception and cognition, persons with PTSD automatically, and often unconsciously, scan the environment for signs of threat. Based on their own trauma experiences and the activation of the fight–flight stress response (i.e., hyperarousal), they have a faster recognition threshold of threat stimuli. Upon perception, or actual recognition of a threat source, affective responses intensify—typically fear, anxiety, anger, or terror. Somatically, the increase in hyperarousal is experienced in physical reactions of muscle tension and increased heart rate, blood pressure, respiration, and sweating. The person is behaviorally ready to deal with fear, anxiety, and the possible need to act in response to the actual or perceived threat. It is important to note that hypervigilance is not an all-or-none phenomenon. Similar to dissociative reactions, there are degrees of hypervigilance as an expression of increased autonomic nervous system arousal. There are also varying levels of conscious awareness (LCA; Wilson et al., 2001) and self-monitoring of internal states of increased arousal and hypervigilant behaviors.

Hyperarousal and Self-Monitoring Difficulties

The problem of self-monitoring of PTSD states of hyperarousal is yet another manifestation of allostatic dysregulation. Persons suffering from PTSD often have a decreased capacity to accurately self-monitor ("read") their internal states of arousal, emotions, and thought patterns. In extreme cases, the failure to accurately monitor and process internal states can lead to the possibility of misinterpreting others' intentions, actions, and verbal expressions and subsequently result in defensive action that includes withdrawal, avoidance, and overt aggression (Wilson et al., 2001).

In extreme states of hypervigilance (as a symptom of PTSD rather than of other mental disorders), the person filters his or her perceptions of the environment through a finely meshed screen that is tightly woven together from the trauma experience. Perception and information processing are then filtered through an ultra-high-grade sieve constructed from the individual trauma encounter, which sifts out irrelevant information and focuses attention on those actions of others or the environment with the highest potential for danger and threat. It must be recognized that as a component of PTSD, hypervigilance is a biologically conditioned (learned) response. Hyperarousal during the trauma was associated with a range of actions that ultimately resulted in survival, albeit with physical or psychological consequences. *Hyperarousal states during the trauma were reinforced by survival itself.* Thus PTSD hypervigilance is an automatic, psychobiologically determined response pattern designed to adapt to the perception, or existence of, threat to the well-being of the organism. It is for this reason that it is very difficult to extinguish a learned survival response. However, extreme hyperarousal may result in misperception of cues and lead to maladaptive responses, including those with potential legal consequences (e.g., self-defense resulting in a criminal assault; see Wilson & Moran, Chapter 21, this volume).

Abnormal Startle Response

The PTSD D5 hyperarousal criterion of exaggerated startle response is perhaps the purest example of a psychobiologically conditioned response. The startle response is an instinctive reaction to unexpected stimuli, such as loud noises, bright flashes of light, and aversive or classically conditioned odors. An exaggerated startle response is an amplified pattern of such reactions, usually with trauma-specific associations that are discernible from the person's history of involvement in the trauma. For example, former combat veterans often manifest exaggerated startle to loud explosion-like noises, the sounds of helicopters, aircraft engines, sandy wind storms, and whistle-like noises associated with mortar rounds or rockets. Further, although exaggerated startle reactions are expectable in patients with PTSD, they may also manifest in unusual, idiosyncratic ways, as in the case of a former torture victim who jumps anxiously at a routine medical examination (Juhler, 1993, in press) or of sexually abused children who become agitated at bedtime. In some situations of torture, medical personnel assist in overseeing torture to ensure its effectiveness and to minimize observable, external scars produced by the process. Exaggerated startle reactions are both generalized and idiosyncratic in nature (Wilson & Drozdek, in press).

In summary, the psychobiological criteria for PTSD presented in the DSM-IV-TR (American Psychiatric Association, 2000) contain four subcategories of hyperarousal phenomena that are important to understand in clinical assessments because the symptoms were not present before the occurrence of the trauma. We can summarize these four psychobiological clusters as: (1) sleep cycle disturbance; (2) cognitive processing deficits (e.g., concentration, attention, memory, information processing, executive functions); (3) perceptual and sensory sensitivity (e.g., startle responses, hypervigilance); and (4) hyperarousal phenomena (hypervigilance, startle response, risk-taking behaviors, sensation seeking, agitation, feeling keyed up, or edgy, etc.).

ACUTE STRESS DISORDER

In DSM-IV (American Psychiatric Association, 1994), acute stress disorder (ASD) was added as a complementary diagnostic category to PTSD. ASD is similar to PTSD except that its onset and offset as a stress-response syndrome occur within 1 month of the traumatic event. ASD is a form of short-term stress-response syndrome and as such reflects a shorter cycle of the disorder

ASD differs from PTSD as a diagnostic entity in several ways relevant to clinical assessments. First, its duration is shorter and does not have the PTSD subtype specifiers of delayed onset, chronic or acute (i.e., symptoms less than 3 months). Second, to be diagnosed with ASD, a person needs to manifest only *one* symptom from each cluster of the core PTSD triad: (1) reexperiencing, (2) avoidance and numbing, or (3) hyperarousal. Third, ASD, unlike PTSD, has a separate diagnostic category for dissociative symptoms. In the DSM-IV-TR (American Psychiatric Association, 2000), the 'B' criteria for ASD states "either while experiencing or after experiencing the distressing event, the individual has three (or more) of the following dissociative symptoms," which include: "(1) a subjective sense of numbing, detachment, or absence of emotional responsiveness; (2) a reduction in awareness of his or her surroundings (e.g., 'being in a daze'); (3) derealization; (4) depersonalization; and (5) dissociative amnesia (i.e., inability to recall an important aspect of the trauma)" (p. 471). Thus, *only* for the dissociative cluster of symptoms for ASD must the person manifest three of the five forms of dissociation listed to have a positive diagnosis.

ASD AND DISSOCIATIVE PROCESSES

Several aspects of the criteria for ASD require further examination. First, the B set of diagnostic criteria for *dissociative symptoms* uses the words "distressing event" rather than "traumatic event." It also states that the dissociative symptoms may occur during the event (i.e., "while experiencing") or after its termination ("after experiencing"). The proximity of the dissociative reaction to the traumatic or distressing event reflects what are known as *peritraumatic dissociation* and posttraumatic dissociation (Wilson et al., 2001).

Moreover, Marmar, Weiss, and Metzler (1997) have provided conceptual and clinical clarity to the understanding of peritraumatic dissociation:

> One fundamental aspect of the dissociative response to trauma concerns immediate dissociation at the time the traumatic event is unfolding . . . dissociation at the time of trauma may take the form of altered time sense, with time being experi-

enced as slowing down or rapidly accelerated; profound feelings of unreality that the event is occurring, or that the individual is the victim of the event; experiences of depersonalization; out-of-body experiences; altered pain perception; altered body image or feelings or disconnection from one's body; tunnel vision; and other experiences reflecting immediate dissociative responses to trauma. (p. 44)

PTSD VERSUS ASD: DIAGNOSTIC INCONSISTENCIES IN DISSOCIATIVE CRITERIA

The distinction between pre- and posttraumatic forms of dissociation in response to trauma or distressing events is quite useful, as it helps in assessing how the person coped with the distressing situation. *Peritraumatic dissociation reflects the individual's need to control the degree of threat experienced at the time of the event by using dissociation to cope with perceived danger*. In this regard, dissociation is an ego defense designed to alter awareness of potential harm (Chu & Bowman, 2000). Posttraumatic dissociation is a form of reexperiencing trauma, as noted in the PTSD B3 criteria, or as a response to current life situations involving the perception of threat. However, it is important to point out a contradiction within DSM-IV-TR (American Psychiatric Association, 2000) because *different sets* of criteria are being used to differentiate ASD from PTSD. PTSD does not require any dissociative symptoms following the traumatic event to establish a positive diagnosis. ASD requires three symptoms to make the diagnosis.

Space limitations do not permit a further analysis of the discrepancies in the diagnostic criteria for PTSD and ASD. It should be noted that persons suffering from either type of stress disorder (i.e., ASD or PTSD) can exhibit dissociative symptoms. As noted by Marmar et al. (1997), peritraumatic dissociative symptoms involve perceptual and cognitive alterations in time, space, person, location, emotions, body image, and reality in general.

ASD was included in DSM-IV (American Psychiatric Association, 1994) to be conceptually congruent with a diagnostic sense that there is a stress-response continuum that may be acute or chronic in nature. Without ASD as a diagnostic subtype of PTSD as an anxiety disorder, there is no correct way to diagnose disruptive, clinically significant impairments in functioning that have an onset and offset within a short period of time.

COMPLEX PTSD AND POSTTRAUMATIC DAMAGE TO THE SELF

A scientific awareness has been emerging that the diagnostic criteria for ASD and PTSD are "skeletal structures" of a much larger set of psychological impacts to organismic functioning in posttraumatic states. The core triad of PTSD symptoms define the primary modalities of the psychobiology of the stress-response syndrome, which has been extraordinarily useful in understanding various parameters of the disorder. Our knowledge of PTSD prevalence, gender differences, chronicity, neurobiological changes in brain morphology, and assessment technologies has advanced the front line of scientific knowledge (Friedman, 2000; Wilson et al., 2001). Moreover, it has long been recognized that trauma's impact on persons is more than an aggregate of symptoms that manifest as posttraumatic changes in behavior patterns and coping adaptation.

Understanding and assessing PTSD in a holistic framework includes a sensitive understanding of how the inner self-processes of the person are affected by trauma. Traumatic events, especially those involving acts of interpersonal assault, violence, abuse or prolonged coercive internment under degrading conditions, attack the bases of the self and systems of personal meaning. The results of traumatic injury to the self and personhood are deleterious, diverse, and, in some cases, pathologically lethal. Our understanding of persons with dissociative identity disorders, war veterans, interned political prisoners, prisoners of war, rape victims, Holocaust survivors, and those who have suffered repeated, prolonged, and multiple forms of abuse have provided clinical descriptions of the various ways that trauma damages the inner self, the very "soul" of the person (Krystal, 1968; Lifton, 1967; Niederland, 1968; Wilson et al., 2001; Ulman & Brothers, 1988; Herman, 1999). Such terms as "soul death," "broken spirits," "soul bruising," "walking dead," "catanoid state," "empty shells," and "vacuum states" have been used to characterize traumatic damage to the self that extends beyond the mere presence of the core triad of PTSD symptoms (Krystal, 1988; Lifton, 1967; Simpson, 1993; Gabbard, 1992; Wilson, 2003a). The self-structure is a central organizing component of personality (Stern, 1985) and has both *structural* and *functional* dimensions that are critical to understanding responses to trauma. Extreme trauma attacks the individual's core self, resulting in structural damage to the organization of self. As a consequence, self-dissolution, dissociative processes, fragmentation in ego processes, and a loss of self-sameness in continuity in identity may be evident. Wilson (2002, 2003a, 2003b, in press) has identified 11 separate typologies of posttraumatic self-configurations that exist on a continuum from severe pathology (e.g., the inert self) to optimal health (e.g., the integrated self). This typology also includes related aspects of posttraumatic pathology and personality processes and illustrates the wide range of possible ways in which self-transformation occurs following trauma.

It is not possible to describe and assess how the self is damaged by trauma without understanding the inner world of traumatization (Kalsched, 1996). Descriptions of complex PTSD have abounded in many sources published on the severe effects of traumatization dating back to the early Greeks (Friedman, 2000). Judith Herman (1992) reviewed some of the major categories that made up her description of complex PTSD—including suicidality, self-mutilation, dissociation, substance abuse, depression, psychosomatic complaints, character and identity changes, and disruptions in intimacy, sexuality, and patterns of interpersonal relationships. Herman (1992, 1999) notes quite correctly that "concepts of personality developed in *ordinary circumstances* are frequently applied to survivors without an understanding of the deformation of personality which occur under conditions of coercive control" (p. 93, emphasis added). Viewed in another way, we have no separate psychology of how trauma affects the self and personality processes in lifespan development. Traditional theories of personality have a useful but limited relevance to understanding assaults on the self-structure in situations of repeated, prolonged, or extreme abuse and trauma. For example, who would consider a death camp an ordinary life experience? Or surviving years of secretive childhood sexual or physical abuse? Or being a torture victim of a political regime? Or the perpetrator and recipient of trauma in prolonged combat exposure under conditions of guerrilla warfare? Or being a wrongfully convicted murderer living for years in prison on death row and later exonerated? Herman (1992) suggests that the misapplication of personality disorders is among the most common diagnostic errors for trauma survivors whose personality characteristics and self-structures have been altered and sometimes warped by extreme stress experiences. This diagnostic insufficiency is typically the case in clinical assessments in which an inadequate trauma history fails to establish the level of optimal functioning prior to the traumatic event.

IMPACT OF PTSD ON THE SELF, EGO PROCESSES, AND IDENTITY

How is the inner core of self-esteem and personal identity damaged by trauma? Trauma's impact on the self-structure, ego processes, and identity is a complex intrapsychic phenomenon of critical importance to a holistic–dynamic understanding of PTSD. Wilson et al. (2001) and Wilson (2002a, 2003a, in press) have reviewed the various conceptualizations of trauma's impact on the self and its functional properties. Based on the works of Freud (1916/1957), Lifton (1967, 1979, 1993), Krystal (1968, 1988), Kalsched (1996, 2003), Ulman and Brothers (1988), Niederland (1968), Putnam (1997), Erikson (1968) and others, it was possible to extract similarities and consistencies in clinical findings concerning posttraumatic damage to the self. In particular, Wilson (2002b, 2002c, 2003b) notes that six core dimensions of the self are affected by traumatic events: (1) coherency, (2) connection, (3) continuity, (4) energy, (5) autonomy, and (6) vitality. Each of these dimensions of the self can be adversely affected by trauma and can result in varying degrees of self-dissolution, disintegration, fissility, disunion, dissociation, fracturing, or annihilative effects. Moreover, it is historically interesting to note that Freud (1916/1957) believed that "*a person is brought so completely to a stop by a traumatic event which shatters the foundation of his life that he abandons all interest in the present and remains permanently absorbed in mental concentration upon the past*" (p. 342, emphasis added). Clearly, Freud understood the potential transformative power of trauma, especially to ego processes, as a protection against harm (see *Beyond the Pleasure Principle* [Freud, 1920/1959] for a complete discussion). Similarly, Erik Erikson (1968) developed the concept of *identity diffusion* from his therapeutic work with World War II veterans and stated, "Most of our patients had neither been shell-shocked nor became malingerers, but through the exigencies of war lost a sense of personal sameness and historical continuity. . . . *I spoke of a loss of ego-identity*" (1968, p. 17, emphasis added).

In his pioneering studies of Hiroshima survivors of the first atomic bomb, Robert J. Lifton (1967, 1979, 1993) spoke of how the self-structure fragmented and dissolved for many survivors of the bombing in 1945. Lifton spoke of *psychic numbing*: a loss of capacity of the self to experience emotions and life experiences. He also noted that survivors showed distinct changes in their sense of continuity in time, space, and future orientation. Lifton (1967) observed, for example, that some bombing survivors believed they were "walking dead," living in penance in a Buddhist hell. He reported that they experienced a loss of continuity and future orientation, as well as a sense of fragmented personal and physical integrity. In his psychoformative theory of the self, Lifton (1976) suggested that self-alteration could be expressed as stasis, separation, and *self-discontinuity* in posttraumatic states. Nearly identical observations were made by William Niederland (1968) in his clinical studies of Holocaust survivors, in which impairments to personal identity and self-function were paramount issues in recovery. More recently, studies of survivors of the terrorist attacks on the World Trade Center in 2001 now show similar findings on self-changes (Cardenas, Williams, Wilson, Fanouraci, & Singh, 2003).

Many other areas of traumatic stress research support the undeniable deleterious impact of trauma for aspects of self-functioning. Space limitations restrict our analysis, but research on dissociative identity disorders (DIDs), childhood sexual abuse, torture victims, rape victims, refugees, prisoners of war, and battered women have all confirmed that traumatic events can cross-cut all dimensions of the self-structure and result in self-fragmentation, discontinuity, loss of drive, loss of autonomy and vigor, and loss of the will to thrive (Chu & Bowman, 2000).

POSTTRAUMATIC DAMAGE TO IDENTITY, EGO PROCESSES, AND THE SELF-STRUCTURE

Wilson and colleagues (2001) presented a detailed, tetrahedral model of PTSD with five symptom clusters that include the core injuries of the PTSD triad, as well as injuries to the self-structure, attachment, intimacy, and interpersonal relations that *were not present before the traumatic event*. In terms of PTSD and the self-structure, they identified 13 symptoms that are manifestations of traumatic injury to the self-structure, ego processes, personal identity, and personality processes:

1. Narcissistic and other personality characteristics that reflect damage to the self-structure associated with trauma.
2. Demoralization, dispiritedness, dysphoria, and existential doubt as to life's meaning.
3. Loss of ego coherence and dissolution of the self-structure.
4. Loss of a sense of sameness and continuity to ego identity or capacity for ego stability.
5. Fragmentation of ego identity and identity disturbance (e.g., identity diffusion).
6. Shame, self-doubt, loss of self-esteem, guilt, and self-recrimination.
7. Fluctuating ego states; proneness to dissociation and lack of ego mastery.
8. Hopelessness, helplessness, and self-recrimination; masochistic and self-destructive tendencies.
9. Suicidality; patterns of self-destructiveness or self-mutilation.
10. Chronic feelings of uncertainty and vulnerability; levels of depression, helplessness, and hopelessness.
11. Existential personal or spiritual angst; dread, despair, and a sense of futility in living.
12. Loss of spirituality, essential vitality, willingness to thrive, religious/cosmic belief systems, and so forth.
13. Misanthropic beliefs, cynicism, and a view of the world as unsafe, dangerous, untrustworthy, and unpredictable.

Posttraumatic damage to the self-structure may be manifested in degrees of injury, impairment, or deficits anywhere on the continuum of fragmentation to integration *of the structure itself (i.e., coherence, connection, continuity, vitality, autonomy, energy)*. In extreme cases of PTSD, the entire self-structure dissolves (Goodwin, 1993, 1999; Kalsched, 2003; Jung, 1953–2000). Extreme fragmentation of the self-structure caused by traumatic injuries may result in a loss of energy to thrive, a loss of autonomy and "free" self-regulation, a loss of self-continuity with the past, a loss of a meaningful sense of connection to others, and a loss of the capacity for intimacy. The person with severe PTSD may manifest a profound loss or altered sense of continuity in personal identity; the threads of self-sameness with the flow of one's past dissipate, leaving a sense of interrupted life sequence (Wilson, 1980, 1981, 1994a, 1994b, 1995). The inner core of the self may be experienced as empty or dead or as existing in an abyss of nothingness.

The 13 symptoms of PTSD identified by Wilson et al. (2001) are useful to clinical assessments because they employ the same criteria that were used for the B, C, and D PTSD symptoms in the DSM-IV-TR (American Psychiatric Association, 2000); that is, these symptoms of traumatic injury to the fabric of the self-structure and its functional capacities *were not present before the trauma*. The symptoms are manifestations of allostatic psychobiological adaptations to traumatic stress impact on the *inner agency of the self*. Trauma produces changes in psychological functions that were not present in the same functional or structural manner as before the stressful event. *As reexperiencing, avoidance, and hyperarousal symptoms have a specific and traceable relationship to the precipitating trauma, so do the symptoms of altered self-functions*. Furthermore, these symptom manifestations are not only directly caused and/or correlated with trauma exposure, but there are also not more viable, logical, or meaningful explanations for their presence in the repertoire of posttraumatic adaptive behaviors of the person.

IMPACT OF PTSD ON ATTACHMENT, INTIMACY, AFFILIATIVE BEHAVIORS, AND INTERPERSONAL RELATIONS

How does trauma affect the nature and quality of interpersonal relationships? As noted in DSM-IV-TR (American Psychiatric Association, 2000) under the "associated descriptive features and mental disorders," other symptoms of complex PTSD are also important to clinical assessment and treatment protocols. The diagnostic manual lists such symptoms as interference in relationships, marital conflict, and poor job performance (p. 465). Although these are useful observations, it is possible to gain greater conceptual and diagnostic clarity by specifying the domain of PTSD symptoms that represent traumatic damage to attachment, intimacy, sexuality, and interpersonal relationships. Wilson et al. (2001) list 13 symptoms for this criterion that were not present before the trauma:

1. Alienation: social, emotional, personal, cultural, spiritual.
2. Mistrust, guardedness, secretive behaviors, non-self-disclosure, reticence toward social encounters.
3. Detachment, isolation, withdrawal, estrangement, and feelings of emptiness.
4. Anhedonia: loss of pleasure in living; loss of sensuality, sexuality, feeling, capacity for joy.
5. Object relations deficits; loss of capacity for healthy connectedness to others.
6. Self-destructive or self-defeating interpersonal relationships which are repetitive in nature.
7. Impulsiveness, sudden changes in residence, occupation, or intimate relationships.

8. Impaired sensuality, sexual drive, capacity for sexuality or loss of libidinal energy in general.
9. Inability to relax; discontent with self-comfort activities and an inability to receive nurturing, affection, or physical touching from others.
10. Unstable and intense interpersonal relationships whose origin is in trauma experiences.
11. Problems with establishing or maintaining boundaries in relationships based on trauma experiences.
12. Anxiety over abandonment or loss of loved ones, which is either conscious or unconscious in nature and based in traumatic experiences.
13. Repetitive self-defeating interpersonal relationships which reflect unmetabolized patterns of attachment behavior from abusive developmental experiences.

These symptom clusters are manifestations of trauma's adverse impact on *interpersonal* and *intrapersonal* functioning. Traumatic impact on the domain of affiliative and attachment behaviors creates problems with: (1) healthy boundary maintenance, (2) trust of others, (3) repetitive self-defeating relationships, (4) impulsiveness in areas of sexuality, friendships, and economic consumption, (5) personal, social, and cultural alienation, (6) geographical isolation from others, (7) self-care, (8) fears of abandonment, (9) intense, unstable relationships, (10) secretiveness, guardedness, or an unwillingness to self-disclose, and (11) impaired capacity for enjoyment of work, play, exercise, sensual relations, and sex drive.

BEYOND COMPLEX PTSD: ORGANISMIC IMPACTS OF TRAUMATIC STRESS

The complexity of PTSD and personality functioning allows a summary of the organismic nature of these phenomena as prolonged stress-response syndromes that are manifestations of allostatic adaptive processes (Wilson et al., 2001). As such, they are direct manifestations of changes in the primary psychological substrata (see Figure 1.1).

Holistic Stress Response Syndromes

PTSD and self-impairments are holistic stress-response syndromes and function synergistically in their psychodynamics. Trauma impacts on the organism are multidimensional and affect psychological systems of functioning (e.g., memory, learning, information processing, self-esteem, personality development, interpersonal relations, motivational striving, system of meaning and belief, etc.).

Synergistic Dynamics

A holistic, dynamic understanding of allostatic processes indicates that there are five distinct but interrelated sets of symptom clusters that make up ASD, PTSD, and complex PTSD: (1) reliving; (2) avoidance and numbing; (3) increased physiological reactivity (hyperarousal); (4) changes in self-structure, personal identity, and ego processes; (5) changes in affiliation, attachment, intimacy, and interpersonal relationships. *For each of the five clusters of symptoms, there are a discernible set of symptom indicators of posttraumatic changes in baseline organismic functioning that were not present before the trauma*. These symptom manifestations are synergistic. Changes in one cluster produce changes in the others, which can be described as a tumbling, cascade set of effects. The five clusters have *reciprocal interaction effects* with one another, creating cycles or episodes of symptom manifestation until a steady state of allostatic stabilization is achieved.

New Organismic Baseline in PTSD

The five clusters of PTSD-related symptoms reflect organismic shifts in adaptive functioning, a new baseline (i.e., set point) of functioning after trauma. The new baseline of functioning applies to each set of symptom clusters, as well as to the integrated posttraumatic functioning of the organism as a whole (Wilson et al., 2001).

Periodicity in PTSD Symptom Clusters

The variability in manifestations of PTSD symptom clusters consists of allostatic alterations in symptom functions. It is possible for some symptom patterns (e.g., avoidance) to persevere longer than others. Symptom patterns may be episodically activated through conditioned learning and may evoke psychobiological response patterns. Other symptom patterns (e.g., self-dissolution) are manifestations of a relatively permanent injury to the organism. PTSD has permutations in the severity, duration, intensity, and frequency of symptom manifestation in all five dimensions of the syndrome. Thus there is variability in periodicity in PTSD symptom manifestation.

Severe and Prolonged Stress-Related Damage to the Core Psychological Processes

The most severe damage in PTSD occurs to the two core structures of the syndrome: (1) neurobiological responses of the adrenergic system and (2) structural components of the self. Damage to the genetically driven and biologically hardwired, instinctive components of the stress-response system reflects allostatic loads described by McEwen (1998) as: (1) repeated hits (i.e., recurrent or prolonged exposure to stressors); (2) lack of capacity for adaptation;

(3) prolonged stress response; and (4) inadequate response or system failure, that is, the capacity of the neurohormonal engineering mechanisms to begin to fail. In severe PTSD, prolonged activity of the neurobiological components becomes deleterious to the organism, as repeated demands on the system to function effectively may not allow sufficient time and resources for reparative maintenance of the system itself. Empirical research demonstrates that prolonged stress responses, without relief and allostatic restabilization, are associated with changes in the cardiovascular, endocrine, and other systems of the body (McEwen, 1998; Bremner, 2002).

In an analogous way, damage or prolonged stress to the core dimensions of the self-structure (i.e., coherence, continuity, connection, vitality, energy, autonomy) may result in severe personality damage in terms of: (1) self-esteem; (2) personal identity and sense of self-identity; (3) loss of striving in life; (4) suicidality and self-destructiveness; (5) fragmentation in ego processes and self-components (e.g., alternate personalities in DID); (6) capacity for intimate relationships; (7) changes in systems of meaning, beliefs, values, and faith.

Etiology, Clinical Assessment, and Lifespan Development

An organismic approach to PTSD enables assessment of a broader, more encompassing set of psychological and psychosocial functions associated with the syndrome. These include, but are not limited to: (1) understanding of the etiology of the disorder in five subsystems and functioning affected by trauma; (2) understanding of the changes in pretraumatic baseline functioning to a new, allostatic set point in organismic functioning; (3) assessment of profile configurations in terms of frequency, periodicity, severity, intensity, and duration of symptoms within and among the five interrelated clusters of symptoms; (4) knowledge of how core, inner dimensions of the self are altered in ways that are associated with posttraumatic self-typologies that fall along a continuum of fragmentation (i.e., loss of structural coherence) to integration and transformation (i.e., unity transcendence, resilience); and (5) understanding of how trauma affects biosocial functioning in terms of epigenetic development and personality functioning in the life cycle.

Diagnoses: PTSD and Axis I and Axis II Mental Disorders

The clinician assessing PTSD, especially for purposes of formulating a treatment plan, or in forensic evaluations (see Chapter 21, this volume) must attempt to obtain as complete a picture of the patient's functioning as possible. To do this requires taking a comprehensive trauma history and determining whether or not there is a prior history of abuse, victimization, or a preexisting Axis I or Axis II mental disorder. A five-step decision-making process to gain information as to the pretrauma level of functioning and psychobiological stress response set point of adaptation is recommended.

CONSIDERATIONS IN THE DIFFERENTIAL DIAGNOSIS OF PTSD

1. *Premorbidity.* Is there any psychiatry history prior to the traumatic event that would suggest or document an Axis I or Axis II clinical disorder?

2. *Substance abuse.* Is there any history of drug or alcohol abuse prior to the traumatic event?

3. *Changes in personality and behavior.* Are there identifiable and independently verifiable changes in personality and behavior that were not present before the trauma but are posttraumatically manifest as personality processes? If so, are the changes discernible in the self-structure and ego processes of the individual?

4. *Transient behavioral and personality changes.* Are there transient changes in personality and behavior that reflect allostatic dysregulations in behavior as attempts at coping with trauma in proximity to the event (e.g., one month to one year posttrauma)?

5. *Interaction of premorbidity, trauma, and PTSD.* If a preexisting Axis I or Axis II disorder exists, to what extent does it contribute to the current symptoms, personality processes, and forms of coping? It is important to determine in what ways, if any, a preexistent psychiatric disorder or history influences the clinical presentation of PTSD and the processing of the trauma experience.

6. *Multiple diagnoses.* PTSD can coexist with any Axis I or Axis II clinical disorder. There are multiple combinations of comorbid diagnoses possible with PTSD. These combinations may present complex and difficult assessment and treatment issues.

CONCLUSION

In conclusion, the analysis of PTSD as a prolonged stress response syndrome has enabled us to gain a panoramic, wide-lens view of the disorder. In the aftermath of trauma, the psychobiological nature of the human stress response involves the characteristic development of reactions, symptoms, and integrated syndromes of adaptive functioning. Traumatic events activate primary biological and psychological processes of the organism that control the mechanisms of adaptive responses. PTSD is a synergistic syndrome, and the symptom clusters that develop have reciprocal, interactive influences on each other. As an organismic stress response, PTSD involves five clusters of symptoms that develop from the two primary psychobiological substrates of the underlying neurohormonal engineering systems of the body. The five PTSD clusters are epiphenomenal manifestations of the psychobiological substrates and include reexperiencing phenomena, avoidance and numbing, hyperarousal states, impaired self-function, and effects on interpersonal relations.

These integrated symptom clusters are unique to PTSD as a psychiatric disorder because they: (1) were not present before the traumatic event and (2) are specific manifestations of the normal, adaptive stress response pattern in a prolonged and potentially impairing way to psychological functioning. Once ASD or PTSD develops, various forms of behavioral adaptations may become evident in the person's repertoire of coping and adaptive capacities. These behavioral adaptations configure in dysregulated affects, personality alterations, altered interpersonal relations, and psychosocial functioning until recovery, restabilization, and healing occur.

REFERENCES

American Psychiatric Association. (1980). *Diagnostic and statistical manual of mental disorders* (3rd ed.). Washington, DC: Author.

American Psychiatric Association. (1987). *Diagnostic and statistical of mental disorders* (3rd ed., rev.). Washington, DC: Author.

American Psychiatric Association. (1994). *Diagnostic and statistical manual of mental disorders* (4th ed.). Washington, DC: Author.

American Psychiatric Association. (2000). *Diagnostic and statistical manual of mental disorders* (4th ed., text rev.). Washington, DC: Author.

Blank, A. S. (1985a). Irrational reactions to PTSD and Vietnam veterans. In S. M. Sonnenberg, A. S. Blank, Jr., & J. A. Talbott (Eds.), *The trauma of war: Stress and recovery in Vietnam veterans* (pp. 69–99). Washington, DC: American Psychiatric Press.

Blank, A. S., Jr. (1985b). The unconscious flashback to the war in Vietnam veterans: Clinical mystery, legal defense, and community problem. In S. M. Sonnenberg, A. S. Blank, Jr., & J. A. Talbott (Eds.), *The trauma of war: Stress and recovery in Vietnam veterans* (pp. 293–309). Washington, DC: American Psychiatric Press.

Bremner, J. D. (2002). *Does stress damage the brain?* New York: Norton.

Breslau, N. (1998). Epidemiology of trauma and posttraumatic stress disorder. In R. Yehuda (Ed.), *Psychological trauma* (pp. 1–27). Washington, DC: American Psychiatric Press.

Cardenas, J., Williams, K., Wilson, J. P., Fanouraki, G., & Singh, A. (2003). PTSD, major depressive symptoms, and substance abuse following September 11, 2001 terrorist attacks, in a midwestern university population. *International Journal of Emergency Mental Health, 5*(1), 15–28.

Chu, J. A., & Bowman, E. S. (2000). Trauma and dissociation: 20 years of study and lessons. *Journal of Trauma and Dissociation, 1*(1), 5–21.

Erikson, E. H. (1968). *Identity, youth and crisis*. New York: Norton.

Freud, S. (1959). Beyond the pleasure principle. In J. W. Strachey (Ed. and Trans.), *The standard edition of the complete psychological works of Sigmund Freud*. New York: Norton. (Original work published 1920)

Freud, S. (1957). The future prospects of psycho-analytic therapy. In J. W. Strachey (Ed. and Trans.), *The standard edition of the complete psychological works of Sigmund Freud* (Vol. 11, pp. 139–151). London: Hogarth Press. (Original work published 1910)

Freud, S. (1957). The introductory lecture on psychoanalysis. In J. W. Strachey (Ed. and Trans.), *The standard edition of the complete psychological works of Sigmund Freud*. New York: Norton. (Original work published 1916)

Friedman, M. J. (1994). Neurobiological sensitization models of posttraumatic stress disorder: Their possible relevance to multiple chemical sensitivity syndrome. *Toxicology and Industrial Health*, *10*, 449–462.

Friedman, M. J. (2000). *Posttraumatic stress disorder: The latest assessment and treatment strategies*. Kansas City, MO: Compact Clinicals.

Gabbard, G. O. (1992). Commentary on "dissociative" processes and transference–countertransference paradigms in the psychoanalytically oriented treatment of adult survivors of childhood sexual abuse. *Psychoanalytic Dialogues*, 2, 37–47.

Goodwin, J. M. (1993). *Rediscovering childhood trauma*. Washington, DC: American Psychiatric Press.

Goodwin, J. (1999). The body finds its voice (Part 4). In J. Goodwin & R. Attias (Eds.), *Splintered reflections*. New York: Basic Books.

Green, B., & Schnurr, P. (2000). Trauma and physical health. *Clinical Quarterly*, *9*(1), 3–5.

Green, B., Wilson, J. P., & Lindy, J. (1985). Conceptualizing posttraumatic stress disorder: A psychosocial framework. In C. R. Figley (Ed.), *Trauma and its wake: The study and treatment of posttraumatic stress disorders* (Vol. I, pp. 53–69). New York: Brunner/Mazel.

Herman, J. (1992). *Trauma and recovery*. New York: Basic Books.

Herman, J. (1999). Complex PTSD. In M. Horowitz (Ed.), *Essential papers on posttraumatic stress disorder*. New York: New York University Press.

Janet, P. (1890). *L' automatisme psychologique*. Paris: Felix Alcan.

Juhler, M. (1993). Medical diagnosis and treatment of torture survivors. In J. P. Wilson & B. Raphael (Eds.), *International handbook of traumatic stress syndromes* (pp. 763–767). New York: Plenum Press.

Juhler, M. (in press). Surgical approach to victims of torture and PTSD. In J. P. Wilson & B. Drozdek (Eds.), *Broken spirits: The treatment of traumatized asylum seekers, refugees, war and torture victims*. New York: Brunner-Routledge.

Jung, C. G. (1928). The therapeutic value of abreaction. In *Collected works* (Vol. 16).

Jung, C. G. (1953–2000). *Collected works* (Vols. 1–20). In H. Read, M. Fordham, & G. Adler (Eds.) R. F. C. Hull (Trans.). Princeton, NJ: Princeton University Press.

Kalsched, D. (1996). *The inner world of trauma: Archetypal defenses of the personal spirit*. London: Routledge.

Kalsched, D. (2003). Daimonic elements in early trauma. *Journal of Analytical Psychology*, *48*(2), 145–176.

Kessler, R. C., Sonnega, A., Bromet, E., Hughes, M. H., & Nelsen, C. B. (1995). Posttraumatic stress disorder in the National Comorbidity Survey. *Archives of General Psychiatry*, *52*, 1048–1060.

Krystal, H. (1968). *Massive psychic trauma*. New York: International Universities Press.

Krystal, H. (1988). *Integration and healing*. Hillsdale, NJ: Analytic Press.

Lifton, R. J. (1967). *Death in life: The survivors of Hiroshima*. New York: Simon & Schuster.

Lifton, R. J. (1976). *The life of the self*. New York: Simon & Schuster.

Lifton, R. J. (1979). *The broken connection: On death and the continuity of life.* New York: Basic Books.
Lifton, R. J. (1993). From Hiroshima to the Nazi doctors: The evolution of psychoformative approaches to understanding traumatic stress syndromes. In J. P. Wilson & B. Raphael (Eds.), *International handbook of traumatic stress syndromes* (pp. 11–25). New York: Plenum Press.
Marmar, C. R., Weiss, D. S., & Metzler, T. J. (1997). The peritraumatic dissociative experiences scale. In J. P. Wilson & T. M. Keane (Eds.), *Assessing psychological trauma and PTSD* (pp. 412–428). New York: Guilford Press.
McEwen, B. (1998). Protective and damaging effects of stress mediators. *Seminars of the Beth Israel Deaconess Medical Center, 338*(3), 171–179.
McFarlane, A. C. (2001). Dual diagnosis and treatment of PTSD. In J. P. Wilson, M. J. Friedman, & J. D. Lindy, *Treating psychological trauma and PTSD* (pp. 237–254). New York: Guilford Press.
Miller, J. G. (1978). *Living systems.* New York: McGraw-Hill.
Niederland, W. (1968). Clinical observations of the survivor syndrome. *International Journal of Psycho-Analysis, 49,* 313–315.
North, C. S., & Pfefferbaum, B. (2002). Research on the mental health effects of terrorism. *Journal of the American Medical Association, 288*(5), 633–636.
Putnam, F. W. (1997). *Dissociation in children and adolescents: A developmental perspective.* New York: Guilford Press.
Pynoos, R., & Nader, K. (1993). Issues in the treatment of posttraumatic stress in children. In J. P. Wilson & B. Raphael (Eds.), *International handbook of traumatic stress syndromes* (pp. 527–535). New York: Plenum Press.
Schnurr, P., & Green, B. (2004). *PTSD and physical health.* Washington, DC: American Psychological Association Press.
Simpson, M. (1993). Traumatic stress and the bruising of the soul: The effects of torture and coercive interrogation. In J. P. Wilson & B. Raphael (Eds.), *International handbook of traumatic stress syndromes* (pp. 667–685). New York: Plenum Press.
Stern, D. (1985). *The interpersonal world of the infant.* New York: Basic Books.
Ulman, R. B., & Brothers, D. (1988). *The shattered self.* Hillsdale, NJ: Analytic Press.
Wang, S., Wilson, J. P., & Mason, J. (1996). Stages and decompensation in combat-related PTSD: A new conceptual model. *Integrative Physiological and Behavioral Science, 31*(3), 236–253.
Williams, M. B., & Somers, J. (2002). *Simple and complex PTSD.* New York: Haworth Press.
Wilson, J. P. (1980). Conflict, stress and growth: The effects of war on psychosocial development among Vietnam veterans. In C. R. Figley & K. S. Leventman (Eds.), *Strangers at home: Vietnam veterans since the war.* New York: Praeger Press.
Wilson, J. P. (1981, January). *Cognitive control mechanisms in stress response syndromes and their relation to different forms of the disorder.* Paper presented at the Hospital and Community Psychiatry Conference, San Diego, CA.
Wilson, J. P. (1988). Understanding the Vietnam veteran. In F. Ochberg (Ed.), *Post-traumatic therapy and victims of violence* (pp. 227–254). New York: Brunner/Mazel.
Wilson, J. P. (1989). *Trauma, transformation and healing: An integration approach to theory, research and posttraumatic theory.* New York: Brunner/Mazel.

Wilson, J. P. (1994a). The historical evolution of PTSD diagnostic criteria: From Freud to DSM-IV. *Journal of Traumatic Stress*, *7*, 681–689.

Wilson, J. P. (1994b). The need for an integrative theory of posttraumatic stress disorder. In M. B. Williams (Ed.), *Handbook of PTSD therapy*. New York: Greenwood.

Wilson, J. P. (1995). Traumatic events and posttraumatic stress disorder and prevention. In B. Raphael & G. Barrows (Eds.), *Handbook of studies on preventive psychiatry* Amsterdam: Elsevier Press.

Wilson, J. P. (2002a, October). *The abyss experience and catastrophic stress*. Paper presented at the Conference on Terrorism and Weapons of Mass Destruction, Philadelphia, PA.

Wilson, J. P. (2002b, October). *The abyss experience and the trauma complex*. Paper presented at the Conference on Mental Health Response to Weapons of Mass Destruction: Terrorist Attacks, Philadelphia, PA.

Wilson, J. P. (2002c, November). *An organismic, holistic model of complex PTSD*. Paper presented at the annual meeting of the International Society for Traumatic Stress Studies, Baltimore, MD.

Wilson, J. P. (2003a, June). *PTSD and self-transformation*. Paper presented at the International Institute of Psychotraumatology, Dubrovnik, Croatia.

Wilson, J. P. (2003b, February). *Target goals and interventions for PTSD: From trauma to the abyss experience*. Paper presented at the World Congress on Stress, Trauma and Coping, Baltimore, MD.

Wilson, J. P. (in press) Broken spirits. In J. P. Wilson & B. Drozdek (Eds.), *Broken spirits: The treatment of traumatized asylum seekers, refugees, war and torture victims*. New York: Brunner-Routledge.

Wilson, J. P., & Drozdek, B. (Eds.). (in press). *Broken spirits: The treatment of traumatized asylum seekers, refugees, war and torture victims*. New York: Brunner-Routledge

Wilson, J. P., Friedman, M. J., & Lindy, J. D. (2001). *Treating psychological trauma and PTSD*. New York: Guilford Press.

Wilson, J. P., & Keane, T. M. (Eds.). (1997). *Assessing psychological trauma and PTSD*. New York: Guilford Press.

Wilson, J. P., & Raphael, B. (1993). *International handbook of traumatic stress syndromes*. New York: Plenum Press.

Wilson, J. P., & Zigelbaum, S. D. (1986). PTSD and the disposition to criminal behavior. In C. R. Figley (Ed.), *Trauma and its wake* (Vol. II, pp. 305–321). New York: Brunner/Mazel.

World Health Organization. (1992). *The ICD-10 classification of mental and behavioral disorders: Clinical descriptions and diagnostic guidelines*. Geneva: Author.

CHAPTER 2

Assessing Acute Stress Disorder

RICHARD A. BRYANT

In recent years, increasing attention has been given to the psychological reactions that occur in the initial period after trauma exposure. The desire to identify people who may require mental health assistance in the initial aftermath of trauma has raised questions about the optimal means of identifying those people who are in need. This chapter reviews recent developments in the assessment of acute stress reactions and particularly focuses on assessment of acute stress disorder (ASD). This review outlines the rationale for acute stress disorder, critiques the evidence for this diagnosis, discusses available measurement tools for acute stress disorder, highlights the limitations of current approaches, and suggests directions for more accurate means of acute stress assessments.

WHAT IS ACUTE STRESS DISORDER?

In 1994 the fourth edition of the *Diagnostic and Statistical Manual of Mental Disorders* (DSM-IV; American Psychiatric Association, 1994) introduced the ASD diagnosis to describe stress reactions in the initial month after a trauma. DSM-IV stipulated that posttraumatic stress disorder (PTSD) could only be recognized at least one month after a trauma because of concerns that earlier diagnostic decisions would incorrectly pathologize transient stress reactions. This requirement led to a nosological gap because people distressed by a traumatic event could not be readily described in existing diagnostic categories. In response to a proposal that DSM-IV should recognize the initial psychological reactions to trauma, the ASD diagnosis was introduced to describe stress reactions that occur in the initial month.

DSM-IV stipulates that ASD can occur after a fearful response to experiencing or witnessing a threatening event (cluster A). The requisite symptoms to meet criteria for ASD include three dissociative symptoms (cluster B), one reexperiencing symptom (cluster C), marked avoidance (cluster D), marked anxiety or increased arousal (cluster E), and evidence of significant distress or impairment (cluster F). The disturbance must last for a minimum of 2 days and a maximum of 4 weeks (cluster G), after which time a diagnosis of PTSD should be considered. The primary differences between the criteria for ASD and for PTSD are the time frame and the former's emphasis on dissociative reactions to the trauma. ASD refers to symptoms manifested during the period from 2 days to 4 weeks posttrauma, whereas PTSD can be diagnosed only after 4 weeks. The diagnosis of ASD requires that the individual has at least three of the following: (1) a subjective sense of numbing or detachment, (2) reduced awareness of his or her surroundings, (3) derealization, (4) depersonalization, or (5) dissociative amnesia.

WHAT ARE WE ASSESSING IN THE ACUTE PHASE?

The ASD diagnosis was intended to serve two functions. The first goal was to fill the diagnostic gap that existed in the initial month following trauma. That is, the ASD diagnosis was intended to describe posttraumatic stress reactions that occur in the initial month after trauma exposure. Strong evidence indicates that most people who are recently exposed to a traumatic experience show a broad array of posttraumatic stress reactions in the initial weeks after trauma. The literature reports high rates of emotional numbing (Feinstein, 1989; Noyes, Hoenk, Kuperman, & Slymen, 1977), reduced awareness of one's environment (Berah, Jones, & Valent, 1984; Hillman, 1981), derealization (Cardeña & Spiegel, 1993; Noyes & Kletti, 1977; Sloan, 1988; Freinkel, Koopman, & Spiegel, 1994), depersonalization (Noyes et al., 1977; Cardeña & Spiegel, 1993; Sloan, 1988; Freinkel et al., 1994), dissociative amnesia (Feinstein, 1989; Cardeña & Spiegel, 1993; Madakasira & O'Brien, 1987), intrusive thoughts (Feinstein, 1989; Cardeña & Spiegel, 1993; Sloan, 1988), avoidance behaviors (Cardeña & Spiegel, 1993; North, Smith, McCool, & Lightcap, 1989; Bryant & Harvey, 1996), insomnia (Feinstein, 1989; Cardeña & Spiegel, 1993; Sloan, 1988), concentration deficits (Cardeña & Spiegel, 1993; North et al., 1989), irritability (Sloan, 1988), and autonomic arousal (Feinstein, 1989; Sloan, 1988). These incidence rates indicate that psychological distress is very common in the weeks after a traumatic experience.

A number of studies have now reported the incidence of ASD following a range of traumatic events. ASD rates have been reported of between 13 and 21% following motor vehicle accidents (Harvey & Bryant, 1998b; Holeva, Tarrier, & Wells, 2001), 14% following mild brain injury (Harvey & Bryant, 1998a), between 16 and 19% following assault (Brewin, Andrews, Rose, & Kirk, 1999; Harvey & Bryant, 1999a), 16% following traumatic loss (Green, Krupnick, Stockton, & Goodman, 2001), 10% following burns (Harvey &

Bryant, 1999a), between 6 and 12% following industrial accidents (Creamer & Manning, 1998; Harvey & Bryant, 1999a), 33% following a mass shooting (Classen, Koopman, Hales, & Spiegel, 1998), and 7% following a typhoon (Staab, Grieger, Fullerton, & Ursano, 1996) Overall, the reported incidence of ASD is generally lower than the rate of acute PTSD (minus the duration criterion; Feinstein, 1989; Rothbaum, Foa, Riggs, Murdock, & Walsh, 1992). This pattern probably reflects the more stringent criteria for the ASD diagnosis, in particular the requirement that three dissociative symptoms be present (Harvey & Bryant, 2002).

In terms of describing acute trauma reactions, the ASD diagnosis appears somewhat limited because of its focus on PTSD-type symptoms. The trend for the incidence of ASD to be lower than the incidence of PTSD in the initial month suggests that the ASD diagnosis is more restrictive. It is for this reason that some commentators have criticized the ASD diagnosis for not adequately encompassing the range of acute trauma responses. It has been suggested that a more appropriate way to identify initial distress following trauma exposure is to follow the definition of acute stress reactions in the tenth edition of the *International Classification of Diseases* (ICD-10; World Health Organization, 1992). Whereas the ASD diagnosis describes posttraumatic stress reactions that persist beyond 48 hours, the ICD-10 approach focuses on transient reaction that occurs in the initial 48 hours and encompasses a broad range of anxiety and depressive reactions. Specifically, ICD-10 recognizes generalized anxiety, withdrawal, narrowing of attention, apparent disorientation, anger or verbal aggression, despair or hopelessness, overactivity, and excessive grief. This broadness reflects the divergence in the underlying assumptions about the course of the two disorders. Whereas ASD is conceived of as a pathological response to trauma, ICD conceptualizes acute stress reactions as transient. Moreover, the ICD approach of including anxiety and depressive responses is regarded by some commentators as a more useful approach to describing the range of initial reactions often observed in the initial aftermath of trauma (Solomon, Laor, & McFarlane, 1996). Although the DSM-IV and ICD-10 approaches are conceptually different, the discrepancies between these two diagnostic systems highlight the problem in the DSM-IV approach of trying to serve two functions in the single diagnosis. That is, by attempting to both describe acute stress reactions and also identify those reactions that will develop into chronic PTSD, the ASD diagnosis appears to be adopting a restrictive approach in describing acute reactions that do not develop into chronic PTSD.

PREDICTING PTSD

The second goal of the ASD diagnosis is to discriminate between recent trauma survivors who are experiencing transient stress reactions and those who are suffering reactions that will persist into long-term PTSD (Koopman, Classen, Cardeña, & Spiegel, 1995). Although acute stress reactions are very common, there is also strong evidence that the majority of these stress responses are transient. That is, the majority of people who initially display distress naturally adapt to their experience in the following months. For example, whereas 94% of rape victims displayed PTSD symptoms 2 weeks posttrauma, this rate dropped to 47% after 11 weeks (Rothbaum et al., 1992). In another study, 70% of women and 50% of men were diagnosed with PTSD at an average of 19 days after an assault; the rate of PTSD at 4-month follow-up dropped to 21% for women and 0% for men (Riggs, Rothbaum, & Foa, 1995). Similarly, half of a sample that met criteria for PTSD shortly after a motor vehicle accident had remitted by 6 months, and two-thirds had remitted by 1 year posttrauma (Blanchard et al., 1996). A similar pattern was observed in community studies of residents of New York following the terrorist attacks on the World Trade Center. Whereas 8.8% of residents reported PTSD within 1 month after the attacks (Galea, Resnick, et al., 2002), the rate dropped to 3.8% after 4 months (Galea, Ahern, Resnick, Kilpatrick, & Vlahov, 2002). These patterns suggest that the normative response to trauma is the initial experiencing of a range of PTSD symptoms but with remission of the majority of these reactions in the following months.

The ASD diagnosis, as an attempt to identify people who would develop PTSD at an early stage, was strongly influenced by the perspective that dissociative reactions are a crucial mechanism in posttraumatic adjustment. Tracing its origins to Janet (1907), this perspective argues that dissociative responses following trauma lead to psychopathological responses because they impede access to and processing of memories and emotions associated with the traumatic experience (van der Kolk & van der Hart, 1989). The reasoning behind this rationale was that numerous studies have reported that dissociative reactions at the time of the trauma are highly predictive of posttraumatic stress symptoms (e.g., Koopman, Classen, & Spiegel, 1994; Marmar et al., 1994; McFarlane, 1986; Shalev, Orr, & Pitman, 1993; Solomon & Mikulincer, 1992).

In regard to the predictive ability of the ASD diagnosis, 10 prospective studies (Brewin et al., 1999; Bryant & Harvey, 1998; Harvey & Bryant, 1998a, 1999b, 2000; Holeva et al., 2001; Kangas, Henry, & Bryant, in press; Creamer, O'Donnell, & Pattison, 2004; Schnyder, Moergeli, Klaghofer, & Buddeberg, 2001; Staab et al., 1996) have assessed the relationship between ASD in the initial month after trauma and subsequently assessed PTSD. Table 2.1 presents a summary of the 10 studies in terms of (1) the proportion of people who initially had ASD and who subsequently developed PTSD, and (2) the proportion of people who eventually developed PTSD who initially met criteria for ASD. In regard to people who initially display ASD symptoms, a significant number of studies have found that approximately three-fourths of trauma survivors who display ASD symptoms subsequently develop PTSD (Brewin et al., 1999; Bryant & Harvey, 1998; Harvey & Bryant, 1998b). These studies suggest that the ASD diagnosis is performing reasonably well in predicting people who will develop PTSD. The lower rates of PTSD following

TABLE 2.1. Summary of Prospective Studies of Acute Stress Disorder

Trauma type	Study	Proportion of people with ASD who develop PTSD	Proportion of people with PTSD who had ASD
MVA	Harvey & Bryant (1998b)	78%	39%
Brain injury	Bryant & Harvey (1998)	83%	40%
Assault	Brewin et al. (1999)	83%	57%
MVA	Holeva et al. (2001)	72%	59%
MVA	Creamer et al. (2004)	30%	34%
MVA	Schnyder et al. (2001)	34%	10%
Typhoon	Staab et al. (1996)	30%	37%
Cancer	Kangas, Henry, & Bryant (in press)	53%	61%
MVA	Harvey & Bryant (1999b)	82%	29%
Brain injury	Harvey & Bryant (2000)	80%	72%

Note. MVA, motor vehicle accident.

ASD in some studies may be attributed to methodological factors in these studies. For example, both the Creamer et al. (2004) and the Schnyder et al. (2001) studies adopted strict exclusion criteria that may have limited the identification of ASD in these studies.

The utility of the ASD diagnosis is less promising, however, when one considers the proportion of people who eventually developed PTSD and who had initially displayed ASD. Across studies, the minority of people who eventually developed PTSD initially met criteria for ASD. This convergence across studies suggests that, whereas the majority of people who develop ASD are at high risk for developing subsequent PTSD, many other people who will develop PTSD do not initially meet ASD criteria. One probable reason that people who are at high risk for PTSD may not meet ASD criteria is the requirement that three dissociative symptoms be displayed. In one prospective study, 60% of people who met all ASD criteria except for the dissociation cluster met PTSD criteria 6 months later (Harvey & Bryant, 1998b), and 75% of these people still had PTSD 2 years later (Harvey & Bryant, 1999b). This pattern suggests that emphasizing dissociation as a key factor in predicting subsequent PTSD will result in many high-risk individuals being neglected. This conclusion is reinforced by increasing evidence that peritraumatic dissociation is not necessarily related to development of subsequent PTSD (Marshall & Schell, 2002).

The prospective studies of ASD and PTSD should be interpreted in the context of a range of methodological factors (for a review, see O'Donnell, Creamer, Bryant, Schnyder, & Shalev, 2003). These studies have varied markedly in terms of populations, assessment procedures, and inclusion criteria. For example, whereas some studies have diagnosed ASD with tools that have been specifically developed to index ASD (Bryant & Harvey, 1998; Harvey & Bryant, 1998b), others have derived ASD diagnoses on the basis of different measures that purportedly indexed symptoms that are comparable to those of ASD (Brewin et al., 1999; Staab et al., 1996). Additionally, these studies have adopted variable approaches to excluding different participants on the grounds that they may not be appropriate for an ASD diagnosis. For example, some studies have excluded people with brain injury because of the difficulty discriminating amnesia caused by traumatic brain injury from dissociative amnesia (e.g., Creamer et al., 2004). These procedural discrepancies may contribute to varying incidence of ASD. The sensitivity and specificity of any measure can fluctuate according to prevalence rates observed in a target population. For example, sensitivity of a test can drop markedly when the prevalence rate decreases (Baldessarini, Finkelstein, & Arana, 1983). The importance of validating measures of PTSD in different populations that have varying prevalence rates has been previously demonstrated (Gerardi, Keane, & Penk, 1989). It needs to be recognized that the current evidence about the relationship between ASD and PTSD may be limited because of variability across studies in terms of prevalence rates, inclusion criteria, and assessment methods.

CONTROVERSIES ABOUT ASD

It should be noted that the construct of ASD has been widely debated on both conceptual and empirical grounds (see Bryant & Harvey, 2000; Butler, 2000; Keane, Kaufman, & Kimble, 2000; Koopman, 2000; Marshall, Spitzer, & Liebowitz, 2000; Simeon & Guralnik, 2000; Spiegel, Classen, & Cardeña, 2000). The ASD diagnosis has been criticized for a range of reasons. First, the ASD diagnosis was introduced with very little evidence to support its inclusion. Even those who supported the introduction of the ASD diagnosis recognized that the alleged relationship between ASD and PTSD was "based more on logical arguments than on empirical research" (Koopman et al., 1995, p. 38). Second, the ASD diagnosis was one of the few diagnoses that were included without being subjected to the empirical or peer-review scrutiny given to other potential diagnoses that were considered for inclusion in DSM-IV (Bryant, 2000). Third, the emphasis on dissociation as a necessary response to trauma has been criticized because there is inadequate evidence to warrant requirement that dissociation be present in trauma survivors who will subsequent develop PTSD (Bryant & Harvey, 1997; Marshall et al., 2000). Fourth, the notion that we need a distinct diagnosis to predict another very similar diagnosis has been questioned (Bryant, 2000). Fifth, some commentaries have suggested that the ASD diagnosis may pathologize transient stress reactions (Marshall, Spitzer, & Liebowitz, 1999). Sixth, distinguishing between two diagnoses (ASD and PTSD) that have comparable symptoms on the basis of the duration of these symptoms may not be justified (Marshall et al., 1999). Seventh, it was suggested that the broader conceptualization adopted by ICD-10 was more useful for clinicians than the more focused DSM-IV criteria (Marshall et al, 1999; Solomon et al., 1996).

MEASUREMENT TOOLS FOR ASD

There are currently three major measures for ASD. The first measure to be developed was the Stanford Acute Stress Reaction Questionnaire (SASRQ). The original version of the SASRQ (Cardeña, Classen, & Spiegel, 1991) was a self-report inventory that indexed dissociative (33 items), intrusive (11 items), somatic anxiety (17 items), hyperarousal (2 items), attention disturbance (3 items), and sleep disturbance (1 item) symptoms, and different versions of this measure have been employed by the authors across a range of studies (Cardeña & Spiegel, 1993; Classen et al., 1998; Freinkel et al., 1994; Koopman et al., 1994). Each item asks respondents to indicate the frequency of each symptom on a 6-point Likert scale (0 = "not experienced"; 5 = "very often experienced") that can occur during and immediately following a trauma. The SASRQ possesses high internal consistency (Cronbach's alpha = .90 and .91 for dissociative and anxiety symptoms, respectively) and concurrent validity with scores on the IES (r = .52–.69; Koopman et al., 1994; Cardeña, Koopman, Classen, Waelde, & Spiegel, 2000). Different versions of the SASRQ have been employed in a number of studies conducted by the authors (Classen et al., 1998; Freinkel et al., 1994; Koopman et al., 1994). The current version of the SASRQ (Cardeña et al., 2000) is a 30-item self-report inventory that encompasses each of the ASD symptoms. At this stage, the SASRQ has not been validated against independent clinician diagnoses of ASD. Although SASRQ scores are predictive of subsequent posttraumatic stress symptomatology, there is limited data concerning SASRQ scores and subsequent PTSD diagnostic status.

The Acute Stress Disorder Interview (ASDI; Bryant, Harvey, Dang, & Sackville, 1998) is a structured clinical interview that is based on DSM-IV criteria. The ASDI contains 19 dichotomously scored items that relate to the dissociative (cluster B, five items), reexperiencing (cluster C, four items), avoidance (cluster D, four items), and arousal (cluster E, six items) symptoms of ASD. Summing the affirmative responses to each symptom provides a total score indicative of acute stress severity (range 1 to 19). The ASDI possesses good internal consistency (r = .90), test–retest reliability (r = .88), sensitivity (91%), and specificity (93%) relative to independent clinician diagnoses of ASD. The ASDI has also been used in a range of prospective studies that have identified people exposed to recent trauma who subsequently develop PTSD (Bryant & Harvey, 1998; Harvey & Bryant, 1998b, 1999b, 2000).

The Acute Stress Disorder Scale (ASDS; Bryant, Moulds, & Guthrie, 2000) is a self-report inventory that is based on the same items described in the ASDI. Each item on the ASDS is scored on a 5-point scale that reflects degrees of severity. It was validated against the ASDI on 99 civilian trauma survivors assessed between 2 and 10 days posttrauma. The researchers used a formula to identify ASD. The ASDS possessed good sensitivity (95%) and specificity (83%). Test–retest reliability was evaluated on 107 bushfire survivors 3 weeks posttrauma, with a readministration interval of 2 to 7 days. Test–retest reliability of the ASDS scores was strong (r = .94). Predictive ability of the ASDS was investigated in 82 trauma survivors who completed the ASDS and were subsequently assessed for PTSD 6 months posttrauma. A cutoff score of 56 on the ASDS predicted 91% of those who developed PTSD and 93% of those who did not. The major limitation of the ASDS in predicting PTSD, however, was that one-third of people who scored above the cutoff did not develop PTSD.

PROBLEMS IN ASSESSING ASD

Certain problems are inherent in measures of ASD. The construct of these measures assumes that there is some gold standard against which the measure can be validated. As discussed, the ASD diagnosis is based on theoretical constructs that lack strong empirical support. Underpinning this notion is the finding that the symptom clusters of the ASD diagnosis are not supported by factorial analysis. A confirmatory factor analysis of 420 responses on the ASDS attempted to fit the responses into the model generated by the four symptom clusters of ASD (Bryant & Bird, 2003). Although numerous models were attempted, none of the tested models adequately explained the data. The observed patterns suggested that acute stress reactions tend to load on a single construct of distress and that reactions do not conform to the factors described by the current ASD criteria. Development of measures also relies on related measures or constructs to establish concurrent validity or construct validity (Haynes, Wilner, & Kubany, 1995). The absence of these measures in ASD results in measures being developed that attempt validation by comparing them against the same items that were driven by the questionable DSM-IV construction of the diagnosis. The tendency for current measures of ASD to demonstrate construct validity by comparing the measures against existing PTSD scales (e.g., Impact of Event Scale) reinforces the notion that ASD has questionable distinction from PTSD.

The development of reliable measures is difficult in the context of ASD because of the rapidly changing nature of acute stress reactions. In contrast to the reasonably stable nature of most psychiatric diagnoses, the ASD diagnosis is susceptible to marked changes within the initial days and weeks after trauma exposure. Although DSM-IV stipulates that the ASD diagnosis can be established 2 days after trauma exposure, there is no empirical basis to justify this time frame. It is very probable that the sooner one diagnoses ASD after trauma exposure, the more likely it is that one will confuse a psychopathological response with a transient stress reaction. There is some evidence from a study of civilians involved in the Gulf War that many people experience immediate posttraumatic stress reactions in the initial days after trauma exposure but that these reactions subsequently remit (Solomon et al., 1996). Although there is insufficient evidence to direct the optimal time frame for identifying psychopathological stress reactions, it is very likely that the DSM-IV prescription of 2 days after trauma exposure is too soon for accurate identification of people who will subsequently develop PTSD.

Accurate assessment of ASD is also difficult because of the vague temporal parameters associated with the prescribed dissociative symptoms. DSM-IV stipulates that the dissociative symptoms may occur "while experiencing or after experiencing the distressing event" (American Psychiatric Association, 1994, p. 431). That is, DSM-IV regards transient and persistent dissociative responses as equivalent responses to trauma. There are several reasons to question the equivalence of these responses. Dissociation that occurs at the time of the trauma may serve a protective function, because reduced awareness of the experience may limit encoding of a threatening experience (Horowitz, 1986). In this context, it is noteworthy that transient dissociative responses are reportedly common during traumatic experiences and may not be indicative of subsequent psychopathology (Cardeña & Spiegel, 1993). Moreover, dissociative experiences are commonplace in community samples (Hilgard, 1977; Kihlstrom, Glisky, & Angiulo, 1994). There is considerable experimental evidence that dissociative responses can be elicited under conditions of stress in nonclinical populations. For example, presenting experimental participants with a threatening object can lead to reduced awareness of many features of that experience (Kramer, Buckhout, & Eugenio, 1990; Maas & Kohnken, 1989). Further, novice skydivers reported elevated levels of dissociation during the skydive, and these reactions were associated most strongly with levels of panic (Sterlini & Bryant, 2002). This observation accords with the proposition that peritraumatic dissociation reflects a compensatory mechanism to marked physiological arousal (Friedman, 2000). This view is also consistent with evidence that dissociative reactions are commonly reported during panic attacks (Krystal, Woods, Hill, & Charney, 1991). It is possible that one reason for the mixed findings concerning the relationship between acute dissociation and subsequent PTSD is the confusion between transient and persistent dissociation. Information processing models of trauma response posit that persistent dissociation forms a type of cognitive avoidance that may impede access to and resolution of traumatic memories and may contribute to ongoing psychopathology (Foa & Hearst-Ikeda, 1996). Overall, this evidence suggests that dissociative responses during trauma exposure may reflect a number of nonpathological reactions that are not necessarily predictive of subsequent disorder.

DIFFERENTIAL DIAGNOSIS

It is important to note that differential diagnosis of ASD can be difficult because many people recently exposed to trauma may suffer ASD-type reactions for medical reasons. Many individuals who may potentially qualify for a diagnosis of ASD may also sustain traumatic brain injury or experience serious medical conditions. Brain injury is a very common occurrence in trauma-exposed populations, including survivors of assault, motor vehicle accidents, combat, and industrial accidents. The utility of the ASD diagnosis for people after brain injury is indicated by evidence that approximately 80% of people with ASD after brain injury subsequently develop PTSD (Bryant & Harvey, 1998; Harvey & Bryant, 2000). The dissociative symptoms of reduced awareness, depersonalization, derealization, and amnesia are commonly reported during posttraumatic amnesia after brain injury (Grigsby, 1986; Grigsby & Kaye, 1993; Gronwall & Wrightson, 1980). In addition, insomnia, irritability, and concentration deficits, which are common hyperarousal symptoms in ASD, are also common following brain injury (Bohnen & Jolles, 1992). Although there are some suggestions concerning differential diagnosis of dissociative and organic amnesia (Sivec & Lynn, 1995), there are currently no reliable means to differentiate between the overlapping ASD and postconcussive symptoms. The differential diagnosis is particularly difficult when there are no external indications of brain injury (e.g., lacerations or bruising) following acceleration/deceleration injuries (e.g., motor vehicle accidents). Many hospitalized patients will also experience impaired consciousness as a result of sedation or coma, and these impaired states can include reduced awareness, depersonalization, derealization, numbing, and amnesia. It is important in the acute phase after trauma that states associated with medical conditions or substance use are not confused with severe stress reactions.

FUTURE DIRECTIONS

The current evidence challenges the utility of the ASD diagnosis as an accurate means of identifying people recently exposed to trauma who will subsequently develop PTSD or other psychiatric disorders. Although the evidence does suggest that the majority of people who do satisfy ASD criteria are very likely to suffer subsequent PTSD, too many people who are at high risk for PTSD are not identified using the ASD criteria. Recent attempts to improve our capacity to identify people who will suffer long-term PTSD are focusing on biological and cognitive indices that may provide more sensitive markers of people who will suffer more than a transient stress reaction following trauma.

Attempts to identify biological markers of high risk have emerged from models that posit that fear conditioning and progressive neural sensitization in the weeks after trauma lead to increased activation of the sympathetic nervous system and subsequent development of PTSD (Pitman, Shalev, & Orr, 2000). It is possible that the persistent activation of the sympathetic nervous system develops secondary to elevated sensitivity of limbic networks (Post, Weiss, & Smith, 1995), reduced extinction of conditioned fear responses (Charney, Deutch, Krystal, Southwick, & Davis, 1993), or sensitization of the hypothalamic–pituitary–adrenocortical axis in which reduced cortisol fails to contain sympathetic activity (Yehuda, 1997). In support of these proposals, there is initial evidence that elevated resting heart rate in the first week after trauma (Bryant, Harvey, Guthrie, & Moulds, 2000; Shalev et al., 1998) and lower cortisol levels (Delahanty, Raimonde, & Spoonster, 2000; McFarlane, Atchison, & Yehuda, 1997) are predictive of subsequent PTSD development.

Recent cognitive models of trauma response have proposed that the transition from acute stress reaction to chronic PTSD is mediated by people's cognitive styles in the ways that they manage their memories of a trauma. For example, Ehlers and Clark (2000) suggest that PTSD can be explained in terms of (1) excessively negative appraisals of the trauma and its aftermath and (2) a disturbance of autobiographical memory that is characterized by poor elaboration and contextualization, strong associative memory, and strong perceptual priming. Consistent with this proposition, people with ASD (who are at high risk for developing PTSD) exaggerate both the probability of future negative events occurring and the adverse effects of these events, compared with participants without ASD (Smith & Bryant, 2000; Warda & Bryant, 1998). Evidence exists that negative appraisals in the initial period after trauma exposure predict subsequent PTSD (Ehlers, Mayou, & Bryant, 1998; Engelhard, van den Hout, Arntz, & McNally, 2002). Initial evidence shows that the attributions of responsibility for a trauma that trauma survivors make in the acute posttrauma phase influence subsequent PTSD (Andrews, Brewin, Rose, & Kirk, 2000; Delahanty et al., 1997). Research also shows that how people manage their retrieval of personal memories initially after trauma significantly predicts subsequent PTSD (Harvey, Bryant, & Dang, 1998).

Overall, there is initial evidence that a range of biological and cognitive factors may increase our ability to identify people recently exposed to trauma who will subsequently develop chronic PTSD. In this sense, the ASD diagnosis has been a significant watershed in our understanding of acute stress reactions because it has initiated an unprecedented amount of research on factors that mediate the transition from initial to chronic posttraumatic stress reactions. As future research looks beyond simple diagnostic categories as a means of identifying people who are at high risk of developing PTSD, we will develop more sensitive evidence-based means to guide our assessment of people in the initial period following trauma.

REFERENCES

American Psychiatric Association. (1994). *Diagnostic and statistical manual of mental disorders* (4th ed.). Washington, DC: Author.

Andrews, B., Brewin, C. R., Rose, S., & Kirk, M. (2000). Predicting PTSD in victims of violent crime: The role of shame, anger, and blame. *Journal of Abnormal Psychology*, *109*, 69–73.

Baldessarini, R. J., Finkelstein, S., & Arana, G. W. (1983). The predictive power of diagnostic tests and the effect of prevalence of illness. *Archives of General Psychiatry*, *40*, 569–573.

Berah, E. F., Jones, H. J., & Valent, P. (1984). The experience of a mental health team involved in the early phase of a disaster. *Australian and New Zealand Journal of Psychiatry*, *18*, 354–358.

Blanchard, E. B., Hickling, E. J., Barton, K. A., Taylor, A. E., Loos, W. R., & Jones-Alexander, J. (1996). One-year prospective follow-up of motor vehicle accident victims. *Behaviour Research and Therapy*, *34*, 775–786.

Bohnen, N., & Jolles, J. (1992). Neurobehavioral aspects of postconcussive symptoms after mild head injury. *Journal of Nervous and Mental Disease*, *180*, 183–192.

Brewin, C. R., Andrews, B., Rose, S., & Kirk, M. (1999). Acute stress disorder and posttraumatic stress disorder in victims of violent crime. *American Journal of Psychiatry*, *156*, 360–366.

Bryant, R. A. (2000). Acute stress disorder. *PTSD Research Quarterly*, *11*, 1–7.

Bryant, R. A., & Bird, K. (2003). *Confirmatory factor analysis of acute stress disorder.* Manuscript submitted for publication.

Bryant, R. A., & Harvey, A. G. (1996). Initial post-traumatic stress responses following motor vehicle accidents. *Journal of Traumatic Stress*, *9*, 223–234.

Bryant, R. A., & Harvey, A. G. (1997). Acute stress disorder: A critical review of diagnostic issues. *Clinical Psychology Review*, *17*, 757–773.

Bryant, R. A., & Harvey, A. G. (1998). Relationship of acute stress disorder and posttraumatic stress disorder following mild traumatic brain injury. *American Journal of Psychiatry*, *155*, 625–629.

Bryant, R. A., & Harvey, A. G. (2000). New DSM-IV diagnosis of acute stress disorder [Letter to the editor]. *American Journal of Psychiatry*, *157*, 1889–1890.

Bryant, R. A, Harvey, A. G., Dang, S., & Sackville, T. (1998). Assessing acute stress disorder: Psychometric properties of a structured clinical interview. *Psychological Assessment*, *10*, 215–220.

Bryant, R. A., Harvey, A. G., Guthrie, R., & Moulds, M. (2000). A prospective study of acute psychophysiological arousal, acute stress disorder, and posttraumatic stress disorder. *Journal of Abnormal Psychology*, *109*, 341–344.

Bryant, R. A., Moulds, M., & Guthrie, R. (2000). Acute Stress Disorder Scale: A self-report measure of acute stress disorder. *Psychological Assessment*, *12*, 61–68.

Butler, L. D. (2000). New DSM-IV diagnosis of acute stress disorder [Letter to the editor]. *American Journal of Psychiatry*, *157*, 1889.

Cardeña, E., Classen, C., & Spiegel, D. (1991). *Stanford Acute Stress Reaction Questionnaire.* Stanford, CA: Stanford University Medical School.

Cardeña, E., Koopman, C., Classen, C., Waelde, L. C., & Spiegel, D. (2000). Psychometric properties of the Stanford Acute Stress Reaction Questionnaire (SASRQ): A valid and reliable measure of acute stress. *Journal of Traumatic Stress*, *13*, 719–734.

Cardeña, E., & Spiegel, D. (1993). Dissociative reactions to the San Francisco Bay Area earthquake of 1989. *American Journal of Psychiatry*, *150*, 474–478.

Charney, D. S., Deutch, A. Y., Krystal, J. H., Southwick, S. M., & Davis, M. (1993). Psychobiologic mechanisms of posttraumatic stress disorder. *Archives of General Psychiatry*, *50*, 294–305.

Classen, C., Koopman, C., Hales, R., & Spiegel, D. (1998). Acute stress disorder as a predictor of posttraumatic stress symptoms. *American Journal of Psychiatry*, *155*, 620–624.

Creamer, M., & Manning, C. (1998). Acute stress disorder following an industrial accident. *Australian Psychologist*, *33*, 125–129.

Creamer, M., O'Donnell, M. L., & Pattison, P. (2004). The relationship between acute stress disorder and posttraumatic stress disorder in severely injured trauma survivors. *Behaviour Research and Therapy, 42*(3), 315–328.

Delahanty, D. L., Herberman, H. B., Craig, K. J., Hayward, M. C., Fullerton, C. S., Ursano, R. J., & Baum, A. (1997). Acute and chronic distress and posttraumatic stress disorder as a function of responsibility for serious motor vehicle accidents. *Journal of Consulting and Clinical Psychology, 65*, 560–567.

Delahanty, D. L., Raimonde, A. J., & Spoonster, E. (2000). Initial posttraumatic urinary cortisol levels predict subsequent PTSD symptoms in motor vehicle accident victims. *Biological Psychiatry, 48*, 940–947.

Ehlers, A., & Clark, D. (2000). A cognitive model of posttraumatic stress disorder. *Behaviour Research and Therapy, 38*, 319–345.

Ehlers, A., Mayou, R. A., & Bryant, B. (1998). Psychological predictors of chronic PTSD after motor vehicle accidents. *Journal of Abnormal Psychology, 107*, 508–519.

Engelhard, I. M., van den Hout, M. A., Arntz, A., & McNally, R. J. (2002). A longitudinal study of "intrusion-based reasoning" and posttraumatic stress disorder after exposure to a train disaster. *Behaviour Research and Therapy, 40*(12), 1415–1424.

Feinstein, A. (1989). Posttraumatic stress disorder: A descriptive study supporting DSM-III-R criteria. *American Journal of Psychiatry, 146*, 665–666.

Foa, E. B., & Hearst-Ikeda, D. (1996). Emotional dissociation in response to trauma: An information-processing approach. In L. K. Michelson & W. J. Ray (Eds.), *Handbook of dissociation: Theoretical and clinical perspectives* (pp. 207–222). New York: Plenum Press.

Freinkel, A., Koopman, C., & Spiegel, D. (1994). Dissociative symptoms in media witnesses of an execution. *American Journal of Psychiatry, 151*, 1335–1339.

Friedman, M. (2000). What might the psychobiology of PTSD teach us about future approaches to pharmacotherapy? *Journal of Clinical Psychiatry,61*(Suppl. 7), 44–51.

Galea, S., Ahern, J., Resnick, H., Kilpatrick, D., & Vlahov, D. (2002, November). Posttraumatic stress disorder and depression in New York City after 9/11. Paper presented at the annual meeting of the International Society of Traumatic Stress Studies, Baltimore, MD.

Galea, S., Resnick, H., Kilpatrick, D., Bucuvalas, M., Gold, J., & Vlahov, D. (2002). Psychological sequelae of the September 11 terrorist attacks in New York City. *New England Journal of Medicine, 346*, 982–987.

Gerardi, R., Keane, T. M., & Penk, W. (1989). Utility, sensitivity and specificity in developing diagnostic tests of combat-related post-traumatic stress disorder (PTSD). *Journal of Clinical Psychology, 45*, 691–701.

Green, B. L., Krupnick, J. L., Stockton, P., & Goodman, L. (2001). Psychological outcomes associated with traumatic loss in a sample of young women. *American Behavioral Scientist, 44*, 817–837.

Grigsby, J. (1986). Depersonalization following minor closed head injury. *International Journal of Clinical Neuropsychology, 8*, 65–69.

Grigsby, J., & Kaye, K. (1993). Incidence and correlates of depersonalization following head trauma. *Brain Injury, 7*, 507–513.

Gronwall, D., & Wrightson, P. (1980). Duration of post-traumatic amnesia after mild head injury. *Journal of Clinical Neuropsychology, 2*, 51–60.

Harvey, A. G., & Bryant, R. A. (1998a). Acute stress disorder following mild traumatic brain injury. *Journal of Nervous and Mental Disease, 186*, 333–337.

Harvey, A. G., & Bryant, R. A. (1998b). Relationship of acute stress disorder and posttraumatic stress disorder following motor vehicle accidents. *Journal of Consulting and Clinical Psychology, 66*, 507–512.

Harvey, A. G., & Bryant, R. A. (1999a). Acute stress disorder across trauma populations. *Journal of Nervous and Mental Disease, 187*, 443–446.

Harvey, A. G., & Bryant, R. A. (1999b). A two-year prospective evaluation of the relationship between acute stress disorder and posttraumatic stress disorder. *Journal of Consulting and Clinical Psychology, 67*, 985–988.

Harvey, A. G., & Bryant, R. A. (2000). A two-year prospective evaluation of the relationship between acute stress disorder and posttraumatic stress disorder following mild traumatic brain injury. *American Journal of Psychiatry, 157*, 626–628.

Harvey, A. G., & Bryant, R. A. (2002). Acute stress disorder: A synthesis and critique. *Psychological Bulletin, 128*, 892–906.

Harvey, A. G., Bryant, R. A., & Dang, S. (1998). Autobiographical memory in acute stress disorder. *Journal of Consulting and Clinical Psychology, 66*, 500–506.

Haynes, S. N., Wilner, N., & Kubany, E. S. (1995). Content validity in psychological assessment: A functional approach to concepts and methods. *Psychological Assessment, 7*, 238–247.

Hilgard, E. R. (1977). *Divided consciousness: Multiple controls in human thought and action*. New York: Wiley-Interscience.

Hillman, R. G. (1981). The psychopathology of being held hostage. *American Journal of Psychiatry, 138*, 1193–1197.

Holeva, V., Tarrier, N., & Wells, A. (2001). Prevalence and predictors of acute stress disorder and PTSD following road traffic accidents: Thought control strategies and social support. *Behavior Therapy, 32*, 65–83.

Horowitz, M. J. (1986). *Stress response syndromes* (2nd ed.). New York: Aronson.

Janet, P. (1907). *The major symptoms of hysteria*. New York: Macmillan.

Kangas, M., Henry, R. A., & Bryant, R. A. (in press). The relationship between acute stress disorder and posttraumatic stress disorder following cancer. *Journal of Consulting and Clinical Psychology*.

Keane, T. M., Kaufman, M., & Kimble, M. O. (2000). Peritraumatic dissociative symptoms, acute stress disorder, and posttraumatic stress disorder: Causation, correlation, or epiphenomenona. In L. Sanchez-Planell & C. Diez-Quevedo (Eds.), *Dissociative states* (pp. 21–43). Barcelona, Spain: Springer-Verlag.

Kihlstrom, J. F., Glisky, M. L., & Angiulo, M. J. (1994). Dissociative tendencies and dissociative disorders. *Journal of Abnormal Psychology, 103*, 117–124.

Koopman, C. (2000). New DSM-IV diagnosis of acute stress disorder [Letter to the editor]. *American Journal of Psychiatry, 157*, 1888.

Koopman, C., Classen, C., Cardeña, E., & Spiegel, D. (1995). When disaster strikes, acute stress disorder may follow. *Journal of Traumatic Stress, 8*, 29–46.

Koopman, C., Classen, C., & Spiegel, D. (1994). Predictors of posttraumatic stress symptoms among survivors of the Oakland/Berkeley, Calif., firestorm. *American Journal of Psychiatry, 151*, 888–894.

Kramer, T., Buckhout, R., & Eugenio, P. (1990). Weapon focus, arousal, and eyewitness memory: Attention must be paid. *Law and Human Behavior, 14*, 167–184.

Krystal, J., Woods, S., Hill, C. L., & Charney, D. S. (1991). Characteristics of panic attack subtypes: Assessment of spontaneous panic, situational panic, sleep panic, and limited symptom attacks. *Comprehensive Psychiatry*, *32*, 4474–4480.

Maas, A., & Kohnken, G. (1989). Eyewitness identification. *Law and Human Behavior*, *11*, 397–408.

Madakasira, S., & O'Brien, K.F. (1987). Acute posttraumatic stress disorder in victims of a natural disaster. *Journal of Nervous and Mental Disease*, *175*, 286–290.

Marmar, C. R., Weiss, D. S., Schlenger, W. E., Fairbank, J. A., Jordan, K., Kulka, R. A., & Hough, R. L. (1994). Peritraumatic dissociation and posttraumatic stress in male Vietnam theater veterans. *American Journal of Psychiatry*, *151*, 902–907.

Marshall, G. N., & Schell, T. L. (2002). Reappraising the link between peritraumatic dissociation and PTSD symptom severity: Evidence from a longitudinal study of community violence survivors. *Journal of Abnormal Psychology*, *111*, 626–636.

Marshall, R. D., Spitzer, R., & Liebowitz, M. R. (1999). Review and critique of the new DSM-IV diagnosis of acute stress disorder. *American Journal of Psychiatry*, *156*, 1677–1685.

Marshall, R. D., Spitzer, R., & Liebowitz, M. R. (2000). New DSM-IV diagnosis of acute stress disorder. *American Journal of Psychiatry*, *157*, 1890–1891.

McFarlane, A. C. (1986). Posttraumatic morbidity of a disaster. *Journal of Nervous and Mental Disease*, *174*, 4–14.

McFarlane, A. C., Atchison, M., & Yehuda, R. (1997). The acute stress response following motor vehicle accidents and its relation to PTSD. In R. Yehuda & A. C. McFarlane (Eds.), *Psychobiology of posttraumatic stress disorder* (pp. 433–436). New York: New York Academy of Sciences.

North, C. S., Smith, E. M., McCool, R. E., & Lightcap, P. E. (1989). Acute postdisaster coping and adjustment. *Journal of Traumatic Stress*, *2*, 353–360.

Noyes, R., Hoenk, P. R., Kuperman, S., & Slymen, D. J. (1977). Depersonalization in accident victims and psychiatric patients. *Journal of Nervous and Mental Disease*, *164*, 401–407.

Noyes, R., & Kletti, R. (1977). Depersonalizaton in response to life-threatening danger. *Comprehensive Psychiatry*, *18*, 375–384.

O'Donnell, M., Creamer, M., Bryant, R. A., Schnyder, U., & Shalev, A. (2003). Posttraumatic stress disorder following injury: An empirical and methodological review. *Clinical Psychology Review*, *23*(4), 587–603.

Pitman, R. K., Shalev, A. Y., & Orr, S. P. (2000). Posttraumatic stress disorder: Emotion, conditioning and memory. In M. D. Corbetta & M. Gazzaniga (Eds.), *The new cognitive neurosciences* (2nd ed., pp. 1133–1147). New York: Plenum Press.

Post, R. M., Weiss, S. R. B., & Smith, M. (1995). Sensitization and kindling: Implication for the evolving neural substrates of posttraumatic stress disorder. In M. J. Friedman, D. S. Charney, & A. Y. Deutch (Eds.), *Neurobiological and clinical consequences of stress: From normal adaptation to posttraumatic stress disorder* (pp. 203–224). Philadelphia: Lippincott-Raven.

Riggs, D. S., Rothbaum, B. O., & Foa, E. B. (1995). A prospective examination of symptoms of posttraumatic stress disorder in victims of nonsexual assault. *Journal of Interpersonal Violence*, *10*, 201–214.

Rothbaum, B. O., Foa, E. B., Riggs, D. S., Murdock, T., & Walsh, W. (1992). A prospective examination of post-traumatic stress disorder in rape victims. *Journal of Traumatic Stress*, *5*, 455–475.

Schnyder, U., Moergeli, H., Klaghofer, R., & Buddeberg, C. (2001). Incidence and prediction of posttraumatic stress disorder symptoms in severely injured accident victims. *American Journal of Psychiatry, 158*, 594–599.

Shalev, A. Y., Orr, S. P., & Pitman, R. K. (1993). Psychophysiologic assessment of traumatic imagery in Israeli civilian patients with posttraumatic stress disorder. *AmericanJournal of Psychiatry, 150*, 620–624.

Shalev, A. Y., Sahar, T., Freedman, S., Peri, T., Glick, N., Brandes, D., et al. (1998). A prospective study of heart rate responses following trauma and the subsequent development of PTSD. *Archives of General Psychiatry, 55*, 553–559.

Simeon, D., & Guralnik, O. (2000). New DSM-IV diagnosis of acute stress disorder [Letter to the editor]. *American Journal of Psychiatry, 157*, 1888–1889.

Sivec, H. J., & Lynn, S. J. (1995). Dissociative and neuropsychological symptoms: The question of differential diagnosis. *Clinical Psychology Review, 15*, 297–316.

Sloan, P. (1988). Post-traumatic stress in survivors of an airplane crash-landing: A clinical and exploratory research intervention. *Journal of Traumatic Stress, 1*, 211–229.

Smith, K., & Bryant, R. A. (2000). The generality of cognitive bias in acute stress disorder. *Behaviour Research and Therapy, 38*, 709–715.

Solomon, Z., Laor, N., & McFarlane, A. C. (1996). Acute posttraumatic reactions in soldiers and civilians. In B. A. van der Kolk, A. C. McFarlane, & L. Weisaeth (Eds.), *Traumatic stress: The effects of overwhelming experience on mind, body, and society* (pp. 102–114). New York: Guilford Press.

Solomon, Z., & Mikulincer, M. (1992). Aftermaths of combat stress reactions: A three-year study. *British Journal of Clinical Psychology, 31*, 21–32.

Spiegel, D., Classen, C., & Cardeña , E. (2000). New DSM-IV diagnosis of acute stress disorder [Letter to the editor]. *American Journal of Psychiatry, 157*, 1890–1891.

Staab, J. P., Grieger, T. A., Fullerton, C. S., & Ursano, R. J. (1996). Acute stress disorder, subsequent posttraumatic stress disorder and depression after a series of typhoons. *Anxiety, 2*, 219–225.

Sterlini, G., & Bryant, R. A. (2002). Hyperarousal and dissociation: A study of novice skydivers. *Behaviour Research and Therapy, 40*, 431–437.

van der Kolk, B. A., & van der Hart, O. (1989). Pierre Janet and the breakdown of adaptation in psychological data. *American Journal of Psychiatry, 146*, 1530–1540.

Warda, G., & Bryant, R. A. (1998). Cognitive bias in acute stress disorder. *Behaviour Research and Therapy, 36*, 1177–1183.

World Health Organization. (1992). *The ICD-10 classification of mental and behavioural disorder: Diagnostic criteria for research* (10th rev.). Geneva: Author.

Yehuda, R. (1997). Sensitization of the hypothalamic–pituitary–adrenal axis in posttraumatic stress disorder. *Annals of the New York Academy of Science, 821*, 57–75.

PART II

Assessment Methods

CHAPTER 3

Standardized Self-Report Measures of Civilian Trauma and PTSD

FRAN H. NORRIS
JESSICA L. HAMBLEN

This chapter reviews 24 standardized self-report measures for traumatic stress that are suitable, with some modification, for use with adults by professional or lay interviewers or in paper-and-pencil questionnaires. Each scale is described in terms of its content, number of items, and response formats and is evaluated in terms of the available evidence regarding its reliability and validity. We also describe the population or populations on whom the scale was validated. We note strengths and weaknesses but stop short of recommending one scale for all situations. In fact, our assumption is that different scales may be more or less suitable for different purposes in different contexts involving traumatic stress responses.

Because measures of combat-related trauma are described elsewhere in this volume, this chapter focuses on scales that are suitable for studying civilian trauma in clinical or community populations. These populations may include veterans of military service but are not limited to them. The measures described herein are those that either have been significant to this field historically or appear quite promising for future research. In deciding which scales warranted inclusion in this chapter, we relied heavily on the published literature and, to a lesser extent, on information gained from networking with investigators working in this area. The selected scales make up a reasonable cross-section of standardized self-report measures available in the field today.

The scales reviewed here fall into two broad categories: seven that measure DSM-IV posttraumatic stress disorder (PTSD) criterion A, or trauma histories, and 17 that measure DSM-IV PTSD criteria B–D, or symptom histories. The chapter is organized accordingly. Researchers and practitioners should plan on selecting one scale from each category to fully capture the phenomenon of trauma.

DSM-IV PTSD CRITERION A: ASSESSING TRAUMATIC EVENTS

Over the past two decades, the definition of a traumatic event has changed considerably. These changes in definition have a significant impact on what events qualify for PTSD and must be considered when determining what trauma exposure measure to use. In DSM-III, a trauma was defined as a "recognizable stressor that would evoke significant symptoms of distress in almost anyone" (American Psychiatric Association, 1980, p. 238). In 1987, the DSM-III-R definition of trauma was revised to mean an event that is "outside the range of usual human experience and that would be markedly distressing to almost anyone" (American Psychiatric Association, 1987, p. 250). These two definitions were intended to capture catastrophic events that happen with low frequency and to exclude more common events such as simple bereavement, chronic illness, business loss, and marital conflict. The current DSM-IV (American Psychiatric Association, 1994) defines a traumatic event as one in which both of the following were present: "(1) the person experienced, witnessed, or was confronted with an event or events that involved actual or threatened death or serious injury, or a threat to the physical integrity of self or others (criterion A1), and (2) the person's response involved intense fear, helplessness, or horror" (criterion A2; pp. 427–428). Thus the current definition has been expanded to include events that would not have been considered in earlier versions because of their frequency, such as personal illness. On the other hand, the definition has been made narrower by requiring a subjective response of fear, helplessness, and horror. Some controversy continues to exist among experts as to exactly which events should be characterized as traumatic.

In this section, we review seven scales in which criterion A is the sole or primary focus. Most scales do not assess criterion A2. The scales are the Traumatic Stress Schedule (TSS; Norris, 1990), the Traumatic Events Questionnaire (TEQ; Vrana & Lauterbach, 1994), the Trauma History Questionnaire (THQ; Green, 1996), the Stressful Life Events Screening Questionnaire (SLESQ; Goodman, Corcoran, Turner, Yuan, & Green, 1998), the Traumatic Life Events Questionnaire (TLEQ; Kubany et al., 2000), the Life Stressor Checklist—Revised (LSC-R; Wolfe, Kimerling, Brown, Chrestman, & Levin 1996), and the Brief Trauma Questionnaire (BTQ; Schnurr, Vielhauer, Weathers, and Findler 1999). Because of our focus on brief measures that can be self-administered, we excluded some measures that are seriously worthy of consideration in situations in which a more in-depth assessment (e.g., Potential Stressful Events Interview; Kilpatrick, Resnick, & Freedy, 1991) or clinician administration (e.g., Evaluation of Lifetime Stressors; Krinsley, Gallagher, Weathers, Kaloupek, & Vielhauer, 1997) is feasible.

Also excluded from this chapter were measures that detail the experiences of specific trauma populations, such as adult survivors of child abuse (e.g., Briere, 1992), refugees (Mollica et al., 1995), or victims of natural disasters (e.g., Norris & Kaniasty, 1992). Their exclusion should be taken neither as a criticism nor as a statement that such measures are unimportant. Rather, we excluded them because such instruments almost inevitably need to be tailored to the specific event, population, and context and thus are difficult to describe or evaluate in a standardized way. The scales described here screen for the occurrence of potentially traumatic events more broadly. They are best used to supplement more targeted assessments of a focal event or experience. In clinical practice, one of these measures could be used to identify experiences that might subsequently be probed for greater detail in a less structured way.

For each scale, we note which events are specifically assessed and provide evidence for the scale's reliability and validity where such data exist. For self-reported trauma histories, reliability evidence has typically taken the form of test–retest correlations. Internal consistency (e.g., Cronbach's alpha) is not applicable to event measures because the experience of one event does not necessarily imply the experience of another. It should be noted, however, that length restrictions prevent us from providing the exact wording of the events. For any scale of interest, we recommend obtaining the specific instrument to determine whether the wording is appropriate for the intended use.

Validity is difficult to establish unequivocally for these scales. To the extent that face validity may be counted, construct validity has been used most often; that is, checklists of events typically "seem" reasonable. Criterion validity is virtually impossible to establish because no external standard of accuracy exists. Concurrent validity is sometimes evidenced when similar estimates of trauma prevalence are yielded by different scales (see Resnick, Falsetti, Kilpatrick, & Freedy, 1996). In our opinion, content validity could receive much more attention than it has in the development of these scales. Any list of life events, traumatic or otherwise, is a sample representing a larger population of life events. Bruce Dohrenwend (e.g., Dohrenwend, Krasnoff, Askenasy, & Dohrenwend, 1978) must be credited with directing researchers' attention to the fact that decisions made in constructing the list will ultimately determine the kinds of inferences and generalizations that can be made. He raised two basic and related questions: How do we define the events to be sampled? And, what is the population of events from which the sample is to be drawn? Life-event-scale developers seldom have described *explicitly* the population of events that the items on their scales purportedly represent. Some consensus among researchers is implicit in these measures: If we exclude the contributions of open-ended or "catch-all" items, no trauma scales reviewed here are so broad as to include all events demanding readjustment (e.g., moving to a new place) or even all undesirable life events (e.g., losing a job). Yet consensus still has not emerged with regard to just where to draw the line between traumatic events and other undesirable events. This is a critical issue for content validity, which, like construct validity, is often established more on conceptual than on empirical grounds (Wilson, 1994).

Traumatic Stress Schedule

Among the earliest published self-report measures was the Traumatic Stress Schedule (TSS), developed by Fran Norris (1990) as a short screening instrument for assessing traumatic stress in the general population. The format of the scale followed from two basic assumptions: first, that it was important to assess rates of impairment within specific event-defined populations (e.g., crime victims) in addition to assessing those rates within the population at large; and second, that it is important to quantify stressful experiences generically, using descriptors such as life threat, loss, and scope that are not unique to any one event.

In selecting the items for the scale, Norris relied on the DSM-III-R (American Psychiatric Association, 1987) definition of criterion A, in which the defining feature was that events should be beyond the realm of normal human experience. For research purposes, she proposed a more restricted definition of the relevant event population as that involving "violent encounters with nature, technology, or humankind" (p. 1706). She defined a violent event as one that (1) is marked by extreme and/or sudden force, (2) involves an external agent, and (3) is typically capable of arousing intense fear or aversion. The events were selected to provide a reasonable cross-section of this population of events. The scale, as initially published, assessed eight potentially traumatic events: (1) robbery, a theft involving force or threat of force; (2) physical assault; (3) sexual assault, that is, forced unwanted sexual activity of any kind; (4) loss of a loved one through accident, homicide, or suicide; (5) personal injury or property loss as a result of fire, severe weather, or disaster; (6) being forced to evacuate or otherwise learning of an imminent danger or hazard in the environment; (7) having a motor vehicle accident serious enough to cause injury to one or more passengers; and (8) "some other terrifying or shocking experience." The current version has 10 items; fire was separated from disaster, and serving in combat was added. For each stressor, six dimensions are assessed: loss (the tangible loss of persons or property), scope (the extent to which persons other than the respondent were affected by the incident), threat to life and physical integrity (including actual physical injury), blame, familiarity, and four probes assessing posttraumatic stress reactions. This last dimension of posttraumatic stress shifted the focus from assessing the characteristics of the stressor to assessing the response to that stressor, and it can be used as a brief stress measure for each endorsed event.

The event portion of this scale has performed well in research (see Norris, 1992). Norris and Perilla (1996) reported a test–retest correlation of .88 between English and Spanish versions completed by 53 bilingual volunteers 1 week apart. Estimates of exposure to trauma have been strikingly stable across purposive and random community samples. Excluding events that were the focus of these studies, such as Hurricanes Hugo and Andrew, sample frequencies of exposure to one or more traumatic events (using an "ever" time frame) have ranged from 62 to 75%, with an average of 69%. Quite reasonably, higher frequencies (82%) emerged in a study of family members of homicide victims in inner-city Atlanta (M. Thompson, personal communication, March 24, 1995). The symptom portion of this scale is moderately reliable (alpha =.76) and may be useful as a quick screen for posttraumatic stress, but we do not recommend its use as a measure of PTSD. It does not assess all 17 criterion symptoms and assesses neither duration of distress nor functional impairment. The scale does not include an assessment of A2.

The strength of this scale is that is a brief measure that assesses criterion A1 events only. It is alone in establishing equivalence between English and Spanish versions. The probes provide information on experiences that cross particular events (e.g., number of life-threatening events). In addition, the symptom portion of this measure can be used as an indication of posttraumatic stress. The scale does not provide information on age at time of trauma, does not ask specifically about childhood events, and does not query about fear, helplessness, or horror.

Traumatic Events Questionnaire

The Traumatic Events Questionnaire (TEQ), developed by Scott Vrana and Dean Lauterbach (1994), assesses 11 specific traumatic events: (1) combat, (2) large fires/explosions, (3) serious industrial/farm accidents, (4) sexual assault/rape (forced unwanted sexual activity), (5) natural disasters, (6) violent crime, (7) adult abusive relationships, (8) physical/sexual child abuse, (9) witnessing someone being mutilated, seriously injured, or violently killed, (10) other life-threatening situations, and (11) violent or unexpected death of a loved one. Two nonspecific questions, "other event" and "can't tell," complete the scale. Probes assess dimensions such as life threat and injury after any affirmative response.

Over a 2-week test–retest interval, very high reliability for the total scale was observed (.91) in a sample of 51 students (Lauterbach & Vrana, 1996). In another student sample (*N* = 440), 84% reported at least one event, which is higher than other rates that have been reported in the literature. Endorsement of "catch-all" events was especially high: 30% had some other life threatening experience, 23% had some other event, and 9% endorsed "can't tell." Specific events also showed high prevalence rates. A particularly striking statistic was that almost half (49%) of Vrana and Lauterbach's (1994) sample reported having experienced a violent or unexpected death of a loved one. This scale defined the event population to include unexpected natural deaths, as well as those due to violence from technology or humankind. This expansion is consistent with the present wording of criterion A1 in DSM-IV.

Like the TSS, this measure provides a good, quick screen for traumatic events. Criterion A1 is asked about specifically for each item. The inclusion of events about which the respondent "can't tell" is interesting and constitutes both a strength (comprehensiveness) and shortcoming (the researcher can't tell if the event meets criterion). The scale does not inquire about age at time of trauma or assess for criterion A2.

Trauma History Questionnaire

The Trauma History Quesionnaire (THQ) was developed by Bonnie Green and her associates at Georgetown University (Green, 1996). The THQ aims to provide a comprehensive assessment of exposure and to be suitable for both research and clinical populations. The scale has 24 items: (1) mugging, (2) robbery—a theft by force, (3) break-in with respondent present, (4) break-in with respondent absent, (5) serious accident at work, in a car, or somewhere else, (6) natural disaster with respondent or loved ones in danger, (7) disaster of human origin with respondent or loved ones in danger, (8) toxin exposure, (9) other serious injury, (10) other situation in which respondent feared being killed or injured, (11) witnessed serious injury or death, (12) handled/seen dead bodies, (13) close friend or family member murdered or killed by a drunk driver, (14) spouse, romantic partner, or child died, (15) respondent had serious or life-threatening illness, (16) someone close experienced serious or life-threatening illness, injury, or unexpected death, (17) combat, (18) forced intercourse, oral, or anal sex, (19) forced touching of private parts, (20) other unwanted sexual contact, (21) aggravated assault, (22) simple assault, (23) beaten, spanked, or pushed hard enough to cause injury, and (24) any other extraordinarily stressful situation or event. Each event is followed by probes assessing the number of times that event has occurred and the respondent's age at the time.

Green (1996) provided reliability data collected from 25 female participants that were tested twice over a 2–3 month interval. Excluding the total severe-threat index that received a stability coefficient of only .14, test–retest correlations ranged from .54 for total bereavement to .92 for total crime. Scale means were higher in an outpatient sample than in a university sample, which provides some additional evidence of validity. Green's take on the population of relevant events is the broadest of all those reviewed here, as this scale includes deaths and illnesses of significant others, even if expected and due to natural causes, which many would argue should not qualify as meeting criterion A1. This strategy was chosen because, in the research, respondents who provided affirmative responses were interviewed in more detail about their experiences. Two-thirds of the students in Green's pilot study ($N = 423$) reported that someone close to them had become seriously ill at some time, making the frequency for this one event as high as the total frequency across events obtained using the TSS.

In the past few years, the scale has been used in a variety of populations, including cancer, epilepsy, and chronic pain patients, battered women, persons with serious mental illness, and adult offspring of Holocaust survivors. The strengths of this measure include its comprehensiveness and careful wording. This measure includes a range of both traumatic and stressful life events. Additional information is available about the frequency of the event and the age at time of trauma. There is no assessment of fear, helplessness, or horror.

Traumatic Life Events Questionnaire

The Traumatic Life Events Questionnaire (TLEQ) was described by Edward Kubany and colleagues (2000). The scale was designed for both clinical and research purposes. The present version, expanded from the experimental version described by Norris and Riad (1997), assesses the occurrence of 23 events: (1) natural disaster, (2) motor vehicle accident involving injury or death, (3) other accident involving injury or death, (4) combat, (5) sudden and unexpected death of a close friend or loved one due to accident, illness, suicide, or murder, (6) loved one surviving life-threatening illness, accident, assault, (7) life-threatening illness, (8) mugging or robbing by someone with a weapon, (9) physical assault by an acquaintance or stranger, (10) witnessing someone being attacked or assaulted, (11) being threatened with death or bodily harm, (12) childhood physical abuse, (13) witnessing severe family violence, (14) physical abuse from intimate partner, (15) childhood sexual touching by someone at least 5 years older (probes for force, penetration), (16) childhood sexual touching by someone less than 5 years older, (17) adolescent unwanted sexual activity (probes for force, penetration), (18) adulthood unwanted sexual activity (probes for force, penetration), (19) sexual harassment, (20) stalking, (21) miscarriage, self or partner, (22) abortion, self or partner, and (23) other extremely disturbing or distressing experience. As with the THQ, many would argue that some of the events included would not qualify as meeting criterion A1, such as sexual harassment or abortion. This scale provides a good match to criterion A2 by including a probe after each experienced event that reads, "Did you experience intense fear, helplessness, or horror when it happened?" Additional questions ask about frequency, injury, whether any of the events occurred within the past 2 months or 12 months, and which event caused the most distress. There is also a brief version of the scale that assesses for the same events but with fewer probes.

Kubany et al. (2000) described the results in a series of five studies. The first four were conducted using the earlier 16-item version; the last study was conducted using the expanded 21-item version. In the first study, the authors generated a preliminary version of the measure and sent it to seven published experts in the area. On average, the reviewers believed that the items were worded "very well" and sampled the range of events "very well." In Study 2, 49 patients completed the TLEQ twice, over a 60-day interval. When assessed item by item, test–retest percent agreements averaged 83%. Kappas varied widely because some of the events assessed were extremely rare. The stability was lowest for items assessing "other" accidents and childhood sexual abuse by someone less than 5 years older. In Study 3, 51 veterans completed the

TLEQ two times. The length of the interval varied from 5 to 45 days, with a median of 13 days. The results were quite similar to those of the second study; percent agreements averaged 84%. In Study 4, 62 undergraduate students completed the standard self-report version of the TLEQ. One week later, they were interviewed using a structured measure with similar content. Percent agreements were again high for most items. There were no significant differences in proportions disclosing traumatic experiences across the two modalities. In Study 5, 42 members of a support group for battered women completed the 21-item TLEQ 2 weeks apart. Overall percent agreement was 86%.

This scale provides information on a range of potentially traumatic events and is unusual in that it assesses for both criteria A1 and A2. The authors have done an exceptional job of researching the scale's psychometric qualities. The scale has some novel inclusions, such as sexual harassment, abortion, and miscarriage, although there is some debate as to whether these events should be included as criterion A1 events.

Stressful Life Events Screening Questionnaire

The Stressful Life Events Screening Questionnaire (SLESQ) is a 13-item self-report screening measure designed to assess lifetime exposure to potentially traumatic events (Goodman et al., 1998). Trauma was defined according to DSM-IV as an event that involves actual or threatened death or serious injury or a threat to physical integrity of self or others. The SLESQ was designed to be brief. The measure provides more detail on interpersonal trauma than does the TSS but less information about exposure to hazards such as fire or disasters. The events are: (1) life-threatening illness, (2) life-threatening accident, (3) robbery/mugging (4) loss of loved one because of accident, homicide, suicide, (5) forced intercourse, oral, or anal sex, (6) attempted forced intercourse, oral, or anal sex, (7) unwanted sexual touching, (8) childhood physical abuse, (9) domestic violence, (10) threats with weapons, (11) being present when another person was killed, injured, or assaulted, (12) other injury or life threat, and (13) other extremely frightening or horrifying event. For each experienced event, the questionnaire asks for the respondent's age at the time of the trauma. Probes vary across events to provide more detail on the nature of the event.

Psychometric data were collected from a sample of 140 college students assessed twice 2 weeks apart (Goodman et al., 1998). At least one event was reported by 72% of the respondents, a rate similar to others reported in the literature. The correlation between the total number of events reported at Time 1 and the total number reported at Time 2 was .89. Kappas for specific events averaged .73. The least reliably assessed events (i.e., kappa < .60) were attempted rape, witnessing injuries or trauma to others, other injury/life threat, and other extreme event.

The SLEQ is a brief, carefully researched measure of trauma that would be useful in many situations. This scale provides information on age at time of trauma, frequency, and life threat. The measure includes an "other" category. However, there is no assessment of criterion A2.

Life Stressor Checklist—Revised

The Life Stressor Checklist—Revised (LSC-R) was designed to screen for events that would meet DSM-IV criterion A, as well as for some events that are stressful but unlikely traumatic. The measure has a special focus on events that may be relevant to women, such as abortion, but can also be used with men. Developed by Wolfe et al. (1996), it assesses 30 events, including: (1) serious disaster, (2) serious accident, (3), witnessing a serious accident, (4), close family member being sent to jail, (5), being sent to jail, (6) being in foster care or put up for adoption, (7) parents separating or divorcing, (8) separation or divorce, (9) serious financial problems, (10) serious physical or mental illness, (11) emotional neglect, (12) physical neglect, (13) abortion/miscarriage, (14) separation from child against one's will, (15) severe physical or mental handicap of one's child, (16) primary responsibility for someone with severe mental or physical handicap, (17) sudden or unexpected death of someone close, (18) death of someone close, (19) witnessing family violence, (20) seeing a robbery, mugging, or attack, (21) being robbed, mugged, or attacked, (22) physical abuse, (23) physical assault, (24) sexual harassment, (25) forced genital touching before age 16, (26) forced genital touching after age 16, (27) forced intercourse before age 16, (28) forced intercourse after age 16, (29) "other," (30) being seriously upset by any of these events happening to someone close, even though the respondent did not see it. For each endorsed event, respondents are asked between two and five follow-up questions, depending on the event, including: How old were you when it happened/started; How old were you when it ended; Did you believe that you/someone else could be killed or seriously harmed; At the time, did you experience feelings of fear, helplessness, or horror, and how much has it affected your life in the past year? Thus this measure explicitly assesses for both criteria A1 and A2.

McHugo et al. (2004) provided psychometric data for an adapted version of the measure, collected as part of the Women, Co-Occurring Disorders, and Violence Study. Primary differences between the LSC-R and the adapted version used in the study include: the omission of the A2 probe, the addition of several stressors (homelessness and unwanted sex for money or goods), and the rewording of a few items (such as combining abortion and miscarriage). Data were collected on 2,729 women, who were recruited into the study if they had a diagnosis of both mental and substance use disorders and if they reported experiencing physical or sexual abuse during their lifetimes. A test–retest sample was completed on a subset of 186 women who completed the measure on average 7 days later. Kappas ranged from a low of .52 for physical abuse to a high of .97 for miscarriage and averaged .70. Percent agreement ranged from a low of 79% for serious physical or mental illness to a high of 98% for miscarriage.

The Life Stressor Checklist is the longest measure reviewed in this chapter, because it encompasses both potentially traumatic and other seriously stressful life events. This scale asks about age at time of event, assesses for criteria A1 and A2, and asks about how much the event has affected the person in the past year. It is particularly sensitive to the stressors of women and has been shown to be well tolerated in consumer samples.

Brief Trauma Questionnaire

The Brief Trauma Questionnaire (BTQ), developed by Paula Schnurr and colleagues (1999), assesses 10 traumatic events: (1) combat, (2) serious car accident, (3) major natural or technological disaster, (4) life-threatening illness, (5) physical punishment as child, (6) physical assault, (7) unwanted sexual contact, (8) other situation in which respondent was seriously injured or feared being seriously injured or killed, (9) violent death of close friend or family member, and (10) witnessing a situation in which someone was seriously injured or killed or in which respondent feared someone might be seriously injured or killed.

Although the psychometrics of the BTQ are only currently being established, it is included here as a promising new measure. One of its strengths is that it includes explicit assessment of criterion A1. For all endorsed traumatic events, respondents are asked if they thought their lives were in danger or if they thought they might be seriously injured or were in fact injured. Perceived life threat as measured by the BTQ has been shown to be related to higher dissociation scores (Morgan, Hazelett, Wang, Richardson, Schnurr, & Southwick, 2001). In a study of more than 400 military veterans from World War II and the Korean conflict, interrater reliability was established on a subset of interviews (Schnurr, Spiro, Vielhauer, Findler, & Hamblen, 2002). Kappa coefficients for the presence of trauma that met DSM criterion A1 were above .70 (range .74–1.00) for all events except for illness (.69) and "other life-threatening events" (.60).

The BTQ is a brief measure of trauma that explicitly assesses for criterion A1. It does not inquire about criterion A2, age at time of trauma, or childhood events. Preliminary data look promising.

Summary

Table 3.1 summarizes the descriptions of these seven measures of potentially traumatic events. For each scale, the table lists the number of event items included in the scale, the type of data provided, evidence of stability, the population that the measure was developed on, and whether or not the scale assesses for criteria A1 and A2. Evidence of validity was not included because none of these scales are especially well validated, nor are any apparently especially weak in this regard. General guidelines are provided for considering which scales may be the most useful in different settings.

TABLE 3.1. Summary Descriptions of Seven Standardized Self-Report Measures of Trauma Exposure

Scale	Number of event items	Evidence of stability	Population developed on	Assesses for criterion A1	Assesses for criterion A2
Traumatic Stress Schedule	10	TR, total no. = .88	Multicultural	Yes	No
Traumatic Events Questionnaire	11	TR, total no. = .91	Undergraduates	Yes	No
Trauma History Questionnaire	24	TR, by type = .54–.92	Female undergraduates	Partial	No
Traumatic Life Events Questionnaire	17	*M* agreement, by type = 83%	Variety	Partial	Yes
Stressful Life Events Screening Questionnaire	13	TR, total no. = .89 *M* kappa, by type = .73	Undergraduates	Yes	No
Brief Trauma Questionnaire	10	Kappa, by type = .60–1.0	Veterans	Yes	No
Life Stressor Checklist—Revised	30	Agreement, by type = 79–98%	Women	Partial	Yes

Note. Tr, test–retest; na, data not available.

Perhaps the most basic issue to consider in comparing the measures is how well they satisfy criteria A1 and A2. In terms of criterion A1, all of the scales include a range of traumatic events, but they differ in the definitional boundaries of the relevant population of events. The TSS appears to use the most objective and restricted definition. Other measures, such as the THQ, TLEQ, and LSC-R, use a broader definition and include events that are arguably not traumatic and would not satisfy criterion A1. Decisions regarding how broadly or narrowly to define the relevant domain of events depend on the assessor's intent. For example, clinicians may find that the broader measures can better inform their clinical work, whereas researchers may prefer a more restricted range of included events.

A second important issue is assessment of criterion A2. Only the TLEQ and the LSC-R explicitly ask respondents about whether their subjective reactions to the event included fear, helplessness, or horror. In some cases, the inclusion of A2 may not be an issue. For example, event checklists are often used to screen for trauma exposure by identifying a single or most upsetting experience, and then additional questions are used to determine if the event meets criteria A1 and A2. However, if the assessor needs to know how many criterion A traumas the respondent has experienced, it is essential that both criteria A1 and A2 be assessed for each event. It should be noted that many of these measures were structured so that the event is a gate question, followed by additional probes if answered affirmatively. In such cases, it would not be difficult to add a probe that explicitly assesses A2.

A third issue to consider is whether the range of traumatic events being assessed is sufficient. Clearly, scales with more items have a greater likelihood of identifying traumatic events. However, they take longer to administer, and some include items that would not qualify as traumatic. Multipurpose surveys may find it difficult to include one of the longer scales. Also, some measures give more attention to certain types of events. For example, for studying long-term consequences of childhood trauma, measures that explicitly differentiate child abuse from adulthood assault are recommended. A review of the items in the longer scales shows that it is usually exposure to sexual assault and domestic violence that receives additional explicit attention, and this may be very useful in many contexts.

One issue that requires additional consideration is the use of "catch-all" events that compromise specificity. All of the reviewed scales used this technique. The reasoning behind the inclusion of these items is clear. It would be too difficult, costly, and unacceptable to researchers to enumerate every traumatic event that might conceivably occur. Such items also give respondents the chance to report experiences that were important to them, which can be informative, as well as helpful in building rapport. On the other hand, these items may be tapping into personal crises and failures that are not truly in the domain of traumatic life events.

Norris and Riad (1997) reviewed the responses to this open-ended question provided by persons who participated in their study of Hurricane Andrew. Of 404 respondents, 36 (9%) reported some other "shocking or terrifying experience" on the TSS. Fourteen people told of events that clearly qualified as traumatic, according to DSM-III-R definitions, but these events were not asked about directly (or specifically enough) in other TSS questions (e.g., being at the scene of a bank robbery, in a train accident, threatened with a gun). Five told of events that should have been picked up by other items but for some reason were not. For these 19 respondents (roughly half), the item served its purpose: catching other trauma histories not elsewhere recorded. An additional six people described life-threatening or very serious illnesses experienced by themselves (going blind temporarily, surgery) or loved ones (grandfather's cancer) that qualify under DSM-IV PTSD criteria, although they were not in the domain of experiences Norris was initially attempting to capture with the TSS. Three people mentioned deaths due to natural causes of loved ones, and seven told of other unfortunate (husband convicted of murder, son in prison) or unusual (paranormal) experiences. Thus roughly 28–44% of the events captured by this item (2–3% of the total sample) would not qualify under more restrictive definitions. When reviewing the literature across these scales, it is striking that catch-all items seem to have even higher rates of endorsement on longer measures. Compared with 9% of Norris and Riad's (1997) sample, 23% of Vrana and Lauterbach's (1994) sample reported some other event. Even in Green's (1996) sample, 14% reported some other event, although the THQ asked about 23 specific events, including serious illnesses of respondent and others and deaths of close family members, regardless of cause. When affirmative answers were explored in subsequent interviews, Green found that few of the events qualified as criterion A events (personal communication, April 12, 1995).

A related issue with these items was highlighted by Vrana and Lauterbach's (1994) finding that a high percentage of TEQ respondents rated the "other event" as their very worst. This finding may reflect an intrinsic bias wherein participants primarily note another event *if* it was their subjective worst. Conceivably, all respondents have experienced undesirable changes in their lives, but they do not always bring these to mind. The issue here is again one of content validity. If "traumatic events" and "undesirable events" are synonymous terms, these scales need to be expanded to capture the range of undesirable events that have been important in life events research more generally (e.g., Dohrenwend et al., 1978). In our opinion, it is better for measures of PTSD criterion A to focus more specifically on a clearly defined population of events. This is not to say that other events are not important in the lives of individuals but simply that they are beyond the domain of concern for these measures. In many studies, it is advisable to include a scale of normative life events, in addition to a scale of traumatic life events. Perhaps this is analogous to developing a scale for anxiety rather than or in addition to a scale of depression or generalized distress. To summarize, these catch-all questions seem necessary, but the responses they elicit may be seriously compromising the content validity of all of the measures that were reviewed here. Regardless of which scale is selected, the researcher or clinician should probe for content of these events.

Finally, although we were unable to detail the exact wording of each question on the reviewed measures, such wording is nonetheless quite important. Overall, we believed the included measures were careful and clear in their wording. One lesson from earlier research that has clearly been learned is that items must include behavioral descriptions of events. For example, not one of these measures used the term "rape." Instead, each referred to unwanted or forced sexual activity. Wording of prospective measures should be reviewed prior to use.

Thus determining what measure is best really depends on the intended purpose. The TSS, TEQ, and BTQ are brief screens for traumatic stress, which may increase their appeal to researchers focusing on many constructs in addition to trauma, whereas the THQ and TLEQ aim to provide comprehensive trauma histories and may be more suitable for research in which length of the instrument is not an issue. The SLESQ provides an exceptional amount of information about sexual trauma and interpersonal violence. Still other measures, such as the LSC-R, may be most suitable for occasions on which the researcher or clinician does not wish to confine the domain of concern to trauma per se but seeks to include other seriously stressful events, such as divorce. Sources for obtaining these seven measures are provided in Appendix 3.1.

DSM-IV PTSD CRITERIA B–D: INTRUSTION, AVOIDANCE, AND AROUSAL

In this section, we review 17 scales that purport to measure symptomatic criteria for PTSD. We describe each scale in terms of its length and format, provide some background regarding its development, and evaluate its psychometric properties. Rules for establishing reliability and validity are developed much better for symptom measures than for event measures, which raise the standards by which these symptom scales are judged. Regarding reliability, it is usually important for symptom measures to establish both internal consistency and stability over time. Validity data for symptom scales usually takes the form of criterion validity or construct validity. Sometimes, criterion validity is established in terms of a scale's correlations with more established measures in the field. A PTSD scale should correlate highly—but not too highly—with measures of general psychopathology and should correlate most highly with other measures of posttraumatic stress. Most highly regarded is evidence that the scale can correctly classify subjects into diagnostic groups, determined by some independent criterion. Statistics are usually provided regarding the measure's sensitivity (the proportion of cases correctly classified) and specificity (the proportion of noncases correctly classified). Construct validity is important as well. In this case, validity is usually established by showing that scale scores differ across groups having different objective trauma histories. Sometimes, construct validity is examined by exploring how well the observed factor structure of the scale conforms to theoretical predictions.

The difficulty of creating a measure that is both sensitive and specific to PTSD should not be taken lightly, because the disorder is composed of a broad, if unique, constellation of psychological symptoms. In the tradition of the American Psychiatric Association's DSM, these symptoms are grouped into three clusters. DSM-IV PTSD criterion B is the reexperiencing of the trauma. Intrusive symptoms, such as thinking about the event when the individual does not intend to, having nightmares or flashbacks, or being suddenly reminded of the event by environmental stimuli are extremely common experiences following traumatic life events. Criterion C encompasses avoidance and a numbing of responsiveness to the external world. Often, trauma victims avoid people and places that remind them of the event, feel estranged from other people, or lose interest in things they formerly enjoyed. Criterion D refers to a varied collection of symptoms indicative of increased arousal. Being jumpy, easily startled, or hyperalert, having trouble sleeping or concentrating, or feeling easily angered characterize criterion D. To satisfy DSM-IV criteria for PTSD, the person must show at least one intrusion symptom, three avoidance symptoms, and two arousal symptoms.

The measures that are included here are not the only self-report measures of PTSD but are those that appear to be the most commonly used in recent research. These measures reflect varying strategies for assessing PTSD. Perhaps now the most common strategy is to create measures that map directly onto the 17 criterion symptoms included in DSM-IV. Such measures include the National Women's Study PTSD Module (Kilpatrick, Resnick, Saunders, & Best, 1989); the Posttraumatic Stress Diagnostic Scale (Foa, Cashman, Jaycox, & Perry, 1997), which evolved from Foa's earlier PTSD Symptom Scale (Foa, Riggs, Dancu, & Rothbaum, 1993); the PTSD Checklist (PCL) developed by Weathers, Litz, Herman, Huska, and Keane (1993); the Davidson Trauma Scale (Davidson et al., 1997); the Purdue PTSD Scale (Lauterbach & Vrana, 1996); the PTSD Interview (Watson, Juba, Manifold, Kucala, & Anderson, 1991); the Screen for Posttraumatic Stress Symptoms (Carlson, 2001); and the Self-Rating Interview for PTSD (Hovens, Bramsen, & van der Ploeg, 2002). The second strategy has been to develop scales that assess symptoms of posttraumatic stress continuously and in a manner less rigidly tied to DSM guidelines. The Posttraumatic Symptom Scale (Holen, 1990), the Penn Inventory (Hammarberg, 1992), the Trauma Symptom Checklist—40 (Briere & Runtz, 1989), and the Trauma Symptom Inventory (Briere, 1995) are examples here. The Impact of Event Scale (IES) is described by Weiss (Chapter 7, this volume) so will not be included, though this is the group of scales with which it would belong. The third strategy has been to derive PTSD subscales from larger symptom inventories that are commonly used in clinical practice and research. Examples here are the Minnesota Multiphasic Personality Inventory (MMPI; Keane, Malloy, & Fairbank, 1984) and the Symptom Checklist—90 (SCL-90;

Saunders, Arata, & Kilpatrick, 1990; Ursano, Fullerton, Kao, & Bhartiya, 1995) PTSD scales. This strategy is most useful in settings in which MMPI and SCL-90 data are being collected and in which it would be difficult to add a measure specifically focused on PTSD. A fourth strategy has been to develop measures that are tailored to assess culturally relevant outcomes. The Harvard Trauma Questionnaire (Mollica et al., 1992) is the premiere example of this approach. We also included the Revised Civilian Mississippi Scale (Norris & Perilla, 1996) under this strategy rather than the second because it was established so as to be equivalent in English and Spanish. The remainder of this chapter is organized according to this scheme.

PTSD SCALES THAT CLOSELY FOLLOW DSM SYMPTOM CRITERIA

National Women's Study PTSD Module

The National Women's Study (NWS) PTSD Module developed by Dean Kilpatrick and colleagues (1989) was revised from the version of the Diagnostic Interview Schedule (DIS) used in the National Vietnam Veterans Readjustment Survey. Designed for use by lay interviewers, the measure begins with 20 symptom items that span the range of symptoms associated with PTSD. Questions are first answered yes or no. Then, dates of first and last experiences of that symptom are recorded for all affirmative responses. None of the items is anchored to the specific event or events experienced. This characteristic of the scale makes it easy to administer to people with multiple or complex trauma histories. Another advantage of this assessment approach is that the respondent is not required to attribute the symptom to a specific experience, a characteristic for which the original DIS was criticized (Solomon & Canino, 1990). However, open-ended probes are used to assess symptom content in specific instances. For example, if an individual reports nightmares, he or she is asked what the nightmares are about. After the symptom questions, the scale assesses amnesic experiences, timing and co-occurrence of symptoms, and functional impairment. The scale has typically been scored to yield dichotomous measures of lifetime and current PTSD rather than to yield a continuous measure of PTSD symptomatology.

Because of the dichotomous nature of the scoring algorithms, data regarding the scale's reliability and validity have taken the form of kappa coefficients. Resnick, Kilpatrick, Dansky, Saunders, and Best (1993) reported that stability over a 1-year interval for lifetime PTSD was adequate (kappa = .45). Data collected from clinical cases as part of the DSM-IV field trials provided evidence of concurrent validity. Kappa coefficients of agreement between a PTSD diagnosis made on the basis of this module and the Structured Clinical Interview for DSM-III-R (SCID) were .71 for current PTSD and .77 for lifetime PTSD. These analyses also indicated that the NWS Module had high sensitivity for lifetime (.99) and current (.96) PTSD. Specificity was somewhat lower: .79 for lifetime and .80 for current PTSD.

Posttraumatic Stress Diagnostic Scale

The Posttraumatic Stress Diagnostic Scale (PTDS) was developed by Edna Foa and her colleagues (1997) to address the various shortcomings of preexisting self-report measures. It follows DSM-IV closely. The PTSD Symptom Scale (Foa et al., 1993) that was described in Norris and Riad (1997) was the precursor to the PTDS. The PTDS is a measure of current (previous month) PTSD anchored to the single event that "bothers" the respondent the most. Thus the PTDS actually begins with a 12-item checklist of traumatic events followed by a question that asks the respondent to identify the single event that has disturbed him or her the most in the previous month. Criteria A1 and A2 are then assessed by 4 dichotomous questions regarding physical injury, threat, terror, and helplessness. This section is followed by 17 symptom items answered on a 4-point Likert scale of frequency during the previous month. The scale concludes with 9 questions that address functional impairment. An excellent feature of the scale is that it yields both dichotomous (diagnostic) and continuous scores.

Foa et al. (1997) presented impressive validation data, derived from a sample of 248 men and women, of whom 110 composed a retest sample. Participants were excluded from the retest sample if they selected a different event that bothered them the most, which was not uncommon. Internal consistency was high for each symptom cluster B–D (alphas = 78–.84) and for the total scale (alpha = .92). Test–retest reliability coefficients over 2–3 weeks were likewise high for each cluster (*r*'s = .77–.85) and for the total scale (*r* = .83). When scored continuously, the PTDS correlates highly with other symptom measures, such as the Beck Depression Inventory (BDI; Beck, Ward, Mendelsohn, Mock, & Erbaugh, 1961) (.79) and the IES—Revised, Intrusion subscale (Weiss & Marmar, 1997) (.78). Respondents in the initial sample were classified as meeting diagnostic criteria for PTSD using the SCID-PTSD module. The PTDS and SCID yielded the same diagnosis 82% of the time (kappa = .65). The sensitivity of the PTDS was .89, specificity .75.

Foa's scale has a number of excellent features. It provides both a DSM-IV diagnosis and a severity scale. It is both internally consistent and stable when used to study the aftermath of the same trauma over a 2- to 3-week interval. Moreover, it showed good agreement with SCID diagnosis. The high correlations with depression raise questions regarding discriminant validity, but this shortcoming reflects a general issue with the PTSD diagnosis rather than an issue specific to this scale.

PTSD Checklist

The PTSD Checklist, Civilian Version (PCL-C) was developed by Frank Weathers and his colleagues at the National Center for PTSD (1993). The scale consists of 17 questions that now correspond to DSM-IV. Respondents are asked how often they have been bothered by each symptom in the previous month on a 5-point severity scale. According to the authors, the questions may be worded generically to refer to "stressful experiences in the past" (PCL-C) or to describe reactions to a specific event (PCL-S). Initial psychometric data were derived by using a military version of the PCL (PCL-M) in a sample of Vietnam veterans, in which the prevalence of PTSD was high. Internal consistency coefficients were very high for the total scale (.97) and for each subscale (.92–.93). Test–retest reliability over 2–3 days was .96. The PCL-M correlated highly with the Mississippi Scale for Combat-Related PTSD (Keane, Caddell, & Taylor, 1988) (.93), the PK scale of the MMPI (.77), and the Impact of Event Scale (.90). In this sample, the PCL-M was quite predictive of PTSD as assessed with the SCID; a cutoff score of 50 had a sensitivity of .82, a specificity of .83, and a kappa of .64. (The reader should note that cutoff scores may vary depending on the prevalence of disorder in a sample.)

Other researchers have also presented evidence supporting the reliability and validity of the PCL-C or PCL-S. In a sample of 40 motor vehicle accident and sexual assault victims, of whom 18 had PTSD on the Clinician-Administered PTSD Scale (CAPS), Blanchard, Jones-Alexander, Buckley, and Forneris (1996) found an alpha of .94 and an overall correlation between total PCL-S and CAPS scores of .93. They found that a score of 44 (rather than 50) maximized diagnostic efficiency (sensitivity of .94, specificity of .86, overall efficiency of .90). In a sample of individuals in France who had experienced a variety of events, Ventureya, Yao, Cottraux, Note, and De May-Guillard (2002) reported excellent internal consistency (.86) and test–retest reliability (.80) for the total PCL-S score. Using the cutpoint of 44 recommended by Blanchard et al. (1996), the PCL-S showed a sensitivity of .97, a specificity of .87, and an overall diagnostic efficacy of .94.

The PCL appears to have much to recommend it. Because it was developed by the National Center for PTSD, it is in the public domain. It is reliable, and the M and S versions map directly onto DSM criteria. The M and S versions have been shown to correlate highly with clinician-administered measures. Less information is available about version C—the civilian version that does not identify a specific event—and the reader should be cautious about generalizing psychometric findings from one version of the scale to another. Also, the published cutpoints should be used with caution, as they were derived from samples with high prevalence rates of current PTSD and may not be appropriate for samples with lower rates.

Davidson Trauma Scale

The Davidson Trauma Scale (DTS) was developed by Jonathan Davidson and his colleagues (1997) as a self-rating scale for PTSD that is reliable, valid, and sensitive to treatment effects in a variety of trauma survivors. The scale assesses 17 symptoms that correspond to DSM-IV, and each is rated for both frequency and severity on 5-point scales using a past-week time frame. The response formats vary somewhat across questions, making the format for the scale longer than similar 17-item PTSD scales.

Davidson et al. (1997) showed that the scale was quite reliable. In a large sample, composed of participants in various studies, alpha coefficients for internal consistency were very high (.97–.99) for the frequency, severity, and total scales. The test–retest correlation over a 2-week interval was .86 in a small clinical sample that had been rated as showing no change on an independent measure of clinical improvement. In a sample of 129 participants, of whom 67 met SCID criteria for PTSD, a total score of 40 most accurately predicted diagnosis, having a sensitivity of .69, a specificity of .95, and an overall efficiency of .83. Among 102 participants who were administered the CAPS, the DTS correlated .78 with the total CAPS score and .64 with the Impact of Event Scale. An interesting feature of Davidson's analysis was his consideration of whether scores on the scale changed given clinical treatment and improvement. Those who improved during treatment had pre- and postscores of 74 and 40, respectively, whereas those who did not improve had pre- and postscores of 87 and 86, respectively.

Purdue PTSD Scale—Revised

The Purdue PTSD Scale was developed a number of years ago by Don Hartsough and his students at Purdue University (e.g., Wojcik, 1988). Dean Lauterbach and Scott Vrana (1996) revised and regenerated this scale for use in heterogeneous event populations. The Revised Purdue Scale (PPTSD-R) corresponds to DSM-III-R criteria. Like Foa's measure, the PPTSD-R anchors reporting of symptoms to a single worst event identified by a screen for traumatic experience. Respondents report how often they have experienced each symptom in the previous month on a 5-point scale, from *not at all* to *often*. The scale can be scored either continuously or dichotomously.

Lauterbach and Vrana (1996) described three studies undertaken to assess the reliability and validity of the PPTSD-R. Both women and men were well represented in all studies. In the first, 440 undergraduates who had experienced a variety of traumatic events were tested once. All subscales appeared internally consistent. Alphas were .91, .84, .79, and .81 for the total, reexperiencing, avoidance, and arousal scales, respectively. In the second study, 51 undergraduates were tested twice over a 2-week interval. Test–retest correlations were .72, .48, .67, and .71, respectively.

As for validity data, the Purdue Scale correlated highly with both the IES (.66) and the Civilian Mississippi Scale (.50) in the larger sample. These correlations were stronger than those between the scale and general measures of distress, such as the BDI (.37–.39), providing preliminary support for convergent and discriminant validity. These relations were examined further by adding a third group of 35 students receiving psychology services to the sample. Reexperiencing and arousal scores were significantly higher (1) among persons reporting a traumatic event on the TEQ than among persons not reporting an event, (2) among patients than among nonpatients, and (3) among patients seeking treatment because of a traumatic event than among patients seeking treatment for other reasons. However, whereas avoidance scores differed between patient and nonpatient groups, they did not differ between trauma and no-trauma groups.

In summary, this scale has a number of good features. It was developed for use in heterogeneous samples. As the authors correctly noted at the time of its publication, very few scales had been developed and validated on a broad cross-section of trauma survivors. (This is less true today.) In addition to this strength, the scale is internally consistent and correlates with other measures of trauma exposure and outcome in meaningful ways. However, before the scale can be recommended without reservations, two issues must be resolved. One is the lack of stability in the reexperiencing subscale. It is not altogether clear that respondents were thinking about the same event on the two testing occasions, which could deflate test–retest coefficients. The second issue is the sensitivity of the avoidance measure. Scores on this subscale did not differ between respondents reporting a traumatic event and respondents who did not. In traumatized populations, criterion C is satisfied less often than criteria B or D and therefore has a strong impact on classification (e.g., Solomon & Canino, 1990; Norris, 1992).

PTSD-Interview

Charles Watson and his colleagues (1991) developed the PTSD—Interview (PTSD-I) for use with veteran populations, but the scale could easily be applied to other groups. Seventeen items were generated that reflect PTSD symptoms as outlined in DSM-III-R. Each question is answered on a 7-point scale, from *no* to *extremely* or *never* to *always*. The scale can be scored continuously or dichotomously. The authors recommend that any symptom receiving a score of 4 or higher be counted toward PTSD diagnosis but note that users could substitute higher or lower values, depending on the purpose of the assessment. It was designed to be suitable for use by lay interviewers.

Watson et al. reported that the scale has a test–retest reliability coefficient, over 1 week, of .95. This was tested in a sample of 31 veterans, 30 of whom had been in combat. The scale was also internally consistent (alpha = .92).

The scale appears to have substantial validity in veteran populations. Watson et al. (1991) administered the PTSD-I and the Modified DIS-PTSD module (a structured interview) to 53 patients and 8 staff members at a VA medical center. Although the DIS-PTSD measure has been criticized (Weiss, 1993), the authors noted that the issues pertain to its utility with the general population rather than with clinical samples. The correlations between PTSD-I items and their DIS counterparts averaged .77. Using the DIS as the standard, the kappa was .84, which is quite high. The PTSD-I showed a sensitivity of .89, a specificity of .94, and an overall hit rate of 92%. Watson et al. (1994) examined the convergent validity of the scale in a sample of 80 help-seeking veterans. Scored continuously, the PTSD-I correlated .84 with the

Mississippi Scale for Combat-Related PTSD and .79 with the MMPI-PTSD scale; validity coefficients were equal to the Mississippi and superior to the MMPI-PTSD scale. Scored dichotomously, kappa coefficients were .59 and .60. There was about 80% agreement between the PTSD-I and each of the other two scales regarding who did or did not qualify as a case; the three scales' concordances with one another did not differ significantly in this case.

Watson et al.'s scale originally had 20 items. The first question asked whether the interviewee had experienced an unusual or extremely distressful event. By current standards in the field, a single item would not provide an adequate assessment of PTSD criterion A; thus users of this scale would be wise to supplement the PTSD-I with a trauma history or screener. (In later research, e.g., Watson et al., 1994, it appears that the authors may have revised this aspect of the scale so as to provide a list of catastrophic experiences, but this list was not detailed or published.) Two final questions determine whether symptoms have been present for at least 1 month.

All in all, this scale has many good features. It is flexible in scoring and appears to be reliable and valid. Although developed initially for veterans, it was subsequently used with a variety of trauma populations, including medical trauma victims, auto accident victims, and women who have been sexually or physically assaulted (Watson, personal communication, April 19, 1995). The scale also has been translated into French and Spanish.

Screen for Posttraumatic Stress Symptoms

The Screen for Posttraumatic Stress Symptoms (SPTSS) was developed by Eve Carlson (2001) to provide a measure that does not require the respondent to focus on a single event—or any event, for that matter. Thus the scale may be particularly useful when respondents are likely to have experienced multiple traumas, a situation that is not at all uncommon. Although the SPTSS was not intended to provide a diagnosis of PTSD, its items match the 17 DSM-IV criteria except that the symptom is not linked to a particular traumatic stressor. Participants rate their experience of each symptom on an 11-point scale using a past-2-week time frame. The scale is scored as the mean of all items, and thus scores have a potential range of 0 to 10.

In a study of 136 adult psychiatric inpatients, Carlson obtained an alpha of .91 for the total scale, which is indicative of high internal consistency. She also presented considerable evidence of validity. Scores on the SPTSS were higher among participants who had experienced a traumatic event than among participants who had not, and, within the subset of participants who had experienced trauma, scores were far higher for those who met criteria for PTSD on a structured interview than for those who did not. A total SPTSS score of 4 had high sensitivity (.94) though lower specificity (.60). Specificity may have been difficult to establish because of the psychiatric status of participants, and thus further research with community populations is needed.

Self-Rating Inventory for PTSD

The 22-item Self-Rating Inventory for PTSD (SRIP) was developed by J. E. Hovens and colleagues (2002) as a shortened version of an earlier 52-item measure. Like Carlson's SPTSS, the SRIP was developed to assess current symptoms without identifying specific traumatic experiences. Some questions refer to "past events," and others make no reference to events at all. Each item on the SRIP assesses distress over the previous 4 weeks using a 4-point scale from *not at all* to *extremely*. Psychometric data for the 22-item version were collected from several samples of trauma survivors, older adults, peacekeepers, and medical students in the Netherlands. The total scale is highly internally consistent, with alphas ranging from .90 to .94 across samples. Test–retest correlations were also high, ranging from .60 to .97, depending on the length of the interval between tests (the shorter the interval, the higher the correlation). In the trauma survivor sample that was administered other scales measuring PTSD, the SRIP correlated highly with the Civilian Mississippi Scale and MMPI-PTSD scales. In this same sample of survivors, 41 of 76 had PTSD according to the CAPS. Using the CAPS as the criterion, a SRIP cutoff score of 52 had a sensitivity of 86%, specificity of 71%, and efficiency of 78%. However, in a sample of older adults (van Zelst et al., 2003), which had a very low rate of current PTSD, a score of 52 was not at all sensitive (23%) to PTSD as assessed by the Composite International Diagnostic Interview (CIDI). In this case, a score of 39 was superior (sensitivity = 74%, specificity = 81%). This research illustrates our earlier point quite well—that cutpoints developed in clinical samples may not work well in community samples and should be applied with caution. The scale may also be scored according to DSM criteria. Both Dutch and English versions of the SRIP are available from the authors.

OTHER SCALES OF POSTTRAUMATIC STRESS

Post-Traumatic Symptom Scale

One of the earliest measures developed in the field was the Post-Traumatic Symptom Scale (PTSS) developed by Are Holen (1990) for use in studying survivors of the 1980 North Sea oil rig disaster. The scale has both 10- and 12-item versions and has been administered by using a dichotomous yes–no response format, as well as by using a 7-point frequency scale. The scale uses a past-week time frame. The scale does not map onto DSM criteria precisely but does provide a brief assessment of a variety of posttraumatic stress symptoms, including depressed mood, unstable mood, guilt, and tension, as well as selected criterion symptoms, such as sleep difficulties, nightmares, startle, and fears of reminders.

When used with the dichotomous response format, the 10-item and 12-item versions both have alphas of .85, which is good for a scale of this length. When used with the 7-point response format, the alpha increases to .90. The scale correlates more highly with the Global Severity Index of the SCL-90 (.83, .84) than it does with the Impact of Event Scale (.70 , .69). This finding is appropriate given that the scale does not purport to assess PTSD alone.

Penn Inventory for PTSD

The Penn Inventory was developed by Melvyn Hammarberg (1992). The scale has 26 items. Each item is composed of four sentences, scored 0–3, that represent different levels (severity or frequency) of a feeling or thought. The respondent selects the sentence that best describes himself or herself. Although developed for veterans initially, the wording of the scale is not specific to the military.

Hammarberg examined the reliability and validity of the instrument in three phases. The first employed a sample of 83 participants: 28 inpatient combat veterans diagnosed with PTSD, 24 combat veterans who had previously been diagnosed with PTSD but were now at least 6 months into posttreatment, 15 age-matched veterans without PTSD, and 16 age-matched nonveterans without PTSD. The scale was found to be quite reliable, in terms of both internal consistency (alpha of .94) and stability over a 5-day interval ($r = .96$). Mean scale scores differed between groups who had PTSD at the time of testing or previously and the groups who did not have PTSD. However, inpatient and posttreatment groups did not differ. Using a score of 35 as the cutpoint, the scale demonstrated a sensitivity of .90 and a specificity of 1.0.

In the second phase, 98 new participants were selected and assigned to the same four categories: 39 inpatient combat veterans diagnosed with PTSD, 26 combat veterans who had previously been diagnosed with PTSD but were now at least 6 months into posttreatment, 17 age-matched veterans without PTSD, and 16 age-matched nonveterans without PTSD. The scale again demonstrated high internal consistency with an alpha of .94. Results of between-group tests replicated the findings of Phase 1: PTSD participants differed significantly from participants without PTSD, but inpatients did not differ from former patients. Again using a cutoff of 35, sensitivity was .98 and specificity was .94, for an overall hit rate of .97.

Hammarberg's (1992) third phase involved a wider range of psychiatric cases, including 39 veteran patients with PTSD, 18 veteran inpatients with a diagnosis other than PTSD, and 19 survivors of an oil rig disaster, of whom 16 were diagnosed as having PTSD. The groups without PTSD showed significantly lower means on the Penn Inventory than did groups with PTSD. With respect to the veterans in the sample, the Penn again showed excellent sensitivity (.97), although specificity (.61) was lower this time. The Mississippi Scale was also included in this phase of the study and performed similarly. The overall hit rates of the Penn and Mississippi were .86 and .88, respectively. Both performances seem excellent when it is recalled that the scales were discriminating between different groups of psychiatric patients. With respect to the disaster victims, sensitivity was .94 and specificity was 1.0. The high prevalence of PTSD in this group needs to be kept in mind when interpreting these results. Yet they provide evidence that the scale could function effectively with trauma populations other than combat veterans.

Kutcher, Tremont, Burda, and Mellman (1994) administered the Penn Inventory, Combat Mississippi, and MMPI-2-PTSD Scale to 109 inpatient veterans, of whom 54 had been diagnosed as having PTSD. Correlations of the Penn with the other two measures were .78 and .72, respectively, showing good convergent validity. However, as did Hammarberg (1992), these investigators found the Penn to correlate more highly with depressive symptomatology than would be ideal for showing good divergent validity. The BDI's correlation with the Penn (.82) was higher than its correlations with the Mississippi (.65) or the MMPI-2-PTSD scale (.68). Showing a specificity of only .33 in this study, the Penn Inventory was less successful than the Mississippi at discriminating PTSD patients from veterans with other psychiatric diagnoses.

Trauma Symptom Checklist—40

John Briere and Marsha Runtz (1989) created the Trauma Symptom Checklist (TSC) for use in clinical research with adult survivors of childhood sexual abuse. The TSC originally had 33 items divided into five subscales: anxiety, depression, dissociation, post-sexual-abuse trauma, and sleep disturbance. Briere and Runtz established that the original scale was adequately reliable, with the exception of the sleep disturbance scale. The scale was then expanded to improve this subscale and to add a subscale for sexual problems. This version has 40 items. Subjects rate the relevance of each item to their own experience on a 5-point scale from *not at all true* to *very often true*. The reporting period is 2 months.

Using data collected from a large sample (*N* = 2,963) of professional women, Elliott and Briere (1992) determined that the TSC-40 has high internal consistency (alpha = .90). The revision was effective in improving the internal consistency of the Sleep Disturbance subscale (alpha = .77). The scale related to sexual problems also performed well (alpha = .73). Elliott and Briere also showed that the scale discriminates between women who have and have not been abused as children. This difference held strongly for all subscales, as well as for the total scale. Similarly, Gold, Milan, Mayall, and Johnson (1994) administered the TSC-40 to 669 female college students, divided into groups with no sexual assault or abuse (*N* = 438), childhood sexual assault/abuse (*N* = 96), adulthood sexual assault/abuse (*N* = 89), and both childhood and adulthood sexual assault/abuse (*N* = 31). Groups differed in meaningful ways except on the sleep disturbance subscale.

Trauma Symptom Inventory

For clinical purposes, or for whenever a longer measure is acceptable, Briere (1995) developed the Trauma Symptom Inventory (TSI). The TSI is not a measure of PTSD per se, but rather a global measure of trauma sequelae. It is unique among the measures reviewed here in using a time frame for reporting symptoms of 6 months. The TSI has a total of 100 items, scored on a 4-point scale, and contains 10 clinical scales: Anxious Arousal (AA; 8 items, alpha = .86), Depression (D; 8 items, alpha = .91), Anger/Irritability (AI; 9 items, alpha = .90), Intrusive Experiences (IE; 8 items, alpha = .89), Defensive Avoidance (DA; 8 items, alpha = .90), Dissociation (DIS; 9 items, alpha = .82), Sexual Concerns (SC; 9 items, alpha = .87), Dysfunctional Sexual Behavior (DSB; 9 items, alpha = .85), Impaired Self-Reference (ISR; 9 items, alpha = .88), and Tension Reduction Behavior (TRB; 8 items, alpha = .74). In addition, the inventory includes three validity scales. The scale can be self-administered by anyone with a fifth-grade reading level or higher. Norms and *T*-scores were derived on the basis of a large mail-survey sample ($n = 836$) that was approximately representative of the U.S. population in terms of sex, ethnicity, and state of residence.

Briere (1995) provided confirmatory factor analyses as evidence of the inventory's construct validity. Although the factors were highly interrelated, these analyses justify conceptualizing the scale in terms of three higher order constructs. Four of the scales—IE, DA, DIS, and ISR (34 items total)—may be considered as manifestations of traumatic stress, whereas three of the scales—AI, D, and AA (25 items total)—are best viewed as manifestations of generalized dysphoria. The remaining subscales appear to reflect a third factor, Self, that may be more specific to the experience of sexual trauma and dysfunction. Also to assess construct validity, respondents in the national survey were categorized as having experienced childhood or adulthood disaster or interpersonal violence and compared with respondents who had not experienced trauma. All four trauma types were significantly associated with elevated TSI scores. Studies that have been conducted with clinical samples have yielded similar results (Briere, Elliott, Harris, & Cotman, 1995). However, it should be noted that the TSI does not tie the experience of symptoms to any specific stressor.

PTSD SCALES DERIVED FROM ESTABLISHED SYMPTOM INVENTORIES

MMPI-PTSD (PK) Scale

A different approach to developing measures of PTSD has been to derive new subscales for symptom inventories that are commonly used in clinical practice. The best known among these empirically (as opposed to rationally) derived measures is the MMPI-PTSD (PK) Scale developed by Terry Keane and colleagues (1984). The scale was modified slightly when the MMPI-2 was released. The original PK scale had 49 items, whereas the MMPI-2 version has 46 (see Lyons & Keane, 1992). The items were selected because they discriminated between veterans who did and did not have diagnoses of PTSD. Items are dichotomous, but the scale provides a continuous measure of symptomatology.

Herman, Weathers, Litz, Joaquim, and Keane (1993) provided strong evidence of scale reliability. In their studies, the alpha was .95, and test–retest reliability, over 2–3 days, was .94. Notwithstanding its excellent reliability, the validity of the scale has been challenged. Because it draws from available items in the MMPI, the PK scale does not explicitly measure all PTSD symptoms as defined in DSM-IV. However, Watson, Juba, Anderson, and Manifold (1990) found that the scale correlates highly and equally well with various diagnosed symptoms such as intrusive memories, flashbacks, detachment, arousal, and cognitive interference. These were important data for establishing the scale's validity, because otherwise high scores may have indicated the presence of some, but not necessarily all, criterion symptoms. An area of much debate in the literature has been the determination of the scale value that provides the optimal cutpoint for discriminating cases from noncases. Keane et al. (1984) originally suggested a cutpoint of 30, but other investigators subsequently suggested using much lower values (see Watson et al., 1990). Based on a series of psychometric studies (Herman et al., 1993), a score of 23 was recommended. This value yielded a sensitivity of .79 and a specificity of .71 in veteran samples.

The PK scale has been used primarily with veterans. Reliability and validity data derived from veteran populations need to be viewed with caution when the scale is used with other populations. Nonetheless, there is nothing specific to combat or military experience in the wording of the MMPI items and thus no reason why the scale could not be equally applicable to other groups. Data from several studies support this conclusion. Koretsky and Peck (1990) administered the original 49-item MMPI-PTSD scale to 18 adults diagnosed as having civilian trauma and 27 controls who had a variety of psychiatric conditions. Using a cutoff score of 19, the scale correctly classified 89% of the PTSD cases and 85% of the other cases. The scale performed equally well in a second sample of 15 PTSD patients and 9 other psychiatric cases. Dutton, Hohnecker, Halle, and Burghardt (1994) compared scores obtained from forensic and clinical samples of battered women. Quite reasonably, both groups were very distressed, as measured by the PK scale: The mean of 22 in the clinical sample approached the currently recommended cutpoint, and the mean of 28 in the forensic sample exceeded it. However, the two groups' means were not different significantly, whereas their IES and CR-PTSD means were. Neal, Busuttil, Rollins, Herepath, Strike, and Turnbull (1994) examined the convergent validity of the scale in a heterogeneous sample of 70 trauma victims; many participants had service-related trauma, but others were victims of assaults, accidents, or childhood abuse. The MMPI-PTSD scale correlated highly with CAPS measures of endorsed symptoms (r = .84) and symptom intensity (r = .85) and with the IES (.79). On the other hand, correlations were equally high with a measure of general distress (.82). On the basis of CAPS diagnoses of PTSD, a cutoff score of 21 successfully classified 80% of the cases (sensitivity .83, specificity .79.) The IES performed slightly better in this same study. In Hovens and van der Ploeg's (1993) study of 53 psychiatric inpatients in the Netherlands, trauma victims and patients with no trauma differed significantly from one another on their MMPI-PK scores. These differences were of comparable strength to those found for the Civilian Mississippi Scale and greater than those found for the SCL-90. These two scales were highly correlated (*r* = .89), suggesting high concurrent validity.

All in all, the MMPI-PK scale has performed reasonably well in both veteran and civilian samples, although the shifting cutpoints should be noted. However, there is little evidence that the measure is superior to shorter scales presently available. Using the PK scale may therefore make the most sense in settings in which the MMPI is administered routinely.

Symptom Checklist—90 PTSD Scales

CR-PTSD

A similar approach was taken by Ben Saunders and his colleagues at the Crime Victims Research and Treatment Center (1990). The Symptom Checklist—90 (SCL-90; Derogatis, 1977) is a commonly used 90-item self-report symptom inventory. The 90 items are categorized into nine subscales measuring somatization, depression, anxiety, phobic anxiety, hostility, obsessive–compulsive behavior, paranoid ideation, interpersonal insensitivity, and psychoticism. All items are scored on a 5-point scale (0 = *not at all*, 4 = *extremely*). Using items on the SCL-90-R, Saunders et al. derived a 28-item scale that discriminated between crime victims with and without PTSD. Originally named the SCL-PTSD, it later became known as the CR-PTSD scale.

The CR-PTSD has high internal consistency, as evidenced in its alpha of .93. Arata, Saunders, and Kilpatrick (1991) compared the CR-PTSD scale with the IES in a sample of 266 women with a history of criminal victimization. The rate of PTSD was 7.5%. Victims with and without PTSD differed greatly on both the CR-PTSD and IES scales. The CR-PTSD scale was only moderately correlated with the IES (.44), suggesting that the two measures might be tapping different aspects of the same phenomenon. Regression analyses confirmed this impression: The SCL scale made a unique contribution to the prediction of caseness over and above the contribution of the IES. The unique contribution of the CR-PTSD scale was actually somewhat greater than the unique contribution of the IES. Of the 20 cases, the IES correctly classified 17, compared to 15 for the CR-PTSD. This difference in sensitivity was not statistically significant. Of the 246 noncases, the IES correctly classified 207, compared with 223 for the CR-PTSD. This difference in specificity was significant, with the SCL appearing superior. These results need to be viewed with some caution because the validation sample was not completely independent of the derivation sample. Dutton et al. (1994) found forensic and clinical samples of battered women to differ significantly on the CR-PTSD scale, but the difference was no greater than that obtained for the Global Severity Index (GSI) of the SCL-90. The difference was equivalent to that found for the IES Avoidance subscale but smaller than the two groups' difference on the IES Intrusion subscale.

Like the MMPI-PK scale, an advantage of the CR-PTSD scale is that it can be administered, and often is, without knowledge of trauma history. Also like the MMPI, the SCL-90 is used in many settings anyway, so the PTSD subscale can be scored at no additional cost. However, its precision as a measure of posttraumatic stress is uncertain.

SCL-Supplemented PTSD

Robert Ursano and his colleagues (1995; see also Fullerton et al., 2000) also created a PTSD measure for the SCL-90. Theirs was rationally rather than empirically derived, that is, 31 items were selected on their apparent relevance and then assigned to categories B, C, and D. To provide coverage of criterion symptoms that were not well measured, they added 12 items, such as nightmares, feelings of reliving something unpleasant, avoidance, and hyperalertness. An advantage of this scale over Saunders et al.'s SCL-90 PTSD scale is that DSM guidelines, rather than a cutpoint, can be used to classify respondents as "probable PTSD" or not.

The scale alpha was .77 in a sample of motor vehicle accident survivors (Fullerton et al., 2000). Validity was assessed by comparing results obtained using this scale with results obtained using the MMPI-PTSD scale and a score of 19 as the cutpoint. In four community samples of disaster victims, sensitivity averaged 67% and specificity 91%. Overall, 88% were classified correctly. The scale was also related highly to the IES. Given its similar measurement strategy and controversy over optimum cutpoint, the MMPI PTSD may not have been the best choice as a criterion measure for the purpose of documenting the precision of this scale as a measure of PTSD. Fullerton et al. (2000) reported correlations in the range of .19 and .50 between the SCID and their measure. Importantly, Fullerton and colleagues also demonstrated that the sensitivity and specificity of the measure varied considerably depending on the scoring rule used, the percentage of PTSD in the sample, and whether the PTSD being assessed was of an acute or chronic nature.

SCALES DEVELOPED FOR CULTURALLY SPECIFIC OR CROSS-CULTURAL RESEARCH

Revised Civilian Mississippi Scale

The Civilian Mississippi Scale for PTSD was one of the earliest self-report scales for assessing posttraumatic stress. The Mississippi Scale for Combat-Related PTSD measured self-reported symptoms of posttraumatic stress in veteran populations. Because of its excellent psychometric characteristics, Terry Keane and other researchers associated with the Veterans Administration subsequently developed a civilian form of the scale. The scale had 35 items when used in the National Vietnam Veterans Readjustment Survey (NVVRS; Kukla et al., 1990). Four items were subsequently added. The original 35 items fall into four categories, three that align with criteria for PTSD and a fourth that taps self-persecution (guilt and suicidality). Whereas the Mississippi Scale for Combat-Related PTSD elicited information about symptoms experienced "since I was in the military," the civilian form elicits frequency of symptoms "in the past." Vreven, Gudanowski, King, and King (1995) presented psychometric data from a sample of 668 civilians who participated in the NVVRS. They found the civilian form of the Mississippi Scale to have high internal consistency (.86) but questionable discriminant validity (see also Lauterbach, Vrana, King, and King, 1995). In an analysis of the factor structure of the original Civilian Mississippi Scale, Inkelas, Loux, Bourque, Widawski, and Nguyen (2000) found that the positively worded items grouped together into a single factor, regardless of the criterion they might be assumed to reflect. The total scale was more internally consistent when these items were removed.

Fran Norris and Julia Perilla (1996) revised the Civilian Mississippi in a number of ways, partly to shorten the scale but also to sharpen its focus on posttraumatic stress. The Revised Civilian Mississippi Scale (RCMS) has 30 items. Twenty-eight were selected from the 39-item form. Two intrusion items were selected from the TSS because they had received high endorsement in previous research with victims of traumatic events (Norris, 1992). Other changes concerned question formats. As noted, Kukla et al.'s (1990) civilian form elicits frequency of symptoms "in the past." Another reason this scale may act more as a general measure of distress than as a scale of posttraumatic stress is that this wording is not tied very closely to specific trauma experiences. Norris and Perilla (1996) therefore argued (see also the discussion of Vreven et al., 1995) that it would be better to elicit feelings surrounding a specific stressful event rather than to refer vaguely to feelings "in the past." They also divided the 30 items into two parts: The first 18 items "anchored" the symptom to a specific event (e.g., "Since the event, unexpected noises make me jump"); the last 12 items did not ("I am able to get emotionally close to others"). Another change they made was to score all items on the same 5-point scale (1 = *not at all true*; 5 = *extremely true*). This eases administration considerably when data are being collected by lay interviewers or by self-administration.

Norris and Perilla (1996) developed equivalent Spanish and English versions of the RCMS, using back translation and centering (Brislin, Lonner, & Thorndike, 1973), and conducted a study to assess the instruments' cross-language stability. Participants were 53 bilingual volunteers who completed paper-and-pencil instruments twice, with a 1-week interval between tests. The total scale was reasonably consistent internally, with alphas in the bilingual sample of .86 and .88 for the English and Spanish versions, respectively. Norris and Perilla also presented data from a study involving 404 victims of Hurricane Andrew. This time, the data for the English (n = 299) and Spanish

(n = 94) versions of the RCMS were provided by different respondents, assigned according to their own language preference. Both versions of the scale again were found to have good internal consistency. Alphas were .92 and .88 for the Spanish and English versions, respectively. Norris, Perilla, and Murphy (2001) also used the RCMS to compare the structure of PTSD across samples of disaster victims from the United States (Hurricane Andrew) and Mexico (Hurricane Paulina). In an analysis that excluded the noncriterion symptoms, a 4-factor measurement model (Intrusion, Avoidance, Numbing, Arousal) fit the data of the U.S. and Mexican samples equally well. Norris et al. (2001) also administered the RCMS to a subset of respondents in a larger epidemiological study of trauma in Mexico, in which PTSD was assessed by using the CIDI (version 2.1). When RCMS symptoms were dichotomized as absent (*not* or *slightly true*) or present (*somewhat*, *very*, or *extremely true*) and counted according to DSM-IV criteria, this measure yielded the same diagnosis as the CIDI 84% of the time. Given that the RCMS was not intended for use in clinical settings, this amount of agreement is sufficient to suggest that the scale is valid as a measure of posttraumatic stress.

Altogether, the RCMS has some shortcomings relative to other, more recently developed diagnostic scales, but it performs well as a continuous measure of posttraumatic stress and stands out in terms of its validation for use with Spanish-speaking populations.

Harvard Trauma Questionnaire

The Harvard Trauma Questionnaire (HTQ) was developed by Richard Mollica and his colleagues (1992). Both traumatic events and symptoms are included in the questionnaire. In the first section, 17 items describe a range of stressors experienced by refugees, such as torture, rape, murder, and lack of food or water. For each item, the respondent notes whether he or she has (1) not experienced, (2) heard about, (3) witnessed, or (4) personally experienced that stressor. The symptom portion consists of 30 items, 16 of which correspond to DSM-IV criteria and 14 of which tap other aspects of distress as it is expressed in Indochinese culture. Items are scored on a 4-point scale from *not at all* = 1 to *extremely* = 4, and the investigators now recommend scoring the scale as the mean item value (Mollica, personal communication, April 18, 1995). The HTQ is available in Khmer, Lao, and Vietnamese, in addition to English. Linguistic equivalence was established using back translation and centering.

The HTQ is important to review here because it illustrates an approach to the cross-cultural assessment of trauma and PTSD. The investigators (Mollica et al., 1995) note that it is important to *adapt* rather than merely translate the questionnaire for each trauma population and culture. According to Mollica, the "core" PTSD section should be kept equivalent across languages, but the remaining symptom questions should vary so that they are specific and relevant to the culture of respondents. These items should be identified by ethnographic studies, clinical experience, key informants, and healers in the setting of interest (Mollica et al., 1995).

Mollica et al. (1992) examined the reliability and validity of the Cambodian, Lao, and Vietnamese versions of the instrument in a sample of 91 Indochinese refugees, of whom 34 were men and 57 were women, and of whom 55 were Cambodian, 20 Laotian, and 16 Vietnamese. Reliability was very high: The symptom portion of the HTQ yielded an alpha of .96 and a test–retest correlation of .92, with a 1-week interval between tests. To assess criterion validity, research participants were divided into groups on the basis of independent diagnoses. The PTSD group (n = 65) showed significantly higher symptom scores than the non-PTSD group (n = 26). A cutpoint of 75 (mean item value of 2.5) was found to maximize classification accuracy. Sensitivity was .78, specificity was .65, and the overall hit rate was .75. These initial studies provided the tools used in a large-scale study (Mollica, Poole, & Tor, 1998) involving a random sample of nearly 1,000 Cambodian refugees living in camps along the Thai–Cambodian border. Approximately one-third of the sample had PTSD scores in the clinical range (2.5+), and two-thirds had depression scores in the clinical range. Most relevant to the purpose of this chapter were the exceptionally strong relations between traumatic experiences and symptom scores. Rates of PTSD varied from 14% among refugees reporting four or fewer trauma events to 81% among refugees reporting 25 or more trauma events. The relative odds ratio was 38.9 in the most traumatized group. Rates of depression varied from 45 to 93%. In this case, the relative odds ratio was 21.8 in the most traumatized group. These data are instructive in showing that posttraumatic stress symptoms were more specifically associated with the cumulative amount of trauma, whereas depressive symptoms were more pervasive among the refugees.

SUMMARY

Table 3.2 summarizes the information available on these 17 scales. Sources for obtaining these measures are shown in Appendix 3.1. All of the scales reviewed here show acceptable reliability and validity, although some test creators have documented these attributes more completely than have others. Undoubtedly, clinician-administered interviews will remain the "gold standard" in the field. Yet, as a group, these self-report measures performed well when contrasted directly with them. In Table 3.2, we have reserved the descriptor of "strong" validity for those scales that have shown sensitivity and specificity in clinical samples within studies that have been subjected to peer review. This crude summary may give undue weight to criterion validity at the expense of construct validity, which is excellent among many of the scales whose validity is described only as moderate in Table 3.2. Even more important, these data on clinical validity need to be interpreted most cautiously. Much of it resulted from researchers identifying a scale score cutpoint in a sin-

TABLE 3.2. Summary Descriptions of 17 Standardized Self-Report Measures of Posttraumatic Stress

Scale	Number of items	Evidence of stability	Evidence of consistency	Evidence of validity	Reporting period	Anchored to identified event
NWS Module	20+	Kappa = .45	na	Strong	Lifetime	No
PTDS	17	*r* = .83	.92	Strong	Past month	Yes
PCL	17	*r* = .96	.97	Strong	Past month	Varies
Davidson TS	34	*r* = .86	.97	Strong	Past week	Yes
Purdue PTSD-R	17	*r* = .71	.91	Moderate	Past month	Yes
PTSD-Interview	20	*r* = .95	.92	Strong	Lifetime	Yes
SPTSS	17	na	.91	Moderate	Past 2 weeks	No
SRIP	22	.60–.97	.90–.94	Strong	Past 4 weeks	No
PTSS	10–12	na	.85–.90	Moderate	Past week	No
Penn Inventory	26	*r* = .96	.94	Moderate–strong	Past week	No
TSC-40	40	na	.90–.92	Moderate	2 months	No
TSI	100	na	.74–.90	Moderate–strong	6 months	No
MMPI-PTSD	46	*r* = .94	.95	Moderate–strong	Not explicit	No
CR-PTSD	28	na	.93	Moderate	Past 2 weeks	No
SCL-Supplemented PTSD	43	na	na	Moderate	Past 2 weeks	No
Revised Civilian Mississippi	30	*r* = .84	.86–.92	Moderate–strong	Varies	Partially
HTQ	16 + 14	*r* = .92	.96	Moderate–strong	na	Partially

Note. na, data not available.

gle sample that was sensitive and specific to PTSD. Such data establish only that the measure in question *can* predict caseness; they do not establish that the identified cutpoint is appropriate for other samples and populations.

With so many adequate symptom measures available, how should the reader decide which measure to use? The answer to this question is found by considering the wide array of choices these scales offer for measuring post-traumatic stress. Some, but not all, are in the public domain. Some scales adhere closely to DSM-IV criteria; others take a broader sweep. Some are relatively short, whereas others are relatively long. Some take advantage of available clinical data, such as the MMPI or SCL-90; most require additional assessment materials. Most assess current symptoms, whereas a few assess symptoms over the lifetime or since a specific event. Some require the specification of a single or most stressful event, but some refer broadly to past events. Thus a person who is studying reactions to a variety of traumatic events that cannot easily be distinguished but who has few constraints in terms of cost or time of administration may make one choice of measure, whereas a person who is studying a specific event but who needs a brief measure that is available at no cost may make a different choice; yet both choices are equally valid and defensible.

Before leaving this point, we need to acknowledge that the extent to which a PTSD measure must be anchored to a specific traumatic experience is among the points of most controversy in trauma assessment. On the one hand, when symptoms are not tied to a specific stressor, it is difficult to establish for certain that the respondent met criterion A (see the first part of this chapter) or even that the various symptoms pertain to an event at all. (For example, trauma is certainly not the only source of irritability.) On the other hand, epidemiological research has shown quite clearly that it is not uncommon for people to experience multiple events, and victims may not be cognizant of the reason they feel a certain way. There are experts who advocate for each point of view quite strongly, and whichever approach the researcher decides on, it is reasonable to expect at least some criticism from proponents of the other perspective. The best way to manage this dilemma is to acknowledge the issue and to be clear about the reasons for deciding on one measurement approach or the other.

In the first edition of this volume, Norris and Riad (1997) noted that progress in the measurement of civilian trauma had lagged behind that related to military trauma. That statement may no longer be true. That there are now numerous reliable and valid self-report measures of PTSD should aid epidemiological and community-based studies immensely over the next few years. Notwithstanding the quality of these measures, we believe there is still room for improvement in the methods used to validate them. Systematic research comparing various self-report measures in representative community samples, as well as clinical and survivor samples, is needed. Perhaps it is our own bias, but we were disappointed in the lack of attention to diversity in validation samples in this literature. The SRIP was unusual in having been evaluated in a sample of older adults. Excluding the Revised Civilian Mississippi Scale and HTQ, little attention was given to potential ethnic or cross-cultural differences in symptom expression. We concluded this chapter with the HTQ because it illustrates a forward-thinking approach that balances cross-cultural standardization with cultural specificity in developing assessment tools. In our increasingly global and mobile society, cross-cultural equivalence and relevance are extremely important issues for psychometricians to address in future research.

In summary, we believe that future progress in this area would be served best by efforts to refine and cross-validate the existing measures of PTSD. Can we, if only for awhile, forego the temptation of generating new, but largely similar, scales? We hope the answer to this question is yes. As measurement becomes more standardized, we can build a database that elucidates the prevalence and nature of PTSD across different populations and events.

APPENDIX 3.1. Sources for Obtaining Standardized Self-Report Scales

Scale and contact person	Affiliation and e-mail	Telephone
Brief Trauma Questionnaire Paula Schnurr	National Center for PTSD (NCPTSD) White River Junction, VT *Paula.P.Schnurr@Dartmouth.edu*	(802) 296-5132
Civilian Mississippi—Revised Fran Norris	Dartmouth Medical School/ NCPTSD *Fran.Norris@Dartmouth.edu*	(802) 296-5132
Davidson Trauma Scale Jonathan Davidson	Duke University Medical Center *tolme@acpub.duke.edu*	(919) 684-2880
Harvard Trauma Questionnaire Richard Mollica	Harvard Program in Refugee Trauma *rmollica@partners.org*	(617) 876-7879
Life Stressor Checklist—Revised Rachel Kimerling	NCPTSD/ Palo Alto VAMC *Rachel.Kimerling@med.va.gov*	(650) 493-5000 X 23218
MMPI-PTSD Terence Keane	Boston University/ NCPTSD Boston VAMC *Terry.Keane@med.va.gov*	(617) 278-4551
NWS PTSD Module Heidi Resnick	Crime Victims Research and Treatment Center Medical University of South Carolina *Resnickh@musc.edu*	(843) 792-2945
Penn Inventory Melvyn Hammarberg	University of Pennsylvania *mhammarb@ccat.sas.upenn.edu*	(215) 898-0981

Scale and contact person	Affiliation and e-mail	Telephone
PTSD Checklist Frank Weathers	Auburn University *weathfw@auburn.edu*	(334) 844-6495
PTSD-Interview Charles Watson	St. Cloud MN, DVAMC	(570) 824-3521 X 7818
Posttraumatic Stress Diagnostic Scale Edna Foa	University of Pennsylvania, Department of Psychiatry *Foa@mail.med.upenn.edu*	(215) 746-3327
Post-Traumatic Symptom Scale Are Holen	Norwegian University of Science and Technology *are.holen@ntnu.no*	47-7-355-1513
Purdue PTSD Scale—Revised Scott Vrana	Virginia Commonwealth University *srvrana@saturn.vcu.edu*	(804) 828-6273
Screen for Posttraumatic Stress Symptoms Eve Carlson	NCPTSD/Menlo Park, CA *Eve.Carlson@med.va.go*	
Self-Rating Inventory for Posttraumatic Stress Disorder J. E. Hovens	Delta Psychiatric Teaching Hospital *hans.hovens@deltabouman.nl*	31-10-503-1512
SCL-PTSD (CR-PTSD) Ben Saunders	National Crime Victims Research and Treatment Center Medical University of South Carolina *Saunders@musc.edu*	(843) 792-2945
SCL-Supplemented PTSD Robert Ursano	Uniformed Services University School of Medicine *rursano@usuhs.mil*	(301) 295-3293
Stressful Life Events Screening Questionnaire Lisa Goodman	Boston College *goodmalc@bc.edu*	(617) 552-1725
Trauma History Questionnaire Bonnie Green	Georgetown University Medical School *Bgreen01@georgetown.edu*	(202) 687-6529
Traumatic Events Questionnaire Dean Lauterbach	Eastern Michigan University *dlauterba@emich.edu*	(734) 487-0785
Traumatic Life Events Questionnaire Edward Kubany	NCPTSD/ Honolulu DVAMC *edward.kubany@med.va.gov* or *kubany@hawaii.rr.com*	(808) 284-4497

Scale and contact person	Affiliation and e-mail	Telephone
Traumatic Stress Schedule Fran Norris	Dartmouth Medical School and NCPTSD *Fran.Norris@Dartmouth.edu*	(802) 296-5132
Trauma Symptom Checklist–40 John Briere	Department of Psychiatry, Keck School of Medicine, University of South Carolina *www.johnbriere.com/psych_tests.htm*	1-800-331-Test
Trauma Symptom Inventory John Briere	Department of Psychiatry, Keck School of Medicine, University of South Carolina *www.johnbriere.com/psych_tests.htm*	1-800-331-Test

REFERENCES

American Psychiatric Association. (1980). *Diagnostic and statistical manual of mental disorders* (3rd ed.). Washington, DC: Author.

American Psychiatric Association. (1987). *Diagnostic and statistical manual of mental disorders* (3rd ed., rev.). Washington, DC: Author.

American Psychiatric Association. (1994). *Diagnostic and statistical manual of mental disorders* (4th ed.). Washington, DC: Author.

Arata, C., Saunders, B., & Kilpatrick, D. (1991). Concurrent validity of a crime-related posttraumatic stress disorder scale for women with the Symptom Checklist—90—Revised. *Violence and Victims*, *6*, 191–199.

Beck, A. T., Ward, C. H., Mendelsohn, M., Mock, J., & Erbaugh, J. (1961). An inventory for measuring depression. *Archives of General Psychiatry*, *4*, 561–571.

Blanchard, E., Jones-Alexander, J., Buckley, T., & Forneris, C. (1996). Psychometric properties of the PTSD Checklist (PCL). *Behaviour Research and Therapy*, *34*, 669–673.

Briere, J. (1992). *Child abuse trauma: Theory and treatment of the lasting effects.* Newbury Park, CA: Sage.

Briere, J. (1995). *Trauma Symptom Inventory (TSI): Professional manual.* Odessa, FL: Psychological Assessment Resources.

Briere, J., Elliott, D., Harris, K., & Cotman, A. (1995). Trauma Symptom Inventory: Psychometrics and association with childhood and adult victimization in clinical samples. *Journal of Interpersonal Violence*, *10*, 387–401.

Briere, J., & Runtz, M. (1989). The Trauma Symptom Checklist (TSC-33): Early data on a new scale. *Journal of Interpersonal Violence*, *4*, 151–163.

Brislin, R., Lonner, W., & Thorndike, R. (1973). *Cross-cultural research methods.* New York: Wiley.

Carlson, E. (2001). Psychometric study of a brief screen for PTSD: Assessing the impact of multiple traumatic events. *Psychological Assessment*, *8*, 431–441.

Davidson, J., Book, S., Colket, L., Tupler, L., Roth, S., David, D., et al. (1997). Assessment of a new self-rating scale for posttraumatic stress disorder. *Psychological Medicine*, *27*, 153–160.

Derogatis, L. (1977). *SCL-90: Administration, scoring, and procedure manual for the revised version.* Baltimore: John Hopkins University School of Medicine.

Dohrenwend, B. S., Krasnoff, B., Askenasy, A., & Dohrenwend, B. P. (1978). Exemplification of a method for scaling life events: The PERI Life Events Scale. *Journal of Health and Social Behavior, 19,* 205–229.

Dutton, M., Hohnecker, L., Halle, P., & Burghardt, K. (1994). Traumatic responses among battered women who kill. *Journal of Traumatic Stress, 7,* 549–564.

Elliott, D., & Briere, J. (1992). Sexual abuse trauma among professional women: Validating the Trauma Symptom Checklist—40 (TSC-40). *Child Abuse and Neglect, 16,* 391–398.

Foa, E., Cashman, L., Jaycox, L, & Perry, K. (1997). The validation of a self-report measure of posttraumatic stress disorder: The Posttraumatic Diagnostic Scale. *Psychological Assessment, 9,* 445–451.

Foa, E. B., Riggs, D. S., Dancu, C. V., & Rothbaum, B. O. (1993). Reliability and validity of a brief instrument for assessing posttraumatic stress disorder. *Journal of Traumatic Stress, 6,* 459–473.

Fullerton, C., Ursano, R., Epstein, R., Crowley, B., Vance, K., Craig, K., & Baum, A. (2000). Measurement of posttraumatic stress disorder in community samples. *Nordic Journal of Psychiatry, 54,* 5–12.

Gold, S., Milan, L., Mayall, A., & Johnson, A. (1994). A cross-validation of the Trauma Symptom Checklist: The role of mediating variables. *Journal of Interpersonal Violence, 9,* 12–25.

Goodman, L., Corcoran, C., Turner, K., Yuan, N., & Green, B. (1998). Assessing traumatic event exposure: General issues and preliminary findings for the stressful life events screening questionnaire. *Journal of Traumatic Stress, 11,* 521–542.

Green, B. (1996). Trauma History Questionnaire. In B. H. Stamm & E. M. Varra (Eds.), *Measurement of stress, trauma, and adaptation* (pp. 366–368). Lutherville, MD: Sidran Press.

Hammarberg, M. (1992). Penn Inventory for Posttraumatic Stress Disorder: Psychometric properties. *Psychological Assessment, 4,* 67–76.

Herman, D., Weathers, F., Litz, B., Joaquim, S., & Keane, T. (1993, October). *The PK Scale of the MMPI-2: Reliability and validity of the embedded and stand-alone versions.* Paper presented at the annual meeting of the International Society for Traumatic Stress Studies, San Antonio, TX.

Holen, A. (1990). *A long-term outcome study of survivors from a disaster.* Oslo, Norway: University of Oslo Press.

Hovens, J., Bramsen, I., & van der Ploeg, H. (2002). Self-rating inventory for posttraumatic stress disorder: Review of the psychometric properties of a new brief Dutch screening instrument. *Perceptual and Motor Skills, 94,* 996–1008.

Hovens, J., & van der Ploeg, H. M. (1993). Posttraumatic stress disorder in Dutch psychiatric in-patients. *Journal of Traumatic Stress, 6,* 91–102.

Inkelas, M., Loux, L., Bourque, L., Widawski, M., & Nguyen, L. (2000). Dimensionality and reliability of the Civilian Mississippi Scale for PTSD in a postearthquake community. *Journal of Traumatic Stress, 13,* 149–167.

Keane, T. M., Caddell, J. M., & Taylor, K. L. (1988). Mississippi scale for combat-related posttraumatic stress disorder: Three studies in reliability and validity. *Journal of Consulting and Clinical Psychology, 56,* 85–90.

Keane, T., Malloy, P., & Fairbank, J. (1984). Empirical development of an MMPI subscale for the assessment of combat-related posttraumatic stress disorders. *Journal of Consulting and Clinical Psychology*, *52*, 888–891.

Kilpatrick, D., Resnick, H., & Freedy, J. (1991). *The Potential Stressful Events Interview*. Charleston, SC: Medical University of South Carolina, Department of Psychiatry, Crime Victim Research and Treatment Center.

Kilpatrick, D., Resnick, H., Saunders, B., & Best, C. (1989). *The National Women's Study PTSD module*. Charleston, SC: Medical University of South Carolina, Department of Psychiatry, Crime Victim Research and Treatment Center.

Koretsky, M., & Peck, A. (1990). Validation and cross-validation of the PTSD subscale of the MMPI with civilian trauma victims. *Journal of Clinical Psychology*, *46*, 296–300.

Krinsley, K., Gallagher, J., Weathers, F., Kaloupek, D., & Vielhauer, M. (2003). Reliability and validity of the Evaluation of Lifetime Stressors questionnaire. *Journal of Traumatic Stress*, *16*, 399–409.

Kubany, E., Haynes, S., Leisen, M., Owens, J., Kaplan, A., Watson, S., & Burns, K. (2000). Development and preliminary validation of a brief broad-spectrum measure of trauma exposure: The traumatic life events questionnaire. *Psychological Assessment*, *12*, 210–224.

Kulka, R., Schlenger, W., Fairbank, J., Hough, R., Jordan, B. K., Marmar, C., & Weiss, D. (1990). *Trauma and the Vietnam war generation: Report of findings from the National Vietnam Veterans Readjustment Study*. New York: Brunner/Mazel.

Kutcher, G., Tremont, M., Burda, P., & Mellman, T. (1994). *The effectiveness of PTSD self-report measures with an inpatient veteran population*. Paper presented at the annual meeting of the International Society for Traumatic Stress Studies, Chicago, IL.

Lauterbach, D., & Vrana, S. (1996). Three studies on the reliability and validity of a self-report measure of posttraumatic stress disorder. *Assessment*, *3*, 17–25.

Lauterbach, D., Vrana, S., King, D., & King, L. (1995, May). *Psychometric properties of the Civilian Version of the Mississippi PTSD Scale*. Paper presented at the Midwestern Psychological Association, Chicago, IL.

Lyons, J., & Keane, T. (1992). Keane PTSD Scale: MMPI and MMPI-2 update. *Journal of Traumatic Stress*, *5*, 111–117.

McHugo, G., Caspi, Y., Kammerer, N., Mazelis, R., Jackson, E., Russell, L., et al. (2004). *The assessment of trauma history in women with co-occurring mental health and substance use disorders and a history of interpersonal violence*. Unpublished manuscript.

Mollica, R., Caspi-Yavin, Y., Bollini, P., Truong, T., Tor, S., & Lavelle, J. (1992). The Harvard Trauma Questionnaire: Validating a cross-cultural instrument for measuring torture, trauma, and posttraumatic stress disorder in Indochinese refugees. *Journal of Nervous and Mental Disease*, *180*, 111–116.

Mollica, R., Caspi-Yavin, Y., Lavelle, J., Tor, S., Yang, T., Chan, S., et al. (1995). *Manual for the Harvard Trauma Questionnaire*. Brighton, MA: Indochinese Psychiatry Clinic.

Mollica, R., Poole, C., & Tor, S. (1998). Symptoms, functioning, and health functioning in a massively traumatized population: The legacy of the Cambodian tragedy. In B. P. Dohrenwend (Ed.), *Adversity, stress, and psychopathology* (pp. 34–51). New York: American Psychiatric Association Press.

Morgan, C.A., Hazelett, M.G., Wang, S., Richardson, E.G., Schnurr, P., & Southwick, S. (2001). Symptoms of dissociation in humans experiencing acute, uncontrollable stress: A prospective investigation. *American Journal of Psychiatry, 158*, 1239–1247.

Neal, L., Busuttil, W., Rollins, J., Herepath, R., Strike, P., & Turnbull, G. (1994). Convergent validity of measures of posttraumatic stress disorder in a mixed military and civilian population. *Journal of Traumatic Stress, 7*, 447–456.

Norris, F. (1990). Screening for traumatic stress: A scale for use in the general population. *Journal of Applied Social Psychology, 20*, 1704–1718.

Norris, F. (1992). Epidemiology of trauma: Frequency and impact of different potentially traumatic events on different demographic groups. *Journal of Consulting and Clinical Psychology, 60*, 409–418.

Norris, F., & Kaniasty, K. (1992). Reliability of delayed self-reports in disaster research. *Journal of Traumatic Stress, 5*, 575–588.

Norris, F., & Perilla, J. (1996). The Revised Civilian Mississippi Scale for PTSD: Reliability, validity, and cross-language stability. *Journal of Traumatic Stress, 9*, 285–298.

Norris, F., Perilla, J., & Murphy, A. (2001). Postdisaster stress in the United States and Mexico: A cross-cultural test of the multicriterion conceptual model of posttraumatic stress disorder. *Journal of Abnormal Psychology, 110*, 553–563.

Norris, F., & Riad, J. (1997). Standardized self-report measures of civilian trauma and posttraumatic stress disorder. In J. P. Wilson & T. M. Keane (Eds.), *Assessing psychological trauma and PTSD* (pp. 7–42). New York: Guilford Press.

Resnick, H., Falsetti, S., Kilpatrick, D., & Freedy, J. (1996). Assessment of rape and other civilian trauma-related posttraumatic stress disorder: Emphasis on assessment of potentially traumatic events. In T. Miller (Ed.), *Theory and assessment of stressful life events* (pp. 235–271). Madison, CT: International Universities Press.

Resnick, H., Kilpatrick, D., Dansky, B., Saunders, B., & Best, C. (1993). Prevalence of civilian trauma and posttraumatic stress disorder in a representative national sample of women. *Journal of Consulting and Clinical Psychology, 61*, 984–991.

Saunders, B., Arata, C., & Kilpatrick, D. (1990). Development of a crime-related posttraumatic stress disorder scale for women with the Symptom Checklist—90—Revised. *Journal of Traumatic Stress, 3*, 439–448.

Schnurr, P., Spiro, A., Vielhauer, M., Findler, M., & Hamblen, J. (2002). Trauma in the lives of older men: Findings from the normative aging study. *Journal of Clinical Geropsychology, 8*, 175–187.

Schnurr, P., Vielhauer, M., Weathers, F., & Findler, M. (1999). *The Brief Trauma Questionnaire.* White River Junction, VT: National Center for PTSD.

Solomon, S., & Canino, G. (1990). The appropriateness of DSM-III-R criteria for posttraumatic stress disorder. *Comprehensive Psychiatry, 31*, 227–237.

Ursano, R., Fullerton, C., Kao, T., & Bhartiya, V. (1995). Longitudinal assessment of posttraumatic stress disorder and depression after exposure to traumatic death. *Journal of Nervous and Mental Disease, 183*, 36–42.

van Zelst, W., de Beurs, E., Beekman, A., Deeg, D., Bramsen, I., & van Dyck, R. (2003). Criterion validity of the self-rating inventory for posttraumatic stress disorder (SRIP) in the community of older adults. *Journal of Affective Disorders, 76*, 229–235.

Ventureya, V., Yao, S., Cottraux, J., Note, I., & De Mey-Guillard, C. (2002). The validation of the Posttraumatic Stress Disorder Checklist Scale in posttraumatic stress disorder and nonclinical subjects. *Psychotherapy and Psychosomatics*, *71*(1), 47–53.

Vrana, S., & Lauterbach, D. (1994). Prevalence of traumatic events and posttraumatic psychological symptoms in a nonclinical sample of college students. *Journal of Traumatic Stress*, *7*, 289–302.

Vreven, D., Gudanowski, D., King, L., & King, D. (1995). The Civilian Version of the Mississippi PTSD Scale: A psychometric evaluation. *Journal of Traumatic Stress*, *8*, 91–110.

Watson, C., Juba, M., Anderson, P., & Manifold, V. (1990). What does the Keane et al. PTSD Scale for the MMPI measure? *Journal of Clinical Psychology*, *46*, 600–606.

Watson, C., Juba, M., Manifold, V., Kucala, T., & Anderson, P. (1991). The PTSD Interview: Rationale, description, reliability and concurrent validity of a DSM-III-based technique. *Journal of Clinical Psychology*, *47*, 179–185.

Watson, C., Plemel, D., DeMotts, J., Howard, M., Tuorilla, J., Moog, R., et al. (1994). A comparison of four PTSD measures' convergent validities in Vietnam veterans. *Journal of Traumatic Stress*, *7*, 75–82.

Weathers, F., Litz, B., Herman, D., Huska, J., & Keane, T. (1993, October). *The PTSD Checklist (PCL): Reliability, validity, and diagnostic utility*. Paper presented at the annual meeting of the International Society for Traumatic Stress Studies, San Antonio, TX.

Weiss, D. (1993). Structured clinical interview techniques. In J. Wilson & B. Raphael (Eds.), *International handbook of traumatic stress syndromes* (pp. 179–189). New York: Plenum.

Weiss, D. S., & Marmar, C. R. (1997). The Impact of Event Scale—Revised. In J. P. Wilson & T. M. Keane (Eds.), *Assessing psychological trauma and PTSD: A handbook for practitioners* (pp. 399–411). New York: Guilford Press.

Wilson, J. (1994). The historical evolution of PTSD diagnostic criteria: From Freud to DSM-IV. *Journal of Traumatic Stress*, *7*, 681–689.

Wojcik, E. (1988). Disruption to pretrauma social support networks considered as a factor in posttraumatic stress reaction (Doctoral dissertation, Purdue University, 1987). *Dissertation Abstracts International*, *49*, 246B.

Wolfe, J., Kimerling, R., Brown, P. J., Chrestman, K. R., & Levin, K. (1996). Psychometric review of the Life Stressor Checklist—Revised. In B. H. Stamm (Ed.), *Measurement of stress, trauma, and adaptation* (pp. 198–201). Lutherville, MD: Sidran Press.

CHAPTER 4

Structured Clinical Interview Techniques for PTSD

DANIEL S. WEISS

A review of two previous discussions of structured clinical interview techniques (Weiss, 1993, 1997) shows just how much the field of assessment of posttraumatic stress disorder (PTSD) has grown up in the past decade. Whether the field has or has not attained puberty is certainly a debatable matter; both researchers and practitioners might differ about the degree of maturity the field has attained. It is unlikely, however, that any informed consumer, in either the clinical or research domain, would dispute the conclusion that there has been a steady and impressive growth of the breadth of interview techniques and that the evidence base for these techniques has kept apace of the tools themselves.

This progress notwithstanding, some of the basic issues that were problematic in 1993 and 1997 remain problematic, suggesting that the major advances have been technical, not conceptual. For example, clarification of the evidence base for the diagnostic criteria, and convincing evidence that PTSD is a diagnostic entity or taxon (see Meehl, 1995), has not really appeared. The alternative, that PTSD is merely a profile of high scores on several dimensional constructs (e.g., intrusion, avoidance, hyperarousal), all of which normally increase after traumatic exposure and then dissipate, is still a viable alternative conceptualization. Nor has the continuing controversy (see, e.g., Spitzer, 1993) regarding the equivalence of interviews conducted by clinicians and those conducted by lay interviewers (Anthony et al., 1985) been satisfactorily resolved, though clinicians appear to be used less and less often.

The birth of structured interview techniques in psychiatry occurred in the late 1970s and early 1980s, with the publication of the research diagnostic criteria (Williams & Spitzer, 1982) that accompanied the revision of the *Diag-*

nostic and Statistical Manual of the American Psychiatric Association, from the second edition to the third (DSM-III; American Psychiatric Association, 1980). This revision was driven partially by the poor interrater reliability of research studies of psychiatric disorders, both nationally and internationally, and was understood at the time to be due to the emphasis in the DSM-II (American Psychiatric Association, 1968) on an etiological basis for diagnostic entities. This emphasis resulted in many studies in which the phenotypic features of individuals who were given the same diagnosis were sometimes quite heterogeneous, so much so that it was felt that progress in research was being hindered (Kendell, 1983) and the search for understanding of the true nature of the disorders was faltering because of the absence of points of discontinuity established empirically rather than theoretically. Thus the DSM-III took a purely phenotypic stance on diagnostic criteria.

In the attempt to respond to these problems, structured interviews were introduced for use both in clinical studies (e.g., the Schedule for Affective Disorders and Schizophrenia [SADS], Endicott & Spitzer, 1978; the Present State Examination [PSE], Wing, Cooper, & Sartorius, 1974) and in epidemiological studies (e.g., the NIMH Diagnostic Interview Schedule [DIS], Robins, Helzer, Croughan, & Ratcliff, 1981). These efforts generated a spate of studies investigating the reliability (e.g., Williams et al., 1992; Wittchen, 1994; Wittchen, Lachner, Wunderlich, & Pfister, 1998; Wittchen et al., 1991) and validity (e.g., Robins et al., 1981; Spitzer, Endicott, Cohen, & Nee, 1980; Spitzer, Williams, Gibbon, & First, 1992; Wittchen, 1994) of these structured interviews.

This activity has continued, and beginning with DSM-III (American Psychiatric Association, 1980) and with each subsequent edition of the DSM, the New York State Psychiatric Institute group has issued an updated structured diagnostic interview for the major psychiatric disorders that tracks the changed criteria (First, Spitzer, Gibbon, & Williams, 1996; Spitzer, Williams, & Gibbon, 1987a, 1987b; Spitzer et al., 1992; Williams et al., 1992). Similarly, the epidemiological interview field has also seen the introduction of revised and new interview schedules for adults (e.g., Janca, Robins, Cottler, & Early, 1992; Kessler, 1999, 2000; Robins et al., 1988) and children (Shaffer, Fisher, Lucas, Dulcan, & Schwab-Stone, 2000).

This activity established the standards for the state of the art when ruling in or ruling out diagnoses in research settings and activities. A not unexpected outgrowth of this activity was the introduction of structured interview schedules for specific classes of diagnoses (e.g., Steinberg, 1994), as well as specific diagnoses, of which PTSD has probably been the clearest example. The remainder of this chapter comprises a presentation of representative interview schedules specifically designed to be administered by a trained interviewer (usually a clinician), separately for children and adults, and currently in the literature (though there is no claim that this presentation is exhaustive). A discussion of common issues about the diagnostic criteria of PTSD relevant for any of these interviews and some concluding comments about structured interviews and the process of diagnosis follow. The focus on interviews designed to be administered by a trained clinician in a clinical setting means that the so-called epidemiological structured interviews, such as the Composite International Diagnostic Interview (World Health Organization, 1997), are not covered in this chapter.

CLINICAL INTERVIEWS FOR USE WITH CHILDREN

One clear advance since the last edition of this volume (Weiss, 1997) is the wider introduction to the literature of interview schedules designed to be used with children. This is a welcome addition, as the field of PTSD has been largely dominated by work and publications about adults. This advance notwithstanding, it is important to recognize several key issues that are neither problematic nor consequential in the use of structured interviews with adults but that with children have the potential to attenuate the reliability and validity of the results using any one of the interview schedules.

The most obvious of these issues is the level of cognitive development that the child has attained. Though age is customarily a valid proxy of the capacity of a child to understand complex and complicated ideas, in some cases, especially those in which exposure to trauma has been pervasive and long lasting, the child's age may not be as good a marker of his or her level of cognitive development as presumed. To the degree that a very accurate diagnostic assessment is required, clinicians who administer the interview may wish to independently establish the child's cognitive capacity with a standard measure such as the Wechsler Abbreviated Scale of Intelligence (WASI; Wechsler, 1999). This is analogous to establishing a child's or adult's reading level prior to administering a self-report scale that requires a certain level of ability. Especially in forensic settings, the failure to conduct such an ancillary assessment may put the validity of the whole assessment in question.

Other issues have to do with the primary language in the home of the child in cases involving immigrants and refugees; the gender of the interviewer and the gender of the child in situations of alleged or confirmed sexual abuse; and the time elapsed between the traumatic event and the administration of the interview protocol.

Clinician-Administered PTSD Scale for Children

The Clinician-Administered PTSD Scale for Children (CAPS-CA; Nader et al., 1996; Newman & Ribbe, 1996) was among the first of the structured clinical interviews for children and adolescents introduced to the field. When introduced, the CAPS-CA had forms for lifetime and current diagnoses, as well as a 1-week version. The initial material suggested that the interview was developmentally adjusted, appropriate for children ages 7 or 8 and older, and included iconic representations of the separate intensity and frequency rating scales. The iconic representations available to assist the child consisted of smiley faces and variations (e.g., neutral, unhappy) thereof to indicate the intensity ratings of feelings. A series of robot-like figures with increasingly large depictions of a wound or injury indicated how much a problem the item was, and a miniature weekly calendar with an increasing number of X's in each of the day boxes helped to convey the concept of frequency.

The interview scale comprised the 17 DSM-IV (American Psychiatric Association, 1994) PTSD diagnostic criteria, along with another eight associated features: (1) guilt, (2) survivor guilt, (3) shame, (4) reduction in awareness of surroundings, (5) derealization, (6) depersonalization, (7) changes in attachment, and (8) trauma-specific fears (e.g., fearing seeing a perpetrator).

The text of the CAPS-CA attempted to make the description of the diagnostic criteria comprehensible and digestible for children, especially in the domain of the probes and follow-up questions. Nonetheless, despite the attempt to be clear to children, some of the items are hard for a child to understand. For example, criterion 3 in category C, avoidance and numbing—the inability to recall an important aspect of the trauma—requires the inference that a part that is not remembered "ought to be remembered." The youngest children may have difficulty comprehending the complex idea of distress at not remembering, yet they could respond in such a way that the item would be endorsed as written. This issue applies in some degree to all of the child interviews, but it is especially salient with the CAPS-CA because of the separation of frequency and intensity, a distinction that in and of itself may not be easy for the youngest children.

Ultimately, resolution of these concerns is an empirical question, but the validity evidence that would resolve such issues has been very difficult to attain. Perhaps one of the upshots of the more widespread use of the structured interviews for children will be to build an empirical base that leads to the adoption of different criteria for PTSD in children than in adults, should careful research studies emerge to suggest this. Clearly, in the realm of cognition, as opposed to avoidance and hyperarousal, these issues are likely more difficult for children than for adults.

The CAPS-CA was initially offered without a manual, not at all unusual for the first stages of a measure of a specific clinical phenomenon that is difficult and costly to research—for example, the Beck Depression Inventory was initially offered only in a journal article (Beck, Ward, Mendelson, Mock, & Erbaugh, 1961). A recent PsycINFO search specifically targeted at the CAPS-CA revealed only three citations: one study examining hyperarousal and numbing (Weems, Saltzman, Reiss, & Carrion, 2003), another an open trial of citalopram in adolescents (Seedat, Lockhat, Kaminer, Zungu-Dirwayi, & Stein, 2001), and the third an MRI study of the frontal areas and hippocampus (Carrion et al., 2001). Examination of the literature for pure studies of the reliability or validity of the CAPS-CA reveals only the chapter by Newman and Ribbe (1996). Thus at this point it is unclear whether there is continuing development of this measure or whether the empirical concerns raised here will become moot.

Childhood PTSD Inventory

The Childhood PTSD Inventory (Fletcher, 1996) is the least well researched of the three children's structured clinical interviews presented here. A PsycINFO search revealed only a single published journal article (Dubner & Motta, 1999) subsequent to Newman and Ribbe's (1996) chapter, and this paper is not specifically focused on data about the measure. It appears that this structured interview is a matter of historical interest only, if the published record is used to arrive at such judgments.

Children's PTSD Inventory

The Children's PTSD Inventory (CPTSDI; Saigh et al., 2000; Yasik et al., 2001) is an outgrowth of the DSM-III-R–driven Children's Posttraumatic Stress Disorder Inventory (Saigh, 1989a, 1989b), revamped to be consistent with the DSM-IV criteria for PTSD. Designed to be administered to children from ages 7–18, the interview schedule comprises 43 items grouped into five subtests: (1) exposure and situational reactivity—8 items; (2) reexperiencing—11 items; (3) avoidance and numbing—16 items; (4) increased arousal—7 items; and (5) impairment—5 items. Each item is scored dichotomously, for presence or absence.

There are five diagnostic decisions possible from the CPTSDI: (1) no diagnosis; (2) PTSD Negative; (3) acute PTSD; (4) chronic PTSD; (5) delayed onset PTSD. The algorithms and decision rules followed to arrive at any of these diagnoses appeared, at the time of writing, to be available only in the privately printed manual from the author. This absence makes it more difficult than would be ideally desired for potential users to fully evaluate the psychometric data, as the scoring method is absent from the generally available published literature.

With that exception, the CPTSDI is a well-documented structured clinical interview for use with children. Saigh and his colleagues (Saigh et al., 2000; Yasik et al., 2001) present a large body of evidence attesting to the reliability and validity of the interview schedule. Indeed, the empirical evidence for this measure and the rationale for its presentation are couched in the standards established by the group of major professional associations involved in psychological measurement (American Educational Research Association, American Psychological Association, & National Council on Measurement in Education, 1999), and the data accumulated and presented is consistent with these standards.

Saigh and colleagues (2000) reported coefficients of internal consistency ranging from .53 to .89 for the subtests and .95 for the overall diagnostic level. Intraclass correlation coefficients (ICC; Shrout & Fleiss, 1979), the proper statistic to use to index interrater reliability, were very high (though the form of the ICC used is not presented, and if a different and perhaps more appropriate form were used, it might result in a lower value), and the kappa coefficient (Cohen, 1960), indexing chance-corrected interrater agreement, was .96. This coefficient is so high that it may be due partly to the heterogeneity of the sample studied. The test–retest stability—probably the most important of all the coefficients—was a kappa of .91 for the present/absent diagnosis and an ICC of .88 for the sum of items endorsed.

Another positive aspect of the CPTSDI is the decision to ask about the DSM-IV symptoms in child-friendly language rather than more narrowly presenting the criteria. In so doing, the inventory has adopted the position that the interviewer's clinical inference about the presence or absence of the criterion symptom will be a function of the child's responses to questions that tap the experience of the child, rather than the child's agreement with the more sophisticated (or stilted) presentation of the DSM-IV–oriented terms. In the Saigh et al. (2000) article, however, it is clear that Saigh and colleagues do not require expert clinical training as a prerequisite for administering the interview. Resolution of this awaits further study and data. This decision may be what has allowed this structured interview to perform as it did, as approximately 47% of the children in the sample used by Saigh et al. (2000) were in elementary school.

Yasik et al. (2001) present further supportive data regarding the characteristics of the CPTSDI, including positive data about diagnostic efficiency and confirming results regarding convergent and divergent validity. The presence of data regarding divergent validity is atypical, and its presence is a very welcome addition to the evidence base supporting the measure (e.g., CPTSDI scores are correlated with CBCL Internalizing but not Externalizing scores). The limits of the evidence base are also well appreciated in the presentation.

It is hoped that additional data will not only focus on larger samples with a wider range of traumatic events but will also begin to present data and information separately by age group. The average age of the individuals studied is about 12 years; it would be important to know what the characteristics of the CPTSDI are in participants who are in the 7- to 9-year range only. These data could increase the user's confidence that the data collected on older children apply equally well to the youngest. Searches of the literature databases revealed considerably greater use for the CPTSDI than for either of the interviews presented here.

CLINICAL INTERVIEWS FOR USE WITH ADULTS

The original work with structured clinical interviews for PTSD was conducted with and for adults. The most widely used initial structured clinical interview to assess PTSD was the module targeted to that disorder in the Structured Clinical Interview for DSM-III-R (SCID; Spitzer et al., 1992), the revision of the Structured Clinical Interview for DSM-III (Spitzer & Williams, 1985), which did not contain a module for PTSD. Though the publication of the SCID for DSM-III-R did not appear until 1992, the PTSD module was in use as early as 1986 in early work on the National Vietnam Veterans Readjustment Study (NVVRS; Kulka et al., 1990; Weiss et al., 1992) in the clinical examination component.

At the same time, however, the Anxiety Disorders Interview Schedule (ADIS; Blanchard, Gerardi, Kolb, & Barlow, 1986) was also being used for the diagnosis of PTSD. It too was revised (ADIS-R; di Nardo & Barlow, 1985; di Nardo, Moras, Barlow, Rapee, & Brown, 1993), but the revision did not increase its use in studies of PTSD, and currently it is rarely used in research on PTSD. A PsycINFO search revealed no published studies on PTSD using the ADIS-R since 1993.

The PTSD literature shows that currently there is a single structured diagnostic interview for adults that has by far the largest share of the market—the Clinician-Administered PTSD Scale (CAPS; Blake et al., 1995; Blake et al., 1990; Weathers, Ruscio, & Keane, 1999). Now considered by most researchers and clinicians to be the interview of choice due to validity data (King, Leskin, King, & Weathers, 1998; Weathers, Keane, & Davidson, 2001; Weathers et al., 1999), the CAPS is almost synonymous with structured clinical interview in the literature on PTSD. A PsycINFO search revealed more than 80 entries, and a search of the PILOTS database revealed more than 250 citations.

Nonetheless, other structured interviews for PTSD are in the literature, with all but one having been introduced roughly contemporaneously with the CAPS. All, however, have been less extensively used and less thoroughly studied.

Structured Clinical Interview for DSM-IV Axis I Disorders (SCID-I), Clinician Version

The Structured Clinical Interview for DSM-IV Axis I Disorders (SCID-I; First et al., 1996) is the most recent addition to the family of the most widely used and researched structured clinical interview for psychiatric disorders as a whole. With this version, the PTSD module is finally included as a "standard" portion of the structured interview. In the DSM-III-R version, the PTSD module was an "optional" module. Though the current generation of SCIDs, now including Axis II as well as Axis I disorders, is more or less the state of the art for establishing diagnoses in the research setting, there is actually a somewhat startling absence of reliability and validity data regarding its use (Werner, 2001). Only weighted kappa across all diagnoses is available: For patient samples it is about .60, but for nonpatient samples it is approximately .37. Data specifically for the PTSD module are not presented, but as a part of the NVVRS (Schlenger et al., 1992; Weiss et al., 1992) clinical examination component, a kappa coefficient of .93 was obtained. In defense of the SCID, however, in many studies (e.g., Foa & Tolin, 2000; Weathers et al., 1999) it is used as the "gold standard" against which other diagnostic interviews are pegged. Consequently, it is hard to know how to establish validity for the SCID itself, given the absence of any two-way pathognomonic indicator of the criteria other than the report by the interviewee of the set of symptoms themselves. This is, of course, one consequence of the phenomenological approach to diagnosis adopted with the DSM-III that uses an evidentiary rather than a definatory approach to a diagnostic entity (see, e.g., Meehl, 1995).

The structure of the SCID is a trichotomous decision for each criterion item for the diagnosis: 2 = present; 1 = subthreshold; and 0 = absent. The numeric ratings have no quantitative value—they are simply codes to indicate the categorical decisions and could as well have been presented as "P," "S," and "A." The diagnosis of PTSD is made when the requisite symptom pattern is present—one reexperiencing, three arousal/numbing, and two hyperarousal symptoms for at least a month, at least 1 month after exposure, where exposure is defined as encompassing an event that is both threatening to self or other and provokes fear, horror, or helplessness.

The SCID has a standard format of "skipouts"—that is, decision rules that allow the interviewer to end administration of any particular module as soon as it is clear that the diagnostic criteria will not be met. In an epidemiological context, this is understandable, especially given how extensive the number of modules is and how intensive completion of any one module needs to be if an individual actually meets the criteria. On the other hand, skipping out will make detailed studies impossible in situations in which there is a desire to understand more about a diagnosis (see, e.g., Keane et al., 1998; Ruscio, Ruscio, & Keane, 2002) or when concluding that someone's lifetime diagnostic status is only partial or in partial remission (see, e.g., Weiss et al., 1992). Thus use of the full SCID or the PTSD module under standard instructions should be undertaken with some caution.

Structured Interview for PTSD

The Structured Interview for PTSD (SI-PTSD) was introduced in 1989 by Davidson and colleagues (Davidson, Smith, & Kudler, 1989). It not only was designed to elicit information about the presence or absence of symptoms, like the SCID, but it also attempted to scale the severity of the experience of each of the symptom categories. The SI-PTSD was designed to provide both lifetime and current diagnostic decisions. The original publication included data from 116 veterans of the Vietnam War, Korean War, and World War II, all of whom were in treatment. In a subsample of 41 patients, the SCID for DSM-III was administered by a separate interviewer. Thirty-seven of 41 diagnoses were in agreement, yielding a kappa coefficient of .79. The diagnostic decisions are made based on the interviewer's assessment that the symptom severity is at least 2 on a 0–4 scale, where 2 means moderate. The items comprising the syndrome can then be summed and used as a continuous variable.

Davidson, Kudler, and Smith (1997) updated the SI-PTSD to the DSM-IV criteria and changed the acronym to SIP. The authors indicated that the interview schedule had also been revised from the original 1989 version to one that was consistent with DSM-III-R, so that the SIP represents a third generation;

but it appears that nothing was published regarding the DSM-III-R modification.

In the most current version, the diagnostic decisions are made based on the interviewer's assessment that the symptom severity is at least 2 on a 0–4 scale, where 2 means moderate. The interview comprises the 17 individual diagnostic criteria of PTSD with two additional items—survival and behavioral guilt. The internal consistency and test–retest stability appear satisfactory, but a factor analysis that yielded seven factors with eigenvalues exceeding 1.00 is worrisome. Though this criterion may not be ideal (see Cliff, 1988), this finding raises some concerns about either the sample on which the analysis was conducted or the interview itself. A PsycINFO and PILOTS search appeared to indicate little use of this structured interview.

PTSD Symptom Scale—Interview

Foa (Foa, Riggs, Dancu, & Rothbaum, 1993) proposed the PTSD Symptom Scale—Interview Version (PSS-I), along with a parallel self-report version, after the introduction of the changed PTSD criteria accompanying DSM-III-R. This semistructured interview was proposed to fill what was perceived as the gap between the SCID for DSM-III-R, which yielded only the categorical PTSD diagnostic decision and other measures of symptom severity (e.g., Horowitz, Wilner, & Alvarez, 1979; Keane, Caddell, & Taylor, 1988) that were not tailored to the new criteria. Oddly, Davidson's SI-PTSD was cited (which, if slightly modified, would have produced the same outcome in the interview domain) but not considered a useful alternative. Therefore, another interview was introduced into the field. The PSS-I is a semistructured interview comprising only the 17 DSM-IV items and designed to "be administered by lay interviewers who are trained to recognize the clinical picture presented by traumatized individuals" (Foa et al., 1993, p. 461). It yields a total symptom score measuring symptom severity, as well as severity scores for reexperiencing, avoidance, and arousal. There are no probes, and the interviewer presents only one brief question for each criterion. The interviewee's responses are scored by the interviewer on a Likert scale ranging from 0 to 3. Its initial version used the word "assault" rather than a more generic term, given the sample studied. Unlike all other interviews, the time frame for the PSS-I was 2 weeks, and designation of the traumatic event and time elapsed since the event is done outside the purview of the PSS-I. The selection of the 2-week interval means that any diagnostic decisions based on the PSS-I are not strictly comparable to other structured interviews, nor to the DSM-III-R criteria themselves, and that the PSS-I can be used only to assess current PTSD, not lifetime criteria.

The data set used to determine reliability and validity in the initial study comprised 46 females who had been sexually assaulted and 72 controls. Estimates of internal consistency were satisfactory for subscales and total score (.85), and the test–retest reliability was approximately .80. Interrater reliability and interrater agreement, indexed by the ICC and kappa, were both very high, .97 and .91. This may well speak to the composition of the sample of two very distinct subgroups. Also presented were appropriate concurrent and convergent validity data. No divergent validity data were offered.

One of the concerns with all structured clinical interviews is the amount of time it takes to administer them. This will vary widely, of course, based on a number of factors: (1) coverage—PTSD only or PTSD and potentially comorbid conditions such as depression, substance abuse, or dissociative disorders; (2) interviewer and interview characteristics, both separately and together in interaction; and (3) the depth and detail of the information elicited. Foa and Tolin (2000) presented an updated examination of the PSS-I partly out of the concern that the version of the CAPS in use at that time (see the next section for more details) was too lengthy and time-consuming. As well, they noted that the PSS-I used combined frequency and intensity anchors for the ratings of severity. The anchors contain explicit instructions: A rating of 3 means "5 or more times per week/very much" (Foa & Tolin, 2000, p. 183). For diagnostic purposes, the decision rule at the item level for the PSS-I is ≥ 1 (once per week or less/a little). As nothing is mentioned about the time frame of symptom ratings, it appears that it remains as before: the past 2 weeks.

Foa and Tolin (2000) explicitly sought to compare the PSS-I with the CAPS. They presented data in a sample of 64 nonveterans, all of whom had been exposed to a PTSD criterion A event; 12 clinic patients; and 52 volunteers who were neither seeking treatment nor presenting because of their response to their exposure. Two separate interviewers administered the PSS-I and the CAPS, and the videotapes were viewed by two other clinicians. The SCID was administered to a subsample of 25 by yet a third interviewer. A total of 22 interviewers were involved in the study.

The results suggested that the PSI and CAPS both functioned well with respect to internal consistency of subscales and total score, interrater agreement of ratings (though intraclass correlations were not used), and, most important, chance-corrected diagnostic agreement. That is, not only did both measures yield good concordance with each other (with the appropriate scoring rule for the CAPS; see the next section), but also there was good concordance with the SCID diagnosis in the subsample. The pattern of subscale correlations was similar in both measures as well. Thus concurrent and convergent validity data for the PSS-I and CAPS were evident. There was no examination of divergent validity.

The main goal, to show that administration of the PSS-I took less time, was also substantiated, though the two comparisons presented suggest a difference of about 10 minutes only. On the one hand, because the average time to complete either of these interviews in this sample was roughly 27 minutes, one could legitimately take the position that the PSS-I is 33% shorter than the CAPS. On the other hand, because the typical research contact with a study participant who will be administered a structured clinical interview to diagnose the presence or absence of PTSD usually comprises a number of other procedures, the 10-minute difference may be a substantially smaller proportion of research contact time than the 33% implies. Users must make their own decisions about the advantages and disadvantages of one approach or the other. A search of the PsycINFO and PILOTS databases appears to show that the decrease in time is not a strong enough feature to generate frequent use, as less than 10 citations occurred in the former with explicit reference to the interview version of the PSS.

The PSS-I does not appear to include a standardized section to elicit details about the traumatic exposure, something that the most current version of the CAPS now does. If the structured clinical interview is the first occasion on which a participant will discuss the traumatic event in depth, it is not clear how this is done with the PSS-I. Moreover, from a strictly process point of view, it is worth considering the message being sent to participants by a study focused on PTSD whose procedures do not particularly encourage exploring the symptomatology.

Clinician-Administered PTSD Scale

Judging by its use as reflected in the literature, the Clinician-Administered PTSD Scale, introduced in 1990 (CAPS; Blake et al., 1990), has evolved into the standard structured clinical interview for arriving at a diagnosis, either current or lifetime, of PTSD, according to the DSM-IV diagnostic criteria. A recent review article by Weathers et al. (2001) is an excellent source of detailed information about the measure.

Initially based on the DSM-III-R criteria and presented as the CAPS-1 and CAPS-2 by Blake and colleagues (1990), the CAPS has undergone exuviation several times. The CAPS-2 used a 1-week symptom status frame and was intended for situations in which repeated frequent measurement was necessary. These designations were recast into the CAPS-DX (i.e., Diagnostic version) and the CAPS-SX (i.e., Symptom Status version) with the reconfiguration for the DSM-IV criteria. The CAPS has also been translated into German (Schnyder & Moergeli, 2002), but it is unclear how much of the evidence base for the English version directly applies.

In its most recent incarnation (Weathers et al., 2001), in addition to minor modifications, four major changes were made. The first was the addition of a protocol for assessing exposure, the second was a rewording to equilibrate the intensity ratings, the third was rating of the linkage between a symptom and the traumatic event identified in the exposure section (see Solomon & Canino, 1990), and the fourth was a major revision of the associated items, retaining the two guilt items and adding items regarding dissociative features, in the hopes of making the CAPS applicable to acute stress disorder. As a consequence, inclusion of these items may contribute to the growing body of knowledge regarding peritraumatic dissociation, recently identified as the strongest single predictor of PTSD (Ozer, Best, Lipsey, & Weiss, 2003). As with the CPTSDI, these changes were approached from the perspective of the test standards that guide the field.

During the period between the introduction of the original CAPS-1 and the current version, two important empirical contributions were made to its evidence base. One was a confirmatory factor analysis (King et al., 1998) that yielded factors of reexperiencing, hyperarousal, and—instead of a combined third factor of avoidance and numbing—a separate factor for each. As in all construct validity situations, one cannot know if this result raises questions about the measure, about the diagnosis it is seeking to replicate, or about both. As usual, further research is required.

The other contribution was a detailed examination of a set of decision rules used to make a dichotomous diagnostic decision of presence or absence of PTSD (Weathers et al., 1999), as the basic structure of the CAPS is a Likert-type rating of frequency (0–4) and a separate rating of intensity (0–4) for each symptom—indeed, as described previously, one of the most recent changes was to make these anchors more consistent. Thus completing the CAPS does not, like the SCID, automatically yield a diagnostic decision of present or absent. Instead, deciding that an individual does or does not meet the criteria for PTSD requires deciding for each criterion item whether the frequency and intensity ratings, whose separation in the CAPS many regard as an important and useful advance over previous interviews, together take it over the threshold for a global decision of absence or presence. The original decision rule, termed F1/I2, was simple: Frequency had to be ≥ 1 (once or twice a month) and intensity had to be ≥ 2 (moderate), and then the DSM algorithm was applied (1-3-2). This rule was not empirically derived, though it was no less reasonable than having the clinician make the distinction between "present" and "subthreshold" on the SCID, where the weighting of frequency and intensity is done implicitly by the clinician. In fact, the separation of frequency and intensity in the CAPS was (and is) an explicit attempt to become clearer and more explicit about how the decision of presence/absence was made for any criterion item.

Weathers and colleagues (Weathers et al., 1999) evaluated nine different rules, some of which were measure based (e.g., frequency [≠ 0] + intensity [≠ 0] ≥ 3) and others of which were more empirically based (e.g., the lowest combination of frequency and intensity ratings that 60% of a panel of expert clinicians rated as making the symptom unequivocally present). Extensive analyses in several samples on the interrater reliability, test–retest stability, and prevalence of PTSD given the different scoring rules generated two important findings. First, the stability and interrater reliability did not vary much as a function of decision rule and were supportive of the measure. Second, the different scoring rules yielded considerably different results regarding prevalence (what proportion ended up meeting the diagnostic criteria), with the highest rates being roughly double the lowest. As the authors point out, this latter finding makes it very important that any research report using the CAPS to establish lifetime or current diagnosis of PTSD present the decision rule that was used to arrive at a positive diagnosis.

That the CAPS also generates scores that can be used as indicators of the severity of each symptom (the sum of the intensity and frequency ratings) and the severity of the whole range of symptoms (the sum of those sums) is, of course, a strength of this structured interview, because it generates continuous variables that can be used in correlation and regression analyses and in assessments of symptom change (hopefully reduction) as a function of treatment, and in so doing makes the detection of small but meaningful effects possible in a way that the SCID PTSD module cannot. Simultaneously, however, it makes findings regarding prevalence such as those noted previously possible, so that in addition to the standard sources of variability of interviewer effects and sample effects, which affect every structured interview, there is in theory (and probably in practice) this additional source variability. This additional source of variability is not inherent in the CAPS, but its presence requires reiteration of the message of Weathers and colleagues (1999, p.142): "investigators should always explicitly describe and defend their choice of a CAPS scoring rule." Given the several versions of the CAPS that have been in the field, it is probably wise to advise investigators to always be explicit about what version of the CAPS they used and which of the variations of administration described by Weathers and colleagues was used. This will help to facilitate clearer conclusions in the field, as well as making other research activities such as meta-analyses more easy to accomplish and more meaningful to utilize.

SUMMARY AND CONCLUSIONS

Just as in psychopharmacology—in which there is no one SSRI that is strictly superior to all the others in efficacy, effectiveness, side effects, time of onset, and continuation of therapeutic effect—so too, in the arena of structured clinical interviews, there is no interview that is strictly superior to all the others. This state of affairs is partly due to the recognition that within the broad goal of producing a current diagnosis of PTSD, different interviews attempt to achieve different outcomes (e.g., speed versus accuracy). As well, because not all researchers or clinicians have the same goals and objectives when they choose a structured interview to use, any blanket recommendation would overlook this variability and result in a less-than-ideal choice.

The bedrock of the process of research on human beings is informed consent. Participants should be informed, in as much detail as is required, about the potential risks and benefits of participating in any research project prior to agreeing to participate. A major goal of this chapter has been to provide the analogue to informed consent for clinicians and researchers who are considering employing a structured clinical interview for the diagnosis of PTSD.

One component of informed consent involves making clear that what is known up to this point may not directly or strictly apply to the circumstances of the study in which an individual will participate. So too with the evidence base presented for the various structured clinical interviews—the results may not be directly applicable to the situation in which the clinician or researcher plans to use that interview.

The issue that is likely to be of more importance than any other is the setting in which the interview will be used, because this will have implications for the base rate of the phenomenon to be identified—PTSD. The accuracy, or sensitivity and specificity, of the structured interview is not necessarily a fixed attribute but can be expected to vary depending on not only the base rate of the phenomenon—what percent have PTSD—but also on the clinical characteristics of the no-diagnosis group (e.g., SCID kappas of .60 and .37). If that group comprises volunteers and is considered against treatment seekers, then an interview may perform better than if the no-diagnosis group comprises those with PTSD in partial remission or with partial PTSD (a distinction not possible to make without lifetime symptom information) or those having a normal stress response after exposure. A decision rule for diagnosis on a continuous measure is just another term for a cutting score. Almost 50 years ago Meehl and Rosen (1955) noted the impact on validity coefficients of tests using a certain cutting score when the base rate deviated considerably from 50%, and the test itself had only moderate validity—an increase in erroneous decisions.

Since that time a whole new sophisticated technology, signal detection theory and receiver operating characteristics (Kiernan, Kraemer, Winkleby, King, & Taylor, 2001; Kraemer, 1992), has emerged, targeted at identifying optimal cuts along a range of parameters. Kraemer (McKitrick et al., 1999) has also presented a quality receiver operating characteristics (QROC) approach to these issues. The point here is that for the structured interviews that require a decision rule to convert from the continuous severity score to a diagnostic decision (virtually all except the SCID), considerable attention needs to be paid to the setting in which the interview was developed and validated compared with the setting in which it will be used. A specialized outpatient PTSD clinic will have a different base rate from a community sample exposed to the collapse of the World Trade Center buildings. And that community sample itself will have different rates if civilians are compared with emergency service personnel. Continued attention to these issues, as already undertaken by—and continuing to be recommended by—Weathers and colleagues (1991, 2001) with respect to the CAPS, is a vigorous start in the right direction.

A separate but related issue, one that could produce a similar effect, is the training and experience of the interviewer. There appears to be an escalating tendency to suggest that training can be ratcheted down and that lay interviewers are sufficient. The empirical basis for this shift is not clear, and given the findings in the Epidemiologic Catchment Area (Anthony et al., 1985), this tendency may be misguided. In epidemiology, where prevalence is the Holy

Grail, as long as false positives and false negatives cancel each other out, the result is as if there were no diagnostic errors. In clinical situations, however, such inexactitude can have unwanted and harmful consequences for individuals regarding treatment services available or reimbursement for the costs of such treatment. Thus training procedures and continuing monitoring for rater drift are important antidotes for this problem. Ultimately, absent empirical data directly on this matter in PTSD using these interviews, it is unlikely that using as interviewers clinicians who have experience with PTSD and who have had appropriate training in the interview technique will produce less valid results than using less experienced or trained interviewers.

In any event, the necessity of trained clinicians to conduct interviews rather than lay interviewers is an empirical question, just one of many that remain unanswered. Perhaps by the time a subsequent review of structured clinical interview techniques is undertaken, this and other questions will have been addressed empirically, and then there will be no doubt that the field of assessment of PTSD will have moved to the age of majority, steering through the chaotic period of the teens.

REFERENCES

American Educational Research Association, American Psychological Association, & National Council on Measurement in Education. (1999). *Standards for educational and psychological testing*. Washington, DC: Educational Research Association.

American Psychiatric Association. (1968). *Diagnostic and statistical manual of mental disorders* (2nd ed.). Washington, DC: Author.

American Psychiatric Association. (1980). *Diagnostic and statistical manual of mental disorders* (3rd ed.). Washington, DC: Author.

American Psychiatric Association. (1994). *Diagnostic and statistical manual of mental disorders* (4th ed.). Washington, DC: Author.

Anthony, J. C., Folstein, M., Romanski, A. J., Von Korff, M. R., Nestadt, G. R., & Chahal, R. (1985). Comparison of the lay Diagnostic Interview Schedule and a standardized psychiatric diagnosis: Experience in eastern Baltimore. *Archives of General Psychiatry*, *42*, 667–675.

Beck, A. T., Ward, C. H., Mendelson, M., Mock, J., & Erbaugh, J. (1961). An inventory for measuring depression. *Archives of General Psychiatry*, *4*, 561–571.

Blake, D. D., Weathers, F. W., Nagy, L. M., Kaloupek, D. G., Gusman, F. D., Charney, D. S., et al. (1995). The development of a clinician-administered PTSD scale. *Journal of Traumatic Stress*, *8*, 75–90.

Blake, D. D., Weathers, F. W., Nagy, L. M., Kaloupek, D. G., Klauminzer, G., Charney, D. S., et al. (1990). A clinician rating scale for assessing current and lifetime PTSD: The CAPS-1. *Behavior Therapy*, *13*, 187–188.

Blanchard, E. B., Gerardi, R. J., Kolb, L. C., & Barlow, D. H. (1986). The utility of the Anxiety Disorders Interview Schedule (ADIS) in the diagnosis of post-traumatic stress disorder (PTSD) in Vietnam veterans. *Behaviour Research and Therapy*, *24*, 577–580.

Carrion, V. G., Weems, C. F., Eliez, S., Patwardhan, A., Brown, W., Ray, R. D., et al. (2001). Attenuation of frontal asymmetry in pediatric posttraumatic stress disorder. *Biological Psychiatry*, *50*, 943–951.

Cliff, N. (1988). The eigenvalues-greater-than-one rule and the reliability of components. *Psychological Bulletin*, *103*, 276–279.

Cohen, J. (1960). A coefficient of agreement for nominal scales. *Educational and Psychological Measurement*, *20*, 37–46.

Davidson, J. R. T., Kudler, H. S., & Smith, R. (1997). Structured interview for PTSD (SIP): Psychometric validation for DSM-IV criteria. *Depression and Anxiety*, *5*, 127–129.

Davidson, J. R. T., Smith, R., & Kudler, H. S. (1989). Validity and reliability of the DSM-III criteria for posttraumatic stress disorder: Experience with a structured interview. *Journal of Nervous and Mental Disease*, *177*, 336–341.

di Nardo, P. A., & Barlow, D. H. (1985). *Anxiety Disorders Interview Schedule—Revised (ADIS-R)*. Albany, NY: State University of New York at Albany, Phobia and Anxiety Disorders Clinic.

di Nardo, P. A., Moras, K., Barlow, D. H., Rapee, R. M., & Brown, T. A. (1993). Reliability of DSM-III—R anxiety disorder categories: Using the Anxiety Disorders Interview Schedule—Revised (ADIS-R). *Archives of General Psychiatry*, *50*, 251–256.

Dubner, A. E., & Motta, R. W. (1999). Sexually and physically abused foster care children and posttraumatic stress disorder. *Journal of Consulting and Clinical Psychology*, *67*, 367–373.

Endicott, J., & Spitzer, R. L. (1978). A diagnostic interview: The schedule for affective disorders and schizophrenia. *Archives of General Psychiatry*, *35*, 837–844.

First, M. B., Spitzer, R. L., Gibbon, M., & Williams, J. B. (1996). *Structured Clinical Interview for DSM-IV Axis I Disorders (SCID-I), Clinician Version*. Washington, DC: American Psychiatric Association.

Fletcher, K. E. (1996). Psychometric review of the Childhood PTSD Interview. In B. H. Stamm (Ed.), *Measurement of stress, trauma, and adaptation* (pp. 87–89). Lutherville: MD: Sidran Press.

Foa, E. B., Riggs, D. S., Dancu, C. V., & Rothbaum, B. O. (1993). Reliability and validity of a brief instrument for assessing posttraumatic stress disorder. *Journal of Traumatic Stress*, *6*, 459–473.

Foa, E. B., & Tolin, D. F. (2000). Comparison of the PTSD Symptom Scale—Interview Version and the Clinician-Administered PTSD Scale. *Journal of Traumatic Stress*, *13*, 181–191.

Horowitz, M. J., Wilner, N., & Alvarez, W. (1979). Impact of Event Scale: A measure of subjective stress. *Psychosomatic Medicine*, *41*, 209–218.

Janca, A., Robins, L. N., Cottler, L. B., & Early, T. S. (1992). Clinical observation of assessment using the Composite International Diagnostic Interview (CIDI): An analysis of the CIDI Field Trials—Wave II at the St. Louis site. *British Journal of Psychiatry*, *160*, 815–818.

Keane, T. M., Caddell, J. M., & Taylor, K. L. (1988). Mississippi Scale for Combat-Related Posttraumatic Stress Disorder: Three studies in reliability and validity. *Journal of Consulting and Clinical Psychology*, *56*, 85–90.

Keane, T. M., Kolb, L. C., Kaloupek, D. G., Orr, S. P., Blanchard, E. B., Thomas, R. G., et al. (1998). Utility of psychophysiology measurement in the diagnosis of posttraumatic stress disorder: Results from a Department of Veteran's Affairs cooperative study. *Journal of Consulting and Clinical Psychology*, *66*, 914–923.

Kendell, R. E. (1983). The choice of diagnostic criteria for biological research. *Archives of General Psychiatry, 39*, 1334–1339.

Kessler, R. C. (1999). The World Health Organization International Consortium in Psychiatric Epidemiology (ICPE): Initial work and future directions—The Nordic Association for Psychiatric Epidemiology Lecture 1998. *Acta Psychiatrica Scandinavica, 99*, 2–9.

Kessler, R. C. (2000). Psychiatric epidemiology: Selected recent advances and future directions. *Bulletin of the World Health Organization, 78*, 464–474.

Kiernan, M., Kraemer, H. C., Winkleby, M. A., King, A. C., & Taylor, C. B. (2001). Do logistic regression and signal detection identify different subgroups at risk? Implications for the design of tailored interventions. *Psychological Methods, 6*, 35–48.

King, D. W., Leskin, G. A., King, L. A., & Weathers, F. W. (1998). Confirmatory factor analysis of the Clinician-Administered PTSD Scale: Evidence for the dimensionality of posttraumatic stress disorder. *Psychological Assessment, 10*, 90–96.

Kraemer, H. C. (1992). *Evaluating medical tests: Objective and quantitative guidelines*. Newbury Park, CA: Sage.

Kulka, R. A., Schlenger, W. E., Fairbank, J. A., Hough, R. L., Jordan, B. K., Marmar, C. R., et al. (1990). *Trauma and the Vietnam war generation: Report of the findings from the National Vietnam Veterans Readjustment Study*. New York: Brunner/Mazel.

McKitrick, L. A., Friedman, L. F., Brooks, J. O., III, Pearman, A., Kraemer, H. C., & Yesavage, J. A. (1999). Predicting response of older adults to mnemonic training: Who will benefit? *International Psychogeriatrics, 11*, 289–300.

Meehl, P. E. (1995). Bootstraps taxometrics. Solving the classification problem in psychopathology. *American Psychologist, 50*, 266–275.

Meehl, P. E., & Rosen, A. (1955). Antecedent probability and the efficiency of psychometric signs, patterns, or cutting scores. *Psychological Bulletin, 52*, 194–216.

Nader, K. O., Kriegler, J. A., Blake, D. D., Pynoos, R. S., Newman, E., & Weathers, F. W. (1996). *Clinician-Administered PTSD Scale for Children and Adolescents for (DSM-IV)*. Los Angeles and White River Junction, VT: UCLA Trauma Psychiatry Program and National Center for PTSD.

Newman, E., & Ribbe, D. (1996). Psychometric review of the Clinician-Administered PTSD Scale for Children. In B. H. Stamm (Ed.), *Measurement of stress, trauma, and adaptation* (pp. 106–114). Lutherville, MD: Sidran Press.

Ozer, E. J., Best, S. R., Lipsey, T. L., & Weiss, D. S. (2003). Predictors of posttraumatic stress disorder symptoms in adults: A meta-analysis. *Psychological Bulletin, 129*, 52–73.

Robins, L. N., Helzer, J. E., Croughan, J. L., & Ratcliff, K. S. (1981). National Institute of Mental Health Diagnostic Interview Schedule: Its history, characteristics, and validity. *Archives of General Psychiatry, 38*, 381–389.

Robins, L. N., Wing, J., Wittchen, H. U., Helzer, J. E., Babor, T. F., Burke, J., et al. (1988). The Composite International Diagnostic Interview: An epidemiologic instrument suitable for use in conjunction with different diagnostic systems and in different cultures. *Archives of General Psychiatry, 45*, 1069–1077.

Ruscio, A. M., Ruscio, J., & Keane, T. M. (2002). The latent structure of posttraumatic stress disorder: A taxometric investigation of reactions to extreme stress. *Journal of Abnormal Psychology, 111*, 290–301.

Saigh, P. A. (1989a). The development and validation of the Children's Posttraumatic Stress Disorder inventory. *International Journal of Special Education, 4*, 75–84.

Saigh, P. A. (1989b). The reliability and validity of a French version of the Children's Post-Traumatic Stress Disorder Inventory [Fiabilité et validité de l'inventaire des troubles post-traumatiques pour enfants]. *Comportement Humain*, *3*, 29–39.

Saigh, P. A., Yasik, A. E., Oberfield, R. A., Green, B. L., Halamandaris, P. V., Rubenstein, H., et al. (2000). The Children's PTSD Inventory: Development and reliability. *Journal of Traumatic Stress*, *13*, 369–380.

Schlenger, W. E., Kulka, R. A., Fairbank, J. A., Hough, R. L., Jordan, B. K., Marmar, C. R., et al. (1992). The prevalence of post-traumatic stress disorder in the Vietnam generation: A multimethod, multisource assessment of psychiatric disorder. *Journal of Traumatic Stress*, *5*, 333–363.

Schnyder, U., & Moergeli, H. (2002). German version of Clinician-Administered PTSD Scale. *Journal of Traumatic Stress*, *15*, 487–492.

Seedat, S., Lockhat, R., Kaminer, D., Zungu-Dirwayi, N., & Stein, D. J. (2001). An open trial of citalopram in adolescents with post-traumatic stress disorder. *International Clinical Psychopharmacology*, *16*, 21–25.

Shaffer, D., Fisher, P., Lucas, C. P., Dulcan, M. K., & Schwab-Stone, M. E. (2000). NIMH Diagnostic Interview Schedule for Children—Version IV (NIMH DISC-IV): Description, differences from previous versions, and reliability of some common diagnoses. *Journal of the American Academy of Child and Adolescent Psychiatry*, *39*, 28–38.

Shrout, P. E., & Fleiss, J. L. (1979). Intraclass correlations: Uses in assessing rater reliability. *Psychological Bulletin*, *86*, 420–428.

Solomon, S. D., & Canino, G. J. (1990). Appropriateness of DSM-III-R criteria for posttraumatic stress disorder. *Comprehensive Psychiatry*, *31*, 227–237.

Spitzer, R. L. (1993). Psychiatric diagnosis: Are clinicians still necessary? *Comprehensive Psychiatry*, *24*, 399–411.

Spitzer, R. L., Endicott, J., Cohen, J., & Nee, J. (1980). The Psychiatric Status Schedule for epidemiological research: Methodological considerations. *Archives of General Psychiatry*, *37*, 1193–1197.

Spitzer, R. L., & Williams, J. B. W. (1985). *Manual for the Structured Clinical Interview for DSM-III*. New York: New York State Psychiatric Institute, Biometrics Research Department.

Spitzer, R. L., Williams, J. B. W., & Gibbon, M. (1987a). *Structured Clinical Interview for DSM-III-R*. New York: New York State Psychiatric Institute, Biometrics Research Department.

Spitzer, R. L., Williams, J. B. W., & Gibbon, M. (1987b). *Structured Clinical Interview for DSM-III-R, Nonpatient Version*. New York: New York State Psychiatric Institute, Biometrics Research Department.

Spitzer, R. L., Williams, J. B. W., Gibbon, M., & First, M. B. (1992). The Structured Clinical Interview for DSM-III-R (SCID): I. History, rationale, and description. *Archives of General Psychiatry*, *49*, 624–629.

Steinberg, M. (1994). *Structured Clinical Interview for DSM-IV Dissociative Disorders (SCID-D)*. Washington, DC: American Psychiatric Association Press.

Weathers, F. W., Keane, T. M., & Davidson, J. R. (2001). Clinician-Administered PTSD Scale: A review of the first ten years of research. *Depression and Anxiety*, *13*, 132–156.

Weathers, F. W., Ruscio, A. M., & Keane, T. M. (1999). Psychometric properties of nine scoring rules for the Clinician-Administered Posttraumatic Stress Disorder Scale. *Psychological Assessment*, *11*, 124–133.

Wechsler, D. (1999). *Manual for the Wechsler Abbreviated Scale of Intelligence*. San Antonio: TX: Psychological Corporation.

Weems, C. F., Saltzman, K. M., Reiss, A. L., & Carrion, V. G. (2003). A prospective test of the association between hyperarousal and emotional numbing in youth with a history of traumatic stress. *Journal of Clinical Child and Adolescent Psychology*, *32*, 166–171.

Weiss, D. S. (1993). Structured clinical interview techniques. In J. P. Wilson & B. Raphael (Eds.), *The international handbook of traumatic stress syndromes* (pp. 179–187). New York: Plenum Press.

Weiss, D. S. (1997). Structured clinical interview techniques. In J. P. Wilson & T. M. Keane (Eds.), *Assessing psychological trauma and PTSD* (pp. 493–511). New York: Guilford Press.

Weiss, D. S., Marmar, C. R., Schlenger, W. E., Fairbank, J. A., Jordan, B. K., Hough, R. L., et al. (1992). The prevalence of lifetime and partial posttraumatic stress disorder in Vietnam theatre veterans. *Journal of Traumatic Stress*, *5*, 365–376.

Werner, P. D. (2001). Structured Clinical Interview for DSM-IV Axis I Disorders: Clinician Version. In B. S. Plake & J. C. Impara (Eds.), *The fourteenth mental measurements yearbook* (pp. 1123–1125). Lincoln: NE: Buros Institute of Mental Measurements.

Williams, J. B., Gibbon, M., First, M. B., Spitzer, R. L., Davies, M., Borus, J., et al. (1992). The Structured Clinical Interview for DSM-III-R (SCID): II. Multisite test–retest reliability. *Archives of General Psychiatry*, *49*, 630–636.

Williams, J. B., & Spitzer, R. L. (1982). Research diagnostic criteria and DSM-III: An annotated comparison. *Archives of General Psychiatry*, *39*, 1283–1289.

Wing, J. K., Cooper, J. E., & Sartorius, N. (1974). *The description and classification of psychiatric symptoms: An instruction manual for the PSE and CATEGO systems*. London: Cambridge University Press.

Wittchen, H. U. (1994). Reliability and validity studies of the WHO—Composite International Diagnostic Interview (CIDI): A critical review. *Journal of Psychiatric Research*, *28*, 57–84.

Wittchen, H. U., Lachner, G., Wunderlich, U., & Pfister, H. (1998). Test–retest reliability of the computerized DSM-IV version of the Munich-Composite International Diagnostic Interview (M-CIDI). *Social Psychiatry and Psychiatric Epidemiology*, *33*, 568–578.

Wittchen, H. U., Robins, L. N., Cottler, L. B., Sartorius, N., Burke, J. D., & Regier, D. (1991). Cross-cultural feasibility, reliability and sources of variance of the Composite International Diagnostic Interview (CIDI): The Multicentre WHO/ADAMHA Field Trials. *British Journal of Psychiatry*, *159*, 645–653, 658.

World Health Organization. (1997). *Composite International Diagnostic Interview*. Geneva: Author.

Yasik, A. E., Saigh, P. A., Oberfield, R. A., Green, B., Halamandaris, P., & McHugh, M. (2001). The validity of the children's PTSD Inventory. *Journal of Traumatic Stress*, *14*, 81–94.

CHAPTER 5

Systematic Assessment of Posttraumatic Dissociation

The Structured Clinical Interview for DSM-IV Dissociative Disorders

MARLENE STEINBERG

Advances in the systematic assessment of dissociative symptoms and disorders have facilitated new research into these disorders and their relationship to posttraumatic stress disorder (PTSD). This development should be situated within the context of changes in diagnostic taxonomy and nomenclature. For over a century, both the dissociative disorders and PTSD have been recognized as posttraumatic syndromes but have been codified under different psychiatric classifications since the first edition of the *Diagnostic and Statistical Manual of Mental Disorders* (DSM-I; American Psychiatric Association, 1952). From a historical perspective, the dissociative disorders and PTSD are syndromes that share a common sociotemporal context, as well as overlapping symptomatology. In the classificatory schemes of the earliest diagnostic manuals, the dissociative disorders were lumped together under the rubric of "hysteria." With respect to PTSD, the early editions of DSM tended to regard what was then termed "gross stress reaction" as implying a premorbid condition in the patient. It was not until the social upheavals of the early 1970s that PTSD and the dissociative disorders emerged as fields of new interest and concern. The present edition of DSM (DSM-IV-TR; American Psychiatric Association, 2000) has assigned a separate section to the dissociative disorders and classifies PTSD and acute stress disorder as anxiety disorders. What is not clear from the present classificatory arrangement is the overlap in symptomatology and etiology.

Recent research documents the high frequency of dissociative symptoms in individuals with PTSD and the importance of dissociation in the development of PTSD (Birmes et al, 2001; Bremner, Steinberg, Southwick, Johnson,

& Charney, 1993; Brunet et al., 2001; Koopman, Classen, & Spiegel, 1994; Griffin, Resick, & Mechanic, 1997; Johnson, Pike, & Chard, 2001; Marmar et al., 1994; Putnam, 1995; Shalev, Peri, Canetti, & Schreiber, 1996; Tichenor, Marmar, Weiss, Metzler, & Ronfeldt, 1996; Ursano et al., 1999). In fact, individuals who suffer from dissociative symptoms at the time of the trauma (peritraumatic dissociation) are at increased risk for developing chronic posttraumatic stress disorder and experience more severe posttraumatic symptoms. In addition, there appears to be a dissociative subtype of persons with PTSD who experience high peritraumatic dissociation and diminished physiological reactivity as compared with individuals with low dissociation (Griffin et al., 1997).

As both the dissociative disorders and PTSD are posttraumatic syndromes, it is not suprising that they have a number of features in common. The first is etiological. Patients diagnosed with PTSD or a dissociative disorder have histories of trauma. Second, both syndromes are marked by dissociative symptoms, including disturbances in memory and depersonalization or detachment from one's self. Patients with PTSD and dissociative disorders experience persistent time distortions; patients typically report disturbances of memory or temporal continuity and a range of disturbances in identity (Wilson & Drozdek, in press). They may be amnestic for certain aspects of the trauma and hypermnesic for others. Alternately, they may have illusory visions or intrusive images of the past. Flashbacks, in which the patient relives the past trauma as if it were present reality, are a common form of temporal confusion in both patient populations (Steinberg, 1995; Steinberg & Schnall, 2001). Third, the pacing of therapy for trauma survivors requires sensitive treatment of both cognitive and affective distortions. Many patients suffering from PTSD or a dissociative disorder have histories of dysfunction in both employment situations and interpersonal relationships because of their distorted cognitive skills and their emotional hyperreactivity. Kluft (1994) has described the result as "entrapment in a vicious cycle of maladaptive responses and behaviors" (p. 122). Understandably, these common elements have led some researchers to propose that the dissociative disorders and PTSD belong in a common diagnostic category or to postulate an integrative theory that would account for both syndromes. Some have hypothesized that PTSD and the dissociative disorders should be categorized as acute forms of pathological posttrauma adaptations (Wilson, 1994). Others have recommended that PTSD be classified as a dissociative disturbance (American Psychiatric Association's Advisors to Dissociative Disorders Text Revision Work Group).

PTSD AND DISSOCIATION

The link between trauma and dissociative symptoms has been noted by a number of researchers (Allen, 1995, 2001; Braun, 1990; Coons, Cole, Pellow, & Milstein, 1990; Fine, 1990; Kluft, 1988; Putnam, 1985; Putnam, 1995;

Spiegel, 1991; Steinberg, 1995; Steinberg & Schnall, 2001; Terr, 1991). In fact, DSM-IV-TR (American Psychiatric Association, 2000) includes dissociative symptoms within the criteria for both PTSD and acute stress disorder, a new diagnostic category also grouped with the anxiety disorders. In the case of acute stress disorder, criterion B states that "either while experiencing or after experiencing the distressing event, the individual has three (or more) of the following dissociative symptoms: (1) a subjective sense of numbing, detachment, or absence of emotional responsiveness; (2) a reduction in awareness of his or her surroundings; (3) derealization; (4) depersonalization; or (5) dissociative amnesia" (p. 471). For PTSD, Criterion B3 stipulates that "the traumatic event is persistently reexperienced . . . [by] acting or feeling as if the traumatic event were recurring (includes a sense of reliving the experience, illusions, hallucinations, and dissociative flashback episodes, including those that occur on awakening or when intoxicated)" (p. 468). Criterion C3 includes "persistent avoidance of stimuli associated with the trauma . . . [including] inability to recall an important aspect of the trauma" (p. 468).

With respect to psychogenic amnesia, dissociative fugue, and depersonalization disorder, acute episodes of severe stress or trauma typically precede the onset of these dissociative disorders. With respect to dissociative identity disorder, chronic or repetitive trauma, usually inflicted in childhood, is implicated in the development of this syndrome. Kluft's (1984) four-factor theory holds that dissociative identity disorder (DID) develops in persons with (1) a biological capacity to dissociate; (2) overwhelming childhood experiences that cause their dissociative potential to evolve into an entrenched defensive process; (3) a number of normal or abnormal intrapsychic structures that incorporate dissociative processes in the formation of alternate personalities; (4) an absence of countervailing protective, nurturing, or healing experiences with significant others. Also, it appears that the dissociative disorders, particularly DID and dissociative disorder not otherwise specified (DDNOS), represent profound changes in the patient's childhood self-structure, whereas PTSD does not invariably have such an impact (Wilson, 1994). This difference appears to be connected to the childhood origin of dissociative disturbances. Although Kluft (1985) has also noted that initial dissociative splits in the personality may be precipitated by extrafamilial or nonabusive trauma (e.g., severe illness, death of parent, war), the most common form of overwhelming stress in childhood is intrafamilial abuse. On the other hand, PTSD may be produced by a wider variety of traumatic experiences. DSM-IV-TR indicates that PTSD "can develop in individuals without any predisposing conditions, particularly if the stressor is especially extreme" (p. 466). For example, one study of Desert Storm veterans found that exposure to death and the handling of human remains may traumatize "psychologically robust persons" (Sutker, Uddo, Brailey, Allain, & Errera, 1994). It has also been observed that persons vary in their response to traumatic stressors, depending on a number of psychological, social, and situational variables, and that some individuals appear to be more vulnerable than others, either to traumatic experiences in general or to specific trauma. In addition, PTSD patients in the early stages of recovery are at risk for developing severe and chronic PTSD if they are subjected to additional or chronic stressors during this period.

In terms of diagnostic assessment, patients suffering from dissociative disorders often have delayed diagnosis and/or previous misdiagnosis as compared with patients with PTSD. It has been estimated that patients suffering from dissociative identity disorder spend an average of 6.8 years in the mental health care system prior to receiving a correct diagnosis and receive an average of 3.6 previous diagnoses (Putnam, Guroff, Silberman, Barban, & Post, 1986). The long time gap between onset and diagnosis in the dissociative disorders appears to be a by-product of a combination of social, as well as clinical, factors. Many of the stressors that are implicated in PTSD are matters of public knowledge or awareness (e.g., wars, natural disasters, transportation accidents, crime, etc.), such that disclosure on the patient's part is not as likely to be a source of shame. On the other hand, timely identification of dissociative symptoms requires specialized interview strategies, which are not yet routinely performed with trauma survivors (Steinberg, 1994b, 1995; Steinberg & Schnall, 2001). In the case of DID, the intrafamilial abuse that is involved in the majority of cases typically occurs in the privacy of the home and is kept secret from the outside world. As a result, survivors of family abuse may fail to draw connections between present symptoms and past traumas, or they may hesitate to disclose either their symptoms or their history. In these situations, accurate differential diagnosis requires systematic assessment of patients' dissociative symptoms, in addition to their trauma history.

POPULATIONS AT RISK FOR DISSOCIATIVE SYMPTOMS AND DISORDERS

Persons with Known Histories of Trauma

Given increased professional awareness of both the incidence of trauma in the general population and the variety of stressors that can affect people's lives, clinicians have begun to recognize the importance of taking trauma histories. Even in circumstances involving public or collective disasters of one kind or another, such as natural disasters, transportation accidents, or acts of terrorism, a thorough history of patients' experiences is necessary.

Mental health professionals working in facilities with survivors of traumas such as the following should routinely screen their patient populations for dissociative symptoms:

- Veterans Administration or military hospitals
- Rape crisis units
- Trauma centers
- Shelters for battered women
- Emergency responders (e.g., police, fire, paramedics)

- Disaster workers
- Social service agencies and mental health clinics

Persons with Covert Histories of Trauma

Clinicians should also note that there are patient populations who do not present with overt histories of trauma or who may not be perceived to be at risk for PTSD or dissociative disorders. These groups include the following:

Persons with Histories of Amnesia for Their Pasts, Including Traumatic Events

Research using the Structured Clinical Interview for DSM-IV Dissociative Disorders (SCID-D; Steinberg, 1994a) indicates that amnesia may be regarded as the "gateway" symptom of the five core dissociative symptoms in that it affects patients' recall of dissociative episodes, as well as of the narrative of their life history (Steinberg, 1995). Ironically, individuals with severe amnesia will sometimes comment that they cannot remember how much they have forgotten (Kluft, 1984, 1985). Moreover, patients with dissociative disorders will frequently report amnesia for large portions of their later childhood and adolescence, in addition to normal amnesia of early childhood.

Patients with dissociative disorders who have covert histories of trauma are often polysymptomatic in their presentation and/or comorbid with other disorders (Coons, 1980; Kluft, 1991; Putnam et al., 1986; Steinberg, 1994b, 1995; Steinberg & Schnall, 2001; Torem, 1990). It is advisable for clinicians to take comprehensive histories of dissociation in patients who fall into the following categories that are often comorbid with the dissociative disorders:

- Patients with a history of recurrent or atypical depression.
- Patients who have been diagnosed with PTSD.
- Patients previously diagnosed as having "atypical" or "NOS (not otherwise specified)" disorders.
- Patients with a history of eating disorders.
- Patients who have been diagnosed with borderline personality disorder.
- Patients who have been diagnosed with impulse control disorders.
- Patients who have substance abuse disorders.
- Patients who fall into one or more of the following categories:
  1. Meet criteria for more than two psychiatric diagnoses or have a history of fluctuating symptoms leading to a variety of diagnoses.
  2. Endorse hearing voices but are otherwise without symptoms of psychosis.
  3. Have difficulty recalling symptom histories.
  4. Have a history of unsuccessful treatments with a series of therapists.
  5. Are nonresponsive to treatment.

Vicariously Traumatized Persons

It has recently been recognized that persons may manifest symptoms of PTSD through secondhand exposure to the trauma histories of others. Such cases include Holocaust survivors and their children, intimates of rape victims, and mental health professionals who work with trauma survivors, as well as journalists covering war, accidents, or other atrocities (Terr, 1990, 1991; Danieli, 1982, 1985; Krystal, 1988; Danieli, 1982, 1985; Lindy & Wilson, 1994; Kelly, 1988; Pearlman & Saakvitne, 1995). Hodgkinson and Shepherd (1994) report that not only do disaster workers experience high levels of stress at the time of the traumatic event but also that these elevated levels are still present at 12-month follow-up. Detection of vicarious traumatization may require taking a history of traumatic events that may have affected other family members, as well as exposure to trauma through one's employment.

ORGANIZING AND ASSESSING DISSOCIATION: FIVE MEASURABLE COMPONENTS

Definitions of dissociation include those by Nemiah (1991): "the exclusion from consciousness and the inaccessibility of voluntary recall of mental events such as memories, sensations, feelings, fantasies and attitudes"; and DSM-IV-TR: "disruption in the usually integrated functions of consciousness, memory, identity, or perception" (American Psychiatric Association, 2000, p. 519). Although these and other definitions may appear overly broad (Frankel, 1990), the complex nature of dissociation can be organized into five specific and reliable dissociative symptoms: amnesia, depersonalization, derealization, identity confusion, and identity alteration (Steinberg, 1994a, 1994b, 1995, 2000; Steinberg, Rounsaville, & Cicchetti, 1990). The SCID-D allows for clinical investigations of the phenomenology and prevalence of these five core dissociative symptoms and has improved diagnostic accuracy with regard to dissociative disorders (Steinberg, 1994a, 2000). This chapter focuses on the assessment of posttraumatic dissociative symptoms and syndromes using the SCID-D.

The Structured Clinical Interview for DSM-IV Dissociative Disorders (SCID-D)

The SCID-D is a diagnostic tool developed to assess the severity of five core dissociative symptoms (amnesia, depersonalization, derealization, identity confusion, and identity alteration) and to diagnose the dissociative disorders in a standardized manner (Steinberg, 1994a, 2000; Steinberg et al., 1990). The five dissociative symptoms and disorders can be considered universal forms of posttraumatic adaptation; virtually identical manifestations have been noted by investigators using the SCID-D in a variety of populations of trauma survivors, including veterans of war and survivors of child abuse (Boon & Draijer, 1999; Gast, Rodewald, Nickel, & Emrich, 2001; Nijenhuis et al., 1997; Steinberg, 2000; Steinberg & Schnall, 2001). In other words, individuals suffering from PTSD (who have suffered many different types of traumatic experiences) have remarkably similar dissociative symptom profiles as compared with individuals with dissociative disorders (whose trauma primarily consisted of childhood abuse). In addition, virtually identical dissociative symptom descriptions, severity, and symptom clusters have been reported in trauma survivors with dissociative disorders in the United States and abroad (using translated SCID-D versions in Dutch, Norwegian, and Turkish; Boon & Draijer, 1999; Gast et al., 2001; Nijenhuis et al., 1997). The reliable nature of survivors' posttraumatic symptoms as assessed with the SCID-D is consistent with the universality of posttrauma experiences (see Wilson & Drozdek, in press), as well as the cross-cultural reliability and applicability of this clinical interview.

The SCID-D can be used with adolescents, as well as adults (Carrion & Steiner, 2000; Steinberg, 1996a; Steinberg & Steinberg, 1995) and has undergone extensive NIMH-funded field testing for reliability and validity (Steinberg et al., 1990; Steinberg, 2000). Good to excellent reliability for each of the five dissociative symptoms and disorders has been noted in numerous investigations in the United States and abroad (Goff, Olin, Jenike, Baer, & Buttolph, 1992; Boon & Draijer, 1999; Gast et al., 2001; Nijenhuis et al., 1997; Steinberg, 2000).

The SCID-D allows the clinician to make diagnoses of the five dissociative disorders (dissociative amnesia, dissociative fugue, depersonalization disorder, dissociative identity disorder [DID], and dissociative disorder, NOS) based on DSM-IV-TR criteria. Disorders newly included in DSM-IV-TR that consist of predominantly dissociative symptoms, including acute stress disorder and dissociative trance disorder (American Psychiatric Association, 2000, Appendix B) can also be assessed with the SCID-D. The SCID-D uses open-ended questions and embeds DSM criteria throughout the interview. Although the SCID-D is not a trauma questionnaire, its ability to elicit spontaneous descriptions of trauma and dissociation from patients without the use of leading questions makes it a valuable instrument for diagnosis, as well as symptom documentation for psychological and forensic evaluations. Guidelines for the administration, scoring, and interpretation of the SCID-D are described in the *Interviewer's Guide to the SCID-D* (Steinberg, 1994b). In addition to its diagnostic utility, the SCID-D can aid in treatment planning (Steinberg & Hall, 1997) as well as forensic evaluations needing to distinguish between valid versus malingered posttraumatic dissociation. One investigation found that the SCID-D allowed examiners to distinguish individuals with genuine DID from individuals who were simulating DID in 100% of cases (Welburn et al., 2003). For specific guidelines for distinguishing valid versus simulated or malingered dissociative symptoms, see Steinberg, Hall, Lareau, and Cicchetti (2001).

Assessing the Five Core Dissociative Symptoms

Systematic review of the five dissociative symptoms assessed with the SCID-D are presented here. Excerpts from a SCID-D interview of a patient referred to here as "Mary," diagnosed initially as having PTSD, are included to illustrate the varied manifestations of dissociation. Mary was referred for evaluation of her dissociative symptoms and to rule out the presence of a dissociative disorder. She is a 41-year-old divorced Caucasian woman. At present she is employed as an administrative assistant. Mary initially presented for treatment with complaints of depression, intrusive memories of abuse, flashbacks, and difficulty sleeping.

Assessing Amnesia with the SCID-D

Amnesia is usually described as "gaps" in the patient's memory, ranging from minutes to years, and sometimes referred to as "lost time." Patients with severe amnesia are often unable to recall the frequency or duration of their amnestic episodes. In addition, they may "come to themselves" away from home, unable to remember how they got there, or have trouble remembering their names, ages, or other personal information (Kluft, 1984, 1985; Steinberg, 1994b, 1995, 1996b; Steinberg & Schnall, 2001).

The SCID-D is divided into five sections, one for each of the five dissociative symptoms. When the history taking is completed, the interviewer proceeds with the SCID-D questions concerning the symptom of amnesia. Mary describes having had recurrent gaps in her memory, as well as significant distress in connection with her amnesia.

INTERVIEWER: Can you describe your memory gaps?

PATIENT: There are still a lot of portions of my childhood that I don't remember. I don't know if I ever will remember it. At first it was scary. Now I understand that it was a way of survival.

INTERVIEWER: What parts of your childhood do you have trouble remembering?

PATIENT: I can remember just a few minor events from birth up until I was around 13.

INTERVIEWER: Do you still experience memory gaps?

PATIENT: Yes. If you ask me what I did yesterday, I would probably have a difficult time thinking about yesterday. But if you ask me about reading a book, that portion of my memory is like a photographic memory, but with my own life and my own functions and what I did I sometimes have a very difficult time.

Given the extent and ongoing frequency of her gaps in memory, she receives a rating of "severe" for this symptom.

Assessing Depersonalization with the SCID-D

Depersonalization is a symptom that manifests in a variety of ways in trauma survivors. The symptom is initially frightening to many people who experience it; patients describe depersonalization in terms of feeling detached from one's emotions, feeling that the self is strange or unreal, or feeling physically separated from part(s) of one's body (Steinberg, 1994b, 1995, 1996b; Steinberg & Schnall, 2001).

On the depersonalization section of the SCID-D, Mary indicates that she experiences several forms of this symptom, including out-of-body experiences. In one example, Mary describes an episode of depersonalization in which she feels as if she is observing herself from a distance.

INTERVIEWER: Can you describe your experience of watching yourself, as if you were seeing yourself at a distance?

PATIENT: Sometimes it's scary and then other times it's as though you're watching a silent movie. There's no emotion. It's like you're sitting back observing somebody else. It's sometimes comforting because you're not dealing with that situation, someone else is. And then other times it's very frightening.

INTERVIEWER: How often have you had that experience?

PATIENT: Quite often. Daily.

INTERVIEWER: Does the experience of seeing yourself as if you're watching a movie of yourself interfere with your relationships with others?

PATIENT: Definitely.

INTERVIEWER: How does it interfere?

PATIENT: Confusion, not being able to explain to someone what's going on, what you're thinking, talking about, or your feelings, you're disconnected.

Again, Mary's depersonalization receives a rating of "severe," given its high frequency and the resultant dysfunction.

Assessing Derealization with the SCID-D

Just as with depersonalization, the symptom of derealization is common in patients with histories of severe trauma. Derealization in particular includes feelings of estrangement or detachment from the environment or a sense that the environment is unreal. Patients who have experienced recurrent emotional, physical, and/or sexual abuse or other traumatic experiences frequently endorse derealization episodes in which friends, relatives, or their own home seem unreal or foreign to them. Derealization episodes are often associated with traumatic memories, and patients may spontaneously share their traumas when describing intense derealization experiences (Steinberg, 1995, 1996b; Steinberg & Schnall, 2001).

Clinicians involved with the assessment of trauma survivors should note that both depersonalization and derealization symptoms are included in the diagnostic criteria for acute stress disorder and PTSD. Patients with histories of trauma frequently experience derealization in conjunction with flashbacks and age-regressed states, in which the contemporary environment becomes unreal while a past experience is relived.

Mary indicates that her experiences of derealization usually consist of familiar people appearing unfamiliar or unreal. Like many patients endorsing this symptom, she finds the experience to be frightening.

INTERVIEWER: Have you ever felt as if familiar surroundings or people you knew seemed unfamiliar or unreal?

PATIENT: Unfamiliar.

INTERVIEWER: What's that experience like?

PATIENT: Weird. It's strange. You're scared to death sometimes that you're going to get caught. I mean it can happen sometimes at work, when I'm talking to someone and they'll feel unfamiliar, different. I can hear us talking, and I'm having a conversation inside saying, "Come on, let's get your act together, we've got to get through this," and then it's like we all come together and start working and then everything will start calming down.

Because Mary reported that her derealization occurred weekly and caused considerable distress, the interviewer rated this symptom as "severe."

Assessing Identity Confusion with the SCID-D

The remaining two core symptoms assessed by the SCID-D concern the disturbances in personal identity that characterize patients suffering from dissociative disorders. Identity confusion and identity alteration may be distinguished as follows: Identity confusion refers to the subjective sense of internal fragmentation of the self that is not ordinarily perceptible to others (Steinberg, 1994b, 1995, 1996b; Steinberg & Schnall, 2001). The person suffering from identity confusion typically describes experiences of inner warfare or conflict, which generate a subjective feeling of incoherence or instability in the sense of self. The SCID-D's definition of identity confusion (Steinberg 1994a, 1994b) should be distinguished from Erikson's (1968) usage, in which the term refers to weaknesses in the sense of self related to developmental issues in adolescence and early adulthood.

Identity alteration on the SCID-D refers to external behavioral manifestations of personality transformation objectively perceptible to others (Steinberg, 1994b). Unlike identity confusion, it is not a primarily subjective experience. Although some patients suffering from identity alteration may be conscious of their switching, others become aware of it through physical evidence (purchases, documents, etc.) or interpersonal feedback. In addition, identity alteration represents a change from a specific personality or ego state to another, as distinct from a sense of inner incoherence or struggle.

In terms of identity confusion, Mary experiences the symptom as an inner fight.

INTERVIEWER: Have you ever felt as if there was a struggle going on inside of you?

PATIENT: Yes.

INTERVIEWER: Can you describe that experience?

PATIENT: It's like two people having an argument or sometimes more than two people having an argument, somebody wanting to do something and the other's not signing onto it.

INTERVIEWER: Have you ever felt as if there was a struggle going on inside of you about who you really are?

PATIENT: Yeah.

INTERVIEWER: Can you describe that?

PATIENT: OK. I don't know if struggle is the word, but I think we're wondering who we really are and afraid at the same time of do we really want to know who we are.

Assessing Identity Alteration with the SCID-D

The fifth dissociative symptom assessed by the SCID-D, identity alteration, has been previously defined as a person's shift in role or identity, which is observable by others through changes in the person's behaviors (Steinberg, 1994b, 1995; Steinberg & Schnall, 2001). Manifestations of identity alteration include uncontrolled mood swings, acting like a different person, the use of different names, the possession of a learned skill for which one cannot account, and the discovery of strange or unfamiliar personal items in one's possession. These transitions in role or behavior may be connected with amnestic episodes, in which a person is unable to remember events that occurred while experiencing altered identity. Identity alteration in DID is characterized by its complexity and distinctness, by the ability of alters to take control of behavior, and by the interconnection with other dissociative symptoms (Steinberg, 1995).

Identity alteration is the dissociative symptom most likely to be noticed by others in the patient's home or workplace environment because of its behavioral manifestations. This symptom often causes the patient significant distress or anxiety because of its actual or potential effects on employment and interpersonal relationships. Mary described disturbances in her functioning that were related to childlike behavior:

INTERVIEWER: Have you ever felt as if, or found yourself acting as if, you were still a child?

PATIENT: Yes.

INTERVIEWER: What is that experience like?

PATIENT: I have felt that I am a child. There are several children within me at different ages. One child feels like it's the 5-year-old child that was molested; it's very upsetting.

INTERVIEWER: How often do you feel like a child?

PATIENT: Frequently. It sometimes can be daily. It just depends on what's going on.

Mary also acknowledged that she has referred to herself by different metaphorical names, which are descriptions of various emotions that have been compartmentalized.

INTERVIEWER: Have you ever referred to yourself by different names?

PATIENT: Yes. We don't give them names, but titles, I guess.

INTERVIEWER: Can you share some of the names or titles?

PATIENT: There's "rage," every anger that I think I've ever felt has been projected into "rage." I mean it's like she's just taking it all in and the balloon is getting bigger and bigger. It's like filling a balloon with water. There's "the child" that's crying. That one cries uncontrollably, and you can hear her all the time. There is "the guilt." I mean it's like each one has been assigned feelings, and that's why "the protector" comes out and "the zombie," to help protect, I guess.

In order to further explore the severity of Mary's identity disturbance and confirm that Mary's "titles" reflect "distinct identities or personality states" (American Psychiatric Association, 2000, p. 529), the interviewer administered a follow-up section on "Different Names," because the patient had mentioned having different "titles" with distinctive personal characteristics.

A series of questions assesses the degree of volition and distinctness of personality states, drawing on patients' own terminology for their altered state(s) of identity.

INTERVIEWER: Have you ever felt as if your emotions are not in your control?

PATIENT: Depends on who we're talking to, yes. Each emotion has been assigned a personality. So if you ask "the professional," who is usually very in control, she would say she's always in control, but if, if you ask the one with rage that one only experiences rage, the same thing with crying and a sense of humor. All the other emotions that are assigned to typically one being, they've been assigned to different people.

INTERVIEWER: Can you say some more about that?

PATIENT: As an example, the "zombie" comes out when we're under a crisis, when either the "suicidal one" or "rage" pops out and something triggers an emotion that I can't deal with and "the zombie" pops out and there are no feelings, no emotions. And that one is in control until it feels that the others have been able to absorb the pain that they just received and have sorted it out and then the zombie will go away.

Mary affirms that she has distinct visual images of these compartmentalized emotions or "titles" and describes how they recurrently control her behavior. She also reports ongoing dialogues with them. Mary appears to suffer from severe identity alteration.

Assessing Intrainterview Dissociative Cues

The SCID-D includes a postinterview assessment of intrainterview dissociative cues to supplement the patient's verbal information. These cues include a number of verbal and nonverbal behaviors, such as alteration in demeanor, spontaneous age regression, and trancelike appearance, which are suggestive of the presence of dissociative symptoms and/or disorders. The interviewer is to note the presence of these cues during the course of the interview and rate them afterward. Mary's manifestation of intrainterview age regression was observed during the interview and consisted of shifts in her demeanor from a childlike state to a more articulate and mature woman.

Severity Ratings

Severity rating definitions are provided in the *Interviewer's Guide to the SCID-D* (Steinberg, 1994b). They allow the interviewer to determine symptom severity based on the individual's responses to each section of the SCID-D. The severity of each dissociative symptom is assessed through questions concerning the frequency, duration, distress, and dysfunction associated with each dissociative experience (see Table 5.1) .These symptom profiles can be represented iconically in a SCID-D symptom profile graph, as demonstrated by the characteristic profiles of patients with dissociative and nondissociative disorders, respectively (see Figure 5.1).

After the interview, the rater records the five symptom severities and dissociative disorder diagnosis on the summary score sheet, which records this summary information in a visually concise form.

TABLE 5.1. SCID-D Severity Rating Definitions of Depersonalization

Depersonalization—Detachment from one's self, for example, a sense of looking at one's self as if one is an outsider.

A. Mild
- Single episode or rare (total of 1–4) episodes of depersonalization which are brief (less than 4 hours), and are usually associated with stress or fatigue.

B. Moderate (one of the following):
- Recurrent (more than 4) episodes of depersonalization (may be brief or prolonged; may be precipitated by stress).
- Episodes (1–4) of depersonalization which (one of the following):
  - Produce impairment in social or occupational functioning.
  - Are not precipitated by stress.
  - Are prolonged (over 4 hours).
  - Are associated with dysphoria.

C. Severe (one of the following):
- Persistent episodes of depersonalization (24 hours and longer).
- Episodes of depersonalization occur daily or weekly. May be brief or prolonged.
- Frequent (more than 4) episodes of depersonalization that (one of the following):
  - Produce impairment in social or occupational functioning.
  - Do not appear to be precipitated by stress.
  - Are prolonged (over 4 hours).
  - Are associated with dysphoria.

Note. The severity rating definitions are not an inclusive list. The purpose of these definitions is to give the rater a general description of the parameters of the spectrum of dissociative symptoms and their severity. From Steinberg (1994b). Copyright 1994 by Marlene Steinberg. Reprinted by permission.

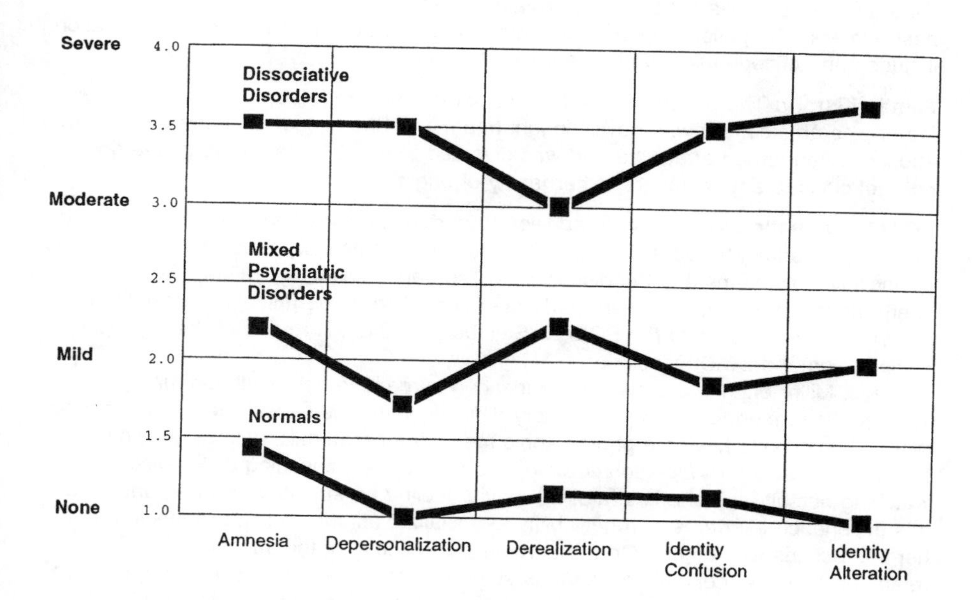

FIGURE 5.1. SCID-D symptom profiles in psychiatric patients and normal controls. Data derived from Steinberg et al. (1990).

Diagnostic Assessment

The constellation of Mary's symptoms meets DSM-IV-TR criteria for a diagnosis of dissociative identity disorder. This case concludes with a sample diagnostic evaluation report, suitable for inclusion in the patient's records and psychological reports (see Figure 5.2).

FIGURE 5.2. Sample SCID-D evaluation report.

Patient: Mary Miller

Date of evaluation: 9/20/03

Referral source: Dana Jones, MD (present therapist)

Reason for referral: Present therapist suspects presence of underlying dissociative disorder.

Information obtained from: Patient and present therapist

Brief summary: The patient is a 41-year-old Caucasian woman, employed as an administrative assistant. She is divorced and lives alone. Ms. Miller has been in outpatient therapy for the past 4 years due to a history of recurrent depression, intrusive memories, and difficulty sleeping. Her referring clinician's diagnosis is PTSD due to a history of childhood trauma and continued reexperiencing symptoms, including flashbacks, along with avoidance of trauma triggers and symptoms of hyperarousal. She has a past history of alcohol abuse and has been abstinent for the past 5 years. The patient reported no major medical problems. Her current medication includes an antidepressant and an antianxiety agent.

Family history: The patient states that her parents seemed depressed and that her father was an alcoholic who never sought treatment. She alleges that she was sexually abused. She married at age 29 and was divorced at age 35. Mary reports she does not feel close to any members of her family of origin.

SCID-D evaluation summary: In addition to performing a routine diagnostic evaluation, I administered the SCID-D in order to systematically evaluate posttraumatic dissociative symptoms and the dissociative disorders (Steinberg, 1994a). Scoring and interpretation of the SCID-D were performed according to the guidelines described in the *Interviewer's Guide to the SCID-D* (Steinberg, 1994b). A review of the significant findings from the SCID-D includes:

Ms. Miller endorsed *amnesia* experienced as gaps in her childhood through age 13. She also reported continued memory difficulties associated with her daily activities, though she reports having a photographic memory for materials such as reading a book. With respect to *depersonalization*, she reported experiencing daily episodes of watching herself as if she is in a silent movie, feeling no emotions. She reported that this experience interferes with her ability to socialize, as she feels disconnected from her interactions with others. On the *derealization* section of the interview, Ms. Miller remarked that she feels that colleagues at work seem unfamiliar, even when they are people she works with every day. She reports experiencing frequent flashbacks of childhood traumas during which she feels that her present surroundings are unreal. She endorsed a high level of *identity confusion*, stating that she experiences it as "two people having an argument or sometimes more than two people having an argument, somebody wanting to do something and the other's not signing onto it" on a daily basis. In terms of *identity alteration*, the patient reported that she has referred to herself by different "titles," which represent compartmentalized personalities with different emotions, behaviors, and functions. She describes the following personality states: "the fat one, the anorexic, the zombie that doesn't feel anything," "rage," and "the child that's crying." She elaborated about how these aspects of herself feel distinct, control her behavior, and engage in recurrent internal dialogues with one another. In addition, I observed intrainterview dissociative cues during the administration of the interview. At times, Ms. Miller appeared to undergo shifts in her demeanor with no apparent external cause, changing from a childish presentation to a more mature one.

Mental status exam: The patient came to the interview casually dressed and was calm and cooperative. She spoke fluently and answered most questions with relevant replies. At times, her affect seemed detached. She denied the presence of psychotic symptoms; likewise, she denied suicidal or homicidal ideation.

Assessment: On the basis of this evaluation, Ms. Miller's symptoms and history are consistent with a primary diagnosis of a dissociative disorder. She suffers from chronic amnesia, depersonalization, derealization, identity confusion, and identity alteration, all at a high level of severity. Her dissociative symptoms, including her identity disturbance that consists of compartmentalized personality states, appear to be sufficiently distinct to meet DSM-IV-TR's criterion A for dissociative identity disorder. These findings are consistent with a diagnosis of dissociative identity disorder.

Recommendation: I would recommend individual psychotherapy aimed at reducing the patient's posttraumatic and dissociative symptoms, consisting of marked amnesia, depersonalization, derealization, identity confusion, and alteration. Focus of treatment remains on optimizing level of functioning while reducing symptoms. Anitidepressant and antianxiety medications may be useful in alleviating some of her associated anxiety and depression.

DIRECTIONS FOR FUTURE SCID-D RESEARCH IN THE DISSOCIATIVE DISORDERS AND PTSD

The SCID-D can be used by researchers, as well as clinicians. In terms of future research, use of the SCID-D should open up a number of new avenues of investigation:

Outcome Studies

At present, no large-scale double-blind study has been done comparing either the relative efficacy of pharmacotherapy and psychotherapy in the treatment of dissociation or the relative efficacy of different forms of psychotherapy. Recent research based on small samples suggests that antidepressent medication may be useful in the treatment of depersonalization (Abbas, Chandra, & Srivastava, 1995; Ratliff & Kerski, 1995; Simeon, Stein, & Hollander, 1998).

Further research is needed using larger samples and double-blind controlled studies.

Researchers interested in pharmacological treatments of symptoms of PTSD and the dissociative disorders, as well as researchers conducting comparative studies of pharmacotherapy and the psychotherapies, can use the SCID-D to record and monitor changes in patients' dissociative symptom severity levels. Because the SCID-D summary score sheet can be used to record the severity, as well as the presence, of dissociative symptoms, it is an effective tool for the establishment of patients' baselines prior to medication trials, as well as for facilitating the matching of patient groups for comparative studies.

Reassessment of DSM Diagnostic Categories

Increasing recognition of the prevalence of the dissociative symptoms and disorders and the high level of misdiagnosis of patients has led a number of researchers to speculate that dissociation may be a more inclusive concept than was previously thought. In particular, the inclusion of three dissociative symptoms (amnesia, depersonalization, and derealization) among the criteria for acute stress disorder and PTSD suggests the wisdom of greater cooperation between specialists in PTSD and clinical researchers in the field of dissociation. Recent research indicating the high prevalence of dissociative symptoms in persons with PTSD suggests a reevaluation of whether PTSD would be more accurately classified along with the dissociative disorders in future editions of DSM.

Recent research confirms that patients with PTSD suffer from a variety of dissociative symptoms. Virtually identical dissociative symptom profiles have been found using the SCID-D in war veterans with PTSD as compared with survivors of childhood trauma with DID and DDNOS (Bremner et al., 1993; Steinberg, 1995; Steinberg & Schnall, 2001). In other words, posttraumatic symptoms of dissociation, when assessed with standardized measures such as the SCID-D, have consistent and characteristic features whether the trauma is related to military combat or to childhood abuse/traumas. Research indicates that the symptoms of PTSD and the dissociative disorders may overlap considerably and that upcoming revisions of DSM should be informed by recent investigations that document the similarity of posttraumatic dissociative experiences in patients with acute stress disorder, PTSD, and the dissociative disorders.

Cost–Benefit Analysis in the Managed Care Era

During the past 10 years, there has been more emphasis on the study of cost–benefit analysis in the mental health care field. Managed care organizations have increased pressure on psychotherapists to demonstrate the effectiveness of specific treatments, as well as cost control. Given researchers' findings that an average of 7 to 10 years elapses between initial assessment of patients with undetected dissociative disorders and proper diagnosis (Coons, Bowman, & Milstein, 1988; Kluft 1991; Putnam et al., 1986), routine screening of patients from populations known to be at risk for the dissociative disorders, such as trauma survivors, is highly cost effective. The costs of SCID-D administration are minor in comparison to the systemic costs of years of misdiagnosis and misdirected treatment. Moreover, patients typically find that the open-ended format of the SCID-D represents the beginning of the actual therapeutic process for them, as well as the establishment of their correct diagnosis; thus their recovery period *after* diagnosis may be effectively shortened as well.

SUMMARY AND CONCLUSION

Because dissociative symptoms and disorders are posttraumatic in etiology and frequently misdiagnosed, it is essential that clinicians use specific interview strategies to evaluate dissociative symptoms in patients with histories of trauma or PTSD. Because accurate diagnostic assessment of posttraumatic syndromes is essential to the implementation of appropriate therapy, it is recommended that use of the SCID-D be included in the clinical training of all mental health professionals (including clinical/counseling psychology, psychiatric residencies, psychiatric nurses, social workers, clergy with graduate training in pastoral counseling.)

With respect to differential diagnosis of the posttraumatic syndromes, research indicates that a subset of patients diagnosed with chronic PTSD suffer from undetected dissociative symptoms and disorders. In addition, a growing body of research documents the importance of dissociation in the development of PTSD, as well as the high frequency of dissociative symptoms in individuals with PTSD (Allen, 2001; Birmes et al., 2001; Bremner et al., 1993; Brunet et al., 2001; Koopman et al., 1994; Griffin et al., 1997; Johnson et al., 2001; Marmar et al., 1994; Putnam, 1995; Shalev et al., 1996; Tichenor et al., 1996; Ursano et al., 1999). Because comprehensive assessment of PTSD demands the use of multiple reliable instruments (Keane, Newman, & Orsillo, 1997), familiarity with the SCID-D assessement process can enhance diagnostic information with respect to the presence and severity of dissociative symptoms and disorders.

As researchers in PTSD and the dissociative disorders continue to study the long-term effects of trauma, as well as the precise relationship between PTSD and dissociation, the SCID-D provides a reliable instrument for diagnosis, symptom documentation, and treatment planning. Given the high frequency of dissociative symptoms in trauma survivors, it is recommended that systematic assessment of dissociative symptoms be included in the evaluation of patients with dissociative symptoms and/or histories of trauma.

ACKNOWLEDGMENT

Preparation of this chapter was supported by NIMH First Independent Research Support and Transition Award No. MH-43352 and NIMH Grant No. RO1-43352 to Marlene Steinberg.

REFERENCES

Abbas, S., Chandra, P., & Srivastava, M. (1995). The use of fluoxetine and buspirone for treatment-refractory depersonalization disorder. *Journal of Clinical Psychiatry*, *56*(10), 484.

Allen, J. (2001). *Traumatic relationships and serious mental disorders*. Chichester, UK: Wiley.

Allen, J. A. (1995). *Coping with trauma*. Washington, DC: American Psychiatric Press.

American Psychiatric Association. (1952). *Diagnostic and statistical manual of mental disorders*. Washington, DC: Author.

American Psychiatric Association. (2000). *Diagnostic and statistical manual of mental disorders* (4th ed., text rev.). Washington, DC: Author.

Birmes, P., Carreras, D., Charlet, J. P., Warner, B. A., Lauque, D., & Schmitt, L. (2001). Peritraumatic dissociation and posttraumatic stress disorder in victims of violent assault. *Journal of Nervous and Mental Disease*, *189*(11), 796–798.

Boon, S., & Draijer, N. (1999). Diagnosing dissociative disorders in the Netherlands: A pilot study with the Structured Clinical Interview for DSM-III-R Dissociative Disorders. *American Journal of Psychiatry*, *148*, 458–462.

Braun, B. G. (1990). Dissociative disorders as sequelae to incest. In R. P. Kluft (Ed.), *Incest-related syndromes of adult psychopathology* (pp. 227–246). Washington, DC: American Psychiatric Press.

Bremner, J. D., Steinberg, M., Southwick, S. M., Johnson, D. R., & Charney, D. S. (1993). Use of the Structured Clinical Interview for DSM-IV Dissociative Disorders for systematic assessment of dissociative symptoms in posttraumatic stress disorder. *American Journal of Psychiatry*, *150*, 1011–1014.

Brunet, A., Verdun, P. Q., Weiss, D. S., Metzler, T. J., Best, S. R., Neylan, T. C., et al. (2001). The Peritraumatic Distress Inventory: A proposed measure of PTSD criterion A2. *American Journal of Psychiatry*, *158*(9), 1480–1485.

Carrion, V., & Steiner, H. (2000, March). Trauma and dissociation in delinquent adolescents. *Journal of the American Academy of Child and Adolescent Psychiatry*, *39*, 353–359.

Coons, P. M. (1980). Multiple personality: Diagnostic considerations. *Journal of Clinical Psychiatry*, *41*, 330–336.

Coons, P. M., Bowman, E. S., & Milstein, V. (1988). Multiple personality disorder: A clinical investigation of 50 cases. *Journal of Nervous and Mental Disease*, *176*(5), 519–527.

Coons, P. M., Cole, C., Pellow, T., & Milstein, V. (1990). Symptoms of posttraumatic stress and dissociation in women victims of abuse. In R. P. Kluft (Ed.), *Incest-related syndromes of adult psychopathology* (pp. 205–226). Washington, DC: American Psychiatric Press.

Danieli, Y. (1982). *Therapists' difficulties in treating survivors of the Nazi Holocaust and their children*. Unpublished doctoral dissertation, New York University.

Danieli, Y. (1985). The treatment and prevention of long-term effects and intergenerational transmission of victimization: A lesson from Holocaust survivors and their children. In C. R. Figley (Ed.), *Trauma and its wake* (pp. 278–294). New York: Brunner/Mazel.

Erikson, E. H. (1968). *Identity: Youth and crisis.* New York: Norton.

Fine, C. G. (1990). The cognitive sequelae of incest. In R. P. Kluft (Ed.), *Incest-related syndromes of adult psychopathology* (pp. 161–182). Washington, DC: American Psychiatric Press.

Frankel, F. H. (1990). Hypnotizability and dissociation. *American Journal of Psychiatry, 147*(7), 823–829.

Gast, U., Rodewald, F., Nickel, V., & Emrich, H. (2001). Prevalence of dissociative disorders among psychiatric inpatients in a German university clinic. *Journal of Nervous and Mental Disease, 189*(4), 249–257

Goff, D. C., Olin, J. A., Jenike, M. A., Baer, L., & Buttolph, M. L. (1992). Dissociative symptoms in patients with obsessive–compulsive disorder. *Journal of Nervous and Mental Disease, 180*(5), 332–337.

Griffin, M. G., Resick, P. A., & Mechanic, M. B. (1997). Objective assessment of peritraumatic dissociation: Psychophysiological indicators. *American Journal of Psychiatry, 154*(8), 1081–1088.

Hodgkinson, P. E., & Shepherd, M. A. (1994). The impact of disaster support work. *Journal of Traumatic Stress, 7*(4), 587–600.

Johnson, D. M., Pike, J. L., & Chard, K. M. (2001). Factors predicting PTSD, depression, and dissociative severity in female treatment-seeking childhood sexual abuse survivors.*Child Abuse and Neglect, 25*(1), 179–198.

Keane, T. M., Newman, E., & Orsillo, S. M. (1997). Assessment of military-related posttraumatic stress disorder. In J. Wilson & T. Keane (Eds.), *Assessing psychological trauma and PTSD* (pp. 267–290). New York: Guilford Press.

Kelly, L. (1988). *Surviving sexual violence.* Minneapolis: University of Minnesota Press.

Kluft, R. P. (1984). Multiple personality in childhood. *Psychiatric Clinics of North America, 7*(1), 121–134.

Kluft, R. P. (1985). Childhood multiple personality disorder: Predictors, clinical findings, and treatment results. In R. P. Kluft (Ed.), *Childhood antecedents of multiple personality.* Washington, DC: American Psychiatric Press.

Kluft, R. P. (1988). The dissociative disorders. In J. Talbott, R. Hales, & S. Yudofsky (Eds.), *American Psychiatric Press textbook of psychiatry* (pp. 557–585). Washington, DC: American Psychiatric Press.

Kluft, R. P. (1991). Multiple personality disorder. In A. Tasman & S. Goldfinger (Eds.), *Psychiatric update* (Vol. 10). Washington, DC: American Psychiatric Press.

Kluft, R. P. (1994). Countertransference in the treatment of multiple personality disorder. In J. P. Wilson & J. D. Lindy (Eds.), *Countertransference in the treatment of PTSD* (pp. 122–150). New York: Guilford Press.

Koopman, C., Classen, C., & Spiegel, D. (1994) Predictors of posttraumatic stress symptoms among survivors of the Oakland/Berkeley, California, firestorm. *American Journal of Psychiatry, 151*, 888–894.

Krystal, H. (1988). *Integration and self-healing: Affect, trauma, alexithymia.* Hillsdale, NJ: Analytic Press.

Lindy, J. D., & Wilson, J. P. (1994). Empathic strain and countertransference roles:

Case illustrations. In J. P. Wilson & J. D. Lindy (Eds.), *Countertransference in the treatment of PTSD* (pp. 62–82). New York: Guilford Press.

Marmar, C. R., Weiss, D. S., Schlenger, W. E., Fairbank, J. A., Kulka, R. A., & Hough, R. L. (1994). Peritraumatic dissociation and posttraumatic stress in male Vietnam theater veterans. *American Journal of Psychiatry, 151*(6), 902–907.

Nemiah, J. C. (1991). Dissociation, conversion, and somatization. In A. Tasman & S. Goldfinger (Eds.), *American Psychiatric Press review of psychiatry* (Vol. 10). Washington, DC: American Psychiatric Press.

Nijenhuis, E. R. S., Spinhoven, P., Van Dyck, R., Van der Hart, O., de Graaf, A. M. J., & Knoppert, E. A. M. (1997). Dissociative pathology discriminates between bipolar mood disorder and dissociative disorder [Letter to the editor]. *British Journal of Psychiatry, 170*, 581.

Pearlman, L., & Saakvitne, K. (1995). Treating therapists with vicarious traumatization and secondary traumatic stress disorders. In C. R. Figley (Ed.), *Compassion fatigue: Coping with secondary traumatic stress disorder in those who treat the traumatized* (Vol. 23, pp. 150–177). New York: Brunner/Mazel.

Putnam, F. W. (1985). Dissociation as a response to extreme trauma. In R. P. Kluft (Ed.), *Childhood antecedents of multiple personality* (pp. 65–97). Washington, DC: American Psychiatric Press.

Putnam, F. W. (1995). Traumatic stress and pathological dissociation. In G. P. Chrousos, & R. McCarty (Ed.), *Annals of the New York Academy of Sciences: Vol. 771.* Stress: Basic mechanisms and clinical implications (pp. 708–715). New York: New York Academy of Sciences.

Putnam, F. W., Guroff, J. J., Silberman, E. K., Barban, L., & Post, R. M. (1986). The clinical phenomenology of multiple personality disorder: Review of 100 recent cases. *Journal of Clinical Psychiatry, 47*, 285–293.

Ratliff, N., & Kerski, D. (1995). Depersonalization treated with fluoxetine. *American Journal of Psychiatry, 152*(11), 1689–1690.

Shalev, A. Y., Peri, T., Canetti, L., & Schreiber, S. (1996). Predictors of PTSD in injured trauma survivors: A prospective study. *American Journal of Psychiatry, 153*(2), 219–225.

Simeon, D., Stein, D., & Hollander, E. (1998). Treatment of depersonalization disorder with clomipramine. *Biological Psychiatry, 44*(4), 302–303.

Spiegel, D. (1991). Dissociation and trauma. In A. Tasman & S. Goldfinger (Eds.), *American Psychiatric Press review of psychiatry* (Vol. 10, pp. 261–275). Washington, DC: American Psychiatric Press.

Steinberg, M. (1994a). *Structured Clinical Interview for DSM-IV Dissociative Disorders—Revised (SCID-D-R).* Washington, DC: American Psychiatric Press.

Steinberg, M. (1994b). *Interviewer's guide to the Structured Clinical Interview for DSM-IV Dissociative Disorders—Revised (SCID-D-R).* Washington, DC: American Psychiatric Press.

Steinberg, M. (1995). *Handbook for the assessment of dissociation: A clinical guide.* Washington, DC: American Psychiatric Press.

Steinberg, M. (1996a). Diagnostic tools for assessing dissociation in children and adolescents. In D. Lewis (Ed.), *Child and adolescent psychiatric clinics of North America* (pp. 333–349). Philadelphia: Saunders.

Steinberg, M. (1996b). *The clinician's guide to the assessment of dissociative symptoms and disorders* [Audiotape and Manual]. North Tonawanda, NY: Multi-Health Systems.

Steinberg, M. (2000, Spring). Advances in the clinical assessment of dissociation: The SCID-D-R. *Bulletin of the Menninger Clinic, 64*(2), 146–163.

Steinberg, M., & Hall, P. (1997). The SCID-D diagnostic interview and treatment planning in dissociative disorders. *Bulletin of the Menninger Clinic, 61*, 108–120.

Steinberg, M., Hall, P., Lareau, C., & Cicchetti, D. (2001). Recognizing the validity of dissociative symptoms and disorders using the SCID-D-R: Guidelines for clinical and forensic evaluations. *Southern California Interdisciplinary Law Journal, 10*(2), 225–242.

Steinberg, M., Rounsaville, B. J., & Cicchetti, D. V. (1990). The Structured Clinical Interview for DSM-III-R Dissociative Disorders: Preliminary report on a new diagnostic instrument. *American Journal of Psychiatry, 147*(1), 76–82.

Steinberg, M., & Schnall, M. (2001). *The stranger in the mirror: Dissociation—The hidden epidemic.* New York: HarperCollins.

Steinberg, M., & Steinberg, A. (1995). Systematic assessment of dissociative identity disorder in adolescents using the SCID-D: Three case studies. *Bulletin of the Menninger Clinic, 59*, 221–231.

Sutker, P. B., Uddo, M., Brailey, K., Allain, A. N., & Errera, P. (1994). Psychological symptoms and psychiatric diagnoses in Operation Desert Storm troops serving graves registration duty. *Journal of Traumatic Stress, 7*(2), 159–171.

Terr, L. C. (1990). *Too scared to cry: Psychic trauma in childhood.* New York: Harper & Row.

Terr, L. C. (1991). Childhood traumas: An outline and overview. *American Journal of Psychiatry, 148*(1), 10–20.

Tichenor, V., Marmar, C. R., Weiss, D. S., Metzler, T. J., & Ronfeldt, H. M. (1996). The relationship of peritraumatic dissociation and posttraumatic stress: Findings in female Vietnam theater veterans. *Journal of Consulting and Clinical Psychology, 64*(5), 1054–1059.

Torem, M. S. (1990). Covert multiple personality underlying eating disorders. *American Journal of Psychotherapy, 65*(3), 357–368.

Ursano, R. J., Fullerton, C. S., Epstein, R. S., Crowley, B., Vance, K., Kao, T. C., & Baum, A. (1999). Peritraumatic dissociation and posttraumatic stress disorder following motor vehicle accidents. *American Journal of Psychiatry, 156*, 1808–1810.

Welburn, K., Fraser, G., Jordan, S., Cameron, C., Webb, L., & Raine, D. (2003). Discriminating dissociative identity disorder from schizophrenia and feigned dissociation on psychological tests and structured interview. *Journal of Trauma and Dissociation, 4*(2), 109–130.

Wilson, J. P. (1994). The need for an integrative theory of posttraumatic stress disorder. In M. B. Williams (Ed.), *Handbook of PTSD therapy.* New York: Greenwood.

Wilson, J. (in press). The broken spirit: Posttraumatic damage to the self. In J. Wilson & B. Drozdek (Eds.), *The treatment of asylum seekers and refugees with PTSD.* New York: Brunner-Routledge.

CHAPTER 6

The Peritraumatic Dissociative Experiences Questionnaire

CHARLES R. MARMAR
THOMAS J. METZLER
CHRISTIAN OTTE

EMPIRICAL STUDIES OF TRAUMA AND DISSOCIATION: A BRIEF OVERVIEW

Although the topic had receded into relative obscurity for much of the 20th century, we have witnessed an intense reawakening of interest in the role of dissociation in the understanding of human responses to catastrophic events. The theoretical contributions and clinical observations of Janet, which had been largely eclipsed by developments within modern ego psychology, self psychology, and more recently in neurobiology, have enjoyed a resurgence of interest. Putnam (1989) and van der Kolk and van der Hart (1989a, 1989b) have provided contemporary reinterpretations of the contributions of Janet to the understanding of traumatic stress and dissociation.

Paralleling the resurgence of interest in theoretical studies of trauma and dissociation, a proliferation of research studies have addressed the relationship of trauma and general dissociative tendencies. Hilgard (1970) observed that students rated as highly hypnotizable reported more frequent histories of childhood punishment than their peers with low hypnotizability. She speculated that a heightened hypnotic capacity might confer protection against reexperiencing painful childhood memories. Chu and Dill (1990) reported that psychiatric patients with a history of childhood abuse reported higher levels of dissociative symptoms than those without histories of childhood abuse. Carlson and Rosser-Hogan (1991), in a study of Cambodian refugees, reported a strong relationship between the amount of trauma the refugees had experienced and the severity of both traumatic stress symptoms and general dissociative tendencies. They reported the following:

1. Retrospective studies support a strong relationship between early physical or sexual abuse and later dissociative phenomenology.
2. Repeated and severe childhood abuse is more strongly associated with adult dissociative phenomena than are isolated instances of abuse.
3. Dissociation at the time of childhood trauma may be a mechanism to cope with overwhelming traumatic events.
4. Adults with posttraumatic stress disorder (PTSD) have higher levels of hypnotizability than adult patients without PTSD.

Following on Hilgard's original observations concerning trauma and hypnotizability, Stutman and Bliss (1985) reported that veterans in a non-patient population who had high levels of PTSD symptoms were more hypnotizable than their counterpart veterans who were low in PTSD symptoms. Spiegel, Hunt, and Dondershine (1988) compared the hypnotizability of Vietnam combat veterans with PTSD with that of patients with generalized anxiety disorders, affective disorders, and schizophrenia, as well as with a normal comparison group. The group with PTSD was found to have higher hypnotizability scores than both the psychopathological and normal controls. Hypnotizability scores in childhood have been shown to have stable trait-like characteristics, raising the possibility that traumatized individuals with higher levels of pretrauma-exposure hypnotizability may be more prone to developing PTSD. It is also possible that chronic PTSD results in changes in level of hypnotizability. Prospective studies are required to disentangle these possibilities.

Empirical studies have supported a strong relationship among trauma, dissociation, and personality disturbances. Herman, Perry, and van der Kolk (1989) found a high prevalence of traumatic histories in patients with borderline personality disorder. Level of adult dissociative symptoms was better predicted by childhood traumatic history than by even borderline personality diagnosis. Ogata and colleagues (1990), in a study of trauma and dissociation in borderline personality disorder, found a higher frequency of childhood abuse in participants with borderline personality disorder than in depressed controls.

A profound relationship has been reported for childhood trauma and dissociative identity disorder (DID). In discussing the causes of DID, Kluft (1993) proposes a four-factor theory: (1) inherent capacity to dissociate, (2) traumatic life experiences that overwhelm the adaptational capacities of the child to utilize nondissociative defenses, (3) the role of the environment in shaping the development of fragmented aspects of personality development, and (4) an inadequate availability of restorative experiences by protective others. Kluft proposes that the dissociative processes that underlie multiple personality development continue to serve a defensive function for individuals who have neither the external or internal resources to cope with traumatic experiences.

Coons and Milstein (1986) reported that 85% of a series of 20 patients with DID had documented allegations of childhood abuse. Similar observations have been made by Frischolz (1985) and by Putnam, Guroff, Silberman, Barban, and Post (1986). The nature of the childhood trauma in many of these cases is notable for its severity, multiple elements of physical and sexual abuse, threats to life, bizarre elements, and profound rupture of the sense of safety and trust when the perpetrator is a primary caretaker or another close relationship.

PERITRAUMATIC DISSOCIATION: ACUTE DISSOCIATIVE RESPONSES TO TRAUMA

The studies reviewed clearly demonstrate the relationship between traumatic life experience and general dissociative response. One fundamental aspect of the dissociative response to trauma concerns immediate dissociation *at the time the traumatic event is unfolding*. Trauma victims, not uncommonly, will report alterations in the experience of self, time, place, and meaning, which confer a sense of unreality to the event as it is occurring. Dissociation during trauma may take the form of altered time sense, with time being experienced as slowing down or rapidly accelerated; profound feelings of unreality that the event is occurring, as though the event were a dream, a movie or a play; experiences of depersonalization; out-of-body experiences; bewilderment, confusion, and disorientation; altered pain perception; altered body image or feelings of disconnection from one's body; tunnel vision; and other experiences reflecting immediate dissociative responses to trauma. We have designated these acute dissociative responses to trauma as "peritraumatic dissociation" (Marmar, Weiss, Schlenger, et al., 1994; Marmar, Weiss, Metzler, Ronfeldt, & Foreman, 1996; Weiss, Marmar, Metzler, & Ronfeldt, 1995; Marmar, Weiss, & Metzler, 1998; Tichenor, Marmar, Weiss, Metzler, & Ronfeldt, 1996; Marmar et al., 1999).

Although actual clinical reports of peritraumatic dissociation date back nearly a century, systematic investigation has occurred more recently. Spiegel (1993) reviewed studies of detachment experiences at the time of trauma, one feature of peritraumatic dissociation. Noyes and Kletti (1977) surveyed 101 survivors of automobile accidents and physical assault. They reported feelings of unreality and altered experience of the passage of time during the accident in 72% of participants, automatic behaviors in 57%, sense of detachment in 52%, depersonalization in 56%, sense of detachment from one's body in 34%, and derealization in 30%. Hillman (1981) reported on the experiences of 14 correctional officers held hostage during a violent prison riot. The hostages described employing dissociative perceptual alterations to cope with the terror and pain of their experience, including time distortion and psychogenic anesthesia to protect against overwhelming pain. Wilkinson (1983) investigated the psychological responses of survivors of the Hyatt Regency Hotel skywalk collapse in Kansas City, Missouri, in which 114 people died and 200 were injured. Survivors commonly reported depersonalization and derealization experiences at the time of the structural collapse. Siegel (1984) studied 31 kidnapping victims and terrorist hostages and reported that, during the hostage experience, 25.8% experienced alterations in body imagery and sensations, depersonalization, and disorientation, and 12.9% experienced out-of-body experiences.

Holen (1993), in a long-term prospective study of survivors of a North Sea oil rig disaster, found that the level of reported dissociation during the trauma was a predictor of subsequent PTSD. Cardeña and Spiegel (1993) reported on the responses of 100 graduate students from two different institutions in the Bay Area following the 1989 Loma Prieta earthquake. At the time the earthquake was occurring, the participants reported experiencing derealization and depersonalization; time distortion; and alterations in cognition, memory, and somatic sensations. These results suggest that among nonclinical populations, exposure to catastrophic stress may trigger *transient dissociative phenomena*. Koopman, Classen, and Spiegel (1994) investigated predictors of posttraumatic stress symptoms among survivors of the 1991 Oakland Hills firestorm. In a study of 187 participants, dissociative symptoms at the time the firestorm was occurring more strongly predicted subsequent posttraumatic symptoms than did anxiety and the subjective experience of loss of personal autonomy.

These independently replicated clinical and research findings point toward an important vulnerability role for *peritraumatic dissociation* as a risk factor for subsequent PTSD. These findings were at first surprising, given the prevailing clinical belief that dissociative responses to trauma at the time of occurrence of life-threatening or otherwise terrifying events conferred a sense of distance and safety to the victim. For example, an adult survivor of childhood incest reported that during the experience of being sexually abused, she would leave her body and view the assault from above, with a feeling of detachment and compassion for the helpless little child who was being sexually assaulted. Although out-of-body and other peritraumatic dissociative responses at the time of traumatic stress occurrence may defend against even more catastrophic states of helplessness, horror, and terror, dissociation at the time of trauma is one of the most important risk factors for the subsequent development of chronic PTSD. Possible causal relationships between peritraumatic dissociation and the heightened risk for PTSD are discussed in the later section titled "Mechanisms for Peritraumatic Dissociation."

THE PERITRAUMATIC DISSOCIATVE EXPERIENCES QUESTIONNAIRE: A MEASURE OF IMMEDIATE DISSOCIATIVE RESPONSES TO TRAUMATIC EVENTS

Based on the important clinical and early research observations on peritraumatic dissociation as a risk factor for chronic PTSD, we embarked on a series of studies to develop a reliable and valid measure of peritraumatic dissociation. We designated this measure the Peritraumatic Dissociative Experiences Questionnaire (PDEQ; Marmar, Weiss, & Metzler, 1998). The first version of the PDEQ was a rater version, consisting of nine items addressing dissociative experiences *at the time the traumatic event was occurring*: (1) moments of losing track or blanking out; (2) finding oneself acting on "automatic pilot"; (3) a sense of time changing during the event; (4) the event seeming unreal, as in a dream or play; (5) a feeling of floating above the scene; (6) feeling disconnected from body or body distortion; (7) confusion as to what was happening to oneself and others; (8) not being aware of things that happened during the event that normally would have been noticed; and (9) not feeling pain associated with physical injury.

In a first study with the PDEQ, the relationship of peritraumatic dissociation and posttraumatic stress was investigated in male Vietnam theater veterans (Marmar, Weiss, Schlenger, et al., 1994). Two hundred and fifty-one male Vietnam theater veterans from the Clinical Examination Component of the National Vietnam Veterans Readjustment Study were examined to determine the relationship of war-zone stress exposure, retrospective reports of dissociation during the most disturbing combat trauma events, and general dissociative tendencies with PTSD case determination. Peritraumatic dissociation was assessed with a rater version of the PDEQ. Total score on the PDEQ was strongly associated with level of posttraumatic stress symptoms, level of stress exposure, and general dissociative tendencies.

Total PDEQ score was weakly associated with general psychopathology as assessed by the 10 clinical scales of the MMPI-2. Logistical regression analyses supported the incremental value of dissociation during trauma, over and above the contributions of level of war-zone stress exposure and general dissociative tendencies, in accounting for PTSD case determination. These results provided initial support for the reliability and validity of the rater version of the PDEQ and for a trauma dissociation linkage hypothesis. Retrospective reports of greater dissociation during traumatic stress exposure were associated with greater likelihood of meeting criteria for current PTSD.

In a first replication of this finding, the relationship of peritraumatic dissociation with symptomatic distress was determined in emergency services personnel exposed to traumatic critical incidents (Weiss et al., 1995; Marmar, Weiss, Metzler, Ronfeldt, & Foreman, 1996). A total of 367 emergency services personnel who had responded to either a large-scale mass disaster operation or a smaller critical incident were investigated, including police, firefighters, EMT/paramedics, and California Department of Transportation workers. One hundred and fifty-four of the EMS workers had been involved in the 1989 Interstate-880 Nimitz Freeway collapse that occurred during the Loma Prieta Bay Area earthquake. A variety of predictors of current symptomatic distress were measured, including level of critical-incident exposure, social support, psychological traits, locus of control, general dissociative tendencies, and peritraumatic dissociation. Findings demonstrated that levels of current symptomatic distress were positively associated with degree of exposure to the critical incident and negatively associated with levels of adjustment. After controlling for both exposure and adjustment, symptomatic distress could still for the most part be predicted by social support, experience on the job, locus of control, general dissociative tendencies, and dissociative experiences at the time of the critical incident. The two dissociative variables, total score on the Dissociative Experience Scale (DES; Bernstein & Putnam, 1986) and total score on the PDEQ, were strongly predictive of symptomatic response, even after controlling for exposure, adjustment, and the three other predictors.

Initial assessments in this study were conducted approximately 2 years after the Loma Prieta earthquake. At follow-up, on average 3.5 years after the earthquake, we examined the longitudinal course and predictors of continuing distress in 332 emergency services personnel (Marmar et al., 1999). We found that despite modest improvement, rescue workers were at risk for chronic symptomatic distress. Peritraumatic dissociation accounted for significant increments in current PTSD symptoms, over and above exposure, adjustment, years of service, locus of control, social support, and general dissociative tendencies. Greater exposure and greater PDEQ scores were the best predictors of continuing distress.

In an extension and replication of our findings with male Vietnam veterans, we studied the relationship of peritraumatic dissociation and posttraumatic stress in female Vietnam theater veterans (Tichenor et al., 1996). Part of the impetus for this study was to assess the relationship of peritraumatic dissociation with posttraumatic stress response in a female sample, as the two earlier studies had focused primarily on male participants. Seventy-seven female Vietnam theater veterans were investigated using the rater version of the PDEQ. Total score on the PDEQ was found to be associated strongly with posttraumatic stress symptomatology, as measured by the Impact of Event Scale, and also positively associated with level of stress exposure and general dissociative tendencies, the latter measured by the DES. Scores on the PDEQ were unassociated with general psychiatric symptomatology as assessed by the 10 clinical scales of the MMPI-2. As in the two earlier studies, PDEQ scores were predictive of posttraumatic stress symptoms above and beyond the level of stress exposure and general dissociative tendencies. The findings provide further support for the reliability and validity of the PDEQ and provide additional support for a linkage between trauma and dissociation, building on our earlier findings with male Vietnam War veterans and emergency services personnel.

We have also investigated the relationship of peritraumatic dissociation with current posttraumatic stress response in participants exposed to the 1994 Los Angeles area Northridge earthquake (Marmar, Weiss, Metzler, & Ronfeldt, 1994). The sample comprised 60 adult men and women who had lived close to the epicenter of the earthquake and were working for a large private insurance company. A self-report version of the PDEQ was used to assess dissociation at the time of the earthquake occurrence. As in the earlier studies with male and female veterans and emergency services personnel, reports of dissociation at the time of the traumatic event were predictive of current posttraumatic stress response symptoms after controlling for the level of exposure.

We next examined the relationship of peritraumatic dissociation and posttraumatic distress in a cross-sectional survey of police officers serving in the New York, Oakland, and San Jose police departments (Brunet et al., 2001). The PDEQ was revised for this study, deleting one item—"not feeling pain associated with physical injury"—because of low frequency of occurrence and concerns that analgesia at the time of injury may be mediated by neurohormonal rather than dissociative responses. Based on clinical reports from participants in our earlier studies, we added two new items: "feeling confused, that is having difficulty making sense of what was happening" and "feeling disoriented, that is being uncertain about where you were or what time it was." In a sample of 702 police officers, internal consistency for the revised 10-item version was high (coefficient alpha = .85). Univariate analyses revealed that greater PDEQ scores were associated with greater cumulative PTSD symptoms related to the self-identified worst critical incident occurring in the line of duty ($r = .43$; $p < .001$).

This article focuses on the development of the Peritraumatic Distress Inventory (PDI), a companion measure to the PDEQ. The PDI assesses level of terror, horror, helplessness, grief, anger, and panic at the time of critical incident occurrence. Of interest, PDEQ and PDI scores were strongly positively associated ($r = .59$; $p < .001$). This finding supports the view that greater peritraumatic dissociation does not protect against peritraumatic emotional distress but rather is associated with greater dysphoric arousal at the time of exposure. Although they were strongly positively correlated in this sample of urban police officers, both PDEQ and PDI independently contributed to the prediction of current PTSD symptom levels after controlling for the effects of the other.

Across these studies the PDEQ has been demonstrated to be internally consistent; strongly associated with measures of traumatic stress response, with a measure of general dissociative tendencies, and with level of stress exposure; and, in our studies of male and female veterans, unassociated with measures of general psychopathology. These studies support the reliability and convergent, discriminant, and predictive validity of the PDEQ.

INDEPENDENT STUDIES USING THE PDEQ

Strengthening these findings are multiple independent studies utilizing the PDEQ by investigators in other PTSD research programs. Bremner and colleagues (1992), utilizing selective items from the PDEQ as part of a measure of peritraumatic dissociation, reported a strong relationship of peritraumatic dissociation with posttraumatic stress response in an independent sample of Vietnam War veterans. In the first prospective study with the PDEQ, Shalev, Peri,

Canetti, and Schreiber (1996) examined the relationship of PDEQ ratings gathered in the first week following trauma exposure with posttraumatic stress symptomatology at 5 months. In this study of acute physical trauma victims admitted to an Israeli teaching hospital emergency room, PDEQ ratings at 1 week predicted stress symptomatology at 5 months, over and above exposure levels, social supports, and Impact of Event Scale scores in the first week. This study is noteworthy in that it is the first finding with the PDEQ in which ratings were gathered prospectively. Retrospective ratings of peritraumatic dissociation made months, years, or decades after the occurrence of traumatic events are subject to the bias that greater current distress may result in greater recollection of dissociation at the time of traumatic stress occurrence. Shalev and colleagues' findings are therefore important in supporting the earlier findings utilizing retrospective ratings of peritraumatic dissociation.

Ursano and colleagues (1999) examined the relationship between peritraumatic dissociation and PTSD in motor vehicle accident victims. They found that the most common peritraumatic dissociative symptom was time distortion, present in 56.6% of the 122 participants. Participants with peritraumatic dissociation were 4.12 times more likely to have acute PTSD and 4.86 times more likely to develop chronic PTSD. The relative risk was independent of risk associated with the presence of PTSD before the accident. In a related publication from the same study, Fullerton and colleagues (2000) reported that younger participants were more likely to experience peritraumatic dissociation, as were those with an injured passenger. Being single and Caucasian were also associated with greater peritraumatic dissociation. After adjusting for age and passenger injury, prior major depression was related to greater peritraumatic dissociation. Those who were younger and reported a history of major depression had the greatest number of peritraumatic dissociation experiences.

In a more detailed analysis of gender differences in PTSD from the same data set of 122 participants following motor vehicle accidents, Fullerton and colleagues (2001) reported that although the risk for acute PTSD was 4.64 times greater for women, men and women had similar frequencies of peritraumatic dissociation. In multiple logistic regression analysis, gender was no longer a significant predictor of PTSD after adjusting for peritraumatic dissociation. However, there was a highly significant gender-by-peritraumatic-dissociation interaction. Women with peritraumatic dissociation were 7.55 times more likely than men with peritraumatic dissociation to develop PTSD. Of those with peritraumatic dissociation, 59.6% of women but only 16.3% of men developed PTSD. Given that women are twice as likely as a men to develop PTSD during their lifetimes (Kessler, Sonnega, Bromet, Hughes, & Nelson, 1995), the importance of peritraumatic dissociation as a mediator of gender as a risk factor is highlighted by this finding.

Bernat, Ronfeldt, Calhoun, and Arias (1998) studied 937 college students who identified lifetime experiences of traumatic events and who, in response to their most stressful event, completed measures of exposure, PTSD symptoms, and peritraumatic reactions. After controlling for vulnerability factors and exposure characteristics, both peritraumatic dissociation and peritraumatic emotional and physical reactions were strongly associated with PTSD symptom levels. Of interest, PDEQ levels were strongly positively associated with both peritraumatic physical and emotional reactivity, consistent with the findings of Brunet and colleagues showing that greater emotional distress and physical manifestations of anxiety are strongly associated with greater peritraumatic dissociation.

Birmes and colleagues (2001) studied 48 French crime victims within 24 hours of traumatic exposure. The participants were followed to assess acute stress responses 2 weeks after the assault and posttraumatic stress at 5 weeks. Higher levels of peritraumatic dissociation and acute stress following violent assault were found to be risk factors for early PTSD.

In one of the first truly prospective longitudinal studies of risk factors for PTSD, Hodgins, Creamer, and Bell (2001) studied 233 junior police officers in Australia. Participants were assessed using a self-report methodology during academy training and again 12 months later. At 1-year follow-up, general psychological health problems were predicted by personality style, gender, and trait dissociation. In contrast, PTSD symptom levels at follow-up were more strongly predicted by severity of incident exposure and by PDEQ scores. The strongest predictor of posttraumatic stress symptoms was peritraumatic dissociation.

In a second prospective longitudinal study, Engelhard, van den Hout, Merel, and Arntz (2003) evaluated 1,370 Dutch women volunteers in early pregnancy. Subsequently, 126 experienced pregnancy loss, and they completed self-report measures 1 month and 4 months later. Peritraumatic dissociation at the time of loss was predicted by baseline expectations of lower control over emotions in the event of pregnancy loss, general dissociative tendencies, and lower educational attainment. Peritraumatic dissociation was not predicted by neuroticism, absorption, and prior stressful life events. Greater peritraumatic dissociation predicted greater acute PTSD symptom levels. This relationship was mediated by self-reported memory fragmentation and thought suppression of pregnancy. Peritraumatic dissociation was also predictive of PTSD symptoms at 4 months after pregnancy loss, and this association was mediated by level of acute PTSD symptoms.

Gershuny, Cloitre, and Otto (2003) studied 146 non-treatment-seeking college women who had personally experienced one or more traumatic events. Zero-order correlations revealed that greater peritraumatic dissociation was associated with greater current PTSD symptom severity; greater frequency of lifetime traumatic events; greater nonspecific fear, helplessness, and horror at the time of exposure; greater fear of death at the time of exposure; and greater fear of losing control at the time of exposure. Hierarchal multiple regression analyses indicated that the relationship between peritraumatic dissociation and posttraumatic stress was mediated by fear of death and fear of loss of control at the time of exposure. The authors note that, although the data suggest that dissociation drives panic and panic drives the subsequent risk for PTSD, it is uncertain whether fears about death and losing control are a cause or a consequence of peritraumatic dissociation. Their findings once again highlight the hand-in-glove relationship between peritraumatic dissociation and peritraumatic terror, which are likely to act alone and in interaction to interfere with adaptive emotional and biological processing of traumatic events.

Although most independent studies, including those in Europe and Australia, have been confirmatory, not all have supported the prediction that peritraumatic dissociation accounts for current PTSD symptom levels. Mellman, David, Bustamante, Fins, and Esposito (2001) studied 50 patients admitted to a trauma center and found that early symptoms of heightened arousal and disengagement coping, but not peritraumatic dissociation or a diagnosis of acute stress disorder, were associated with follow-up PTSD severity. Further research is indicated to determine whether specific traumatized populations—including those with injuries severe enough to warrant admission to a physical trauma center, where they frequently receive narcotic analgesics—may have altered recollections or experiences of peritraumatic dissociation.

Marshall and Schell (2002) reported findings from a cross-lagged panel analysis of a sample of young adult survivors of community violence. They utilized a modified 7-item version of the PDEQ, noting high correlations between the modified version and the original PDEQ. Assessments of peritraumatic dissociation in PTSD symptom severity were determined at baseline within days of the assault, at 3-month follow-up, and at 12-month follow-up. Covariance structure modeling, using the EQS software program, was the primary data analytic method. In both the initial and final models, peritraumatic dissociation was strongly associated with PTSD symptom severity within each time point, replicating earlier results. Peritraumatic dissociation at baseline strongly predicted initial PTSD symptom levels at baseline, after controlling for injury severity and neuroticism.

Of interest, in this study the prediction of follow-up PTSD symptom levels from initial peritraumatic dissociation levels was mediated by the level of initial PTSD symptom severity. The latter finding is broadly consistent with an emerging model, which is that peritraumatic dissociation is a marker of immediate unmanageable terrifying arousal, which in turn drives initial PTSD symptom responding because of memory over consolidation and increased fear conditioning. Initial PTSD symptom responding in turn determines long-term PTSD symptomatic status.

The study also found that the average level of peritraumatic dissociation for the group stayed relatively constant over time. However, individuals' recall of peritraumatic dissociative experiences within the first few days following shooting, penetrating, or blunt object injuries differed from subsequent recall at 3 months and at 12 months. This finding raises concerns about the use of retrospective reports of peritraumatic dissociation and underscores the recent trend toward the study of acute stress disorders, with administration of the PDEQ in the immediate aftermath of traumatic events.

MECHANISMS FOR PERITRAUMATIC DISSOCIATION: PSYCHOBIOLOGICAL DYNAMICS

The strong, replicated findings relating peritraumatic dissociation to acute and chronic PTSD raise theoretically important questions concerning the mechanisms that underlie peritraumatic dissociation. Speculation concerning psychological factors underlying trauma-related dissociation date back to the early contributions of Breuer and Freud (1895/1955). In their formulation, traumatic events are actively split off from conscious experience but return in the disguised form of symptoms. The dissociated traumatic memory complexes have an underground psychological life, causing hysterics to "suffer mainly from reminiscences." Janet (1889) proposed that trauma-related dissociation occurred in individuals with a fundamental constitutional defect in psychological functioning, which he designated *la misère psychologique*. Janet proposed that normal individuals have sufficient psychological energy to bind together their mental experiences, including memories, cognitions, sensations, feelings, and volition, into an integrated synthetic whole under the control of a single personal self with access to conscious experience (Nemiah, 1998). From Janet's perspective, peritraumatic dissociation resulted in the coexistence within a single individual of two or more discrete, dissociative streams of consciousness, each existing independently from the others, each with rich mental contents, including feelings, memories, and bodily sensations, and each with access to conscious experience at different times.

Contemporary psychological studies of peritraumatic dissociation have focused on individual differences in the threshold for dissociation. Adult trauma victims who dissociate during their traumas may have experienced childhood or adolescent traumatic events that lower their threshold for dissociation. It is also possible that the threshold for peritraumatic dissociation or generalized dissociative vulnerability is a heritable trait, aggravated by early trauma exposure and correlated with hypnotizability, as suggested by Spiegel and colleagues (1988). Hypnosis has been conceptualized as a structured and controlled form of dissociation (Nemiah, 1985; Speigel & Speigel, 1978). Three critical elements to the hypnotic experience—absorption, compartmentalization of experience, and suggestibility—share much in common with the clinical phenomena of trauma-related dissociation.

Further supporting the linkage between hypnotizability and trauma-related dissociation are the findings of Stutman and Bliss (1985), who found greater hypnotizability in nonpatient veterans who were high in PTSD symptoms when compared with nonpatient veterans who were low in PTSD symptoms. Spiegel and colleagues (1988) compared patients with schizophrenia, generalized anxiety disorder, affective disorders, and PTSD and found that the group with PTSD had higher hypnotizability scores than did the other groups and normal controls. In a study of hypnotizability, clinical dissociation, and trauma in sexually abused girls and control subjects, Putnam, Helmers, Horowitz, and Trickett (1995) reported a positive association of hypnotizability and clinical dissociation in the trauma victims but not in the control participants. This study suggests that high hypnotizability alone, in the absence of trauma, is not a sufficient condition for high levels of dissociation. Taken together, the studies on trauma, dissociation, and hypnotizability suggest that individuals who are constitutionally predisposed to be highly hypnotizable and who additionally experience trauma early in life are those with greatest vulnerability to subsequent dissociation at the time of threat. Further research is required to determine whether Janet's speculation of a genetically determined weakness in the capacity to bind and integrate psychological information may be related to a genetically determined increase in hypnotizability.

Marmar, Weiss, Metzler, and Delucchi (1996) reported on individual differences in the level of peritraumatic dissociation during critical-incident exposure in emergency services personnel. They found the following factors to be associated with greater levels of peritraumatic dissociation: younger age; higher levels of exposure during critical incident; poorer general psychological adjustment; poorer identity formation; lower levels of ambition and prudence, as defined by the Hogan Personality Inventory; greater external locus of control; and greater use of escape/avoidance and emotional self-control coping. Taken together, these findings suggest that emergency services personnel with less work experience, more vulnerable personality structures, higher subjective levels of perceived threat and anxiety at the time of incidence occurrence, greater reliance on the external world for an internal sense of safety and organization, and greater use of maladaptive coping strategies are more vulnerable to peritraumatic dissociation.

Jaycox, Marshall, and Orlando (2003), in a subsequent report of the Marshall and Schell (2002) study discussed previously, assessed predictors of peritraumatic dissociation. PDEQ ratings were obtained on average 10 days after assault. Greater PDEQ scores were strongly associated with greater acute PTSD symptom levels. Only injury severity and neuroticism emerged as predictors of levels of peritraumatic dissociation, although the effects were small. Level of peritraumatic terror and related emotional distress, the strongest predictor of PDEQ levels in our most recent studies of police officers (Brunet et al., 2001; Marmar et al., 2003), was not directly assessed in this study.

A second line of investigation concerning the underlying mechanisms for peritraumatic dissociation focuses on the neurobiology and neuropharmacology of anxiety. A study by Southwick and colleagues (1993) with yohimbine suggests that, in individuals with traumatic stress disorder, flashbacks occur in the context of high-threat arousal states. It is also significant that patients with panic disorder frequently report dissociative reactions at the height of their anxiety attacks (Krystal, Woods, Hill, & Charney, 1991). The effects of yohimbine in triggering flashbacks in patients with PTSD and panic attacks in patients with panic disorder is mediated by a central catecholamine mechanism, as yohimbine serves as an alpha-adrenergic receptor antagonist, resulting in increased firing of locus ceruleus neurons. These observations suggest that the relationship between peritraumatic dissociation and PTSD may, for some individuals, be mediated by high levels of anxiety during the trauma. The possibility that panic-level states of anxious arousal may trigger dissociation in some individuals is consistent with the Moleman, van der Hart, and van der Kolk (1992) report on the general relationship of high arousal and dissociation.

Several studies have examined the relationship between peritraumatic dissociation, acoustic startle, and psychophysiological responses to trauma reminders. Griffin, Resick, and Mechanic (1997) studied 85 female rape victims (mean age 28.7 ± 7.8) who were assessed within 2 weeks after the rape. Measures of heart rate, skin conductance, and nonspecific movement were obtained. The laboratory assessment consisted of 5 minutes of talking about a neutral topic (e.g. " a special meal that you prepared"), 5 minutes rest, and 5 minutes of talking about the rape.

Based on PDEQ scores that rated levels of dissociation during the rape, in contrast to ratings of dissociation during a recounting of the sexual assault in a laboratory assessment, women were assigned to a high- (*N* = 16) or low-dissociation group (*N* = 31). Women in the high-dissociation group were significantly more likely to have PTSD symptoms than those who did not dissociate during the rape. Interestingly, the high-dissociation group showed a smaller autonomic response, as measured by heart rate and skin conductance, to the trauma narrative task but more subjective distress at the end of the assessment than the low-dissociation group.

Kaufman and colleagues (2002) conducted a secondary analysis of a Veteran's Affairs Cooperative Study (Keane et al., 1998). Extreme subgroups of veterans with current PTSD were classified as low (*N* = 118, mean age 43.0 ± 2.7) or high dissociators (*N* = 256, mean age 42.7 ± 3.1) based on a short version of the PDEQ for assessing retrospective reports of dissociation at the time of worst combat incident. Among veterans with current PTSD, high dissociators reported greater PTSD-related symptomatic distress than did low dissociators, but the groups did not differ with respect to physiological reactivity to trauma-related audiovisual and imagery presentations as measured by heart rate, skin conductance, electromyography, and blood pressure. The hypothesis that veterans who reported greater peritraumatic dissociation during combat would experience greater dissociation during the trauma narrative task, and as a result show lower levels of psychophysiological arousal, was not supported.

A third study examined the electromyogram and skin conductance responses to 15 acoustic startle trials in 103 survivors of a life-threatening cardiac event (mean age 61.0 ± 14.0, mean time since cardiac event 37 months; Ladwig et al. 2002). High peritraumatic dissociation was associated with an enhanced response of skin conductance and electromyography and an impaired habituation to acoustic startle in comparison with patients with low dissociation.

Taken together, these studies do not provide consistent support for the view that greater dissociation during the actual traumatic event will be associated with dissociation-mediated lower psychophysiological arousal during a laboratory-based trauma-narrative task. Differences concerning age, gender, type of trauma, type of challenge, and time since trauma might be responsible for these conflicting results. Prospective studies with psychophysiological characterization of participants previous to traumatization are needed to clarify the relationship between arousal and peritraumatic dissociation. Our group is in the process of conducting such a study with police academy trainees. In addition, family history, twin studies, cross-fostering studies, and biological marker studies will be required to determine whether peritraumatic and general dissociative tendencies are characteristics that are inherited or learned early in life. Alternatively, it remains to be demonstrated whether trauma determines greater vulnerability to dissociative responses, both generally and specifically, with respect to peritraumatic responses. It will also be of interest to determine what factors protect against peritraumatic dissociation and to determine prospectively whether such resilience factors reduce the risk of developing subsequent PTSD. Individual differences in level of panic reactions at the time of traumatic exposure may be in part biologically determined and may in turn determine level of peritraumatic dissociation.

TREATMENT OF TRAUMA-RELATED DISSOCIATION

To date, no controlled clinical trials have been reported of psychosocial or pharmacological interventions that directly target trauma-related dissociation. Kluft (1993), in an overview of clinical reports on treatment approaches for trauma-related dissociation, recommends individual, supportive–expressive psychodynamic psychotherapy, augmented as needed with hypnosis or drug-facilitated interviews. For the treatment of the most severe form of trauma-related dissociation, dissociative identity disorder, Kluft (1993), drawing on the work of Braun (1986), outlines nine stages of a supportive–expressive, psychodynamically informed treatment:

1. Establishing a therapeutic alliance involving the creation of a safe atmosphere and secure treatment frame to establish trust and realistic optimism.
2. Preliminary interventions designed to gain access to the more readily reached dissociative aspects of personality, including the establishment of agreements with the alters against terminating treatment abruptly, self-harm, or other self-defeating behaviors.
3. History gathering and mapping of the nature and relationship among alters to define the constellation of personalities.

4. Metabolism of the trauma, which includes the access to and processing of traumatic events related to the development of MPD.
5. Movements toward integration and resolution across the alters by facilitating cooperation, communication, and mutual awareness.
6. Integration–resolution, involving a smooth collaboration among the alters.
7. Learning new coping skills to manage stress without resorting to dissociation.
8. Solidification of gains in working through in the transference, including the management of anxiety related to conflicted sexual, aggressive, and dependency issues as they arise in the relationship with the therapist.
9. Follow-up to assess the stability of the outcome and address new layers of personality that have not emerged in the prior treatment.

Spiegel (1993) proposes eight "C" principles for the psychotherapy of individuals experiencing acute traumatic–dissociative reactions:

1. *Confrontation* with the trauma to counter depersonalization and derealization.
2. *Condensation* of the traumatic experience in the form of the reconstruction of the memory of the traumatic event, including the technical use of hypnosis to relive the experiences and address psychogenic amnesia.
3. *Confession* to address shame and guilt.
4. *Consolation*, an appropriate expression of sympathy for the tragic circumstances that the patient has experienced.
5. *Consciousness*, the bringing into conscious awareness, without dissociation, the traumatic memories and associated feelings.
6. *Concentration*, the use of hypnosis and self-hypnosis to help the patient gain conscious control over disturbing memories.
7. *Control*, the further management of memories and associated affects through flexible experiencing and suppression of traumatic memories rather than dissociation.
8. *Congruence*, the integration of traumatic memories into preexisting self-concepts.

A number of investigators have advocated the use of hypnosis as adjunct to the treatment of trauma-related dissociation. In 1993, van der Hart and Spiegel advocated the use of hypnosis as a way of creating a safe, calm mental state in which the patient has control over traumatic memories, as an approach to the treatment of trauma-induced dissociative states presenting as hysterical psychosis. Batson (1994), in the treatment of DID, advocated the use of hypnosis to create a safe retreat from the terrifying circumstances surrounding trauma. Under hypnosis, the patient can go back to a childhood environment that was associated with safety and security and utilize this safe haven as a nucleus around which to build and integrate previously dissociative aspects of the self. Batson, in agreement with Spiegel and Kluft, emphasized the patients' growing control over the transitions in their dissociative mental states, allowing for retreat from terror and gradual integration.

Contemporary psychodynamic approaches to the treatment of trauma-related dissociation emphasize the establishment of the therapeutic alliance, reconstruction of traumatic memories, working through of problematic weak and strong self-concepts activated by the trauma, and transference interpretation aimed at helping the patient process perceived threats in the relationship with the therapist without resorting to dissociation (Horowitz, 1986; Marmar, 1991; Steinman, 1994; Marmar, Weiss, & Pynoos, 1995). Contemporary psychoanalytic theory emphasizes the complementarity of traumatic and structural models (Nemiah, 1998). The traumatic model addresses the fractionation of the ego into multiple dissociative elements, the pathological use of dissociation as a defense, and the abreaction and integration of dissociated traumatic memories. As the previously dissociative elements are brought in to a more coherent self, Gabbard (1994) advocates the further use of traditional psychodynamic psychotherapy to solidify gains, mourn losses, and resolve conflicts through interpretation.

Recent pharmacological studies with propranolol in the immediate aftermath of traumatic exposure suggest a novel strategy for reducing peritraumatic terror. Greater peritraumatic terror is associated with greater peritraumatic dissociation (Brunet et al., 2001; Marmar et al., 2003). Peritraumatic terror is mediated in part by prolonged states of adrenergic activation that are believed to increase the risk for PTSD through increased fear conditioning (Orr et al., 2000) and the overconsolidation of the memories related to the traumatic event (Southwick et al., 1999). Prolonged adrenergic activation, as reflected by greater peritraumatic tachycardia, was prospectively shown to increase the risk for PTSD (Shalev et al., 1998). In the first and only double-blind controlled study, Pitman and colleagues (2002) have reported that propranolol given within 6 hours of the traumatic event and continued at 80 mg to 160 mg daily for 10 days was superior to placebo for reducing PTSD symptoms at 1 month and for reducing psychophysiological arousal during a trauma-narrative challenge at 2 to 3 months posttrauma.

In a second study, Vaiva, Duqcrocq, Jezequel, Brunet, and Marmar (2003) investigated the efficacy of propranolol prescribed shortly after trauma exposure in the prevention of PTSD symptoms and diagnosis. Eleven patients received 40 mg of propranolol 3 times daily for 7 days, followed by a taper period of 8–12 days. They were compared with 8 patients who refused propranolol but agreed to participate in the study. Though nonrandomized, the two groups did not differ on demographics, exposure characteristics, physical injury severity, or peritraumatic emotional responses. PTSD symptoms were greater at 2-month follow-up in those who declined propranalol treatment ($W = 85$, $p = .037$). Although not specifically targeting peritraumatic dissociation, the hand-in-glove relationship between peritraumatic terror and peritraumatic dissociation suggests that pharmacologically blocking immediate posttrauma panic reactions will modulate peritraumatic dissociation and reduce the risk for PTSD.

FUTURE RESEARCH DIRECTIONS AND PRACTICAL CLINICAL APPLICATIONS OF THE PDEQ

Future research will clarify the relationships among subjective threat appraisal, emotional distress at the time of trauma occurrence, peritraumatic dissociation, activation of central nervous system structures that regulate threat arousal, and psychophysiological arousal in the peripheral nervous system. Trauma victims can be challenged by reminders of their traumatic events and assessed for level of peritraumatic dissociation and changes in central nervous system activity, determined with brain imaging procedures, event-related potential, and peripheral psychophysiological assessment.

Specific treatment interventions for peritraumatic dissociation and dissociative responses that occur in the course of uncovering traumatic memories will depend on rapid identification of those experiencing peritraumatic dissociation and advances in the understanding of the psychological and neurobiological factors underlying trauma-related dissociation. The PDEQ can be used to screen for acute dissociative responses at the time of traumatic stress exposure. As reviewed previously, the use of beta blockers to lower threat arousal levels at the time of traumatic occurrence may mitigate prolonged peritraumatic terror and dissociation and in turn reduce the risk of PTSD. Alpha-adrenergic agonists, beta-blockers, or other nonsedating, antiarousal agents could be provided to emergency services personnel to aid in the modulation of arousal responses to life-threatening or gruesome exposure. Advances in critical-incident stress-debriefing procedures may lead to psychological interventions that lower immediate threat appraisal and consequently reduce the likelihood of sustained peritraumatic dissociation. The PDEQ can be used to determine the effectiveness of novel pharmacological or psychotherapeutic interventions in reducing acute dissociative response to trauma.

The PDEQ can additionally be used as part of a standard assessment battery for individuals presenting with acute or chronic PTSD symptoms. Higher PDEQ scores in acute trauma victims support the need for active intervention. Higher PDEQ scores in those individuals presenting years to decades following traumatic exposure support the validity of subjective complaints of PTSD and also alert the clinician to the risks for reentry into dissociative states during the uncovering phase of exposure therapy. The current 10-item self-report and clinician versions of the PDEQ are included as appendices to this chapter.

APPENDIX 6.1. Peritraumatic Dissociative Experiences Questionnaire—Self-Report Version

Instructions: Please complete the items below by circling the choice that best describes your experiences and reactions *during the* ________________ *and immediately afterward*. If an item does not apply to your experience, please circle "Not at all true."

1. I had moments of losing track of what was going on—I "blanked out" or "spaced out" or in some way felt that I was not part of what was going on.

1	2	3	4	5
Not at all true	Slightly true	Somewhat true	Very true	Extremely true

2. I found that I was on "automatic pilot"—I ended up doing things that I later realized I hadn't actively decided to do.

1	2	3	4	5
Not at all true	Slightly true	Somewhat true	Very true	Extremely true

3. My sense of time changed—things seemed to be happening in slow motion.

1	2	3	4	5
Not at all true	Slightly true	Somewhat true	Very true	Extremely true

4. What was happening seemed unreal to me, like I was in a dream or watching a movie or play.

1	2	3	4	5
Not at all true	Slightly true	Somewhat true	Very true	Extremely true

5. I felt as though I were a spectator watching what was happening to me, as if I were floating above the scene or observing it as an outsider.

1	2	3	4	5
Not at all true	Slightly true	Somewhat true	Very true	Extremely true

6. There were moments when my sense of my own body seemed distorted or changed. I felt disconnected from my own body, or that it was unusually large or small.

1	2	3	4	5
Not at all true	Slightly true	Somewhat true	Very true	Extremely true

7. I felt as though things that were actually happening to others were happening to me—like I was being trapped when I really wasn't.

1	2	3	4	5
Not at all true	Slightly true	Somewhat true	Very true	Extremely true

8. I was surprised to find out afterward that a lot of things had happened at the time that I was not aware of, especially things I ordinarily would have noticed.

1	2	3	4	5
Not at all true	Slightly true	Somewhat true	Very true	Extremely true

9. I felt confused; that is, there were moments when I had difficulty making sense of what was happening.

1	2	3	4	5
Not at all true	Slightly true	Somewhat true	Very true	Extremely true

10. I felt disoriented; that is, there were moments when I felt uncertain about where I was or what time it was.

1	2	3	4	5
Not at all true	Slightly true	Somewhat true	Very true	Extremely true

APPENDIX 6.2. PERITRAUMATIC DISSOCIATIVE EXPERIENCES QUESTIONNAIRE—RATER VERSION

Instructions: I'd like you to try to recall as best you can how you felt and what you experienced at the time [most upsetting event] happened, including how you felt the few minutes just before. Now, I'm going to ask you some specific questions about how you felt *at that time.*

[*Note.* DK = Don't know, 01 = Absent or false, 02 = Subthreshold, 03 = Threshold.]

1. (At that time) Did you have moments of losing track of what was going on; that is, did you "blank out," "space out," or in some other way not feel that you were part of the experience?	DK	01	02	03
2. (At that time) Did you find yourself going on "automatic pilot," that is, doing something that you later realized you had done but hadn't actively decided to do?	DK	01	02	03
3. (At that time) Did your sense of time change during the event; that is, did things seem unusually speeded up or slowed down?	DK	01	02	03
4. (At that time) Did what was happening seem unreal to you, as though you were in a dream or watching a movie or a play?	DK	01	02	03
5. (At that time) Were there moments when you felt as though you were a spectator watching what was happening to you—for example, did you feel as if you were floating above the scene or observing it as an outsider?	DK	01	02	03
6. (At that time) Were there moments when your sense of your own body seemed distorted or changed—that is, did you feel yourself to be unusually large or small, or did you feel disconnected from your body?	DK	01	02	03
7. (At that time) Did you get the feeling that something that was happening to someone else was happening to you? For example, if you saw someone being injured, did you feel as though you were the one being injured, even though that was not the case?	DK	01	02	03
8. Were you surprised to find out after the event that a lot of things had happened at the time that you were not aware of, especially things that you felt you ordinarily would have noticed?	DK	01	02	03
9. (At that time) Were there moments when you had difficulty making sense of what was happening?	DK	01	02	03
10. (At that time) Did you feel disoriented, that is, were there moments when you felt uncertain about where you were or what time it was?	DK	01	02	03

REFERENCES

Batson, R. (1994, November). *Treatment of trauma-related dissociation.* Paper presented at the annual meeting of the International Society for Traumatic Stress Studies, Chicago, IL.

Bernat, J. A., Ronfeldt, H. M., Calhoun, K. S., & Arias, I. (1998). Prevalence of traumatic events and peritraumatic predictors of posttraumatic stress symptoms in a nonclinical sample of college students. *Journal of Traumatic Stress, 11,* 645–664.

Bernstein, E. M., & Putnam, F. W. (1986). Development, reliability, and validity of a dissociation scale. *Journal of Nervous and Mental Diseases, 174,* 727–735.

Birmes, P., Carreras, D., Ducasse, J., Charlet, J., Warner, B., Lauque, D., & Schmitt, L. (2001). Peritraumatic dissociation, acute stress, and early posttraumatic stress disorder in victims of general crime. *Canadian Journal of Psychiatry, 189,* 649–651.

Braun, B. G. (1986). Issues in the psychotherapy of multiple personality. In B. G. Braun (Ed.), *Treatment of multiple personality disorder* (pp. 1–28). Washington, DC: American Psychiatric Press.

Bremner, J. D., Southwick, S., Brett, E., Fontana, A., Rosenheck, R., & Charney, D. S. (1992). Dissociation and posttraumatic stress disorder in Vietnam combat veterans. *American Journal of Psychiatry, 149,* 328–332.

Breuer, J., & Freud, S. (1955). Studies on hysteria. In J. Strachey (Ed. and Trans.), *The standard edition of the complete psychological works of Sigmund Freud* (Vol. 2, pp. 1–311). London: Hogarth Press. (Original work published 1895)

Brunet, A., Weiss, D. S., Metzler, T. J., Best, S. R., Neylan, T. C., Rogers, C., et al. (2001). The Peritraumatic Distress Inventory: A proposed measure of PTSD criterion A2. *American Journal of Psychiatry, 158,* 1480–1485.

Cardeña, E., & Spiegel, D. (1993). Dissociative reactions to the San Francisco Bay Area earthquake of 1989. *American Journal of Psychiatry, 150,* 474–478.

Carlson, E. B., & Rosser-Hogan, R. (1991). Trauma experiences, posttraumatic stress dissociation, and depression in Cambodian refugees. *American Journal of Psychiatry, 148,* 1548–1551.

Chu, J. A., & Dill, D. L. (1990). Dissociative symptoms in relation to childhood physical and sexual abuse. *American Journal of Psychiatry, 147,* 887–892.

Coons, P. M., & Milstein, V. (1986). Psychosexual disturbances in multiple personality. *Journal of Nervous and Mental Disease, 47,* 106–110.

Engelhard, I. M., van den Hout, M. A., Merel, K., & Arntz, A. (2003). Peritraumatic dissociation and posttraumatic stress after pregnancy loss: A prospective study. *Behaviour Research and Therapy, 41,* 67–78.

Frischolz, E. J. (1985). The relationship among dissociation, hypnosis, and child abuse in the development of multiple personality disorder. In R. P. Kluft (Ed.), *Childhood antecedents of multiple personality* (pp. 99–126). Washington, DC: American Psychiatric Press.

Fullerton, C. S., Ursano, R. J., Epstein, R. S., Crowley, B., Vance, K., Kao, T., & Baum, A. (2000). Peritraumatic dissociation following motor vehicle accidents: Relationship to prior trauma and prior major depression. *Journal of Nervous and Mental Disease, 188,* 267–272.

Fullerton, C. S., Ursano, R. J., Epstein, R. S., Crowley, B., Vance, K., Kao, T., et al. (2001). Gender differences in posttraumatic stress disorder after motor vehicle accidents. *American Journal of Psychiatry, 158,* 1486–1491.

Gabbard, G. O. (1994). *Psychodynamic psychiatry in clinical practice: The DSM-IV edition*. Washington, DC: American Psychiatric Press.

Gershuny, B. S., Cloitre, M., & Otto, M. W. (2003). Peritraumatic dissociation and PTSD severity: Do event-related fears about death and control mediate their relation? *Behaviour Research and Therapy*, *41*, 157–166.

Griffin, M. G., Resick, P. A., & Mechanic, M. B. (1997). Objective assessment of peritraumatic dissociation: Psychophysiological indicators. *American Journal of Psychiatry*, *154*(8), 1081–1088.

Herman, J. L., Perry, J. C., & van der Kolk, B. A. (1989). Childhood trauma in borderline personality disorder. *American Journal of Psychiatry*, *146*, 490–495.

Hilgard, E. R. (1970). *Personality and hypnosis: A study of imaginative involvement*. Chicago: University of Chicago Press.

Hillman, R. G. (1981). The psychopathology of being held hostage. *American Journal of Psychiatry*, *138*, 1193–1197.

Hodgins, G. A., Creamer, M., & Bell, R. (2001). Risk factors for posttrauma reactions in police officers: A longitudinal study. *Journal of Nervous and Mental Disease*, *189*, 541–547.

Holen, A. (1993). The North Sea oil rig disaster. In J.P. Wilson & B. Raphael (Eds.), *International handbook of traumatic stress syndromes* (pp. 405–525). New York: Plenum Press.

Horowitz, M. J. (1986). *Stress response syndromes* (2nd ed.). Northvale, NJ: Aronson.

Janet, P. (1889). *L'automatisme psychologique*. Paris: Balliere.

Jaycox, L. H., Marshall, G. N., & Orlando, M. (2003). Predictors of acute distress among young adults injured by community violence. *Journal of Traumatic Stress*, *16*, 237–245.

Kaufman, M. L., Kimble, M. O., Kaloupek, D. G., McTeague, L. M., Bachrach, P., Forti, A., & Keane, T. M. (2002). Peritraumatic dissociation and physiological response to trauma-relevant stimuli in Vietnam combat veterans with posttraumatic stress disorder. *Journal of Nervous and Mental Disease*, *190*, 167–194.

Keane, T. M., Kolb, L. C., Kaloupek, D. G., Orr, S. P., Blanchard, E. B., Thomas, R. G., et al. (1998). Utility of psychophysiology measurement in the diagnosis of posttraumatic stress disorder: Results from a Department of Veteran's Affairs cooperative study. *Journal of Consulting and Clinical Psychology*, *66*, 914–923.

Kessler, R. C., Sonnega, A., Bromet, E., Hughes, M., & Nelson, C. B. (1995). Posttraumatic stress disorder in the National Comorbidity Survey. *Archives of General Psychiatry*, *52*, 1048–1060.

Kluft, R. P. (1993). Multiple personality disorder. In D. Spiegel, R. P. Kluft, M. D. Loewenstein, J. C. Nemiah, F. W. Putnam, & M. Steinberg (Eds.), *Dissociative disorders: A clinical review*. Lutherville, MD: Sidran Press.

Koopman, C., Classen, C., & Spiegel, D. (1994). Predictors of posttraumatic stress symptoms among survivors of the Oakland/Berkeley, California, firestorm. *American Journal of Psychiatry*, *151*, 888–894.

Krystal, J., Woods, S., Hill, C., & Charney, D. S. (1991). Characteristics of panic attack subtypes: Assessment of spontaneous panic, situational panic, sleep panic, and limited symptom attacks. *Comparative Psychiatry*, *32*, 474–480.

Ladwig, K., Marten-Mittag, B., Deisenhofer, I., Hofmann, B., Schapperer, J., Weyerbrock, S., et al. (2002). Psychophysiological correlates of peritraumatic dissociative responses in survivors of life-threatening cardiac events. *Psychopathology*, *35*, 241–248.

Marmar, C. R. (1991). Brief dynamic psychotherapy of post-traumatic stress disorder. *Psychiatric Annals, 21*, 404–414.

Marmar, C. R., Best, S., Metzler, T. J., Chemtob, C. T., Gloria, R., Killeen, A., & Jackson, T. (2003, May). *Impact of the World Trade Center attacks on the New York Police Department.* Paper presented at the annual meeting of the American Psychiatric Association, San Francisco.

Marmar, C. R., Weiss, D. S., & Metzler, T. J. (1998). Peritraumatic dissociation and posttraumatic stress disorder. In J. D. Bremner & C. R. Marmar (Eds.), *Trauma, memory, and dissociation* (pp. 229–252). Washington, DC: American Psychiatric Association.

Marmar, C. R., Weiss, D. S., Metzler, T. J., & Delucchi, K. (1996). Characteristics of emergency services personnel related to peritraumatic dissociation during critical incident exposure. *American Journal of Psychiatry, 153*, 94–102.

Marmar, C. R., Weiss, D. S., Metzler, T. J., Delucchi, K., Best, S. R., & Wentworth, K. A. (1999). Longitudinal course and predictors of continuing distress following critical incident exposure in emergency services personnel. *Journal of Nervous and Mental Disease, 187*, 15–22.

Marmar, C. R., Weiss, D. S., Metzler, T. J., & Ronfeldt, H. M. (1994, January). *Peritraumatic dissociation and posttraumatic stress after the Northridge earthquake.* Paper presented at the annual meeting of the Anxiety Disorders of America, Santa Monica, CA.

Marmar, C. R., Weiss, D. S., Metzler, T. J., Ronfeldt, H. M., & Foreman, C. (1996). Stress responses of emergency services personnel to the Loma Prieta earthquake Interstate 880 freeway collapse and control traumatic incidents. *Journal of Traumatic Stress, 9*, 63–85.

Marmar, C. R., Weiss, D. S., & Pynoos, R. S. (1995). Dynamic psychotherapy of posttraumatic stress disorder. In M. J. Friedman, D. S. Charney, & A. Y. Deutch (Eds.), *Neurobiological and clinical consequences of stress: From normal adaptation to posttraumatic stress disorder.* Philadelphia: Lippincott Williams & Wilkins.

Marmar, C. R., Weiss, D. S., Schlenger, W. E., Fairbank, J. A., Jordan, B.K., Kulka, R. A., & Hough, R. L. (1994). Peritraumatic dissociation and posttraumatic stress in male Vietnam theater veterans. *American Journal of Psychiatry, 151*, 902–907.

Marshall, G. N., & Schell, T. L. (2002). Reappraising the link between peritraumatic dissociation and PTSD symptom severity: Evidence from a longitudinal study of community violence survivors. *Journal of Abnormal Psychology, 111*, 626–636.

Mellman, T. A., David, D., Bustamante, V., Fins, A. I., & Esposito, K. (2001). Predictors of posttraumatic stress disorder following severe injury. *Depression and Anxiety, 14*, 226–231.

Moleman, N., van der Hart, O., & van der Kolk, B. A. (1992). Dissociation and hypnotizability in posttraumatic stress disorder. *Journal of Nervous and Mental Disease, 180*, 271–272.

Nemiah, J. C. (1985). Dissociative disorders. In H. I. Kaplan & B. J. Sadock (Eds.), *Comprehensive textbook of psychiatry* (4th ed., pp. 942–957). Baltimore: Williams & Wilkins.

Nemiah, J. C. (1998). Early concepts of trauma, dissociation, and the unconscious: Their history and current implications. In D. Bremner & C. R. Marmar (Eds.), *Trauma, memory, and dissociation* (pp. 1–26). Washington, DC: American Psychiatric Association.

Noyes, R., & Kletti, R. (1977). Depersonalization in response to life-threatening danger. *Comparative Psychiatry, 18*, 375–384.

Ogata, S. N., Silk, K. R., Goodrich, S., Lohr, N. E., Westen, D., & Hill, E. M. (1990). Childhood sexual and physical abuse in adult patients with borderline personality disorder. *American Journal of Psychiatry, 147*, 1008–1013.

Orr, S. P., Metzger, L. J., Lasko, N. B., Macklin, M. L., Peri, T., & Pitman, R. K. (2000). De novo conditioning in trauma-exposed individuals with and without posttraumatic stress disorder. *Journal of Abnormal Psychology, 109*, 290–298.

Pitman, R. K., Sanders, K. M., Zusman, R. M., Healy, A. R., Cheema, F., Lasko, N. B., et al. (2002). Pilot study of secondary prevention of posttraumatic stress disorder with propranolol. *Biological Psychiatry, 51*, 189–192.

Putnam, F. W. (1989). Pierre Janet and modern views of dissociation. *Journal of Traumatic Stress, 2*, 413–429.

Putnam, F. W., Guroff, J. J., Silberman, E. K., Barban, L., & Post, R. M. (1986). The clinical phenomenology of multiple personality disorder: Review of 100 recent cases. *Journal of Clinical Psychiatry, 47*, 285–293.

Putnam, F. W., Helmers, K., Horowitz, L. A., & Trickett, P. K. (1995). Hypnotizability and dissociativity in sexually abused girls. *Child Abuse and Neglect, 19*, 645–655.

Shalev, A. Y., Peri, T., Canetti, L., & Schreiber, S. (1996). Predictors of PTSD in injured trauma survivors: A prospective study. *American Journal of Psychiatry, 153*, 219–225.

Shalev, A. Y., Sahar, T., Freedman, S., Peri, T., Glick, N., Brandes, D., et al. (1998). A prospective study of heart rate response following trauma and the subsequent development of posttraumatic stress disorder. *Archives of General Psychiatry, 55*, 553–559.

Siegel, R. K. (1984). Hostage hallucinations. *Journal of Nervous and Mental Disease, 172*, 264–272.

Southwick, S. M., Bremner, J. D., Rasmusson, A., Morgan, C. A., III, Arnsten, A., & Charney, D. S. (1999). Role of norepinephrine in the pathophysiology and treatment of posttraumatic stress disorder. *Biological Psychiatry, 46*, 1192–1204.

Southwick, S. M., Krystal, J. H., Morgan, C. A., Johnson, D., Nagy, L. M., Niculaou, A., et al. (1993). Abnormal noradrenergic functioning posttraumatic stress disorder. *Archives of General Psychiatry, 50*, 266–274.

Spiegel, D. (1993). Dissociation and trauma. In D. Speigel (Ed.), *Dissociative disorders: A clinical review*. Lutherville, MD: Sidran Press.

Spiegel, D., Hunt, T., & Dondershine, H. E. (1988). Dissociation and hypnotizability in posttraumatic stress disorder. *American Journal of Psychiatry, 145*, 301–305.

Spiegel, H., & Spiegel, D. (1978). *Trance and treatment: Clinical uses of hypnosis*. New York: Basic Books.

Steinman, I. (1994, November). *Psychodynamic treatment of multiple personality disorder*. Paper presented at the annual meeting of the International Society for Traumatic Stress Studies, Chicago, IL.

Stutman, R. K., & Bliss, E. L. (1985). Posttraumatic stress disorder, hypnotizability and imagery. *American Journal of Psychiatry, 142*, 741–743.

Tichenor, V., Marmar, C. R., Weiss, D. S., Metzler, T. J., & Ronfeldt, H. M. (1996). The relationship of peritraumatic dissociation and posttraumatic stress: Findings in female Vietnam theater veterans. *Journal of Consulting and Clinical Psychology, 64*, 1054–1059.

Ursano, R. J., Fullerton, C. S., Epstein, R. S., Crowley, B., Vance, K., Kao, T. C., & Baum, A. (1999). Peritraumatic dissociation and posttraumatic stress disorder following motor vehicle accidents. *American Journal of Psychiatry, 156*, 1808–1810.

Vaiva, G., Duqcrocq, F., Jezequel, K., Brunet, A., & Marmar, C. R. (2003), Immediate treatment with propranolol decreases PTSD two months after trauma. *Biological Psychiatry, 54*, 947–949.

van der Hart, O., & Spiegel, D. (1993). Hypnotic assessment and treatment of trauma-induced psychoses: The early psychotherapy of H. Breuknik and modern views. *International Journal of Clinical and Experimental Hypnosis, 41*, 191–209.

van der Kolk, B. A., & van der Hart, O. (1989a). Pierre Janet on posttraumatic stress. *Journal of Traumatic Stress, 2*, 265–278.

van der Kolk, B. A., & van der Hart, O. (1989b). Pierre Janet and the breakdown of adaptation in psychological trauma. *American Journal of Psychiatry, 146*, 1530–1540.

Weiss, D. S., Marmar, C. R., Metzler, T. J., & Ronfeldt, H. M. (1995). Predicting symptomatic distress in emergency services personnel. *Journal of Consulting and Clinical Psychology, 63*(3), 361–368.

Wilkinson, C. B. (1983). Aftermath of a disaster: The collapse of the Hyatt Regency Hotel skywalks. *American Journal of Psychiatry, 140*, 1134–1139.

CHAPTER 7

The Impact of Event Scale—Revised

DANIEL S. WEISS

Even though posttraumatic stress disorder (PTSD) was not introduced into the world psychiatric nomenclature until 1978 with the publication of the *International Classification of Diseases, Ninth Revised Edition* (ICD-9; World Health Organization) and the American psychiatric nomenclature until 1980 with the publication of the *Diagnostic and Statistical Manual of Mental Disorders, Third Edition* (DSM-III, American Psychiatric Association), there was already clear recognition of the typical symptomatic response to exposure to traumatic life events (e.g., Horowitz, 1976). The pith of the disorder was the distressing oscillation between intrusion and avoidance. Intrusion was characterized by nightmares, unbidden visual images of the trauma or its aftermath, unbidden thoughts about aspects of the traumatic event, and variations thereof. Avoidance was exemplified by effortful attempts not to think about the event, not to talk about, and to avoid reminders of it, as well as more active attempts to push it out of mind by increasing use of alcohol or drugs, overworking, and other strategies that would divert attention or so exhaust someone that he or she would be spared the intrusive phenomenology. In addition to the frank avoidance, Horowitz (1975; Horowitz & Kaltreider, 1977) also described emotional numbing as a not uncommon sequel to exposure to a traumatic life event. Empirical evidence supporting three of these four phenomena has recently appeared (King, Leskin, King, & Weathers, 1998) in analyses of the most commonly used structured clinical interview for PTSD, the Clinician-Administered PTSD Scale (CAPS; see Weathers, Keane, & Davidson, 2001).

ORIGINAL IMPACT OF EVENT SCALE

In 1979, before DSM-III, Horowitz and colleagues (Horowitz, Wilner, & Alvarez, 1979) published a short self-report measure for assessing the degree of symptomatic response to a specific traumatic exposure as it was manifested in the previous 7 days; it was modestly titled the Impact of Event Scale (IES). (Sadly, many citations and publications using the IES have used the plural of "event," designating it the Impact of Events [sic] Scale, perhaps because when the name of the scale is spoken one cannot easily distinguish between singular and plural. This misnomer has influenced bibliographic information to an unknown extent.) Drawing from his understanding of the response to traumatic stressors, Horowitz (1976) considered responses in the realm of intrusion and avoidance as the primary domains of measurement, noting that measurement of this response had primarily been confined either to experimental physiological measures such as galvanic skin responses or to self-reports on general measures of anxiety, such as the MMPI-derived Taylor Manifest Anxiety Scale (Taylor, 1953).

The original IES loosely assessed the B and C criteria of the diagnosis of PTSD, the signs and symptoms of intrusive cognitions and affects together or oscillating with periods of avoidance, denial, or blocking of thoughts and images. The scale comprised two subscales: Intrusion (the sum of 7 items) and Avoidance (the sum of 8 items). The scale used a somewhat unusual response format: Not at all = 0, Rarely = 1, Sometimes = 3, and Often = 5.

In the initial report of the measure (Horowitz et al., 1979), data supported the existence of homogeneous clusters of items characterized by intrusion and avoidance (Cronbach's [1951] alpha for intrusion = .79, for avoidance = .82). The correlations between subscales of .42 was small enough (only 18% of the variance) to allow for substantial independence of the item subscales. The test–retest reliability in the original study was satisfactory, with coefficients of .87 for intrusion and .79 for avoidance.

CONSTRUCT VALIDATION OF THE IES

Zilberg, Weiss, and Horowitz (1982) conducted an in-depth replication and cross-validation of the psychometric characteristics of the Impact of Event Scale and the accompanying conceptual model of responses to traumatic stress that had given rise to its development. They studied outpatients with pathological grief and compared them to a group who had also experienced the death of a parent but had not sought treatment. Both groups were evaluated at three time points.

The results revealed that all items were endorsed frequently, ranging from 44% to 89% of the pooled sample. This replicated the high relevance of the item pool for responses to traumatic stress. The rank order of items based on frequency of endorsement in the parental-bereavement patient groups was compared with the rank order reported in the initial publication of the IES. A Spearman rank correlation (Spearman, 1904) of .86 ($p < .001$) was obtained. This result suggested that the content of experience following traumatic events as represented in the IES item pool was similar across types of events and patient versus nonpatient populations.

To assess the item assignments to the Intrusion and Avoidance subscales, a factor analysis was conducted. Two factors were extracted using a principal-factors procedure with a varimax rotation. In the case of all items, the loading on its hypothesized factor was higher than it was on the other factor. This was taken as evidence of the coherence of the two subscale item sets. Reliability data were also reported in this cross-validation study. Coefficients of internal consistency were reported for both subscales for all three time points for the two groups both separately and combined. These coefficients ranged from .79 to .92.

This study carefully examined the structure of the relationship between the Intrusion and Avoidance subscales in order to clarify whether a total score or the reporting of subscale scores was preferable. The authors argued that, if the data had produced correlations of the order of .40–.60 in all six of the time-by-group conditions, it would have been difficult to maintain separate subscale scoring solely on empirical grounds. The empirical findings and a conceptual rationale converged to suggest that separate scores be retained. In five of the six conditions, the subscales were substantially correlated, ranging from .57 to .78. There was one striking exception: The patient sample at the pretherapy evaluation point produced a coefficient of only .15. These data suggested that it was potentially misleading to use only a total score.

UPDATE ON PSYCHOMETRICS OF THE ORIGINAL IES AND LITERATURE

Sundin and Horowitz (2002) recently presented an updated status report on the psychometric properties of the original IES, concentrating on published research using the scale. They presented nonweighted averages for coefficient alpha across 18 studies and reported, for Intrusion, alpha = .86, and, for Avoidance, alpha = .82.

Sundin and Horowitz (2002) also presented estimates of stability over time, finding that the longer the time interval, the lower the estimates; but no coefficient was below .51. Not considered was the overall level of symptoms of the different samples, an issue raised by Zilberg et al. (1982); nor was this issue considered when they reported a nonweighted average correlation of the two subscales of .63 (accounting for 40% of the variance) across 18 studies. Evidence that this issue is salient appeared in the review of factor analyses of the 15 items. In these 12 studies, it appeared that only 7 supported the two-factor structure, with 3 obtaining three factors (avoidance and numbing are separate), and 2 finding only a single factor. The latter is what would be expected from samples in which the proportion of those having significant symptomatology is low, a matter described in more detail elsewhere (Weiss, Chapter 4, this volume). A summary of 18 studies presented the correlations between a variety of other measures of symptoms and intrusion and avoidance. Most were appropriate, though it appeared that divergent validity is an issue that requires further study, as the correlations with general symptoms were larger than the average relationship of the two subscales (Sundin & Horowitz, 2002).

The original IES has been the most widely used self-report measure of stress response or PTSD symptoms of reexperiencing and numbing and avoidance. As of May 2001, the PILOTS database reported its use in 1,147 studies; the next most frequent measure was the Beck Depression Inventory (Beck, Ward, Mendelson, Mock, & Erbaugh, 1961). The next most frequent measure of PTSD symptoms was the Mississippi Scale for Combat-Related PTSD (MCS; Keane, Caddell, & Taylor, 1988), with fewer than half of the citations. A search of PsycINFO that targeted only empirical studies revealed 515 citations. Unfortunately, it is not possible to determine, without actually reviewing each article, whether data using the IES were collected or whether it was the IES, not the IES-R, that was actually used in either database in studies after 1996 (see the next section). Despite these minor concerns, it is clear that the IES has made an extremely valuable contribution to the field.

THE INITIAL PILOT WORK ON THE IMPACT OF EVENT SCALE—REVISED

Despite the usefulness of the original IES, complete assessment of the responses to traumatic events required tracking of responses in the domain of hyperarousal symptoms. Beginning with data from a longitudinal study of the response of emergency service personnel to traumatic events, including the Loma Prieta earthquake (e.g., Weiss, Marmar, Metzler, & Ronfeldt, 1995), a set of 7 additional items, with 6 to tap the domain of hyperarousal and 1 to parallel the DSM-III-R (now DSM-IV) diagnostic criteria for PTSD, were developed, piloted, and used. These additional 7 items were interspersed with the existing 7 Intrusion and 8 Avoidance items of the original IES using a table of random numbers to establish placement. The Impact of Event Scale—Revised (IES-R) comprises these 22 items and was originally presented in Weiss and Marmar (1997).

An important consideration in the construction of the revised IES was to maintain comparability with the original version of the measure as much as was possible. Consequently, the 1-week time frame to which the instructions refer in measuring symptomatic response was retained, as was the original scoring scheme of frequency—0, 1, 3, and 5 for the responses of "Not at all," "Rarely," "Sometimes," and "Often." The only modification to the original items that was made was to change the item "I had trouble falling asleep or staying asleep" from its double-barreled status into two separate items. The first is simply "I had trouble staying asleep," and, because of a somewhat higher correlation between it and the remaining intrusion items, it was assigned to represent the original item in the Intrusion subscale. The second item, "I had trouble falling asleep," was assigned to the new Hyperarousal subscale because of its somewhat higher correlation with the other Hyperarousal items, its somewhat lower correlation with the Intrusion items, and its more apparent link with hyperarousal than with intrusion. The six new items comprising the Hyperarousal subscale target the following domains: anger and irritability; jumpiness and exaggerated startle response; trouble concentrating; psychophysiological arousal on exposure to reminders; and hypervigilance. As mentioned, the one new Intrusion item taps the dissociative-like reexperiencing captured in true flashback-like experiences. Weiss and Marmar (1997) present an extensive summary of the internal consistency of the three subscales, all of which were strong; the pattern of item–total correlations; test–retest stability, which was also satisfactory; and communality of the interitem correlations.

Based on the experience with those data, considerations of the insufficiency of frequency as a completely summarizing marker for self-report, and the over weighting of responses of "sometimes" and "often" in the scoring scheme, the following changes were incorporated into the IES-R.

1. The directions were modified so that the respondent is not asked about the frequency of symptoms in the previous 7 days but is instead asked to report the *degree of distress* of the symptom in the previous 7 days.
2. The response format was modified to a 0–4 response format with equal rather than unequal intervals: 0 = Not at all; 1 = A little bit; 2 = Moderately; 3 = Quite a bit; 4 = Extremely.
3. The subscale scoring was changed from the sum of the responses to the mean of the responses, allowing the user to immediately identify the degree of symptomatology merely by examining the subscale scores, as they are presented in the same metric as the item responses—something the original scale did not do.

These changes brought the IES-R into parallel format with the SCL-90-R (Derogatis, 1994), allowing for direct comparison of endorsement of symptom levels across these two instruments. (The complete set of items, instructions, and scoring scheme appear in the appendix to this chapter.)

INTERNATIONAL WORK ON THE IES-R

The IES-R has been of sufficient interest to scholars worldwide to have been translated into many languages. Published translations exist in Chinese (Wu & Chan, 2003), French (Brunet, St.-Hilaire, Jehel, & King, 2003), German (Maercker & Schuetzwohl, 1998), Japanese (Asukai et al., 2002), and Spanish (Baguena et al., 2001). Unpublished versions exist in Dutch (S. Bal, personal communication, September 23, 1998) and Italian (Giannantonio, 2003).

Internal Consistency

A representative presentation of the basic psychometric characteristics of the IES-R translations showed considerable consistency. In the French version, for example, coefficient alpha was .86 for the Intrusion and Avoidance subscales and .81 for the Hyperarousal subscale. For the Chinese version, the corresponding coefficients were .89, .85, and .83. The Japanese version presented coefficients for four different samples: Intrusion (.91, .88, .89, and .91), Avoidance (.88, .81, .84, and .90), and Hyperarousal (.86, .80, .80, and .86). In the aggregate, as well as individually, all the coefficients reveal considerable subscale homogeneity.

Test–Retest Stability

The data regarding stability, a far more important characteristic of reliability than internal consistency, were also consistent and positive. The French translation reported $r = .73$ for the Intrusion subscale, $r = .77$ for the Avoidance subscale, and $r = .71$ for the Hyperarousal subscale. The Chinese translation presented these data: $r = .74$ for Intrusion, $r = .52$ for Avoidance, and $r = .76$ for Hyperarousal. The data collected for the Japanese translation did not examine stability in as differentiated an approach as would have been most desirable. Instead of examining each subscale separately, Asukai et al. (2002) examined only the total score of the three subscales and opted to report a Spearman (1904) rank-order correlation. In a sample of 114 participants, the data yielded $r_s = .86$.

Scale Intercorrelations

Zilberg et al. (1982) showed that the correlations of intrusion and avoidance in the original IES varied as a function of time elapsed since the traumatic event and level of symptomatology. Though the data from the French and Chinese translations (the Japanese translation did not present these data) could not address the correlations in this differentiated manner, they did, nonetheless, report the subscale correlations. In the French version, the correlation of the Intrusion subscale with Avoidance was $r = .62$, and with Hyperarousal was $r = .69$. The correlation of Avoidance with Hyperarousal was $r = .56$. The analogous data in the Chinese version were $r = .76$, $r = .83$, and $r = .75$.

A SAMPLING OF SUBSEQUENT USE OF THE IES-R

Overview

A substantial amount of new data collection using the IES-R has occurred since its appearance in 1997, over and above the translations. More than 70 citations link to IES-R in the PsycINFO database (e.g., Kimerling et al., 1999; Stein & Kennedy, 2001). Regrettably, at the current time the PILOTS database does not index the IES and the IES-R separately. As of this writing, for example, about 25% of the most recent records indexed under the IES in fact employed the IES-R. Subsequently, the PILOTS database has not been an appropriate resource to delineate the scope of the use of the IES-R. If this is rectified in the near future, PILOTS will be the database of choice for searching the literature regarding the IES-R.

It is valuable to present additional relevant empirical data regarding the properties of the IES-R, extending the evidence base supporting the basic psychometric properties of the measure. These findings derive from a study of the impact of traumatic events on a large sample of police officers and a comparison sample.[1] A much more detailed description of the study samples can be found in several studies published from these data (Brunet, Weiss, et al., 2001; Liberman et al., 2002; Pole, Best, Weiss, & Marmar, 2001), but in brief the samples comprised approximately 700 police officers from Oakland, San Jose, and New York and approximately 300 comparison participants similar in age and gender nominated by each officer. In addition to being administered the IES-R about their most distressing traumatic event, officers and their counterparts completed a battery including but not limited to the Mississippi Scale for Combat-Related PTSD, Civilian Version (MCSCV; Keane et al., 1988; Lauterbach, Vrana, King, & King, 1997); SCL-90-R; the Peritraumatic Dissociative Experiences Questionnaire (PDEQ; Marmar, Weiss, & Metzler, 1997); the Peritraumatic Distress Inventory (PDI; Brunet, Weiss, et al., 2001), and the Michigan Alcohol Screening Test (MAST; Selzer, 1971)

Basic Psychometrics

Estimates of internal consistency using coefficient alpha were these: Intrusion alpha = .89, Avoidance alpha = .84, and Hyperarousal alpha = .82, all values showing high uniformity. The average item-total subscale correlations were $r = .52$, $r = .40$, and $r = .45$, respectively. The subscale intercorrelations were similar to but somewhat higher than those reported for the translated ver-

[1] These data were collected with the support of a National Institute of Mental Health grant, Charles R. Marmar, Principal Investigator, Daniel S. Weiss, Co-Principal Investigator.

sions: Intrusion with Avoidance, $r = .71$; Intrusion with Hyperarousal, $r = .81$; and Avoidance with Hyperarousal $r = .65$. These higher coefficients are likely due to the very low base rate of symptoms in both the police samples and the counterpart group. In these data, test–retest data were not collected on the full sample.

The coefficients describing convergent and divergent validity were computed, as were several approaches to describing the communality of the item set. The correlation between the MCSCV and the three subscales of the IES-R were these: Intrusion, $r = .53$; Avoidance, $r = .55$; and Hyperarousal, $r = .57$, showing strong convergent relationships. By contrast, the analogous correlations with the MAST were $r = .09$, $r = .13$, and $r = .09$, showing strong divergent relationships, as there is no reason that symptoms should relate to the propensity toward alcohol abuse. The set of correlations between the three IES-R subscales and the PDEQ, PDI, and the Depression and Global Symptom Index (GSI) scores of the SCL-90 ranged from a low of $r = .31$ for the coefficient between the PDEQ and Hyperarousal to a high of $r = .50$ for the coefficient of Hyperarousal and the GSI of the SCL-90-R. These data make two points. First, the overall pattern is consistent with the validity of the subscales—highest correlations with another measure of PTSD symptoms, lowest correlations with a conceptually unrelated measure, and midrange correlations between variables that should be somewhat related to symptom levels. Second, among the three subscales, in these data at least, the Hyperarousal subscale shows the most differentiated pattern of the three subscales, something that the original scale could not uncover.

EXPLORING HOW THE IES-R ITEMS COHERE

Conceptual Issues

As described previously, an important aspect of the psychometrics of a measure is the communality of its items, typically expressed by the results of a factor analysis. Such results are regularly taken as dispositive of the structure of the measure, with considerably less attention given to the specific methods used in any one analysis or the sample studied. Nevertheless, any result from a factor analysis needs to be interpreted as one among several potential outcomes, outcomes that may or may not converge and lead to similar conclusions. The main goal of factor analysis is to determine more basic information about what goes with what in a set of variables, whether these variables are subscales of an IQ test, a set of measures of therapeutic outcome (e.g., symptoms, social functioning, quality of life), each from the perspective of patient, therapist, and independent evaluator (see, e.g., Strupp & Hadley, 1977) from a treatment trial, or the set of IES-R items. The conclusions one draws regarding the results of a factor analysis depend on a number of factors (see Kim & Mueller, 1978; Tinsley & Tinsley, 1987), all of which potentially modify conclusions but are often glossed over in many presentations, frequently at the request of journal editors who want to conserve precious page space. An important distinction is whether the variables being subjected to an analysis are themselves composites of other variables (e.g., the subscales of the SCL-90-R, each of which have an alpha coefficient of internal consistency) or are themselves the components that form a composite (e.g., the IES-R items, each of which by definition cannot have an alpha coefficient of internal consistency, as it is a single variable). What it means for factor analysis to partition the variability within a variable across the underlying factors is different for composite variables compared with component variables. Thus, although the assumption is that each of the IES-R items has common and unique variance, their unique variance is more likely error than conceptually meaningful variability. Thus, even though the SCL-90-R Depression and Anxiety subscales have common variance, the unique variance is more likely a combination of conceptually meaningful and error variability rather than just the latter. The interpretation of results of factor analyses of the IES-R items needs to take this issue into account.

As well, the extraction method may lead to different results and conclusions. Principal components assumes a reliability of 1.00 and is best understood as an exact mathematical representation of the data set being analyzed, whereas principal factors is targeted to discovering underlying hypothetical structures. A varimax rotation (Kaiser, 1958) requires that the factors be uncorrelated and attempts to assign as much variability of each item as possible to only one factor, so that one set defines the first factor, a second set the second, and so forth. An oblique rotation (Jennrich & Sampson, 1966) allows the resulting factors to be correlated. Obviously, in the IES-R, it is quite reasonable to presume that the underlying factors, whatever they are, are correlated rather than uncorrelated.

International Data

The data from the French translation were subjected to a principal components analysis, and the solution was rotated using the varimax technique. The results of Brunet and colleagues were not definitive. Both a two-factor and a three-factor solution were interpretable. The two-factor solution comprised an Avoidance factor and a combined Intrusion-Arousal factor, similar to the structure found in the Spanish translation data (Baguena et al., 2001). The three-factor solution replicated the three symptom criteria of PTSD: Hyperarousal, Avoidance, and Intrusion. Item loadings (the correlation of the item with the score on the factor) for the set of 22 items were almost completely coherent with each item loading most strongly on its own scale, though there were instances of low communality (the item did not go with any of the others in these data).

In contrast, the Chinese data yielded a single strong factor that accounted for 45% of the variability in the item set. In another contrast, Maercker and Schuetzwohl (1998) concluded that the German data were most consistent with a four-factor result, yielding factors of Intrusion, Avoidance, Hyperarousal, and Numbing, the same result found for the CAPS by King and his colleagues (1998).

The Japanese data used a kind of factor analysis termed "Varclus," marketed by the SAS Institute (1999), that attempts to find groups of variables that are as correlated as possible among themselves and as uncorrelated as possible with variables in other clusters. The key difference is that all variables start in a single cluster, and additional clusters are formed based on parameters set by the user. The paper reporting the Japanese data did not report the extraction method (principal components versus centroid) and forced a three-cluster solution. Nevertheless, for completeness of presentation, the cluster analysis of the Japanese data are presented. The results suggested that a model comprising three clusters of items fit those data best: an intrusion–hyperarousal cluster, an avoidance cluster, and a third cluster of numbing and sleep and cognitive distress. These clusters are not orthogonal. The correlation of cluster 1 and 2 was $r = .74$, of 1 and 3 was $r = .73$, and of 2 and 3 was $r = .62$. These correlations are of roughly the same magnitude as the regular subscales reported previously.

Police and Comparison Group Data

A series of factor analyses was undertaken to explore the communality of the set of 22 IES-R items in this data set, comprising 994 observations after missing data were eliminated. Two extraction and two rotation methods were used in four combinations: (1) principal components (PC) with varimax rotation; (2) principal factors (PF) with varimax rotation; (3) PC with oblique (correlated factors possible) rotation; and (4) PF with oblique rotation. The extraction yielded three eigenvalues greater than 1.0, but as with the data from the French translation, a two-factor solution was also a reasonable model given the percentages of variance accounted for and the scree plot. As well, given the variety of results described previously, presentation of two- and three-factor solutions seems informative and prudent. The first factor accounted for 44% of the variance, the second 7%, and the third 5%. Items with loadings ≥ .40 on more than one factor were singled out for special note, and this item-to-factor correlation was also used to interpret the factors.

In both the PC and PF two-factor varimax solutions (see Tables 7.1 and 7.2), the first factor comprised all six of the Hyperarousal subscale items, with no item having a loading on the second factor. Also loading only on the first factor were five of the eight Intrusion subscale items. Items 1, 9, and 14 were split between the first and second factors. In the PF analysis, the remainder of the second factor was defined by six of the seven Avoidance subscale items. Item 7 failed to load on either factor in this solution. In the PC analysis, item 7 showed a loading of .43 on the second factor.

The oblique rotation solutions for both factor extraction methods improved the separation of items to factors, not surprising as the constructs are

TABLE 7.1. Loadings from Principal Components Extraction

	Varimax		Oblimin	
Item	I	II	I	II
Reminder brought back feelings	.577	.406	.542	.230
Trouble staying asleep	.755	.117	.863	–.187
Things made me think about it	.725	.287	.764	.026
Felt irritable and angry	.637	.307	.651	.088
Avoided letting myself get upset	.129	.534	–.043	.575
Thought when didn't mean to	.647	.364	.641	.151
Felt hadn't happened, wasn't real	.283	.427	.181	.381
Stayed away from reminders	.184	.749	–.057	.804
Pictures popped into my mind	.595	.407	.563	.224
Jumpy and easily startled	.635	.246	.671	.017
Tried not to think about it	.218	.739	–.012	.777
Aware of feelings but didn't deal with them	.463	.600	.334	.508
Feelings were kind of numb	.297	.547	.154	.517
Acting/feeling like back at that time	.552	.410	.511	.246
Trouble falling asleep	.743	.090	.858	–.214
Waves of strong feelings	.704	.356	.713	.116
Tried to remove it from memory	.294	.692	.097	.689
Trouble concentrating	.710	.273	.751	.016
Psychophysiological reactions	.608	.300	.618	.092
Dreams about it	.660	.255	.697	.016
Watchful and on guard	.487	.326	.463	.175
Tried not to talk about it	.248	.712	.034	.734

related. In these solutions, the pattern of loadings was identical. In this case, however, item 7 failed to load on either factor for either extraction method. In the PF analysis the resulting factors correlated $r = .69$; in the PC analysis, $r = .61$.

Tables 7.3 and 7.4 present the results when three factors were extracted and rotated. For the most part, in the varimax rotations, the pattern of loadings for factors 1 and 2 were similar to those in the two-factor solutions. In the PC solution, the third factor comprised both sleep items loading only on this factor, with items 18, 19, and 20 splitting loadings on this and the first factor. By contrast, in the PF solution, the third factor was loaded by only the two sleep items and a split loading of item 18. Though there were also small differences between these two results, the major outcome to note is that the hypervigilance item (21) did not load at all in only the PC analysis; but although it did load on factor 1 in the PF analysis, in the latter, items 5 and 7 did not load on any of the three factors.

In both the three-factor oblique solutions, the PC and PF extractions yielded more dissimilar results. In both, the third factor was fairly clearly defined. In the PC solution, it was defined only by items 19–22, whereas in the PF solution it was clearly defined by items 2, 15 (sleep items), 18 (trouble concentrating), and 20 (dreaming). The PC solution was more simple: Factor 1 was defined by items 1–9 (which loaded exclusively on this factor) and by a split loading of item 16 (waves of feeling). The second factor was loaded by 11–15, 17, and the split item 16. By contrast, in the PF solution, the first factor was defined by item 12 (shared with the second factor) and items 1, 3, 4, 6, 9, 10, 14, 16, and 19. The second factor was defined by items 5, 8, 11, 13, 17, and 22, with the other part of item 12. In the PF solution, the correlations among the three factors were these: 1 and 2, $r = .71$; 1 and 3, $r = .56$; and 2 and 3, $r = .38$. The analogous data for the PC solution were $r = .62$, $r = .56$, and $r = .32$, all somewhat lower.

The main point of these analyses is to demonstrate that conclusions about the communality or underlying structure of a set of variables analyzed by the

TABLE 7.2. Loadings from Principal Axis Extraction

Item	Varimax		Oblimin	
	I	II	I	II
Reminder brought back feelings	.553	.405	.525	.209
Trouble staying asleep	.704	.169	.833	–.173
Things made me think about it	.696	.311	.754	.011
Felt irritable and angry	.597	.331	.616	.091
Avoided letting myself get upset	.188	.411	.049	.417
Thought when didn't mean to	.620	.375	.625	.134
Felt hadn't happened, wasn't real	.294	.365	.208	.300
Stayed away from reminders	.200	.690	–.069	.764
Pictures popped into my mind	.565	.416	.535	.216
Jumpy and easily startled	.573	.293	.604	.056
Tried not to think about it	.233	.682	–.022	.736
Aware of feelings but didn't deal with them	.453	.582	.311	.488
Feelings were kind of numb	.313	.479	.179	.435
Acting/feeling like back at that time	.516	.421	.470	.249
Trouble falling asleep	.682	.152	.812	–.183
Waves of strong feelings	.673	.381	.692	.112
Tried to remove it from memory	.300	.647	.082	.654
Trouble concentrating	.666	.311	.715	.028
Psychophysiological reactions	.553	.336	.556	.122
Dreams about it	.605	.297	.644	.043
Watchful and on guard	.444	.338	.415	.183
Tried not to talk about it	.258	.661	.021	.695

TABLE 7.3. Loadings from Principal Components Extraction

	Varimax			Oblimin		
Item	I	II	III	I	II	III
Reminder brought back feelings	.730	.278	.123	.835	.022	–.140
Trouble staying asleep	.272	.152	.804	.801	–.089	.113
Things made me think about it	.712	.183	.339	.752	.017	.031
Felt irritable and angry	.639	.214	.290	.750	.064	–.046
Avoided letting myself get upset	.239	.498	–.006	.704	–.020	.080
Thought when didn't mean to	.684	.260	.264	.673	.105	–.035
Felt hadn't happened, wasn't real	.273	.400	.167	.655	.054	.186
Stayed away from reminders	.238	.730	.094	.558	–.014	.223
Pictures popped into my mind	.682	.297	.197	.408	.114	.296
Jumpy and easily startled	.533	.184	.387	.338	.178	.196
Tried not to think about it	.180	.743	.199	–.060	.808	.053
Aware of feelings but didn't deal with them	.486	.539	.226	–.149	.800	.238
Feelings were kind of numb	.382	.492	.090	–.055	.777	.095
Acting/feeling like back at that time	.626	.312	.194	.041	.771	–.078
Trouble falling asleep	.197	.146	.859	.142	.496	–.153
Waves of strong feelings	.633	.277	.395	.405	.435	.013
Tried to remove it from memory	.129	.723	.352	.312	.425	–.094
Trouble concentrating	.442	.252	.586	.186	.359	.038
Psychophysiological reactions	.447	.263	.439	.039	.068	.848
Dreams about it	.416	.234	.540	.147	.045	.763
Watchful and on guard	.385	.291	.333	.376	.100	.459
Tried not to talk about it	.183	.720	.236	.358	.090	.419

broad family of techniques of factor analysis should be examined soberly and with considerable caution. The discussion of a set of results needs always to appreciate that the particular results may or may not be replicated by subsequent research or may not be replicating previous research. In neither case is it typically clear what the lack of convergence actually indicates.

CONTINUING ISSUES IN THE USE OF THE IES-R

Event

The IES-R was designed and validated using a specific traumatic event as the reference in the directions to individuals completing the measure. Any use of the measure requires that this issue be made explicit by the person administering the measure and that respondents are clear about what specific event they are reporting on. Events such as "the automobile accident," "the earthquake," "the sexual assault," "the rescue effort at the WTC on 9/11," are all appropriate events. It is not appropriate to use the IES-R to measure such things as "stress on the job," "my divorce," "my boss's criticism," and the like. For specific questions on this issue, refer to the discussion in DSM-IV (American Psychiatric Association, 1994) on the event (p. 424) and the specific language of criterion A for posttraumatic stress disorder (pp. 427–428) and for acute stress disorder (p. 431).

There is some controversy about whether such events as receiving a diagnosis of breast cancer or finding out one is HIV positive is an example of a traumatic event. Individual researchers need to make their own decisions about this and be able to provide a rationale for how it fits the description in DSM. As well, many researchers desire to broaden the referent from a specific event to a class of events: for example, "my abuse as a child," "my service in

TABLE 7.4. Loadings from Principal Axes Extraction

	Varimax			Oblimin		
Item	I	II	III	I	II	III
Reminder brought back feelings	.645	.306	.141	.835	.022	–.140
Trouble staying asleep	.359	.185	.714	.147	.045	.763
Things made me think about it	.688	.223	.295	.801	–.089	.113
Felt irritable and angry	.599	.260	.239	.704	–.020	.080
Avoided letting myself get upset	.221	.383	.074	.142	.496	–.153
Thought when didn't mean to	.638	.293	.241	.752	.017	.031
Felt hadn't happened, wasn't real	.287	.339	.148	.186	.359	.038
Stayed away from reminders	.263	.659	.070	.041	.771	–.078
Pictures popped into my mind	.628	.328	.173	.750	.064	–.046
Jumpy and easily startled	.535	.243	.268	.558	–.014	.223
Tried not to think about it	.225	.680	.155	–.060	.808	.053
Aware of feelings but didn't deal with them	.479	.528	.187	.405	.435	.013
Feelings were kind of numb	.354	.435	.111	.312	.425	–.094
Acting/feeling like back at that time	.582	.343	.147	.673	.105	–.035
Trouble falling asleep	.264	.171	.855	.039	.068	.848
Waves of strong feelings	.639	.315	.313	.655	.054	.186
Tried to remove it from memory	.205	.683	.263	–.149	.800	.238
Trouble concentrating	.504	.293	.445	.376	.100	.459
Psychophysiological reactions	.483	.303	.299	.408	.114	.296
Dreams about it	.472	.275	.391	.358	.090	.419
Watchful and on guard	.408	.305	.224	.338	.178	.196
Tried not to talk about it	.240	.662	.170	–.055	.777	.095

Vietnam," and "my being beaten by my husband." This is a trickier issue, and one that must be decided by the point of the study, but a guiding principle could be this: If the referent for the IES-R would not qualify as an event for DSM-IV because it is too broad, then the referent is not appropriate for the IES-R. Researchers should also be aware of the conundrum created and the difficulties for respondents when some but not other symptoms are present for one instance of a class of events but the other symptoms are present for a different instance. DSM is not specific about this issue, but the vast majority of the data using the IES-R are in reference to a specific incident, so if a class is used as the referent, the data collected will not be comparable to other data in a potentially important way.

Modifications in the Time Frame

The IES-R was designed and validated using a specific time frame of the past 7 days. Any change in this interval likely makes the data collected not comparable to those collected with the standard time frame. Thus such a change is not recommended. Should a researcher decide to do so anyway, she or he should be aware that any write-up of the research should clearly disclose that a nonstandard, modified version of the measure was used and that no reliability or validity data exist for this new, nonstandard measure in the standard IES-R literature. If there are data in other research that used the identical modification, the researcher is, of course, free to cite that research as evidence in support of the characteristics of this modified measure.

Modifications of the Items

Changes or modifications in the wording or content of items raises problems. Such variations may render comparisons of the data collected using such a version problematic, and without further study, problematic in unknown ways. Though this may appear overly fussy, as simple a change as reversing the wording of an item so that the scoring is reflected does not produce a mirror image response distribution. Changing "I was jumpy and easily startled" to "I was not jumpy and easily startled" alters the meaning (if only subtly) as well as the scoring, and requires a different cognitive process to choose a response option. As above, it is appropriate to acknowledge the use of a modified version.

Use with Children

The IES-R was neither developed nor validated with children. Some of the items have content that is probably comprehensible to children below the seventh grade, but at least one item, item 12, comprises a fairly sophisticated internal psychological process concept. The Flesch-Kincaid Grade Level score is 6.6, but the user should be aware that using the measure with children must be considered preliminary or experimental until such time as the literature contains published evidence that the IES-R functions with children in the same way it functions with adults.

Cutting Scores, Cutoffs, and Categorical Uses

There are no "cutoff" points for the IES-R, nor are they envisioned or appropriate, despite analyses that present them (e.g., Asukai et al., 2002). The IES-R is intended to give an assessment of symptomatic status over the previous 7 days with respect to the three domains of PTSD symptoms stemming from exposure to a traumatic stressor. Neither the IES-R, nor the original IES for that matter, was intended to be used as a proxy for a diagnosis of PTSD, and with the very well-developed stable of clinical interviews that were designed to provide diagnoses (Weiss, Chapter 4, this volume), the only reasons to use the IES-R in this fashion is either a misunderstanding of its goals or a choice not to expend the resources (time, funds, good will) to obtain a valid diagnosis.

This issue is neither new nor confined to symptom measures. Nearly 30 years ago, Rotter (1975) attempted to persuade and cajole researchers interested in the construct of internal–external locus of control *not* to conceptualize it as a categorical variable, nor to use it that way. With respect to the IES-R, there are even more substantive issues that weigh against even attempting to set a cutoff score. One of these is the time elapsed since the traumatic event. Early in the course of reaction to traumatic stress, the level of symptoms on the IES-R may suggest the presence of PTSD, but distinguishing the normal course of response to trauma from PTSD is a difficult issue at 5 weeks or 2 months, regardless of the 1-month criterion in the DSM. A review of conjugal bereavement (Windholz, Marmar, & Horowitz, 1985) suggested that 6 months was not out of the ordinary for a period of time during which to recover from the loss. Thus acute PTSD and chronic PTSD might well require different cutoffs, if one were to attempt to select them. A second issue is the severity of the traumatic event; all other things being equal, the more severe, the higher the symptoms. A third issue is reactions accompanying exposure—both peritraumatic emotionality (Brunet et al., 2003) and peritraumatic dissociation (see Ozer, Best, Lipsey, & Weiss, 2003) may well moderate symptoms and symptom report in a way that would ultimately affect diagnosis.

Most important, however, is the impact of the base rate of stress reactions in the sample being studied (firefighters versus women who have been beaten during a sexual assault) and used to determine a fixed cutoff. Indeed, in presenting an update on the CAPS, Weathers and colleagues (2001) carefully and systematically describe the need for a variety of decision rules (which are functionally equivalent to a cutoff score), to make a diagnosis of PTSD. They explicitly consider the choice of cutoff in light of the types of errors different values will produce, minimizing or maximizing false positives or false negatives. It has been well known for more than 5 decades (Meehl & Rosen, 1955) that the base rate of the phenomenon can have a sizeable impact on the validity of any cut score. Thus it is simply inappropriate to require or to attempt to set any cutoff that will universally apply. Consequently, having cutoffs really serves no useful function.

The choice of the anchor points and the utilization of a mean score, rather than a sum (not universally followed in the literature), was an explicit decision to aid users in interpreting scores. For example, an individual's score or a group's mean on the Intrusion subscale of 1.89 would indicate that in the past week the distress from intrusive symptoms for this person or group was close to, but not quite, moderate. For individuals, similar statements regarding the other two subscales can be made. For groups, using the SD will help immensely in making the pattern of scores meaningful. This ability is consistent with the goal that the IES-R set for itself.

Normative Data

Most, but not all, of the issues that pertain to the futility of setting cutting scores apply equally well to the production of normative data. The central issue in establishing normative data for any measure (American Educational Research Association, American Psychological Association, & National Council on Measurement in Education, 1999) is a clear specification of the group (population) to which the normative data apply (see also Wilkinson & Task Force on Statistical Inference, 1999). In the case of measures of PTSD, this task is daunting because defining the normative population is complicated and complex, most saliently because the time elapsed since the traumatic event creates intractable problems. Average scores on the three subscales measured 2 months after exposure will likely be higher than when measured 2 years later (e.g., Zilberg et al., 1982). Unlike measures such as the SCL-90, on which an "average" score on any of the subscales is straightforward because there is no referent event, by definition the IES-R concerns symptomatic status in the preceding week in reference to an event. Thus, how far in the past the event occurred is not fixed and will vary considerably from person to person. Moreover, specification of normative groups—nonpatients, outpatients, inpatients—is understandable in a manner that does not easily translate to measures of PTSD because of the necessity of specifying a traumatic event from which the symptoms arise.

One solution would be to create norms that apply to all individuals who have ever been exposed to a traumatic event. Doing so, however, would not deal with the issue of time elapsed, nor would it deal with individuals who have had multiple exposures (Brunet, Boyer, Weiss, & Marmar, 2001).

A second choice would be to limit the norms to those who carry a current diagnosis of full PTSD. Doing so, however, would exclude a large number of individuals with significant symptomatology but who do not meet current criteria—those with current partial PTSD, those with PTSD in partial remission, and those with lifetime and current partial PTSD (see Weiss et al., 1992). As well, it would not deal with the issue of elapsed time.

A third choice would be to select a single event (e.g., September 11, 2001), fix a point in time, recruit only those with exposure, and carry out the measurements and building of norms. Doing so would take the time elapsed into account. It would not, however, take account of the likely differences between subgroups (e.g., civilians versus emergency personnel workers) in symptomatic response. Additionally, it would create a new dilemma—the norms would then apply only to a single type of traumatic event, thus largely defeating the purpose of creating norms in the first place.

These issues do not merely affect self-report measures of symptoms. The most commonly used interview measure, the CAPS (Weathers et al., 2001), does not provide a set of norms, nor does the SCID PTSD module (First, Spitzer, Gibbon, & Williams, 1996) or the MCS (Keane et al., 1988). Indeed, almost all measures of PTSD symptoms of any form present data regarding internal consistency, stability, and some construct validity (Cronbach & Meehl, 1955), typically only convergent but not divergent relationships. The argument, therefore, that norms are neither particularly useful nor especially meaningful appears to be supported by the virtual absence of norms for any measure of PTSD, either symptoms or diagnosis. Finally, it should be not be overlooked that in the 30-plus years that the original IES has been used in the field, normative data have never been presented.

SUMMARY AND CONCLUSIONS

The IES-R has emerged from infancy into its latent period, now being 6 to 8 years old, depending on whether birth is defined as first use or first publication. In either case, there is an increasing body of evidence that the addition of the Hyperarousal subscale, the change from frequency to a global distress response format, and the change from a stepwise scoring algorithm that produces sums to a smooth Likert scale producing a subscale score of the mean item response have all been positive steps in providing the field with a short, easily understood, ego-syntonic measure of distress from normal stress response to PTSD calibrated over the previous week.

Despite these improvements, there remain important issues to address in the future. The role of time elapsed since the event and subscale scores is a complicated and important issue to research further. Similarly, the relationship between type of sample, base rate of symptoms, and time elapsed since the event also have implications for the communality of items. Some of the items (e.g., item 7, "I felt as if it hadn't happened or wasn't real") should not be expected to display a great deal of communal variance, especially in a sample with a relatively low percentage of individuals having significant levels of symptoms. As a consequence, conclusions about whether items should or should not be included in a measure cannot be made solely on the basis of internal consistency or factor analytic results. The coverage of the content domain (see Haynes, Richard, & Kubany, 1995) is an important feature in measures on which only a few will endorse the item.

Future researchers should continue to accumulate data using the IES-R in the manner in which it has been offered: not to provide a proxy for a diagnosis of PTSD or even to categorize individuals into subgroups, but for its ability to track change over time, to trace the waxing and waning course of symptoms of PTSD, and to give a snapshot of current symptomatic status in the domains of intrusion, avoidance, numbing, and hyperarousal.

APPENDIX 7.1. Impact of Event Scale—Revised

INSTRUCTIONS: Below is a list of difficulties people sometimes have after stressful life events. Please read each item, and then indicate how distressing each difficulty has been for you DURING THE PAST SEVEN DAYS with respect to ________________. How much were you distressed or bothered by these difficulties?

Response Anchors: 0 = Not at all; 1 = A little bit; 2 = Moderately; 3 = Quite a bit; 4 = Extremely.

1. Any reminder brought back feelings about it.
2. I had trouble staying asleep.
3. Other things kept making me think about it.
4. I felt irritable and angry.
5. I avoided letting myself get upset when I thought about it or was reminded of it.
6. I thought about it when I didn't mean to.
7. I felt as if it hadn't happened or wasn't real.
8. I stayed away from reminders of it.
9. Pictures about it popped into my mind.
10. I was jumpy and easily startled.
11. I tried not to think about it.
12. I was aware that I still had a lot of feelings about it, but I didn't deal with them.
13. My feelings about it were kind of numb.
14. I found myself acting or feeling like I was back at that time.
15. I had trouble falling asleep.
16. I had waves of strong feelings about it.
17. I tried to remove it from my memory.
18. I had trouble concentrating.
19. Reminders of it caused me to have physical reactions, such as sweating, trouble breathing, nausea, or a pounding heart.
20. I had dreams about it.
21. I felt watchful and on guard.
22. I tried not to talk about it.

The Intrusion subscale is the MEAN item response of items 1, 2, 3, 6, 9, 14, 16, and 20. Thus scores can range from 0 through 4.

The Avoidance subscale is the MEAN item response of items 5, 7, 8, 11, 12, 13, 17, and 22. Thus scores can range from 0 through 4.

The Hyperarousal subscale is the MEAN item response of items 4, 10, 15, 18, 19, and 21. Thus scores can range from 0 through 4.

REFERENCES

American Educational Research Association, American Psychological Association, & National Council on Measurement in Education. (1999). *Standards for educational and psychological testing*. Washington, DC: Educational Research Association.

American Psychiatric Association. (1980). *Diagnostic and statistical manual of mental disorders* (3rd ed.). Washington, DC: Author.

American Psychiatric Association. (1994). *Diagnostic and statistical manual of mental disorders* (4th ed.). Washington, DC: Author.

Asukai, N., Kato, H., Kawamura, N., Kim, Y., Yamamato, K., Kishimoto, J., et al. (2002). Reliability and validity of the Japanese-language version of the Impact of Event Scale—Revised (IES-R-J): Four studies of different traumatic events. *Journal of Nervous and Mental Disease*, *190*, 175–182.

Baguena, M. J., Villarroya, E., Belena, A., Amelia, D., Roldan, C., & Reig, R. (2001). Psychometric properties of the Spanish version of the Impact of Event Scale—Revised (IES-R) [Propiedades psicometricas de la version espanola de la Escala Revisada de Impacto del Estressor (EIE-R)]. *Analisis y Modificacion de Conducta, 27*, 581-604.

Beck, A. T., Ward, C. H., Mendelson, M., Mock, J., & Erbaugh, J. (1961). An inventory for measuring depression. *Archives of General Psychiatry*, *4*, 561–571.

Brunet, A., Boyer, R., Weiss, D. S., & Marmar, C. R. (2001). The effects of initial trauma exposure on the symptomatic response to a subsequent trauma. *Canadian Journal of Behavioral Sciences*, *33*, 97–102.

Brunet, A., St.-Hilaire, A., Jehel, L., & King, S. (2003). Validation of a French version of the Impact of Event Scale—Revised. *Canadian Journal of Psychiatry*, *48*, 56–61.

Brunet, A., Weiss, D. S., Metzler, T. J., Best, S. R., Neylan, T. C., Rogers, C., et al. (2001). The Peritraumatic Distress Inventory: A proposed measure of PTSD criterion A2. *American Journal of Psychiatry*, *158*, 1480–1485.

Cronbach, L. J. (1951). Coefficient alpha and the internal structure of tests. *Psychometrika*, *16*, 297–334.

Cronbach, L. J., & Meehl, P. E. (1955). Construct validity in psychological tests. *Psychological Bulletin*, *52*, 281–302.

Derogatis, L. R. (1994). *SCL-90-R administration, scoring, and procedures manual* (3rd ed.). Minneapolis: National Computer Systems.

First, M. B., Spitzer, R. L., Gibbon, M., & Williams, J. B. (1996). *Structured Clinical Interview for DSM-IV Axis I Disorders (SCID-I), Clinician Version*. Washington, DC: American Psychiatric Association.

Giannantonio, M. (2003). *Scala di impatto dell'evento rivista*. Retrieved August 18, 2003, from *http://www.psicotraumatologia.com/ies-r.htm*

Haynes, S. N., Richard, D. C. S., & Kubany, E. S. (1995). Content validity in psychological assessment: A functional approach to concepts and methods. *Psychological Assessment*, *7*, 238–247.

Horowitz, M. J. (1975). Intrusive and repetitive thoughts after experimental stress: A summary. *Archives of General Psychiatry*, *32*, 1457–1463.

Horowitz, M. J. (1976). *Stress response syndromes*. New York: Aronson.

Horowitz, M. J., & Kaltreider, N. B. (1977). The response to stress. *Comprehensive Therapy*, *3*, 38–40.

Horowitz, M. J., Wilner, N., & Alvarez, W. (1979). Impact of Event Scale: A measure of subjective stress. *Psychosomatic Medicine*, *41*, 209–218.

Jennrich, R. I., & Sampson, P. F. (1966). Rotation for simple loadings. *Psychometrika*, *31*, 313–323.

Kaiser, H. F. (1958). The varimax criterion for analytic rotation in factor analysis. *Psychometrika*, *23*, 187–200.

Keane, T. M., Caddell, J. M., & Taylor, K. L. (1988). Mississippi Scale for Combat-Related Posttraumatic Stress Disorder: Three studies in reliability and validity. *Journal of Consulting and Clinical Psychology*, *56*, 85–90.

Kim, J.-O., & Mueller, C. W. (1978). *Factor analysis: Statistical methods and practical issues*. Newbury Park, CA: Sage.

Kimerling, R., Calhoun, K. S., Forehand, R., Armistead, L., Morse, E., Morse, P., et al. (1999). Traumatic stress in HIV-infected women. *AIDS Education and Prevention*, *11*, 321–330.

King, D. W., Leskin, G. A., King, L. A., & Weathers, F. W. (1998). Confirmatory factor analysis of the clinician-administered PTSD Scale: Evidence for the dimensionality of posttraumatic stress disorder. *Psychological Assessment*, *10*, 90–96.

Lauterbach, D., Vrana, S., King, D. W., & King, L. A. (1997). Psychometric properties of the Civilian Version of the Mississippi PTSD scale. *Journal of Traumatic Stress*, *10*, 499–513.

Liberman, A. M., Best, S. R., Metzler, T. J., Fagan, J. A., Weiss, D. S., & Marmar, C. R. (2002). Routine occupational work stress as a risk factor for stress reactions among police officers. *Journal of Police Strategies and Management*, *25*, 421–441.

Maercker, A., & Schuetzwohl, M. (1998). Assessment of posttraumatic stress reactions: The Impact of Event Scale—Revised (IES-R) [Erfassung von psychischen Belastungsfolgen: Die Impact of Event Skala—revidierte Version (IES-R)]. *Diagnostica*, *44*, 130–141.

Marmar, C. R., Weiss, D. S., & Metzler, T. J. (1997). The Peritraumatic Dissociative Experiences Questionnaire. In J. P. Wilson & T. M. Keane (Ed.), *Assessing psychological trauma and PTSD* (pp. 412–428). New York: Guilford Press.

Meehl, P. E., & Rosen, A. (1955). Antecedent probability and the efficiency of psychometric signs, patterns, or cutting scores. *Psychological Bulletin*, *52*, 194–216.

Ozer, E. J., Best, S. R., Lipsey, T. L., & Weiss, D. S. (2003). Predictors of posttraumatic stress disorder symptoms in adults: A meta-analysis. *Psychological Bulletin*, *129*, 52–73.

Pole, N., Best, S. R., Weiss, D. S., & Marmar, C. R. (2001). Effects of gender and ethnicity on posttraumatic stress symptoms among urban police officers. *Journal of Nervous and Mental Disease*, *189*, 442–448.

Rotter, J. B. (1975). Some problems and misconceptions related to the construct of internal versus external control of reinforcement. *Journal of Consulting and Clinical Psychology, 43*, 56–67.

SAS Institute. (1999). *SAS/STAT User's Guide*. Cary, NC: Author.

Selzer, M. L. (1971). The Michigan Alcoholism Screening Test: The quest for a new diagnostic instrument. *American Journal of Psychiatry, 127*, 1653–1658.

Spearman, C. (1904). The proof and measurement of association between two things. *American Journal of Psychology, 14*, 72–101.

Stein, M. B., & Kennedy, C. (2001). Major depressive and posttraumatic stress disorder comorbidity in female victims of intimate partner violence. *Journal of Affective Disorders, 66*, 133–138.

Strupp, H. H., & Hadley, S. W. (1977). A tripartite model of mental health and therapeutic outcomes: With special reference to negative effects in psychotherapy. *American Psychologist, 32*, 187–196.

Sundin, E. C., & Horowitz, M. J. (2002). Impact of Event Scale: Psychometric properties. *British Journal of Psychiatry, 180*, 205–209.

Taylor, J. A. (1953). A personality scale of manifest anxiety. *Journal of Abnormal and Social Psychology, 48*, 285–290.

Tinsley, H. E., & Tinsley, D. J. (1987). Uses of factor analysis in counseling psychology research. *Journal of Counseling Psychology, 34*, 414–424.

Weathers, F. W., Keane, T. M., & Davidson, J. R. (2001). Clinician-administered PTSD scale: A review of the first ten years of research. *Depression and Anxiety, 13*, 132–156.

Weiss, D. S., & Marmar, C. R. (1997). The Impact of Event Scale—Revised. In J. P. Wilson & T. M. Keane (Eds.), *Assessing psychological trauma and PTSD* (pp. 399–411). New York: Guilford Press.

Weiss, D. S., Marmar, C. R., Metzler, T. J., & Ronfeldt, H. M. (1995). Predicting symptomatic distress in emergency services personnel. *Journal of Consulting and Clinical Psychology, 63*(3), 361–368.

Weiss, D. S., Marmar, C. R., Schlenger, W. E., Fairbank, J. A., Jordan, B. K., Hough, R. L., et al. (1992). The prevalence of lifetime and partial posttraumatic stress disorder in Vietnam theatre veterans. *Journal of Traumatic Stress, 5*, 365–376.

Wilkinson, L., & Task Force on Statistical Inference. (1999). Statistical methods in psychology journals. *American Psychologist, 54*, 594–604.

Windholz, M. J., Marmar, C. R., & Horowitz, M. J. (1985). A review of the research on conjugal bereavement: Impact on health and efficacy of interventions. *Comprehensive Psychiatry, 26*, 433–447.

World Health Organization. (1978). *Clinical modification of the World Health Organization's manual of the international statistical classification of diseases, injuries, and causes of death* (9th rev. ed.). Geneva: Author.

Wu, K. K., & Chan, K. S. (2003). The development of the Chinese version of Impact of Event Scale—Revised (CIES-R). *Social Psychiatry and Psychiatric Epidemiology, 38*, 94–98.

Zilberg, N. J., Weiss, D. S., & Horowitz, M. J. (1982). Impact of Event Scale: A cross-validation study and some empirical evidence supporting a conceptual model of stress response syndromes. *Journal of Consulting and Clinical Psychology, 50*, 407–414.

CHAPTER 8

The Role of the Rorschach in the Assessment and Treatment of Trauma

TONI LUXENBERG
PATTI LEVIN

Trauma appears to be a deceptively simple concept—something terrible happens, and people continue to be disturbed by it, even after the event itself is complete and in the past. Those who work in the field of trauma have come to realize that trauma is a much more complex, multifaceted concept than originally believed. Individual responses to traumatic events vary widely, as do responses to treatment. No longer do most clinicians believe that there is one penultimate means by which to treat trauma. Rather, the field has been pushed to develop increasingly more sophisticated means of understanding the complexities of individual responses to trauma.

Concomitantly, there has been a growing need to create appropriate treatments that are attuned to the specific needs of the individual, rather than based on a one-size-fits-all approach. No assessment tool appears to be as well suited to such an endeavor as the Rorschach Inkblot Test, constructed not as a means to assess *what* a person has experienced but, rather, to assess each person's unique responses to and subjective perceptions of themselves, others, their experiences, and the world around them. It is precisely this level of information that is necessary in both understanding and ameliorating an individual's reactions to traumatic experiences.

HISTORY OF TRAUMA IN THE 20TH CENTURY

To understand the significance of the Rorschach in assessing traumatic responses and informing treatment planning, it is necessary to first understand how the concept of trauma and its treatment has evolved throughout the 20th century. During World War I, the concept of trauma came to public attention as many returning soldiers exhibited a range of physical and emotional difficulties that were attributed primarily to the concussive effects of bombs. This was believed to be a medical condition, referred to as "shell shock," despite the fact that many of the men who suffered from it had not been directly involved in battle (Myers, 1915). "Shell shock" was little understood and often seen as a sign of cowardice. Treatment was aimed at preparing men, as quickly as possible, to return to the front, often through the use of shaming and intimidation (van der Kolk, Weisaeth, & van der Hart, 1996). In the interim between the two World Wars, physicians began to recognize the psychological nature of these problems. The need for a more comprehensive and compassionate treatment was recognized. Kardiner (1941) labeled the experiences of distressed soldiers as "traumatic war neuroses," and the salutary value of helping individuals to remember and process their traumatic experiences was recognized in at least some military contexts.

With the advent of the Vietnam War, military personnel and mental health workers alike began to recognize and document a consistent constellation of symptoms that was both persistent and disabling. Veterans were noted to exhibit a greatly heightened sensitivity to their environment, massive overreactions to things that were reminiscent of the original trauma(s), and a singular focus on survival that often led to erratic, seemingly incomprehensible behavior (e.g., crawling under objects in response to loud sounds, as if bombs were dropping). The initial diagnosis of posttraumatic stress disorder (PTSD), in fact, was based largely on literature that delineated and explored the psychological functioning of these traumatized men (Shatan, Smith, & Haley, 1977).

When the women's movement in the United States brought the issues of sexual assault, incest, other forms of sexual abuse, and domestic violence to the national forefront, the theoretical concepts developed through work with veterans began to be applied to these populations, as well. Similar symptom presentations were noted, and terms such as "rape trauma syndrome" were coined, in attempts to explore the traumatic responses of hitherto ignored groups—women and children (van der Kolk et al., 1996). At approximately this same time, Horowitz (1978) expanded the field's understanding of trauma by noting what he called the "biphasic" trauma response—or, the alternation of a flooded, reexperiencing state (e.g., nightmares, vivid relivings of traumatic events, dysregulated affect, etc.) with a numb, avoidant state (e.g., feelings of numbness, avoidance of reminders of trauma, avoidance of thoughts about the trauma, etc.).

During the 1980s the sexual abuse of children became a major focus for researchers and clinicians alike in the United States and thus awareness grew of the dynamics unique to certain forms of traumatization that required intervention in their own right. For example, Finkelhor and Browne (1985) delineated four areas of dysfunction typically seen in sexual abuse survivors—traumatic sexualization, betrayal, powerlessness, and stigmatization. They stressed that, although some of these dynamics can occur in other forms of trauma, taken together, they form a unique "profile" requiring intervention. Further, it came to be appreciated that a whole host of internal and external factors were important in determining the extent to which a person was ultimately traumatized (e.g., Feinauer, 1989; Browne & Finkelhor, 1986). For example, a child molested by a stranger on one occasion, through persuasion rather than violence, would typically experience less difficulty and have a more straightforward recovery process than a child repeatedly and forcibly raped by a relative.

In the 1990s, researchers found that some of the sequelae of impersonal traumas (e.g., natural disasters) were different from those of interpersonal traumas (e.g., sexual assault; Briere, 1997). The same distinction was found to be true when comparing single-incident traumas with more violent and/or chronic traumas (e.g., Breslau et al., 1998). The latter forms of trauma in both categories tend to result in more extensive, longer lasting, and more treatment-resistant symptomatology (McFarlane, 1989; Resnick, Yehuda, Pitman, & Foy, 1995; Cassidy & Mohr, 2001). What began to crystallize was an awareness among both clinicians and researchers that there were, in fact, many possible responses to trauma—with the "classic" PTSD diagnosis being only one possible response (van der Kolk & McFarlane, 1996)—depending on a range of factors, including personal characteristics, historical events, age of onset, characteristics of the trauma, and characteristics of the current environment (Carlson, Furby, Armstrong, & Schlaes, 1997). One of the most powerful examples of the latter was the work of Everson, Hunter, Runyon, Edelson, and Coulter (1989), who found that the single most important factor in how well children ultimately coped with being sexually abused by a family member was how their caregivers responded to their disclosures of abuse. In sum, it came to be increasingly appreciated that to be effective, trauma treatment had to take into account these myriad of moderating and mitigating factors.

Currently, it is recognized that traumatic symptoms may ebb and flow over time, sometimes with intrusive, reexperiencing symptomatology being dominant, sometimes with numbing, avoidant symptomatology being dominant, and, quite frequently, with both sets of symptoms being present at the same time. Each of these situations requires a different focus of intervention. There are entire constellations of symptoms that are not covered in the PTSD diagnosis that have significant impact on the treatment of some trauma survivors (van der Kolk, Roth, Pelcovitz, & Mandel, 1993). Thus it becomes crucial to have assessment tools at our disposal that can respond to the enormous complexity within the deceptively simple rubric of "trauma."

THE RORSCHACH

It has been argued that perhaps the most uniquely human quality that separates us from other beings is our need to make meaning—to finds patterns, to impose structure. As humans, we strive to understand our experiences and perceptions, to place them within a meaningful framework that allows us to predict, plan, and, above all, attenuate the anxiety inherent in ambiguity. This was most recently and dramatically demonstrated during the September 11, 2001, terrorist attacks in the United States (Armstrong & Kaser-Boyd, in press). As people struggled to comprehend and deal with the essentially incomprehensible and senseless violence and destruction of the attacks, a frenetic debate began in the media about what the smoke clouds above the World Trade Center towers looked like. Among the top "projected" contenders were the devil, God, and Osama bin Laden, himself (Wells & Maher, 2001).

It is this simple but crucial concept of projection of meaning onto ambiguous stimuli on which the Rorschach Inkblot Test (and, indeed, all projective measures) was based. Developed in 1921 by a Swiss psychiatrist, Hermann Rorschach, the Rorschach consists of 10 standard inkblots, which are presented to an individual in a standardized manner. The person is simply asked what each inkblot might be. Presented with essentially meaningless stimuli, people will almost always impose some form of structure, and in so doing, they will call upon their own knowledge bases, experiences, feelings, biases, outlooks, and defenses. Their end product, therefore, will have much to tell us about their own unique way of taking in, ordering, and processing information and how this is impinged on by factors such as emotion, thinking processes, preoccupations, and so forth.

NORMS/VALIDITY

Initially, the Rorschach was not standardized in any meaningful way, but this began to change in 1925, when five different psychologists, all in the United States, independently developed their own systematized means of administering and scoring the Rorschach. Unfortunately, each of these psychologists (Samuel Beck, Bruno Klopfer, Zygmunt Piotrowski, Marguerite Hertz, and David Rappaport) was guided by distinct and separate theoretical viewpoints. This lack of a universal scoring and interpretive system was highly problematic and led to the Rorschach receiving much criticism. This changed in 1974, when John Exner developed his extensive Comprehensive System, based not on theoretical constructs but rather on careful analyses of the existing systems, including the review of all existing studies (which numbered over 4,000). Exner attempted to distill and consolidate those aspects of existing systems that were the most reliable and the most robustly backed by research and clinical findings. The end result is a highly systematized method of administration, scoring, and interpretation based on a very substantial database of both nonpatient and clinical populations. An individual's answers are coded, scored, and then compared against normative data, resulting in a psychometrically sound instrument (Parker, 1983). In 1999, Hiller, Rosenthal, Bornstein, Berry, and Brunell-Neuleib carried out a meta-analytic study comparing the validity of the Rorschach with that of the Minnesota Multiphasic Personality Inventory (MMPI)—the exemplar of objective, empirically sound assessment instruments. Not only did they demonstrate the validity of a number of Rorschach indices, but they also found that the average effect size of the Rorschach was essentially identical to that of the MMPI—.29 versus .30.

Nevertheless, there remains some controversy about whether or not the Rorschach is a reliable assessment tool (e.g., Garb, 1999). There have been those who assert that there is little evidence of the Rorschach's scientific soundness or even clinical utility (e.g., Hunsley & Bailey, 1999; Garb, Wood, Nezworski, Grove, & Stejskal, 2001). For an excellent, evenhanded, and extensive review on the subject, we refer the reader to Meyer and Archer (2001). We agree with their conclusion that "the Rorschach can validly predict a range of criterion variables and can do so about as well as alternative tests." They also stress that the Rorschach performs better (like all tests) in certain situations than in others. We return to the issue of what use the Rorschach is being put to shortly.

There have been questions in recent years about the applicability of the nonpatient norms developed by Exner (e.g., Shaffer, Erdberg, & Haroian, 1999; Wood, Nezworski, Garb, & Lilienfeld, 2001). Shaffer et al. found that in their sample of 123 nonpatients, there were significant discrepancies between many of the Rorschach variables in their sample and those in Exner's nonpatient sample. As Weiner, Spielberger, and Abeles (2002) point out, however, there were serious problems with the representativeness of the Shaffer et al. sample, as well as with the level of training of their protocol administrators, calling the validity of their findings into question. Wood et al. have also been vocal in their criticism of the Exner norms, basing this criticism on a summary of 32 studies that they carried out. Although they examined the nonpatient control groups in multiple studies, it is clear that this may be a problematic procedure. Combining disparate groups from studies that were not intended to be normative in nature is a questionable research methodology. So too is the high level of inclusion of elderly and college student samples, both of which are known to test in idiosyncratic ways that are often outside of established norms. Further, some of the samples used consisted of current or former psychiatric patients, who clearly have no place in a nonpatient sample. This is in stark contrast to Exner's 1993 nonpatient sample, which, as pointed out by Weiner et al. (2002), was carefully composed of individuals with no psychiatric history *and* evidence of positive social or vocational functioning. It should not be surprising, in fact, that such discrepant samples should provide such different norms.

Although there are good reasons to be very cautious about interpreting the findings from either the Shaffer et al. (1999) or Wood et al. (2001) studies, they clearly underline the need to ensure that the current Rorschach norms are still appropriate for use, and to that end, Exner has been working on a replication study based on a new normative sample (Exner, 2002a). This was further bolstered by Exner's presentation (2002b) at the International Rorschach Conference, at which he reported an update on this study, at the time composed of 300 participants, which had no statistically significant deviation from the existing norms. Thus initial data indicate that the new participants are producing very similar patterns of response when compared with the earlier sample (Weiner et al., 2002), increasing our confidence that Comprehensive System norms are both reliable and valid for nonpatient samples.

One caveat that has become abundantly clear over the course of time is that the Rorschach should not be thought of or treated as a diagnostic test per se, in terms of the criteria laid out by the *Diagnostic and Statistical Manual of Mental Disorders* (American Psychiatric Association, 1994). For example, many researchers have pointed out the Rorschach's failure to accurately diagnose depression, based on the depression index (DEPI) score (e.g., Archer & Krishnamurthy, 1997; Wood, Lilienfeld, Garb, & Nezworski, 2000). This should not be surprising, given that the Rorschach's purpose and strength is not in assessing observable behavior or conscious statements/productions but rather in assessing a person's attitudes, perceptions, and underlying personality characteristics, often at the unconscious level. These go beyond diagnostic criteria but are clearly very important in understanding individuals and in designing effective treatment for them. The use of the Rorschach to deepen understanding of individuals and obtain a personalized view of their functioning, internal structures, and needs is well supported in the literature (e.g., Meyer, 1996; Stricker & Gold, 1999; Viglione, 1999).

WHAT THE RORSCHACH CAN TELL US ABOUT TRAUMA

The Value of Projective Testing in Assessing Trauma

At this time, there are numerous measures available to measure PTSD symptomatology, including the PTSD subscales of the Minnesota Multiphasic Personality Inventory (MMPI; Wilson & Walker, 1990), the Impact of Event Scale (IES; Zilberg, Weiss, & Horowitz, 1982), the Clinician-Administered PTSD Scale (CAPS; Blake et al., 1995), and the Trauma Symptom Inventory (TSI; Briere, Elliot, Harris, & Cotman, 1995). All of these measures, however, are based on the clients' reports of their experiences and symptoms. This fact leaves these measures vulnerable to vagaries of memory, subjectivity, and, in some cases, either the intentional or unconscious manipulation of information.

Such difficulties are, for the most part, avoided in projective testing because the stimuli are ambiguous, and, therefore, the "meaning" of any given answer is unclear. This is especially true in the Rorschach, on which no one answer carries much importance in and of itself. Rather, it is the entire test, viewed in toto, that is important. An individual wishing to please the examiner, therefore, is left to her or his own devices, there being no "clues" within the test itself to guide the answers given. Further, although the Rorschach may well address specific PTSD symptomatology (e.g., intrusive thoughts or feelings), it goes well beyond this, to investigate a person's sense of self, worldview, perceptions of others, use of affect, and so forth. As it becomes clearer that PTSD is only one possible response to trauma, it also becomes increasingly important to have available measures that capture and address the broader range of traumatic symptomatology.

Additionally, one problem that clinicians frequently experience is that their clients do not connect their current difficulties or symptoms with their past traumatic experiences and thus do not report those experiences to the clinician (Scurfield, 1985). Further, van der Kolk and Ducey (1989) have cautioned that there is a great danger of missing the diagnosis of PTSD entirely if a person presents to treatment in a constricted mode, which they suggest may be one of the most common presentations. Alternately, some highly traumatized clients are perfectly aware of the impact of the trauma(s) on them but do not raise the issue of trauma, fearing that their symptoms will worsen beyond what they can bear. Yet another scenario is that clients may have, in order to cope with their traumatic experience(s), compartmentalized those experiences behind a dissociative barrier, where they are not available to their day-to-day conscious mind. In all of these cases, a clinician is severely limited in his or her ability to help or even to understand the client's presentation.

The Rorschach can be a great asset in these situations because it provides information not always tapped by self-report measures and allows clinicians to gain insight into a client's inner experiences without the client having to talk directly about the experiences. This may actually be the safest, most respectful way to explore the trauma of highly flooded, aroused, or symptomatic clients. Importantly, the Rorschach has been found to powerfully evoke traumatic material, even in those individuals who denied experiencing any current impact of the trauma in their daily lives (van der Kolk & Ducey, 1989; Franchi & Andronikof-Sanglade, 1993). Further, the Rorschach has been shown to be helpful in discerning individuals who are consciously attempting to manufacture psychopathology (Seamons, Howell, Carlisle, & Roe, 1981) or who deny existing psychopathology (Grossman, Wasyliw, Benn, & Gyoerkoe, 2002).

It should be noted that Schretlen (1997) reviewed relevant studies and concluded that individuals could, in fact, successfully dissimulate on the Rorschach and not be detected by trained professionals. This conclusion, however, is called into question by several studies in which it was found that malingerers could be discerned from their truly pathological counterparts when attention was paid to their scores on specific variables (e.g., overly dramatic nature of responses, less complex responses, less emotional restraint, etc.; Frueh & Kinder, 1994; Ganellen, Wasyliw, Haywood, & Grossman, 1996). Schretlen is quite right, however, in asserting that malingerers are, at times, able to achieve very similar scores to genuinely disturbed or distressed individuals on select variables. This, clearly, highlights the need to focus on the whole, rather than parts, of response sets.

Unlike objective measures, then, the Rorschach maintains its utility in the face of clients who are not reporting traumatic histories but who have them, clients who are unaware of aspects of their traumatic experiences, clients who are denying pathology, and clients who are malingering. Used appropriately, this is power indeed.

Further, the Rorschach can potentially illuminate several crucial processes in understanding and building effective treatments for trauma survivors. It can help clinicians in understanding how a person's reality testing, management of emotion, focus on the environment, anticipation of good or poor treatment by others, emotional control, thought processes, and perception of neutral stimuli has been affected by trauma. Most of these would be difficult for individuals to report on fully, accurately, and directly in self-reports, or interviewing formats, but they are crucial to planning effective treatment.

Research

The assessment of trauma or any other psychological experience should never rest on a single instrument. Responsible assessment pulls from multiple sources, compares and contrasts information, and arrives at conclusions based on the full clinical picture. The Rorschach is only one piece (albeit a potentially powerful one) in the assessment process, and it should never be taken as a "stand alone" measure. That being said, some researchers have questioned the Rorschach's incremental validity (e.g., Garb et al., 2001; Hunsley & Bailey, 2001), emphasizing that it does not add any information beyond what can be obtained through other measures. This seems an unwarranted conclusion, however, in light of the previously discussed fact that the Rorschach is intended to tap the implicit, internal, and structural realm in a manner that is not exclusively tied to diagnosis. This clearly distinguishes it from many other tests, whose foci are overt, explicit, and, in some cases, diagnosis driven (e.g., the MMPI or Beck Depression Inventory). The point is not that one is better than the other—rather, that both are necessary to gain a full understanding of an individual that is appropriately deep and wide.

The utility of the Rorschach for work with traumatized populations seems especially clear. Given the number of different clinical presentations, all of which fall under the rubric of "trauma," the field is clearly in need of an instrument that can go beyond the diagnosis of PTSD and help clinicians and researchers alike understand the similarities and differences among survivors and to appreciate the structural issues involved in the recovery from trauma.

Before continuing, we must note that we refer to numerous indices on the Rorshcach as being indicative of a range of experiences (e.g., oppositionality, emotionality, depression, etc.). It should be kept in mind that we are speaking of characterological "sets" or tendencies rather than strict diagnostic categories. A person who shows signs of oppositionality on the Rorschach, for example, may or may not meet criteria for oppositional defiant disorder (if a child), conduct disorder (if an adolescent), or antisocial personality disorder (if an adult). Nor should they be diagnosed as such solely on the basis of signs of oppositionality in their Rorschach responses. That would be an inappropriate use of the Rorschach. What is appropriate, however, is to use signs of oppositionality to develop an understanding of the individual's perception of the world (e.g., as hostile, demanding, etc.), their expectational sets (e.g., that they will be treated unfairly), their interpersonal style, and so forth.

The Rorschach has been found to be very responsive to traumatic experience and a sensitive marker of distress. The first study carried out with the Rorschach was done by Shalit (1965) on an Israeli naval ship at sea during a severe storm. In the protocols of 20 service people, a marked increase in inanimate movement (m) was found when compared with their baseline protocols administered prior to leaving shore. The elevation in inanimate movement responses, indicative of helplessness and situational stress, has continued to be one of the most consistent findings in the protocols of traumatized individuals.

There were hints of what was to come in Modlin's (1967) study, in which individuals who had been in accidents and exhibited signs of a "post-accident anxiety syndrome" were studied. Modlin reported that among 40 individuals tested, the average number of responses given was between eight and nine (subsequently deemed invalid by Exner's Comprehensive System), which he interpreted as exhibiting a marked constriction and difficulty mobilizing imaginative processes or approaching affective material. The understanding of this process became more sophisticated as time went on. After the inclusion of the PTSD diagnosis in the psychological nomenclature, van der Kolk and Ducey (1984, 1989) found evidence of both the intrusive and numbing "phases" of trauma in the Rorschach protocols of 14 Vietnam War veterans. Protocols of these veterans were severely constricted, with simple, unelaborated responses that failed to engage in the normal imaginative processes typically stimulated by the Rorschach. van der Kolk and Ducey (1989) interpreted this as "psychic numbing" and also pointed out that a smaller subset of protocols also displayed a marked reliance on use of unstructured color (CF and pure C responses), which was seen as indicating an affectively unmodulated response to the intrusive phase of PTSD. Of note, an almost identical pattern was found by Salley and Teiling (1984) in their study of Vietnam veterans. Like Shalit (1965), van der Kolk and Ducey (1989) also found elevated inanimate movements (m), which they characterized as representing the participants' sense that they were surrounded by "threatening forces" beyond their control, rendering them helpless. Intriguingly, van der Kolk and Ducey (1989) also found evidence for traumatic intrusions in the protocols of these veterans. These individuals reported concrete, and obvious, images related to their war experiences, including many blood and anatomy responses. Sloan, Arsenault, Hilsenroth, Harvill, & Handler (1995) found similar results while working with Persian Gulf War veterans. They created what they called the Combat Content (CC) score, which comprised weapon and specific combat experience percepts.

Similar "biphasic" protocols were found by Cerney (1990), who used the Rorschach to investigate 48 inpatient participants with a range of traumatic experiences. Cerney noted that the women who had been sexually and/or physically abused displayed one of two patterns on their Rorschach responses—either constricted protocols that avoided almost all affect and aggression or responses dominated by color and numerous primitive and aggressive themes. Levin (1990, 1993), interestingly, found signs of biphasic response *within* individual protocols in her sample of 36 individuals traumatized as adults, who had no premorbid psychiatric history. She noted that her participants' FC:CF+C ratios were heavily weighted to the CF+C side, indicating intense affective experience with little cognitive mediation. In these same protocols, however, she also found low affective ratios (Afr), pointing to the avoidance of affectively charged material. It should be noted that the identical pattern of response has been found by other researchers as well (Swanson, Blount, & Bruno, 1990; Hartman et al., 1990; Armstrong, 1991; Kaser-Boyd, 1993).

Levin characterized the positive Hypervigilance Index (HVI), elevated perseveration scores, and trauma-related percepts throughout these protocols as representing the preoccupation and watchfulness associated with traumatic experiences and PTSD. As in past and subsequent studies (Armstrong, 1991; Sloan et al., 1995; Swanson et al., 1990), Levin also found elevated inanimate movement, impaired reality testing (low X+%) that included cognitive slippage (FABCOMS and INCOMS), and shading responses (elevated Y and V, linked with the experience of painful, intrusive affects).

Additional support for the "numbing" phase of traumatic response was found by Hartman et al. (1990), who hypothesized that the low number of responses (*R*) and the elevated Lambda scores (*L*) of their participants were signs of the emotional numbing inherent in PTSD. This was borne out in the low Afr, a measure of affect avoidance. It should be noted, however, that low *R* and high *L* are now commonly conceptualized as being emblematic of cognitive avoidance (Armstrong & Kaser-Boyd, in press). Although they conceptualized the low Afr somewhat differently, Swanson et al. (1990) found similarly depressed Afr scores, as well as impaired reality testing, poor stress tolerance, heightened inanimate movement, and unmodulated affect. The high negative D and Adjusted D (Adj D) scores consistently found among traumatized participants (Salley & Teiling, 1984; Hartman et al., 1990; Levin, 1993; Sloan et al., 1995; Scroppo, Weinberger, Drob, & Eagle, 1998) have been conceptualized as highlighting how coping is undermined by the chronic management of intrusions and sense of helplessness that characterizes a major aspect of traumatic experience.

The Rorschach's Discriminant Ability

The clinician's world is not a simple one. Clinicians are called on not only to diagnose clients but also to choose among competing, and often overlapping, diagnoses, to discern false presentations, and to determine the relative impact of multiple, valid diagnoses on a person's functioning. This level of subtlety can be overwhelming. Fortunately, however, the Rorschach has proven very helpful in drawing such distinctions. Souffrant (1987) used the Rorschach to distinguish between 60 Vietnam veterans with and without PTSD. She was able to do so by considering, in conjunction, two aspects of the Rorschach—elevated inanimate movement and the presence of unmodulated affect, as captured by unstructured color responses. Importantly, the color responses, in and of themselves, were not sufficient to distinguish between those veterans who were suffering from PTSD and those who were not. This, then, was further evidence of the lack of any "magic bullet" that could identify trauma; rather, it emphasized the importance of considering all information.

Leavitt and Labott (1996) were able to use the Rorschach (non-Exner method) to successfully differentiate between women with documented histories of sexual abuse and control participants in their differential use of traumatic contents. Such percepts are now believed to represent trauma-specific intrusions. Likewise, Kamphuis, Kugeares, and Finn (2000) used the Traumatic Content Index (a measure of traumatic intrusions originally developed by Armstrong in 1991) to successfully distinguish between women with documented sexual abuse histories and those without abuse histories. The ability of Armstrong's TC/R scale to do this, based on a ratio of traumatic contents (blood, anatomy, sex, morbid, and aggressive scores) to total responses, is striking in its implications. Those working in the field of trauma have long sought to reliably make increasingly fine distinctions between individuals with actual trauma histories, those individuals who are deliberately fabricating such histories, those individuals who may, for any number of reasons, unconsciously be elaborating past histories of disappointment and hurt beyond that which is accurate, and those individuals who are not reporting such histories but nevertheless have them.

It is imperative to understand, however, that this should not be taken to mean that the Rorschach can or should be used to *diagnose* sexual abuse. This would be an inappropriate use of the Rorschach. What these studies clearly indicate, however, is that the Rorschach may be one useful source of information in assessing the "fit" between a person's testing presentation and past life experiences. This would have equal applicability in highly complex cases in which no trauma history is reported but is suspected and those in which reports of a trauma history may be part of a psychotic disorder, inaccurate, exaggerated, or false. Use of the Traumatic Content Index is very promising as a first step in obtaining objective means to make these difficult and crucial distinctions.

Nichols and Czirr (1986) also used the Rorschach to help distinguish PTSD from psychosis and depression in an elderly population. They indicated that the Rorschach was helpful in making such difficult but important distinctions, because nonpsychotic elderly individuals with PTSD could be distinguished from their psychotic counterparts on the basis of their acceptable form quality (i.e., lack of distortion of percepts) and lack of bizarre responses other than those tied to actual experiences (see Armstrong, 1991). In a very interesting study of 28 battered women who went on to murder their abusive spouses, Kaser-Boyd (1993) found that her participants, like the Vietnam veterans studied by others, had some signs of unconventional perceptual processes but could be distinguished from psychotic individuals based on an absence of special scores accompanying their perceptual distortions and bizarre precepts (many of which were specifically related to their traumatic experiences).

Numerous studies have shown problems in reality testing in traumatized individuals (Armstrong & Kaser-Boyd, in press; Swanson et al., 1990; Hartman et al., 1990; Kayser-Boyd, 1993; Levin, 1990, 1993). The demands of managing the constant traumatic intrusions can, for some individuals, override what is otherwise intact reality testing. This may lead, unfortunately, to a misdiagnosis of thought disorder. This is such a frequent finding that Armstrong (personal communication, 1995) suggested that this phenomenon be labeled a "traumatic thought disorder"—in other words, problems with logical, consensually based reality testing and thinking that are solely tied to traumatic symptomatology, rather than globally disordered thought processes.

The impact of trauma on cognitive processes can be profound. Forced to marshal significant emotional and cognitive resources to manage traumatic symptoms, some individuals become too overwhelmed (particularly in the face of strong emotion) to sort out what has happened to them in the past from what is actually currently happening, as well as their fears about what might happen. This may not be apparent at all in situations that appear to provide no traumatic triggers but become florid in those instances in which they are reminded of their traumatic experiences.

There are several markers on the Rorschach that can suggest that individuals are experiencing problems with their reality testing based on traumatic interference, rather than globally disordered thinking (although it is certainly possible both to be traumatized and to have a true thought disorder or psychosis). Idiosyncracies in thinking are suggested by both M– scores and M none scores, with the latter indicating a tendency to distance oneself from, or detach altogether from, the actual perceptual subjects. Further, X–% is a measure of distorted and inaccurate perceptual processes. Heightened X–% is typically part of the constellation indicative of schizophrenia. Traumatized populations tend toward elevations in Xu% (idiosyncratic ways of viewing the world) rather than frank distortion (X–%). On the other hand, low X+% scores indicate that an individual may become compromised in the face of affectively charged material, particularly when F+% is in the normal range, as the latter score measures perceptual distortion or inaccuracy without affect being a variable. If there are signs of impaired reality testing combined with normative levels of Popular responses and suppressed D scores (indicating significant situational distress), one can be more confident that an individual is experiencing traumatically induced perceptual problems that prevent him or her from responding appropriately to conventional reality, although he or she may be well aware of it (Levin, 1993).

The Rorschach's special scores address unusual thought processes that can occur and "derail" a person's cognitive activity, often referred to as cognitive slippage. Two special scores that are particularly important for understanding traumatically induced cognitions are INCOMS and FABCOMS, both of which deal with the improbable combination of elements that do not actually fit or go together. The elevated rate of these scores in the protocols of traumatized individuals may reflect their responses to the implausible, unsuspected occurrence of a horrific event(s) in their own lives (Levin, 1993).

All of these factors should particularly be examined closely when an individual with a trauma history (or without an acknowledged trauma history) has a positive Schizophrenia Index (SCZI) on the Rorschach but does not actually display any signs of psychosis in his or her day-to-day functioning or interactional patterns or when the clinician is asked: trauma or thought disorder?

Armstrong and Loewenstein (1990) and Scroppo et al. (1998) found that the Rorschach could be used to distinguish between individuals with dissociative disorders and those diagnosed with borderline personality disorder (BPD). This is a very important distinction, as there is often some overlap between the two sets of diagnoses, in terms of both symptomatology and past history. These two groups of individuals, however, have distinct clinical needs, and being able to reliably discern one from the other is critical for effective treatment. These two studies indicate that aspects of the Rorschach can be helpful in making such distinctions. Specifically, high M's (human movement), use of form dimension (FD) and texture responses (T) and high whole-to-part human ratios distinguish individuals with dissociative disorders from their counterparts diagnosed with BPD. This latter whole-to-part human criterion makes sound theoretical sense, when one considers that individuals with BPD are thought to have great difficulty in viewing others as whole, integrated individuals, tending to split them into "good" and "bad" parts, resulting in problematic interpersonal relations. The dissociative cohort had a greater capacity for interpersonal relatedness and greater ability to introspect.

The Rorschach has also been used to successfully track treatment gains gleaned from eye movement desensitization and reprocessing (EMDR) in working with traumatized individuals (Levin, Errbo & Call, 1996; Levin, Lazrove, & van der Kolk, 1999). Levin et al. (1999) used SPECT neuroimaging before and after three sessions of EMDR in a pilot study of individuals diagnosed with PTSD. Similar to the Levin et al. (1996) study, they found that the HVI indices moved, after the course of treatment, from positive to negative, indicating a relaxing of the rigid need for watchfulness and being "on guard" that is associated with PTSD. This was believed to be linked with the participants' increased ability, after treatment, to access their frontal lobe functions, as seen in the SPECT scans (e.g., planning, assessing objects, evaluating incoming information in a structured manner), in the service of distinguishing real threat from false (reliving, PTSD-inspired) threat.

The Rorschach and Dissociative Disorders

Dissociative disorders are generally thought to be linked with extensive, chronic, and intense histories of childhood abuse and trauma. Although the field's understanding of these complex disorders is by no means complete, numerous researchers have sought to better understand, through the Rorschach, the complicated and intricate processes involved in these disorders. Lovitt and Lefkof (1985) assessed three female participants diagnosed with multiple personality disorder (MPD; now known as dissociative identity disorder, or DID). The Rorschach was administered several times to each participant, in an effort to test "host" personalities, as well as predetermined "secondary" personalities. Interestingly, all of the "hosts," or main personalities, displayed ambitent EB styles (more stress-vulnerable), whereas many of the secondary personalities displayed superintroversive EB styles. This same pattern was also found by Armstrong and Loewenstein (1990) and by Scroppo et al. (1998). Seven of the eight personalities in the Lovitt and Lefkof study showed a very unusual combination of unstructured but constricted color responses, suggesting that two normally separate processes were co-occurring. The most remarkable finding, however, was the wide variability among the personalities in terms of different scoring categories, so that the different protocols looked quite dissimilar.

Armstrong increased her original (1991) sample of 14 individuals diagnosed with MPD or a severe dissociative disorder to 119 individuals (Armstrong, personal communication, 1994). Both sets of participants revealed very similar patterns, however. Armstrong reported that the participants in her sample exhibited highly introversive EB styles (with 85% being either introversive or superintroversive), very complex organization (e.g., low *L*, but numerous blends), elevated form dimension responses (FD—seen as the ability to look internally in a detached manner), low Afr, unusual reality testing seen throughout the literature on Rorschach research with trauma-sequelae disorders (Levin & Reis, 1997; Sloan, et al., 1995), and the presence of trauma-related percepts in the protocol, as seen in morbid, blood, sex, aggressive, and anatomy content. Armstrong stressed that although many of the aspects seen in the protocols of individuals with PTSD were seen in the dissociative protocols, the latter appeared to retain the ability to access fantasy as a coping resource and to employ imagination defensively.

There have been some exciting attempts to use the Rorschach as a means of assessing dissociation directly. Leavitt and Labott (1997) and Leavitt (2000) developed a dissociative index on the Rorschach, using non-Exner variables that include: forms being partially obscured, the distance of objects being exaggerated, and "disorientation," which is the perception of percepts as rapidly shifting or changing in some manner. This index correlates well with the Dissociative Experiences Scale (Leavitt & Labott, 1997) and may prove to be a powerful addition to the Rorschach's usefulness in assessing divergent trauma presentations.

THE MULTIFACETED NATURE OF TRAUMA

Research has proven PTSD to be a prevalent psychological disorder that has serious, deleterious, and potentially long-term consequences for an individual's ability to function (Brett, Spitzer, & Williams, 1988; Hidalgo & Davidson, 2000; Davidson, Hughes, Blazer, & George, 1991). It has long been understood, however, that the PTSD criteria, as delineated in DSM (American Psychiatric Association, 1980, 1987, 1994), have not been and are not currently adequate to capture all traumatic symptomatology and responses (Cole & Putnam, 1992; Breslau, Davis, & Andreski, 1991). In fact, in a consensus statement written by leaders in the field (Ballenger et al., 2000), it was stated that the "pure" form of PTSD (i.e., that which is outlined in DSM-IV) is, in fact, unrepresentative of the "typical" PTSD presentation seen in clinical settings. Herman (1992a) was one of the first to put shape to issues that had been discussed by others (e.g., Kroll, Habenicht, Mackenzie, & Yang, 1989; Brown & Fromm, 1986; Herman & van der Kolk, 1987), formally naming and delineating a new diagnostic category, which she called Complex PTSD.

Many have pointed out that the traumatic responses to single-incident, adult-onset traumas tend to be fairly well captured by the PTSD criteria laid out in DSM-IV, whereas responses to chronic, childhood-onset, and interpersonal traumas are less well represented by these same criteria, leaving a sizable "hole" or "blind spot" in our current diagnostic nomenclature for trauma (Herman, 1992b; Deering, Glover, Ready, Eddleman, & Alarcon, 1996; World Health Organization, 1992; van der Kolk, et al., 1996). The DSM-IV PTSD task force concurred, delineating a constellation of symptoms that are not captured in the current PTSD diagnosis but that are highly prevalent in clinical settings among individuals with long histories of trauma (Pelcovitz et al., 1997; van der Kolk et al., 1993). They called this constellation of symptoms disorders of extreme stress, not otherwise specified (DESNOS). Six areas of functioning were identified that are seen as consistently being negatively affected in survivors of complex trauma: (1) affect regulation, (2) attention/consciousness, (3) self-perception, (4) relationships, (5) somatization, and (6) meaning systems (e.g., belief in God). Two different assessment instruments for evaluating complex trauma in clinical settings have been developed since the findings of the task force—the Structured Interview of Disorders of Extreme Stress (SIDES) and the Self-Report Inventory for Disorders of Extreme Stress (SIDES-SR; Pelcovitz et al., 1997; Spinazzola, Blaustein, Kiesel, & van der Kolk, 2001). Further, research has upheld the validity of the clinical picture associated with complex trauma (e.g., Roth, Newman, Pelcovitz, van der Kolk, & Mandel, 1997; Ackerman, Newton, McPherson, Jones, & Dykman, 1998; Zlotnick, Zakriski, Shea, & Costello, 1996).

As discussed, the Rorschach may be able to shed light on some of these areas of dysfunction in those suffering from complex trauma. It is worth stressing again that neither the Rorschach nor any other assessment instrument should be used in isolation. One cannot diagnose complex trauma on the strength of any one instrument. All information needs to be considered as a whole. That being said, however, the Rorschach clearly has the potential to provide a unique view of a person's functioning that is not possible with other measures. It also should be stated at this juncture that the idea to use the Rorschach to specifically address the issue of complex trauma, apart from dissociative disorders, is a relatively new one, and all of the following should be considered to be suggestive in nature. It remains for future research to determine which variables on the Rorschach are most strongly and reliably related to complex trauma. Based on our current state of knowledge, however, there is reason to explore further what role the Rorschach can play in addressing complex trauma.

Those individuals who have experienced complex trauma typically have great difficulty regulating their emotions (Linehan, Tutek, Heard, & Armstrong, 1994). They tend to have more intense emotional reactions than most individuals, often to apparently neutral stimuli, and are frequently prone to unmodulated bursts of anger. They often experience their emotions as being more intense, less controllable, and more frightening than other people do and have great difficulty soothing themselves when distressed (Luxenberg, Spinazzola, Hidalgo, Hunt, & van der Kolk, 2001). These difficulties can be tracked on the Rorschach in several ways.

First, as those familiar with the Rorschach know, this test has an entire section that is devoted entirely to a person's affective experience. More specifically, however, the Rorschach provides us with a very direct measure of how modulated and controlled a person's experience and expression of emotion is. The ratio of FC:CF+C taps precisely this quality. The left side of the ratio (responses in which form is primary and color secondary) is considered to be a representation of modulated emotion, whereas the right side of the equation (responses in which color is primary and form secondary, or in which only color, with no form, is present) is considered to be a representation of increasingly unmodulated, intense, and dysregulating affect. Importantly, the less form a testee uses in her or his color responses, the more unregulated her or his experience and expression of affect is likely to be. Ratios that are heavily weighted to the right, therefore, are much more likely to occur in the protocols of individuals who have experienced complex trauma (Levin & Reis, 1997).

Further, the Rorschach provides us with the Experience Balance (EB) ratio, which is a measure of the extent to which individuals use emotion and/or thinking in their problem-solving and decision-making process. If the EB is weighted to the right (within certain parameters, as defined by Exner), a person is said to have an extratensive style, in which feeling often contributes significantly to the problem-solving process, and displays of affect tend to be more frequent and sometimes less strictly controlled. This finding is what one might expect in individuals who are experiencing significant affect dysregulation (although it should be noted that this finding, in and of itself, is not a sign of pathology and that both introversive and extratensive coping styles are equally efficient at problem solving).

The Rorschach has numerous indicators of painful, troubling affect. Shading responses (elevated Y and one or more V) capture this quality, as well as the Texture response (T), which, when elevated, is thought to represent the presence of painful, unmet needs for nurturance. The existence of any shading blends within a protocol suggests the presence of intensely negative and painful emotion. Although such a finding is generally highly unusual, it would be very interesting to see if such responses are equally unusual among survivors of complex trauma. The presence of shading blends may well be more common among this population, but this waits to be formally evaluated in future research.

In addition, how a testee responds to the full-color cards (which are the last 3 of the series of 10) is thought to be diagnostic in terms of how well someone is coping and prepared to manage arousing material. It has long been known that certain testees, who provided relatively coherent, well-formed responses on the first 7 cards of the test, when confronted with the last 3 cards, suddenly provide rambling, loose answers that make poor use of form and are much more affect laden. This has been thought to represent problems in dealing with emotion and may well be a marker for suggesting that individuals may have a complex trauma presentation, in which affect regulation is known to be a critical difficulty. This may be especially helpful in those individuals who, for whatever reason, are not reporting actual trauma histories. Such individuals could potentially present very differently on the last of the cards from how they presented during the rest of the test, thus signaling that closer examination may be warranted. Finally, the unmodulated anger typically seen in those individuals struggling with complex trauma may be suggested by an elevated number of Space (S) responses, which are linked with the experience of anger and oppositionalism. Too, the presence of sex and blood contents indicate a lack of normal censoring, perhaps related to emotional flooding, ineffective coping, and/or specific trauma-sequelae percepts.

As discussed previously, one of the sine qua nons of trauma may well be the co-existence of the disparate processes of being flooded/overwhelmed and numb/constricted. This dual, "biphasic" process of being overwhelmed with emotion and avoiding emotion simultaneously is exquisitely captured in the Rorschach (Levin, 1993). As noted previously, nowhere is this process so well illustrated as in the common finding among traumatized individuals who show high CF and C responses (intense, unmodulated affect) and also exhibit low Afr ratios (avoidance of emotionally laden material or thoughts). The presence of a significant number of blended responses in otherwise constricted, impoverished protocols; complex organization; and constricted but unmodulated emotion are found in the protocols of dissociative, complex trauma survivors (Armstrong, 1991).

It is important to note that all of these variables under consideration are of little value in and of themselves. It is only when one sees a concatenation of these variables that one might begin to suspect that there are significant issues in that area that require closer examination (see Table 8.1 for an outline of possible trauma-sequelae variables).

Individuals who have experienced complex trauma frequently learn to cope with overwhelming experience by "walling off" portions of that experience. These compartmentalized aspects of experience become insulated from one's everyday level of consciousness, to greater or lesser degrees, providing the individuals with some relief from painful, overwhelming cognition, sensation, and affect (Chu, 1998). This tendency to not integrate all information can lead to memory problems, confusion, unreliable access to certain kinds of information, and overall attentional peculiarities and difficulties (Luxenberg, Spinazzola, & van der Kolk, 2001).

Such difficulties could be apparent in several aspects of the Rorschach. First, the tendency to avoid stimuli, particularly affectively laden stimuli, so that one does not have to think, feel, or be aware of painful material, has been strongly linked with constricted protocols and with low Afr ratios. In the same vein, as discussed previously, individuals having significant problems with dissociation are often found to exhibit introversive or superintroversive styles on the Rorschach (Armstrong, 1991). They appear to place strict controls on their emotional experience, striving to keep their cognitive processes unaffected by feelings, all of which may be occurring unconsciously. Levin (1990, 1993), Hartman et al. (1990), and Sloan et al. (1995) found an unusually large proportion of ambitent EB styles. Ambitents use emotion in their problem solving but do not have a preferential coping style, and they are therefore more stress vulnerable. However, van der Kolk and Ducey (1984, 1989) had one Vietnam veteran subgroup who were highly extratensive, and Scroppo et al. (1998) found more extratensives among their nondissociative participants. The fact that dissociative, but not other, traumatized populations

TABLE 8.1. Rorschach Variables That Might Be Related to Complex Trauma

Affect regulation	Attention/consciousness	Ideation	Relationships and self-perception	Somatization
CF + C > FC	Constricted protocols	X + %, X – %, Xu%, F + %	Positive CDI	An responses
Above condition, combined with low Afr ratio	Low Afr ratio	Special Scores	Elevated AG	Xy responses
Extratensive or super-extratensive EB ratio	Introversive or superintroversive EB ratio	SCZI	Low COP	MOR responses
Elevated Y	Elevated FD	M–	Elevated m	
Elevated V	Presence of "biphasic" or contradictory processes (e.g., CF + C > FC and low Afr)	M none	Elevated HVI	
Elevated T	Dissociation index	#M responses	Greater part or imaginary human contents versus whole or real human contents	
Shading blends	TC/R		a:p ratio weighted to right	
Dramatic response to color cards	Elevated HVI		M– responses	
Sex and blood contents	Presence of trauma percepts		Isolation index	
Negative D	Zd and Zf		Food responses	
Negative Adj D	Elevated PSV		Elevated DEPI	
Space responses			Egocentricity index	
			An, Xy, MOR	

score in the introversive and superintroversive range is a strong indication that something is being measured here that is specific to dissociation, not just trauma.

This is also clearly the case in the dissociation index developed by Leavitt and Labott (1996) and Leavitt (2000) discussed earlier. Using this index, they were able to combine several percepts on the Rorschach to serve as markers for significant dissociation that correlate well with a standardized and widely accepted measure of dissociation. Form dimension (FD) responses (one FD is the norm) indicate the ability to observe oneself or one's experience in a removed, detached fashion, framed more positively as the capacity for perspective or insight. An elevation in form dimension responses may be indicative of more compartmentalized, frank dissociation (Armstrong, 1991).

Complex trauma often results in significantly impaired relationships. Such individuals may repeatedly find themselves in abusive relationships, may expect mistreatment from others, and may not adequately either note or respond to their own internal sense of being mistreated (Lisak, Hopper, & Song, 1996). The Coping Deficit Index (CDI), in part, is a measure of interpersonal difficulties and a lack of a sense of being able to count on others for support. An expectation of violence and/or mistreatment can be seen in those protocols containing a high Aggressive content (AG). This variable becomes even more powerful in illuminating unhealthy relational expectations and experiences when coupled with a very low Cooperative Movement score (COP). Further, expectations of mistreatment can also be seen in elevated Inanimate Movements (m) scores, which have been linked with views of the world as a threatening, foreboding place.

In addition, multiple variables can be looked at to begin to tease out how threatening other humans are viewed as being. The HVI, for example, can be seen, in part, as an index of how interpersonally cautious an individual is and how carefully he or she "scans" for harm in his or her interactions with others. Similarly, a greater use of imaginary human percepts, as opposed to realistic or actual human percepts, may suggest a withdrawal from real relationships and an expectation that humans cannot be safe in the "real world." M– responses, which show clear reality distortions, are yet another indication of problematic interpersonal relationships. Finally, the active-to-passive human-movement ratio (a:p) is a potential measure for vulnerability to revictimization. Individuals who demonstrate highly elevated passive scores may well be indicating that they are not comfortable acting in their own behalf, may have difficulty mobilizing to take action and protect themselves, and are victims awaiting rescue. These factors could, potentially, render them more vulnerable to mistreatment.

It has been noted for some time that chronically traumatized individuals often suffer, along with their psychological difficulties, numerous physical problems, many of which often respond poorly to medical treatment and are experienced more intensely than is typical (Felitti et al., 1998; Berkowitz, 1998). Although the Rorschach is by no means a medical test nor a measure of physical functioning and/or somatization, it nevertheless has two potential avenues for exploring unusual physical issues. The presence of anatomy and X-ray responses (An and Xy) on the Rorschach is thought to represent preoccupation with one's body and its functions. This might be expected to appear in the protocols of individuals who have numerous physical complaints from which they can find little relief and whose doctors inform them that their symptoms are unusual, more intense than is normal, or even functional in origin. In addition, the previously discussed MOR responses are also an indication of the body being viewed as damaged, unreliable, experienced as a "perpetrator" toward its "owner," and something to be despised.

The final category of dysfunction typically linked with complex trauma is that of compromised systems of meaning. It is not at all unusual for chronically traumatized individuals to report that they do not believe that life holds any meaning or purpose. They may become fatalistic in their approach to life, anticipating that, ultimately, things will work out badly and that any efforts on their part will be compromised or undermined completely (Herman, 1992b). Although there are no direct measures of this in the Rorschach, many aspects discussed previously may offer hints that meaning systems have been compromised. A high DEPI, HVI, and coping deficit index (CDI) all suggest a pervasive, negative expectational set toward the external world and circumstances. Many of the factors discussed in regard to relationships could also be seen as hinting at the existence of an overall helplessness and fatalism. This area clearly requires further exploration. We suspect that an area as complex as one's sense of meaning is unlikely to be effectively captured in discrete variables but is, rather, more likely to best be illuminated when considering multiple factors in complex, interactional schemas.

TREATMENT

It is now well known among those clinicians who work with trauma survivors not only that the clinical picture varies from simple to complex trauma but also that the course of treatment for those suffering from "complex PTSD" is typically longer, more complicated, suffused with more risky behavior (e.g., drug abuse, self-injury, suicide attempts, etc.), and more vulnerable to the impact of current life stressors. This means, quite simply, that treatments for simple and complex trauma are different (Luxenberg, Spinazzola, Hidalgo, et al., 2001). The treatment of complex trauma is generally conceptualized as occurring in stages—safety and stabilization; processing of and grieving over traumatic experiences; and reconnection with meaningful activities and people in the world (Brown, Scheflin, & Hammond, 1998; van der Kolk et al., 1996). The phases, of course, are not strictly linear but are thought to represent a general progression. Importantly, treatment varies among the stages. The first stage primarily focuses on symptom reduction and the development of coping skills and affect regulation. The second stage primarily deals with the metabolization of traumatic memories and the integrating of those memories into a meaningful and coherent life narrative. This stage tends to have significant impact on individuals' sense of self and their relationship with others. Finally, in the third stage of treatment, focus shifts to developing meaningful life activities and relationships that firmly embed individuals within a larger familial, social, and cultural context.

Clinicians have long lamented that some clients seem to endlessly remain "stuck" in therapy, whereas others actually seem to worsen with treatment, rather than improve. A dramatic example of this occurred when Pitman and colleagues (1991) actually had to stop a flooding treatment study, due to worsening symptomatology among some of their study participants. In addition, although exposure-based treatments have been shown to be very helpful in relieving the symptoms of a certain portion of trauma survivors (Foa et al., 1999), stringent exclusion criteria and high dropout rates have called into question whether all trauma survivors were being adequately represented in most treatment research studies. In addition, a certain subset of individuals appear to do poorly in exposure treatment (e.g., Vaughan & Tarrier, 1992). Further, researchers have often noted high levels of dysfunction in their participants, even after the completion of "successful" treatment (e.g., Jaycox, Foa, & Morral, 1998). All of these factors have led many clinicians to feel that it is crucial to become more facile at articulating the differences among trauma survivors and to be thoughtful about those differences when designing treatments.

What has become clear over time is that, although some individuals are capable of moving directly into the processing of their traumatic memories, others are not ready to do so, and their symptoms are quite likely either to remain unchanged or to worsen if processing is attempted prematurely. Such individuals need to first work on developing coping skills and affect regulation (i.e., stage 1—safety and stabilization) before they have the necessary "tools" to process their traumas. The treatment literature indicates several factors to be considered in deciding whether someone is ready for exposure-based (i.e., stage 2, processing) treatment or would do better with a skills-based (i.e., stage 1) focus in treatment. Anger problems have been found to be predictive of both treatment dropout and symptom recalcitrance (e.g., Foa, Hearst-Ikeda, & Perry, 1995; Chemtob, Novaco, Hamada, Gross, & Smith, 1997). Further, clients who had difficulty with "mental planning," who felt alienated or damaged, or who could not form coherent narratives of their trauma during treatment have been found to have poor treatment outcomes (Ehlers et al., 1998). Finally, the experience of guilt and shame has been found to predict poor outcome in exposure treatments (Kubany et al., 1995).

Two things should be clear at this point: (1) the overlap between some of the poor treatment outcome predictors for exposure-based therapy and the symptomatology associated with survivors of complex trauma and (2) the potential utility of the Rorschach in discerning those individuals who can profit from the various stages of treatment. Clearly, individuals dealing with complex trauma require a more titrated, stage-oriented approach.

The Rorschach clearly addresses areas that have been suggested in the literature as being indicators of those individuals who need a safety and stabilization focus in their treatment. There are several indicators of anger on the Rorschach, both direct and indirect. Space (S) responses are directly linked with a person's experience of anger toward the environment, whereas aggressive content could potentially represent a negativistic, angry expectational set toward the world. In addition, the factors discussed previously that are associated with affect regulation difficulty (e.g., CFFC+C) may also be helpful in discerning the individuals who may, due to general dysregulation problems, be more vulnerable to bursts of anger.

Further, two factors that have been identified as being linked with poor tolerance for and outcome with exposure-based treatments are a sense of alienation and being damaged. Both are specifically captured on the Rorschach. A high presence of MOR (Morbid) contents is directly related to a view of oneself as being damaged. In addition, the presence of an elevated number of An and Xy responses suggests the possibility of preoccupation with the body and its defects, flaws, and injuries. A sense of alienation is well captured in the Rorschach through low Human contents, high imaginary Human contents, low Human Movement (especially Cooperative Movement), and, most directly, the Isolation index. Similarly, level of interest in human interactions is also measured on the Rorschach through the total number of human contents (H + (H) + Hd + (Hd)). Another factor, difficulty with mental planning, can be assessed in examining the Rorschach's extensive information on cognitive functioning. More specifically, a person's tendency to act without forethought in the face of stress can be examined through the D score, Adj D score, and the EA score. A lack of human movement in a protocol further suggests that a person's capacity to think and plan has been foreclosed. Finally, the presence of guilt and shame can potentially be assessed through examination of a person's vista (V) responses.

Shaping Treatment to Meet Individual Needs

Identifying those individuals who need which form of treatment, is, however, only the first step in treatment planning. Once it is clear that an individual suffers from complex trauma, the question still remains what that individual's specific treatment needs are. Here again the Rorschach can provide us with valuable information. Two of the first, and most fundamental, questions when working with trauma survivors are, How affected by the trauma(s) is this individual? and How sturdy is this individual's coping? The more intense the current impact of the trauma and the more precarious a person's coping, the longer and more involved the safety and stabilization phase of treatment is likely to be, and the more intense the focus on the acquisition of skills and affect management should be.

Assessing Level of Impact of the Trauma

Fortunately, the Rorschach provides us with very clear information about both of these topics. The extent to which individuals are being affected by their trauma can be seen quite directly in the number of "intrusions" they experience during their protocols in the form of trauma-related percepts. Further, the more tenuous the connection between the actual structure on the cards and the trauma percept that the individual defines is, the more powerful or compelling one can consider the intrusive material to be. This can be directly assessed by examination of the number of minus (–) forms used in a protocol, which is one aspect of reality testing. Numerous researchers have worked to develop various indices to assess traumatic content on the Rorschach (e.g., Armstrong, 1991; Sloan et al., 1995). Although one global scale of traumatic content may not be realistic (given the plethora of ways in which a person can be traumatized), it is clear that direct assessment of the content of Rorschach responses can be a rich supply of information about what an individual has experienced and the extent to which these experience(s) are dominating that individual's perception of the world. Other measures of the level of "intrusiveness" that a person experiences can be gleaned from elevated Texture scores (T), blends that include m and Y, shading blends in general, lack of human movement, negative D and Adj D scores, impaired reality testing, hypervigilance, and elevated FM and m scores.

Importantly, the more significantly an individual is experiencing intrusive symptomatology, the more preparatory, stage 1 work he or she will need. Under such circumstances, symptom reduction becomes the focus of the work. High intrusive symptomatology may necessitate psychopharmacological intervention before a person can be emotionally available to do any further work. It should be stressed that if someone is experiencing very frequent and intense intrusions, she or he will not be able to tolerate very much in the way of therapy, and relatively small affective experiences may well be intolerable. This needs to be taken into account in structuring the treatment. Such clients should be taught how to notice when they are becoming overwhelmed (physical, emotional, and behavioral signs), and a great deal of emphasis should be put on helping these clients to build a "library" full of ways to calm and soothe themselves.

If an individual has been traumatized within an interpersonal context (as is almost always the case for those who have experienced complex trauma), another important area in which to assess the impact of trauma on an individual is the interpersonal realm. This clearly is important in terms of a person's functioning in daily life, but it also a crucial component in treatment planning. For example, an individual who is suspicious or guarded requires a different structuring of treatment than does an individual who is open and forthcoming. With the former, the clinician may want to forgo or significantly reduce the history taking, beyond basic necessities, as this may actually cause the client to shut down further. In addition, such a client may respond better to a more client-directed, rather than clinician-directed, approach, at least initially. Further, when working with very guarded clients, it is best to bring up difficult or "loaded" material very judiciously, if at all, given that these clients may find this to be intrusive and/or overwhelming.

One of the most difficult experiences for clinicians working with trauma survivors can be the client's tendency to view others, including the therapist, as perpetrators and to "reenact" their traumatic experiences of being shamed, humiliated, mistreated, and so forth, with well-intentioned others. Although it is important to note that the Rorschach cannot be used as a predictive tool of traumatic reenactment, several factors on the Rorschach may alert the clinician to the possibility of such an occurrence. One should be more concerned, clearly, if all of the suspiciousness variables listed previously are present, particularly if combined with significant anger responses (S). Examination of Pure H responses in comparisons to non–Pure H responses ((H) + Hd + (Hd)) will help to determine to what extent a person's perception of others is realistically, versus imaginally, based or distorted. What is likely to be most critical, however, is the extent to which clients distort reality in the percepts that they define, especially in their human percepts. This is directly captured in minus human movement responses (M–). In short, this suggests the extent to which clients may misinterpret or misperceive experiences with people. A content reading of the M– responses will be very helpful in exploring this further and determining to what extent such distortions are in the direction of danger and threat. If, indeed, a client appears to be vulnerable to misperception of the clinician and others, and if this is borne out by other evidence as well, then the clinician would be wise to do two things: (1) remember, as they listen to their clients' stories, that this tendency to misperceive threat may sometimes be present and (2) talk with the client, in advance of a problem, about how they may, at times, feel that others, including the clinician, are being hurtful to them, due to their old feelings related to their mistreatment rising to the surface. Plans should be laid as to how to deal with such a turn of events.

A strong word of caution is in order. This is quite subtle work. It is absolutely crucial not to invalidate the clients' experience nor to assume that any given situation they relay is being misperceived on their part. This would be a tremendous disservice to clients—as would listening to clients uncritically and not helping them sort out their realistic perceptions from their trauma-based perceptions. If alerted by the Rorschach and other relevant information that a client may tend to view others as being harmful and abusive, then clinicians can know to begin to look for the patterns and the signs that will help them, and ultimately their clients, distinguish between accurate perception and trauma-influenced perception. Such clinicians would also do well to be vigilant about their own emotional experiences while sitting with the client. Clients who present in this way on the Rorschach are quite likely to inspire in the therapist a whole range of disconcerting feelings, and such emotions should be used as clues as to what may be going on internally in the client, in addition to being monitored and dealt with by the clinician.

The therapy outcome studies cited previously (Levin et al., 1996; Levin et al., 1999) using EMDR, in light of the robust research on EMDR's treatment effectiveness with trauma (Shapiro, 2002), as well as the increasing use of EMDR in stage 1 work in the form of resource installation (Korn & Leeds, 2002) and affect management (Omaha, 2000), should be seriously considered by trauma clinicians.

Of final note, group work is often recommended as a powerful intervention for trauma survivors. It is unlikely, however, to be helpful to individuals who currently exhibit the suspiciousness discussed here.

Assessing Individuals' Coping

Those familiar with the Rorschach know that an entire section of the interpretive process is devoted to the exploration of a person's capacity for control and stress tolerance. This, clearly, is a very rich source for understanding a person's level of impulsivity and tendency to become overwhelmed by experience. The coping deficit index (CDI) measures this directly. Further, the D and Adj D scores shed light on how well a person is able to cope with stress and how likely a person is to "lose" the capacity to cope in the face of difficult circumstances. Importantly, although individuals with simple traumas may have similar Adj D scores to their complexly traumatized counterparts, they are likely to show an elevated right side of the EB ratio, which indicates that generally adequate resources are being presently overwhelmed by current, high stressors. A chronically traumatized individual, however, is unlikely to have the elevated right side EB ratio, and he or she may exhibit a depressed EA score as well, indicating a general dearth of coping skills.

Further, the EB ratio can be very helpful in illuminating where precisely an individual may be compromised. A lack of human movement contents (the left side of the ratio), for example, indicates that a person may have become affectively overwhelmed, leading to a "shutdown" in cognition. SumC = 0 (right side of the EB ratio), however, indicates that emotional states are the area of "shutdown" and that the person has become emotionally constricted. It is interesting to note that this ratio could be helpful in sorting out which traumatic "phase" a person is currently most vulnerable to—flooding or numbing.

Plainly, the more indications that there are in a protocol that a person has coping deficits and may be impulsive (e.g., D score, sex and blood contents), the more concerned a clinician should be with the possibility of acting-out behavior. Such a situation would clearly necessitate a heavy concentration on the building and strengthening of coping skills, both inside and outside of therapy. Clients with heavy deficits in this area and heightened impulsivity may need therapy to focus in a very concrete way on behaviors that they can engage in when overwhelmed, to obviate the need for destructive, impulsive forms of coping. Clearly the suicide index (S-CON) should be examined in all cases to determine how likely it may be that clients would use this "ultimate" disordered, impulsive form of coping. Although a low S-CON cannot rule out the possibility of a suicide attempt or completion, a high S-CON certainly raises the level of concern about the likelihood of an attempt or completion.

Another aspect of how well individuals are coping is how facile they are at managing their emotions. This was discussed at length previously. Emotional dysregulation has a direct impact on the structure of treatment. With patients who exhibit such affective lability on the Rorschach, it will be important for the clinician to realize that therapy will need to focus, in part, on teaching the client to titrate and modulate her or his own emotional experience. This often involves helping clients become aware of the full range of feelings, including the moderate range, and teaching them to appreciate gradations of feelings, rather than experiencing their emotions as being either absent or completely overwhelming. In addition, clients who are affectively overwhelmed (or easily become so) often need to be taught thought-stopping techniques to combat their traumatic thinking patterns. Work that focuses on containment and soothing will also be important for such individuals, with a strong emphasis on the clients' learning techniques that they can perform without the therapist, so that the skills truly become internalized.

If the Rorschach indicates that a client is having problems with cognition due to emotional interference, it may become important to work on developing a variety of means by which the client can "activate" his or her thinking. Therapy should explore which methods are most powerful for any individual. Putting things in writing, having lists or plans posted about the home, writing reminders to oneself, or tape-recording messages to oneself may all be ways to help clients remind themselves of all of the planning that has been done in session but that may not be accessible to clients when they become overwhelmed.

We believe that the power of the Rorschach to identify dissociative presentations has been underutilized and merits further exploration and research. The dissociative index discussed previously is an exciting development that should be cross-validated. Identifying dissociative pathology in clients is a critically important process, as clients with unidentified dissociative disorders often do not receive much benefit from treatment. Further, there are a broad range of treatment techniques and approaches that have been found to be helpful to those with dissociative disorders that could be considered, in light of a Rorschach and other relevant information that suggest the presence of serious dissociative symptomatology.

Finally, one of the most challenging, and most important, issues that faces a clinician who is working with survivors of complex trauma is knowing when they are ready to move into the next phase of treatment. Although this process cannot be thought of as absolute and clear-cut, the Rorschach may be very helpful in seeking to determine when a client is ready for the next stage of treatment. Before stage 2 work (processing and integration of traumatic memories) is undertaken, one would want to see significant shifts in those factors that deal with affect regulation, stress tolerance, and coping capacity. If those have not strengthened significantly, the client may not be able to tolerate further processing work. In a similar vein, one would want to see significant, positive shifts in self-concept and perceptions of and interactions with others prior to shifting focus to the third stage of treatment, which is the reintegration with meaningful people and activities.

SUMMARY

The concept of trauma is quite complex, encompassing acute and chronic trauma, interpersonal and impersonal trauma, witnessing and experiencing trauma, and adult and childhood trauma, to name but a few distinctions. As clinicians and researchers have become more sophisticated in their understanding of trauma, they have also come to appreciate the importance of understanding not just what happened to an individual but also how it happened and in what context and how this has affected such variables as the person's view of him- or herself, others, relationships, and the world. This is complex but crucial work, as it is the understanding of these factors that allows clinicians to design the most appropriate and efficient treatments and to tailor those treatments to the individual needs of the client.

Clearly, such subtle work could not be done without assessment tools that go far beyond descriptions of what has happened subjectively to an individual and an exploration of the symptoms associated with PTSD, as laid out in DSM-IV. No instrument is so well suited to this task as the Rorschach Inkblot Test, which can help illuminate a client's attitudes, perceptions, and thinking and emotional patterns.

One of the essential tasks facing clinicians who work with traumatized individuals is that of discriminating between clients who are suffering from trauma or other clinical problems (e.g., borderline personality disorder, thought disorders, etc.) that often can have significant symptom overlap with trauma disorders. Indeed, the work becomes more subtle still when clinicians are called to determine the relative contributions of several actual disorders, including trauma. For example, it is not at all unusual in either of our practices to be asked to determine whether or not a traumatized individual also has a thought disorder and, if so, whether or not some of their symptoms are due to their trauma or to their thought disorder.

In addition, the Rorschach can be potentially very helpful in "catching" trauma when a client is not reporting a history of having been traumatized. This can be useful whether the client does not remember the trauma, remembers the trauma but does not recognize its impact or importance in terms of her or his current functioning, or remembers the trauma but does not wish to reveal or discuss it, often out of fear of being overwhelmed. These are three very different situations clinically, and yet they all could be addressed through an examination of the Rorschach. Enough research has occurred for a number of factors to have been identified that comprise several trauma "profiles" on the Rorschach. Although there is no one magical "marker" of trauma on the

Rorschach, there is a very strong constellation of factors that, taken together, are powerfully suggestive of a traumatic background.

In addition, the Rorschach serves another function for trauma clinicians, which is helping to identify those cases in which malingering or a factitious disorder is present. Although these make up a small percentage of trauma presentations overall, they are not absent from the clinical landscape, and it is crucial to be able to discern when such forces are at play. It is important to note that, as is often the case when working with trauma, the clinical realities are often quite complex. Individuals with actual trauma histories may also have malingering or factitious *components* to their presentation, and the days of either/or choices are long behind us. It becomes crucial to understand when individuals are embellishing or exaggerating real trauma histories, either consciously or unconsciously, so that the needs driving such behavior can be addressed and met in other, more constructive ways. Ignoring a malingering or factitious component in treatment is quite likely to result in a stymied treatment that can extend indefinitely without any real progress being made. The Rorschach is extremely powerful in this area, due to the ability of clinicians to contrast an individual's Rorschach profile with known trauma profiles and catch significant and pervasive discrepancies.

One of the most powerful areas in which the Rorschach can offer invaluable assistance in diagnosis and treatment planning is complex trauma. The Rorschach offers insight directly into the first five of the six areas of dysfunction that have been found to be associated with complex trauma. Nowhere does the information offered by the Rorschach become as important as when designing a powerful and efficient treatment. It can help determine what stage of treatment is appropriate for the client, how long the course of treatment is likely to be, what treatment will need to entail, and what areas should be focused on first.

The interpersonal information that can be gained from the Rorschach is very helpful in terms of assisting the clinician in predicting and preparing for the interpersonal dynamics that may play out during the treatment. The Rorschach allows a clinician not simply to react to potential interpersonal dynamics but to prepare for them and even to prepare the client for them, and thus to anticipate developing effective coping strategies.

In sum, then, the Rorschach is a powerful tool that can be a valuable addition to a trauma clinician's assessment repertoire. It provides the clinician with unprecedented insight into clients' views of themselves, others, and the world around them, while also providing valuable information about if and to what extent clients are suffering from areas of dysfunction associated with their trauma. The clinician is thus able to be sensitive to issues of trauma, even when not reported, as well as to identify protocols that are, in full or in part, discrepant with reported histories of trauma. The clinician is given helpful insight into both understanding the nature of a client's difficulties and planning a powerful treatment with the unique needs of the individual in mind. It is our hope that the continued use of the Rorschach will allow trauma clinicians to come to more accurate and sophisticated understandings of their clients, which will ultimately allow them to be more helpful and efficient in designing powerful treatments that really work.

REFERENCES

Ackerman, P., Newton, J., McPherson, W., Jones, J., & Dykman, R. (1998). Prevalence of posttraumatic stress disorder and other psychiatric diagnoses in three groups of abused children (sexual, physical, and both). *Child Abuse and Neglect*, *22*, 759–774.

American Psychiatric Association. (1980). *Diagnostic and statistical manual of mental disorders*. (3rd ed.). Washington, DC: Author.

American Psychiatric Association. (1987). *Diagnostic and statistical manual of mental disorders*. (3rd ed., rev.). Washington, DC: Author.

American Psychiatric Association. (1994). *Diagnostic and statistical manual of mental disorders*. (4th ed.). Washington, DC: Author.

Archer, R., & Krishnamurthy, R. (1997). MMPI-A and Rorschach indices related to depression and conduct disorder. *Journal of Personality Assessment*, *69*, 517–533.

Armstrong, J. (1991). The psychological organization of multiple-personality-disordered patients as revealed in psychological testing. *Psychiatric Clinics of North America*, *14*, 533–546.

Armstrong, J., & Kaser-Boyd, N. (in press). Projective assessment of psychological trauma. In M. Hilsenroth & D. Segal (Eds.), M. Hersen (Ed.-in-Chief), *Comprehensive handbook of psychological assessment: Vol. 2. Objective and projective assessment of personality and psychopathology*. New York: Wiley.

Armstrong, J., & Loewenstein, R. (1990). Characteristics of patients with multiple personality and dissociative disorders on psychological testing. *Journal of Nervous and Mental Disease*, *178*, 445–454.

Ballenger, J., Davidson, J., Lecrubier, Y., Nutt, D., Foa, E., & Kessler, R. (2000). Consensus statement on posttraumatic stress disorder from the international consensus group on depression and anxiety. *Journal of Clinical Psychology*, *61*, 60–66.

Berkowitz, C. (1998). Medical consequences of child sexual abuse. *Child Abuse and Neglect*, *22*, 541–550.

Blake, D., Weathers, F., Nagy, L., Kaloupek, D., Gusman, F., Charney, D., & Keane, T. (1995). The development of a clinician-administered PTSD scale. *Journal of Traumatic Stress*, *8*, 75–90.

Breslau, N., Davis, G., & Andreski, P. (1991). Traumatic events and posttraumatic stress disorder in an urban population of young adults. *Archives of General Psychiatry*, *48*, 216–222.

Breslau, N., Kessler, R., Chilcoat, H., Schultz, I., Davis, G., & Andreski, P. (1998). Trauma and posttraumatic stress disorder in the community. *Journal of Psychiatry*, *55*, 626–632.

Brett, E., Spitzer, R., & Williams, J. (1988). DSM-III-R criteria for posttraumatic stress disorder. *American Journal of Psychiatry*, *144*, 1232–1236.

Briere, J. (1997). *Psychological assessment of adult posttraumatic states*. Washington, DC: American Psychological Association.

Briere, J., Elliot, D., Harris, K., & Cotman, A. (1995). Trauma Symptom Inventory: Psychometrics and association with childhood and adult victimization in clinical samples. *Journal of Interpersonal Violence*, *10*, 387–401.

Brown, D., & Fromm, E. (1986). *Hypnotherapy and hypnoanalysis*. Hillsdale, NJ: Erlbaum.

Brown, D., Scheflin, A., & Hammond, D. (1998). *Memory, trauma treatment, and the law*. New York: Norton.

Browne, A., & Finkelhor, D. (1986). Impact of child sexual abuse: A review of the research. *Psychological Bulletin*, *99*(1), 66–77.

Carlson, E., Furby, L., Armstrong, J., & Schlaes, J. (1997). A conceptual framework for the long-term psychological effects of traumatic childhood abuse. *Child Maltreatment*, *2*, 272–295.

Cassidy, J., & Mohr, J. J. (2001). Unsolvable fear, trauma, and psychopathology. *Clinical Psychology: Science and Practice*, *8*, 275–298.

Cerney, M. (1990). The Rorschach and traumatic loss: Can the presence of traumatic loss be detected from the Rorschach? *Journal of Personality Assessment*, *55*, 781–789.

Chemtob, C., Novaco, R., Hamada, R., Gross, D., & Smith, G. (1997). Anger regulation deficits in combat-related PTSD. *Journal of Traumatic Stress*, *10*(1), 17–36.

Chu, J. (1998). *Rebuilding shattered lives: The responsible treatment of complex posttraumatic and dissociative disorders*. New York: Wiley.

Cole, P., & Putnam, F. (1992). Effect of incest on self and social functioning: A developmental psychopathology perspective. *Journal of Consulting and Clinical Psychology*, *60*, 174–184.

Davidson, J., Hughes, D., Blazer, D., & George, L. (1991). Posttraumatic stress disorder in the community: An epidemiological study. *Psychological Medicine*, *21*, 713–721.

Deering, C., Glover, S., Ready, D., Eddleman, H., & Alarcon, R. (1996). Unique patterns of comorbidity in posttraumatic stress disorder from different sources of trauma. *Comprehensive Psychiatry*, *37*, 336–346.

Ehlers, A., Clark, D., Dunmore, E., Jaycox, L., Meadows, E., & Foa, E. (1998). Predicting response to exposure treatment in PTSD: The role of mental defeat and alienation. *Journal of Traumatic Stress*, *11*, 457–471.

Everson, M., Hunter, W., Runyon, D., Edelsohn, G., & Coulter, M. (1989). Maternal support following disclosure of incest. *American Journal of Orthopsychiatry*, *59*(2), 197–207.

Exner, J. (1974). *The Rorschach: A comprehensive system*. Oxford, England: Wiley.

Exner, J. (2002a). A new nonpatient sample for the Rorschach comprehensive system: A progress report. *Journal of Personality Assessment*, *78*, 391–406.

Exner, J. (2002b, September). *The new nonpatient sample: An update*. Paper presented at the International Congress of Rorschach and Projective Methods, Rome, Italy.

Feinauer, L. (1989). Comparison of long-term effects of child abuse by type of abuse and by relationship of the offender to the victim. *American Journal of Family Therapy*, *17*(1), 48–56.

Felitti, V., Anda, R., Nordernberg, D., Williamson, D., Spitz, A., & Edwards, V. (1998). Relationship of childhood abuse to many of the leading causes of death in adults: The adverse childhood experiences (ACES) study. *American Journal of Preventative Medicine*, *14*, 245–258.

Finkelhor, D., & Browne, A. (1985). The traumatic impact of child sexual abuse: A conceptualization. *American Journal of Orthopsychiatry*, *55*(4), 530–541.

Foa, E., Dancu, C., Hembree, E., Jaycox, L., Meadows, E., & Street, G. (1999). A comparison of exposure therapy, stress inoculation training, and their combination for reducing posttraumatic stress disorder in female assault victims. *Journal of Consulting and Clinical Psychology*, *67*, 194–200.

Foa, E., Hearst-Ikeda, D., & Perry, K. (1995). Evaluation of a brief cognitive-behavioral program for the prevention of chronic PTSD in recent assault victims. *Journal of Consulting and Clinical Psychology*, *63*, 948–955.

Franchi, V., & Andronikof-Sanglade, H. (1993). Methodological and epistemological issues raised by the use of the Rorschach comprehensive system in cross cultural research. *Rorschachiana*, *18*, 118–133.

Frueh, B., & Kinder, B. (1994). The susceptibility of the Rorschach Inkblot Test to malingering of combat-related PTSD. *Journal of Personality Assessment*, *62*, 280–298.

Ganellen, R., Wasyliw, O., Haywood, T., & Grossman, L. (1996). Can psychosis be malingered on the Rorschach? An empirical study. *Journal of Personality Assessment*, *66*, 65–80.

Garb, H. (1999). Call for a moratorium on the use of the Rorschach inkblot test in clinical and forensic settings. *Assessment*, *6*, 311–318.

Garb, H., Wood, J., Nezworski, T., Grove, W., & Stejskal, W. (2001). Toward a resolution of the Rorschach controversy. *Psychological Assessment*, *13*, 423–448.

Grossman, L., Wasyliw, O., Benn, A., & Gyoerkoe, K. (2002). Can sex offenders who minimize on the MMPI conceal psychopathology on the Rorschach? *Journal of Journal of Personality Assessment*, *78*, 484–501.

Hartman, W., Clark, M., Morgan, M., Dunn, V., Fine, A., Perry, G., & Winsch, D. (1990). Rorschach structure of a hospitalized sample of Vietnam veterans with PTSD. *Journal of Personality Assessment*, *54*, 149–159.

Herman, J. (1992a). Complex PTSD: A syndrome in survivors of prolonged and repeated trauma. *Journal of Traumatic Stress*, *5*, 373–391.

Herman, J. (1992b). *Trauma and recovery*. New York: Basic Books.

Herman, J., & van der Kolk, B. A. (1987). Traumatic antecedents of borderline personality disorder. In B. A. van der Kolk (Ed.), *Psychological trauma* (pp. 111–126). Washington, DC: American Psychiatric Press.

Hildago, R., & Davidson, J. (2000). Posttraumatic stress disorder: Epidemiology and health-related concerns. *Journal of Clinical Psychology*, *61*, 5–13.

Hiller, J., Rosenthal, R., Bornstein, R., Berry, D., & Brunell-Neuleib, S. (1999). A comparative meta-analysis of Rorschach and MMPI validity. *Psychological Assessment, 11*, 278–296.

Horowitz, M. (1978). *Stress response syndromes*. New York: Aronson.

Hunsley, J., & Bailey, J. M. (1999). The clinical utility of the Rorschach: Unfulfilled promises and an uncertain future. *Psychological Assessment*, *11*, 266–277.

Hunsley, J., & Bailey, J. M. (2001). Whither the Rorschach?: An analysis of the evidence. *Psychological Assessment*, *13*, 472–485.

Jaycox, L., Foa, E., & Morral, A. (1998). Influence of emotional engagement and habituation on exposure therapy for PTSD. *Journal of Consulting and Clinical Psychology*, *66*(1), 185–192.

Kamphius, J., Kugeares, S., & Finn, S. (2000). Rorschach correlates of sexual abuse:

Trauma content and aggression indices. *Journal of Personality Assessment, 75,* 212–224.
Kardiner, A. (1941). *The traumatic neuroses of war.* New York: Hoeber.
Kaser-Boyd, N. (1993). Posttraumatic stress disorder in children and adults. *Western State Law Review, 20,* 319–334.
Korn, D., & Leeds, A. (2002). Preliminary evidence of efficacy for EMDR resource development and installation in the stabilization phase of treatment of complex posttraumatic stress disorder. *Journal of Clinical Psychology, 58*(12), 1465–1487.
Kroll, J., Habenicht, M., Mackenzie, T., & Yang, M. (1989). Depression and posttraumatic stress disorder among Southeast Asian refugees. *American Journal of Psychiatry, 146,* 1592–1597.
Kubany, E., Abueg, F., Brennan, J., Owens, J., Kaplan, A., & Watson, D. (1995). Initial examination of a multidimensional model of trauma-related guilt: Applications to combat veterans and battered women. *Journal of Psychopathological Behavioral Assessments, 17,* 253–258.
Leavitt, F. (2000). Texture response patterns associated with sexual trauma of childhood and adult onset: Developmental and recovered memory implications. *Child Abuse and Neglect, 4,* 251–257.
Leavitt, F., & Labott, S. (1996). Authenticity of recovered sexual abuse memories: A Rorschach study. *Journal of Traumatic Stress, 9,* 483–496.
Leavitt, F., & Labott, S. (1997). Criterion-related validity of Rorschach analogues of dissociation. *Psychological Assessment, 9,* 244–249.
Levin, P. (1990). A normative study of the Rorschach and posttraumatic stress disorder (Doctoral dissertation, Massachusetts School of Professional Psychology, 1990). *Dissertation Abstracts International, 51,* 08-B, 4057.
Levin, P. (1993). Assessing PTSD with the Rorschach projective technique. In J. Wilson & B. Raphael (Eds.), *The international handbook of traumatic stress syndromes* (pp. 189–200). New York: Plenum Press.
Levin, P., Errbo, N., & Call, E. (1996, June). *The Rorschach and EMDR.* Paper presented at the International Eye Movement Desensitization Reprocessing Conference, Denver, Colorado.
Levin, P., Lazrove, S., & van der Kolk, B. A. (1999). What psychological testing and neuroimaging tell us about the treatment of posttraumatic stress disorder by eye movement desensitization and reprocessing. *Journal of Anxiety Disorders, 13,* 159–172.
Levin, P., & Reis, B. (1997). Use of the Rorschach in assessing trauma. In J. P. Wilson & T. Keane (Eds.), *Assessing psychological trauma and PTSD* (pp. 529–543). New York: Guilford Press.
Linehan, M., Tutek, D., Heard, H., & Armstrong, H. (1994). Interpersonal outcome of cognitive behavioral treatment for chronically suicidal borderline patients. *American Journal of Psychiatry, 151,* 1771–1776.
Lisak, D., Hopper, J., & Song, P. (1996). Factors in the cycle of violence: Gender rigidity and emotional constriction. *Journal of Traumatic Stress, 9,* 721–743.
Lovitt, R., & Lefkof, G. (1985). Understanding multiple personality disorder with the comprehensive Rorschach system. *Journal of Personality Assessment, 59,* 289–294.
Luxenberg, T., Spinazzola, J., Hidalgo, J., Hunt, C., & van der Kolk, B. A. (2001). Com-

plex trauma and disorders of extreme stress not otherwise specified (DESNOS) diagnosis (Part 2): Treatment. *Directions in Psychiatry, 21*(4), 395–415.

Luxenberg, T., Spinazzola, J., & van der Kolk, B. A. (2001). Complex trauma and disorders of extreme stress not otherwise specified (DESNOS) diagnosis (Part 1): Assessment. *Directions in Psychiatry, 21*(4), 373–393.

McFarlane, A. C. (1989). The aetiology of posttraumatic morbidity: Predisposing, precipitating, and perpetuating factors. *British Journal of Psychiatry, 154*, 221–228.

Meyer, G. (1996). The Rorschach and the MMPI: Toward a more scientifically differentiated understanding of cross-method assessment. *Journal of Personality Assessment, 67*, 558–578.

Meyer, G., & Archer, R. (2001). The hard science of Rorschach research: What do we know and where do we go? *Psychological Assessment, 13*, 486–502.

Modlin, H. (1967). A postaccident anxiety syndrome: Psychosocial aspects. *American Journal of Psychiatry, 123*(8), 1008–1012.

Myers, C. S. (1915). A contribution to the study of shell shock. *Lancet, 188*, 316–320.

Nichols, B., & Czirr, R. (1986). Posttraumatic stress disorder: Hidden syndrome in elders. *Clinical Gerontologist, 5*(3–4), 417–433.

Omaha, J. (2000). *Affect management systems training*. Chico, CA: Keymotion Institute.

Parker, K. (1983). A meta-analysis of the reliability and validity of the Rorschach. *Journal of Personality Assessment, 47*(3), 227–231.

Pelcovitz, D., van der Kolk, B. A., Roth, S., Mandel, F., Kaplan, S., & Resick, P. (1997). Development of a criteria set and a structured interview for disorder of extreme stress (SIDES). *Journal of Traumatic Stress, 10*, 3–16.

Pitman, R., Altman, B., Greenwald, E., Longpre, R., Macklin, M., Poire, R., et al. (1991). Psychiatric complications during flooding therapy for posttraumatic stress disorder. *Journal of Clinical Psychiatry, 52*, 17–20.

Resnick, H. S., Yehuda, R., Pitman, R. K., & Foy, D. W. (1995). Effect of previous trauma on acute plasma cortisol level following rape. *American Journal of Psychiatry, 152*, 1675–1677.

Roth, S., Newman, E., Pelcovitz, D., van der Kolk, B. A., & Mandel, F. (1997). Complex PTSD in victims exposed to sexual and physical abuse: Results from the DSM-IV field trial for posttraumatic stress disorder. *Journal of Traumatic Stress, 10*, 539–555.

Salley, R., & Teiling, P. (1984). Dissociated rage attacks in a Vietnam veteran: A Rorschach study. *Journal of Personality Assessment, 48*, 98–104.

Schretlen, D. (1997). Dissimulation on the Rorschach and other projective measures. In R. Rogers (Ed.), *Clinical assessment of malingering and deception* (2nd ed., pp. 208–222). New York: Guilford Press.

Scroppo, J., Weinberger, J., Drob, S., & Eagle, P. (1998). Identifying dissociative identity disorder: A self-report and projective study. *Journal of Abnormal Psychology, 107*, 272–284.

Scurfield, R. (1985). Posttraumatic stress assessment and treatment: Overview and formulations. In C. Figley (Ed.), *Trauma and its wake: The study and treatment of posttraumatic stress disorder* (pp. 219–256). New York: Brunner/Mazel.

Seamons, D., Howell, R., Carlisle, A., & Roe, A. (1981). Rorschach simulation of mental illness and normality by psychotic and nonpsychotic legal offenders. *Journal of Personality Assessment, 4*(2), 130–135.

Shaffer, T., Erdberg, P., & Haroian, J. (1999). Current nonpatient data for the Rorschach, WAIS-R, and MMPI-2. *Journal of Personality Assessment*, *73*, 305–316.

Shalit, B. (1965). Effects of environmental stimulation of the M, FM, and m responses in the Rorschach. *Journal of Projective Techniques and Personality Assessment*, *29*, 228–231.

Shapiro, F. (2002). EMDR 12 years after its introduction: Past and future research. *Journal of Clinical Psychology*, *58*(1), 1–22.

Shatan, C., Smith, J., & Haley, S. (1977, April). *Johnny comes marching home: DSM III and combat stress.* Paper presented at the annual meeting of the American Psychiatric Association, Toronto, Ontario, Canada.

Sloan, P., Arsenault, L., Hilsenroth, M., Harvill, L., & Handler, L. (1995). Rorschach measures of posttraumatic stress in Persian Gulf War veterans. *Journal of Personality Assessment*, *64*, 397–414.

Souffrant, E. (1987). The use of the Rorschach in the assessment of posttraumatic stress disorder among Vietnam combat veterans (Doctoral dissertation, Temple University, 1987). *Dissertation Abstracts International*, *48*, 04B.

Spinazzola, J., Blaustein, M., Kiesel, C., & van der Kolk, B. A. (2001, May). *Beyond PTSD: Further evidence for a complex adaptational response to traumatic life events.* Paper presented at the annual meeting of the American Psychiatric Association, New Orleans, LA.

Stricker, G., & Gold, J. (1999). The Rorschach: Toward a nomothetically based, idiographically applicable configurational model. *Psychological Assessment*, *11*, 240–250.

Swanson, G., Blount, J., & Bruno, R. (1990). Comprehensive system Rorschach data on Vietnam combat veterans. *Journal of Personality Assessment*, *54*, 160–169.

van der Kolk, B. A., & Ducey, C. (1984). Clinical implications of the Rorschach in posttraumatic stress disorder. In B. A. van der Kolk (Ed.), *Posttraumatic stress disorder: Psychological and biological sequelae* (pp. 29–42). Washington, DC: American Psychiatric Press.

van der Kolk, B. A., & Ducey, C. (1989). The psychological processing of traumatic experience: Rorschach patterns in PTSD. *Journal of Traumatic Stress*, *2*, 259–263.

van der Kolk, B. A., & McFarlane, A. (1996). The black hole of trauma. In B. A. van der Kolk, A. McFarlane, & L. Weisaeth (Eds.), *Traumatic stress: The effects of overwhelming experience on mind, body, and society* (pp. 3–23). New York: Guilford Press.

van der Kolk, B. A., Roth, S., Pelcovitz, D., & Mandel, F. (1993). *Complex PTSD: Results of the PTSD field trial for DSM-IV.* Washington, DC: American Psychiatric Association.

van der Kolk, B. A., Weisaeth, L., & van der Hart, O. (1996). History of trauma in psychiatry. In B. A. van der Kolk, A. McFarlane, & L. Weisaeth (Eds.), *Traumatic stress: The effects of overwhelming experience on mind, body, and society* (pp. 47–76). New York: Guilford Press.

Vaughan, K., & Tarrier, N. (1992). The use of habituation training with posttraumatic stress disorders. *British Journal of Psychiatry*, *161*, 658–664.

Viglione, D. (1999). A review of recent research addressing the utility of the Rorschach. *Psychological Assessment*, *11*, 251–265.

Weiner, I., Spielberger, C., & Abeles, N. (2002). Scientific psychology and the Rorschach inkblot method. *Clinical Psychologist*, *55*, 7–12.

Wells, S., & Maher, J. (2001, September 28). *AP photographer stands by his work.* Retrieved October 2, 2001, from http://9news.com/newsroom/13294.html.

Wilson, J., & Walker, A. (1990). Toward an MMPI trauma profile. *Journal of Traumatic Stress*, *3*(1), 151–168.

Wood, J., Lilienfeld, S., Garb, H., & Nezworski, M. (2000). The Rorschach test in clinical diagnosis. *Journal of Clinical Psychology*, *56*, 395–430.

Wood, J., Nezworski, M., Garb, H., & Lilienfeld, S. (2001). The misperception of psychopathology: Problems with the norms of the comprehensive system of the Rorschach. *Clinical Psychology: Science and Practice*, *8*, 350–373.

World Health Organization. (1992). *The ICD-10 classification of mental and behavioral disorders: Clinical descriptions and guidelines.* Geneva: Author.

Zilberg, N., Weiss, D., & Horowitz, M. (1982). Impact of Event Scale: A cross-validation study and some empirical evidence supporting a conceptual model of stress response syndromes. *Journal of Consulting and Clinical Psychology*, *50*, 407–414.

Zlotnick, C., Zakriski, A., Shea, M., & Costello, E. (1996). The long-term sequelae of sexual abuse: Support for a complex posttraumatic stress disorder. *Journal of Traumatic Stress*, *9*, 195–205.

CHAPTER 9

Epidemiological Methods for Assessing Trauma and PTSD

WILLIAM E. SCHLENGER
B. KATHLEEN JORDAN
JUESTA M. CADDELL
LORI EBERT
JOHN A. FAIRBANK

Since the inclusion in DSM-III (American Psychiatric Association, 1980) of a specific, operational definition of the posttraumatic stress disorder (PTSD) syndrome, there has been a rapid accumulation of knowledge about the epidemiology of the disorder (see Wilson & Raphael, 1993; Saigh & Bremner, 1999). This accumulation has been based on findings from broad-based psychiatric epidemiological studies in the general population, such as the National Comorbidity Study (Kessler, Sonnega, Bromet, Hughes, & Nelson, 1995), and epidemiological studies focused on PTSD among individuals exposed to specific types of trauma, such as combat (e.g., Kulka et al., 1990), criminal victimization (e.g., Resnick, Kilpatrick, Dansky, Saunders, & Best, 1993), natural disasters (e.g., Norris, 1992; Norris, Byrne, Diaz, & Kaniasty, 2002), and so on. The findings from these studies have been reviewed in more detail elsewhere (Fairbank, Schlenger, Saigh, & Davidson, 1995; Fairbank, Ebert, & Caddell, 2001).

The purpose of this chapter is to describe some of the important conceptual and practical issues involved in designing and conducting epidemiological studies of PTSD. By *epidemiological* studies, we mean studies aimed at assessing the prevalence and/or incidence of PTSD in specific population groups, assessing the relationship of PTSD to other psychiatric disorders, and identifying factors associated with the development and course of PTSD.

We focus here on issues germane to *community* studies, rather than *clinical* studies. Community epidemiological studies are aimed at assessing specific exposures and/or outcomes among a specified population, regardless of whether individuals have sought treatment or otherwise come to the attention of the treatment or other (e.g., public health surveillance) systems. Consequently, community studies involve samples selected for reasons *other than their exposure or disease status*. Instead, samples for such studies should be selected in ways that result in their being *representative* of the specific population or subgroup to which inference is to be made (e.g., women, Vietnam veterans, crime victims).

We emphasize community studies of adults in this chapter. Many of the important issues involved in conducting clinical studies are addressed in other chapters in this volume. Although clinical studies are extremely valuable for improving our understanding of those who seek treatment and for designing systems of care that can deliver effective treatment to them, such studies contain an inherent bias that limits their utility for enhancing our understanding of the basic epidemiology of PTSD. That bias arises from the well-established fact (e.g., see Shapiro et al., 1984) that only a relatively small portion of those who meet the diagnostic criteria for a specific psychiatric disorder seek treatment for it in a given time period. The impact of the biases introduced by this self-selection on study findings cannot be *definitively* determined (because the bias cannot be studied in the context of a randomized experiment), which limits the contribution that clinical studies can make to our understanding of the basic epidemiology of psychiatric disorders.

In what follows we describe four major challenges that must be addressed in all community epidemiological studies of PTSD. We begin with some fundamental study design issues, many of which arise from the fact that studies of the prevalence, incidence, or risk factors for a given disorder are *observational* in nature. This fact has important implications for the design of such studies and for our ability to draw causal inferences from them.

We then address issues related to the assessment of exposure to potentially traumatic events (PTEs). By *assessment of exposure,* we mean: How do we determine *whether* a given individual has been exposed to an event that fulfills criterion A of DSM-IV (American Psychiatric Association, 1994) diagnostic criteria for PTSD (i.e., a bona fide traumatic event), and *how much* exposure has the individual received?

We next address issues related to PTSD case identification. By *case identification* we mean: How can we tell whether a given individual meets the diagnostic criteria for PTSD and therefore should be considered a "case"?

Finally, we address ethical issues in community epidemiological studies of PTSD. Because such studies are aimed at assessing the consequences of "disasters" of one kind or another, the potential for research participation to have negative consequences for participants is increased relative to studies of more benign topics.

Our primary goal is to increase the *internal validity* (Cook & Campbell, 1979) of the research. Internal validity (i.e., the "fairness" of study comparisons) is important because classification errors in either exposure or case identification introduce bias and therefore reduce the internal validity of case versus noncase comparisons, which are the heart of epidemiological studies. Such biases can spuriously inflate important relationships or mask them, leading to inaccurate conclusions about prevalence, incidence, risk factors, and so on.

Although we have chosen to emphasize issues of internal validity, we also recognize the importance of *external* validity (i.e., generalizability) in epidemiological studies of PTSD. We have discussed some of the issues of external validity in such studies elsewhere (Kulka & Schlenger, 1993; Kulka et al., 1991; Fairbank, Jordan, & Schlenger, 1996), focusing primarily on the importance of representative (i.e., probability) sampling methods.

STUDY DESIGN

Community epidemiological studies typically involve surveys conducted with probability samples of a specific population, aimed at estimating the prevalence and/or incidence of one or more specific conditions in the population and identifying specific "risk factors" that convey vulnerability to the condition(s). Over the past two decades the prevalence of PTSD has been relatively well documented in community studies that cover a broad range of PTEs (e.g., Kessler et al., 1995) or that focus on a specific PTE (e.g., Resnick, Best, et al., 1993), but the incidence of PTSD and its course have each been less well studied. Additionally, the relationship of PTSD to other psychiatric and substance use disorders has also been well documented, but less attention has been paid to other potentially important comorbidities (e.g., health conditions).

An important reality of studying the epidemiology of PTSD results from the general unpredictability of many of the exposures of interest, that is, the fact that disasters and other large-scale PTEs typically occur with little or no warning. North and Pfefferbaum (2002) have identified a number of issues involved in conducting such studies and offer helpful guidelines and recommendations. In what follows, we address some of the more challenging design problems that arise from two specific characteristics of studies of comparatively sudden and unanticipated large-scale PTEs: the observational nature of the studies and the need for them to be designed and implemented quickly.

Issues Associated with Observational Study Designs

Observational studies are those in which the independent variables are observed as they naturally occur, rather than being assigned or otherwise manipulated in advance by the experimenter. Epidemiological studies following the occurrence of a disaster or other PTE are, of necessity, observational (i.e., researchers cannot randomize people to PTE-exposed vs -nonexposed conditions). As a result, such studies provide the basis for assessment of *associations* among the variables assessed.

But we are most interested in determining whether there are causal relationships between "exposures" and specific "outcomes," not just associations—that is, we want to be able to attribute some or all of the PTSD cases that we find to the specific exposure (e.g., the September 11, 2001, terrorist attacks) that we are studying. One way of strengthening the inferential power of observational studies is to structure the study sample to include one or more quasi-experimental comparison groups, typically of the nonequivalent-comparison-group type. For example, samples for community epidemiological studies of PTSD should always be designed so that they include people with varying levels of exposure to the PTE that is being studied, including an adequately sized "no exposure" group, so that the association of PTSD prevalence with degree of exposure can be documented. This procedure provides a basis for ruling out several alternative hypotheses, for example, that the findings result from measurement bias ("the prevalence is high among exposed persons because the PTSD measure used overestimates PTSD prevalence"). The point is to be sure that the study sample includes groups of adequate size who have varying levels of exposure, so that the study supports empirical documentation of the relationship of exposure to postexposure symptomatology and enables the ruling out of some specific alternative explanations of the findings.

In addition to quasi-experimental comparison groups, it is also wise to assess multiple outcomes, some of which are selected for their ability to demonstrate *discriminant* validity (e.g., to show that exposure is related to PTSD symptoms but not to other symptoms). For example, Schlenger et al. (2002) included screening instruments for PTSD and for nonspecific psychological distress in their study of the psychological aftermath of the September 11 terrorist attacks. The finding that PTSD prevalence in the New York metropolitan area—where the direct exposure was most severe—was three times higher than the prevalence in the rest of the country (a quasi-experimental comparison group) *and* that both in New York and across the country the levels of nonspecific psychological distress (an additional outcome included primarily to assess discriminant validity) were within normal limits added substantial credibility to the study's findings. The credibility results from empirical demonstration that "overendorsement of psychiatric symptoms" was an unlikely explanation of the difference in prevalence between New York and the rest of the nation and that the association of PTE exposure with symptoms was specific to PTSD symptoms.

In addition to being observational, most studies of disasters and other PTEs have *post-only* designs—that is, all assessments occur *after* the fact of the PTE. This is true primarily because of the unpredictability of most PTEs. Post-only quasi-experimental designs are particularly weak with respect to causal inference for a variety of reasons. The most obvious of these are the inability to rule out preexisting disorder (or symptomatology) as an explanation of postexposure symptom levels (i.e., what was the prevalence of PTSD in this population *before* the exposure?) and the opportunity for confounding of self-reports of exposure and symptoms (people with higher postexposure symptom levels may describe their exposure as more severe than people who had the same exposure but were not symptomatic).

A simple, but unsatisfactory, remedy might be to ask participants about symptoms they may have experienced in the period just before the exposure (i.e., provide a retrospective baseline), but it would provide weak evidence because it does not address the problem of confounding with exposure. An alterative involves quasi-experimental comparisons and statistical adjustment. For example, Schlenger et al. (2002) used a least-squares means approach described by Korn and Graubard (1999) to adjust statistically the comparison of prevalence for the New York metropolitan area with the prevalence for the rest of the United States. Doing so allowed adjustment for sociodemographic differences between the two groups and indicated that the prevalence of probable PTSD in New York was 5.1 percentage points higher than in the rest of the United States after adjusting for differences in sociodemographic characteristics. Although not definitive, such findings are consistent with the hypothesis of a substantial impact of the terrorist attacks on people living in the New York metropolitan area.

Issues Associated with Rapid Response

A number of scientific and pragmatic problems result because PTEs are unpredictable, forcing researchers to react quickly and with no advance warning. This typically means assembling interview protocols and sampling procedures very quickly, so that assessments—particularly assessments of exposure—can begin as soon as possible following exposure.

Relatedly, because time is of the essence, studies of disasters and other PTEs must rely on methods that allow rapid sampling and assessment. These can include adding additional modules to a large survey that is ongoing when the PTE occurs, but more frequently it means relying on random digit dialing (RDD) and Internet-based data collection modes.

Research conducted following the terrorist attacks of September 11, 2001, demonstrate some of these issues well. Prior to that time, empirical information about PTEs and their impact had been slow to appear in the literature (i.e., findings typically appeared years after the event). Facilitated by the availability of RDD and Internet-based methods, however, the findings from four large-scale epidemiological studies (Schuster et al., 2001; Galea et al., 2002; Schlenger et al., 2002; Silver, Holman, McIntosh, Poulin, & Gil-Rivas, 2002) were published in top-tier journals within 12 months of the attacks. The ability to respond quickly represents a tremendous advance for the field and also provides an initial empirical database that can inform important short-term policy decisions (e.g., by documenting some aspects of "need").

Although these alternative approaches to face-to-face personal interviews facilitate rapid response, they are not without problems. The most important of these is response rate, which is critical to both the external and internal validity of the studies and is a source of widespread concern among social and health researchers.

Most survey professionals acknowledge a steady decline in survey interview response rates over the past 20 years. This decline is likely related to at least three kinds of factors: (1) increased demand for people to participate in "surveys" (i.e., substantial growth in the number of scientific surveys and opinion polls conducted via telephone, explosive growth in telemarketing, and the difficulty from the potential participant's perspective of distinguishing among these); (2) the development and widespread use of technological barriers (e.g., telephone answering machines and other screening mechanisms) that block contact with sample members; and (3) increased demands on people's time (e.g., increased job demands, increase in two-job families).

At the same time, however, methodologists have been thinking more clearly and in greater detail about nonresponse (at both the person and item levels) and its consequences and developing methods to reduce its impact on study findings. The seminal conceptualization of this problem by Rubin (1976), the details of which were later fleshed out by Little and Rubin (1987) and subsequently extended by Schafer (1997) and others, provides a detailed conceptual framework for understanding the actual threats to validity that occur when data are missing and ways to minimize those threats.

The notions introduced by Rubin of "missing completely at random" (MCAR; distribution of missingness not related to observed or missing data), "missing at random" (MAR; distribution of missingness not related to missing data), and "missing not at random" (MNAR; at least some missingness related to missing data) have helped clarify and improve understanding of the specific nature of the problem and the specific threats each type poses. Although detailed explication of the many implications of this conceptualization are beyond the scope of this chapter, the most important implication is that MCAR and MAR conditions are thought of as "ignorable" missingness, but MNAR is "nonignorable." Additionally, simulation studies have shown that (1) traditional methods for adjusting for missing data—for example, listwise deletion, imputing the mean—introduce bias in the estimates, their confidence intervals, or both; and (2) under conditions of MCAR and MAR, unbiased estimates of parameters and confidence intervals can be produced using new approaches to imputation, even with levels of missingness considered extreme by traditional standards.

A brief summary of the current thinking (Schafer & Graham, 2002) about missingness is that community epidemiological studies can typically be assumed to be at least MAR, but clinical studies cannot. The rationale for this thinking points to the differential "inclusion criteria" of the two types of studies: Participants are included in community epidemiological studies by "luck of the draw" (i.e., random sampling), whereas participants are included in clinical studies because they have a specific disorder and are interested in being treated for it.

Relatively reader-friendly summaries of the current conceptualizations of the problem of missing data and of the advantages of new methods for dealing with nonresponse are provided by Graham, Hofer, and McKinnon (1996) and by Schafer and Graham (2002). Availability of these newer methods and empirical documentation of their effectiveness via simulation makes feasible the compilation of a comprehensive evidence base with respect to the epidemiology of PTSD in the face of the realities of modern life.

One other important issue that emerges because of the need for rapid response has to do with assessment. Briefly, for a variety of practical reasons, telephone and Internet interviews must be short—many experienced survey researchers think that about 30–40 minutes is the practical time limit for telephone and Internet interviews. This restriction has at least two important implications for PTSD studies. First, it means that PTSD case identification will need to be based on screening instruments rather than comprehensive clinical evaluation. This raises questions of validity and mandates the use of screening instruments whose validity (i.e., correspondence with comprehensive clinical diagnosis) has been empirically documented in community populations with characteristics similar to those of the population being studied.

Second, the time limitation typically also means that not all constructs of interest can be measured, even using screening instruments. This creates some difficult a priori judgment calls about which measures to include. Such decisions should always be informed by established findings in the peer-reviewed literature.

ASSESSMENT OF EXPOSURE TO TRAUMA

It is tautological that anyone who meets the criteria for the diagnosis of PTSD has been exposed to one or more PTEs. It is also true, however, that not everyone who has been exposed to a PTE develops PTSD. Additionally, it is also the case that many people are exposed to multiple PTEs across their lifetimes and that individuals who suffer a serious assault, particularly rape, are more likely to develop PTSD following trauma exposure than individuals exposed to other types of events, such as accidents or natural disasters (Breslau et al., 1998; Boudreax, Kilpatrick, Resnick, Best, & Saunders, 1998, Kessler et al., 1995). For these and other reasons, assessment of exposure is an important component of the internal validity of epidemiological studies of PTSD and is critical to the examination of etiology.

Assessment of exposure in community epidemiological studies of PTSD to date has typically relied on retrospective self-reports in the context of a survey interview. That is, most studies have involved structured survey interviews that included questions about various major categories of PTEs to which one might have been exposed in the past (e.g., "Have you ever been . . . ?"). A follow-up set of questions concerning the details of the exposure is then posed to those who indicate having had a given exposure. The interview is typically conducted by a trained survey interviewer who has experience conducting structured interviews but has no clinical expertise and no advanced training or experience in trauma or its assessment.

For example, exposure to combat and other PTEs was assessed comprehensively in the National Vietnam Veterans Readjustment Study (NVVRS; Kulka et al., 1990). Because the NVVRS focused on combat-related PTSD, the survey interview included a comprehensive set of more than 100 questions about the veteran's experience while he or she was in Vietnam. These items addressed specific experiences that may have been stressful (e.g., "How often were you under enemy fire?"; "How often did you experience hand-to-hand combat?"). Using factor analysis, this set of items was combined into specific indices assessing major types of war-zone-stressor exposure (four types for men, six for women), all of which showed good internal consistency reliability (median coefficient alpha = .873). These specific indices were then combined in an overall exposure index that was used to divide Vietnam veterans into high versus low/moderate war-zone stressor-exposure groups for analytic purposes.

Additionally, although the NVVRS was focused on war-zone trauma, Vietnam veterans could have been exposed to other kinds of trauma that could have produced PTSD both before and after their Vietnam experience. Therefore, the NVVRS interview also included questions about other extreme events to which they may have been exposed. To provide a context for participants, the section of the interview that addressed noncombat exposures followed immediately after a set of questions about "stressful life events" (e.g., significant illness, loss of job, divorce, natural death of family member) that participants may have experienced. The rationale for doing so was that if the inquiry was first focused on lower magnitude stressors and then shifted to higher magnitude stressors ("Now I'd like to talk with you about . . . "), the likelihood of "false positive" responses to the extreme-events assessment would be reduced.

Reviewing the details of the NVVRS stressor-exposure assessment serves to underline an important point: Stressor exposure is a multidimensional construct. The point is that there are many different kinds of stressors to which a person may be exposed, and multiple aspects of each exposure that should be assessed (e.g., frequency, severity). Comprehensive assessment of exposure requires specific inquiry about each type of stressor, assessment of qualitative aspects of the exposures that are reported, and assessment of the frequency and intensity of each type of exposure. In addition, beginning by assessing lower magnitude stressors ("stressful life events") may help clarify for respondents the meaning of questions about high-magnitude stressors and thereby contribute to improved validity of the assessment.

A second example of exposure assessment is provided by the recently developed Traumatic Life Events Questionnaire (TLEQ; Kubany et al., 2000). The TLEQ is a brief screening instrument that assesses exposure to a broad range of PTEs, and therefore it provides a broad picture of a person's trauma exposure history. The descriptions of specific exposures were developed via a multistep process that included extensive pretesting, review and input from trauma specialists, and multiple studies that involved diverse populations. The questions about exposures are clear and phrased neutrally, and they are available in both interviewer-administered and self-administered formats. Preliminary studies suggest no mode difference in exposure reporting between the self- and interviewer-administered versions.

A third example of assessing exposure in the context of a community epidemiological study comes from the work of Dean Kilpatrick, Heidi Resnick, and their colleagues (Kilpatrick, Saunders, Veronen, Best, & Von, 1987; Resnick, Kilpatrick, et al., 1993). On the basis of experiences gained through conducting a series of epidemiological studies focusing on noncombat events (particularly sexual assaults), these investigators have developed the Trauma Assessment for Adults (TAA; Resnick, Best, Freedy, Kilpatrick, & Falsetti, 1993), a structured assessment of exposure to extreme events that is available in both interview and self-administered formats. Resnick, Falsetti, Kilpatrick, and Freedy (1996) emphasize a number of important considerations in the assessment of exposure to extreme events, including:

1. Begin by providing a context for the assessment by explaining the nature of extreme events, so that the intent of the specific questions will be clearer and will focus the respondent's attention on the kinds of events of interest.
2. Include behaviorally specific, operational questions (e.g., asking a series of detailed questions about specific sex acts, such as "Has anyone ever made you have anal sex by force or threat of harm?" rather than a global question such as "Have you ever been sexually assaulted?").
3. Assess the broad range of potential events to which respondents may have been exposed.
4. Include assessment of qualitative aspects of the exposure (i.e., details of what happened and the ways in which the event was threatening).
5. Establish the traditional psychometric properties (reliability and validity) of the assessment, using samples that represent the population(s) with which the assessment is intended to be used.

The TAA is a brief version of the more comprehensive Potential Stressful Events Interview (PSE; Kilpatrick, Resnick, & Freedy, 1991), which was developed for use in the DSM-IV PTSD field trial. This trial was conducted to collect information to address specific issues being considered by the committee that drafted the PTSD criteria for inclusion in DSM-IV (American Psychiatric Association, 1994). The PSE includes sections assessing low-magnitude stressors, high-magnitude stressors, and objective and subjective characteristics of reported high-magnitude stressors.

As is always the case, the level of detail provided by the PSE has a price—it is time-consuming to administer. In the context of community epidemiological research, in which exposure is one of multiple important constructs being measured, there is always a trade-off between the scientifically desirable level of detail and the costs (in terms of fiscal resources, respondent burden, etc.) associated with collecting those details. The TAA represents a compromise between the fine detail provided by the PSE (which may be more feasible to use in clinical settings) and the practical demands of community epidemiological studies.

Similarly, Norris (1990, 1992) developed the Traumatic Stress Schedule (TSS) to assess exposure to nine categories of extreme events (and one specific event—Hurricane Hugo) for use in an epidemiological study of exposure to trauma in four cities in the southeastern United States. The TSS assesses lifetime and past-year exposure to these event categories and also includes a five-item stress symptom measure that does not require the respondent to link his or her symptoms to a specific extreme event.

A final example that demonstrates a somewhat different approach to assessing exposure comes from an important longitudinal study of a cohort of young adults enrolled in a large health maintenance organization (HMO) that was conducted by Breslau and her colleagues (Breslau, Davis, Andreski, & Peterson, 1991; Breslau, Davis, & Andreski, 1995). The cohort was assessed in 1989 and again in 1992 for exposure to extreme events and for the presence of PTSD and other psychiatric disorders.

The exposure assessment used by Breslau and her colleagues is more open-ended than the others, in that it begins with a global question about exposure to "terrible experiences" that cites a series of examples ("things like being attacked or raped, being in a fire or flood or bad traffic accident, being threatened with a weapon, or watching someone being badly injured or killed"). Those answering "no" are probed about whether they ever experienced a "great shock because something like that happened to someone close to you," which is another type of potential extreme event. Those answering "yes" to the original question are asked to describe the "worst" such event in their lives, which is coded into specific categories (e.g., combat, rape, physical assault, etc.), then probed for "anything else like this," and then for "any other terrible or shocking experience." As a result, the assessment results in a description of up to three such events.

The preceding represent examples from current practice of state-of-the-art assessment in the context of community epidemiological studies and demonstrate many of the important principles in such assessment. The most important weakness that all of the examples share is that they are *retrospective* methods, usually covering substantial recall periods (e.g., "Have you ever in your life . . . ?"). This limitation is inherent in self-report methods of assessing exposure to trauma and is problematic because it allows for potential confounding of *reaction* to an exposure with *description of* that exposure. In addition, Bromet and Dew (1995) note that cross-sectional, retrospective studies are subject to biases from: selective mortality that might result from the exposure; nonresponse, in which nonexposed individuals may be not motivated and those exposed may be too preoccupied (or angry) to participate; and interviewer bias resulting from the fact that interviewers cannot be blinded to exposure status.

It is important to remember that misclassifications of exposure can occur in both directions—that is, both false positives and false negatives are possible. As an example of a false positive, one participant in the NVVRS reported during the survey interview that he served five tours in Vietnam and was exposed to heavy combat during each. His military record, however, showed that he spent most of his relatively brief stay in the military in a military prison.

Conversely, findings from a study of documented child sexual abuse victims demonstrate that false negatives are also a potential problem. Williams (1994a) interviewed 129 adult women who had been treated for sexual victimization during childhood (on average about 17 years prior to the interview). When interviewed, 38% of the sample did not report the documented incident, even when the interviewer described to them the specific details. Although there may be a variety of interpretations as to why these events were not "remembered" (Loftus, Garry, & Feldman, 1994; Williams, 1994b), it is clear that simply asking someone about exposures does not guarantee accurate assessment.

Confidence in self-reports of exposure can be increased, however, in several ways. First, confidence is increased when those reports can be shown to correspond with independent measures of exposure. For example, the NVVRS team was able to demonstrate good correspondence between the NVVRS self-report measures of exposure and exposure-related information in veterans' military records (Kulka et al., 1990)—for example, those whose military records indicated that they had received the Purple Heart were much more likely to be classified as having had high-stress exposure, based on self-report, than were those who did not, and those whose records indicated that they had a "tactical" military occupational specialty (MOS) were classified as having had higher exposure than those with nontactical MOS's, and so on.

It is important also to remember, however, that independent sources of exposure information often do not provide *definitive* indicators of exposure. Anyone who has ever worked with official records—be they clinical case records, military service records, school records, police records, or others—recognizes that such records are subject to errors of both omission and commission. Nevertheless, such records can be an important source of corroboration in the *construct* (rather than *criterion)* validity sense.

Second, confidence in self-reports is increased by having multiple assessments over time, each of which focuses on a discrete and more limited time period. The multiple-assessment approach is a characteristic of prospective, longitudinal studies, of which Breslau's study of a young adult cohort (Breslau et al., 1995) is an excellent example. Use of multiple assessments helps to control for reporting errors associated with compression of time. This phenomenon, referred to in the survey research literature as "telescoping," occurs when an event is remembered as occurring more recently than it actually did (Sudman & Bradburn, 1973). Telescoping threatens the internal validity of epidemiological studies of PTSD by potentially increasing reports of exposure (i.e., creating "false-positive" exposure reports). In addition, prospective, longitudinal studies provide an excellent vehicle for methodological studies of the validity of exposure assessment.

PTSD CASE IDENTIFICATION

A second important assessment issue in community epidemiological studies is case identification, that is, how one determines who is a "case" and who is not. In clinical studies, patients who are assessed because they are seeking treatment come to the assessment with certain problems, or symptoms, and a "story" to tell (e.g., "I'm here because . . . "). Diagnostic interviews in clinical settings, therefore, often begin with questions such as "Can you tell me why you are here?"; "How I can help you?"; and so on.

In community studies, however, the participant has *not* come to the assessment for the purpose of telling a story. On the contrary, the assessor has approached the participant for the purpose of *learning* his or her story since he or she does not have a "presenting problem" from which to start the assessment process.

A related problem is one that we have come to refer to as "PTSD to what?" The problem arises from several important facts, including: (1) that all people who are exposed to PTEs come to that exposure with a personal history (i.e., they had a life before the exposure); (2) that a large empirical literature documents that prior exposure to PTEs is an important risk factor for development of PTSD following a new exposure; and (3) that a growing empirical literature (Breslau et al., 1998; Boudreaux et al., 1998; Kessler et al., 1995) documents that PTEs are not equally traumatogenic—for example, purposeful violence, such as sexual assault, is more likely to result in PTSD among those exposed than natural disasters, such as a hurricane. The problem, therefore, involves attributing current PTSD symptomatology solely to the new exposure, as it is not clear how well people with multiple severe exposures can do so nor whether the current exposure would have produced PTSD symptoms in the absence of the prior exposures.

Additionally, we focus here on case identification as a *binary* decision—that is, each subject is classified as a "case" or "not a case"—because this is the epidemiological tradition. We recognize, however, that for many psychiatric disorders, including PTSD, subthreshold, or subclinical, phenomena exist that are of interest—that is, people who exhibit some clinically significant symptoms of the syndrome but not enough symptoms to meet the letter of the DSM definition. Weiss et al. (1992) discuss this phenomenon in more detail and presents estimates of the prevalence of "partial PTSD" for Vietnam veterans (see also Weiss, Chapter 4, this volume).

Similarly, although we limit our focus here to identification of cases of PTSD, epidemiological studies of people exposed to a variety of extreme events have demonstrated that: (1) PTSD is often accompanied by comorbid psychiatric disorders, including depressive and substance-use disorders (see Fairbank, Schlenger, Caddell, & Woods, 1993; Fairbank et al., 1995), and (2) other psychiatric disorders, including borderline personality disorder and the dissociative disorders, have been shown to be related to traumatic exposure (see Herman, Perry, & van der Kolk, 1989; Zanarini, Gunderson, Marino, Schwartz, & Frankenburg, 1989; Jordan, Schlenger, Caddell, & Fairbank, 1997). Thus, although we focus here on PTSD as an example, investigators designing epidemiological studies of traumatic exposure will likely want to assess for a broader range of trauma-related and comorbid disorders. Bromet and her colleagues (Neria, Bromet, & Marshall, 2002; Neria & Bromet, 2000) make the important point that some of the current methods for assessing exposure do not provide the opportunity to assess directly the association of exposure with other psychiatric outcomes (e.g., depression) and that this failure is one important limitation to the development of a comprehensive understanding of the consequences of PTE exposure.

Case identification methods that have been used in epidemiological studies of PTSD can be divided into at least four major categories based on the underlying approach taken. These categories are:

1. Survey interview approaches
2. Semistructured clinical interview approaches
3. Psychometric approaches
4. Psychobiological approaches

More detailed descriptions of specific measures, instruments, and methods reflecting these approaches and their psychometric and other properties can be found in various other chapters in this book. In addition, there are research design features that can facilitate case identification. These various approaches are described in the following sections.

The Survey Interview Approach

The survey interview approach to case identification is based on the premise that people can reliably report their experience of specific psychiatric symptoms if the symptoms are described to them briefly in a survey interview setting. Consequently, survey interview approaches use fully structured interviews in which the interviewer simply reads the prescribed questions (e.g., "Have you ever experienced . . . ?") and records the responses, with no interpretation and no unstructured probing. Interviewers in this approach are trained in survey interview techniques but need have no clinical training with respect to the phenomenology of PTSD.

The "parent" of this approach to survey-based psychiatric case identification is the Diagnostic Interview Schedule (DIS; *http://epi.wustl.edu/dis/dishome.htm*; Robins, Helzer, Croughan, & Ratcliff, 1981), a fully structured survey interview developed for use in community epidemiological studies, specifically for the National Institute of Mental Health's (NIMH) Epidemiologic Catchment Area (ECA) program (Regier et al., 1984). The DIS supports diagnosis of a variety of specific psychiatric disorders, including PTSD, and has been revised to maintain correspondence with DSM criteria. Although the DIS (currently DIS-IV) assesses psychiatric disorders of adults, a version targeting psychiatric disorders in children and adolescents—the Diagnostic Interview Schedule for Children (DISC; *www.c-disc.com*; Costello, Edelbrock, Kalas, Kessler, & Klaric, 1982; Shaffer, Fisher, Lucas, Dulcan, & Schwab-Stone, 2000)—has also been developed separately.

Using the DIS as the starting point, the World Health Organization (WHO) developed the Composite International Diagnostic Interview (CIDI 2.1; *www3.who.int/cidi/index.htm*; Robins, Wing, Wittchen, & Helzer, 1988) to incorporate diagnostic criteria from the *International Classification of Diseases* (ICD-10; World Health Organization, 1992). The current versions of both the DIS and WHO CIDI ask whether the respondent has experienced any of 13 (DIS) or 9 (CIDI) specific events or any other extremely stressful event and whether someone close to him or her has experienced such an event. If multiple events are endorsed, the interviewer asks which event was the worst and when that event occurred. For symptoms that can be linked by content to a specific event (e.g., dreams, intrusive recollections), the respondent is asked whether the symptom is related to the specific event. For other symptoms (e.g., sleep disturbance, irritability), the respondent is asked whether the symptom began subsequent to the event.

An alternative variation of the CIDI, which became known as the University of Michigan CIDI (UM-CIDI; *www.hcp.med.harvard.edu/ncs*), was developed for use in the National Comorbidity Study (NCS; Kessler et al., 1994), a community epidemiological study of psychiatric disorders in a nationally representative household sample that was also sponsored by NIMH. The PTSD assessment of the UM-CIDI began by asking about exposure to 10 specific events and "any other very stressful event" and whether any of these events had happened to someone close to the respondent (Kessler et al., 1995). A newer, alternative version of the CIDI, the National Comorbidity Study Replication Survey (NCS-R; also *www.hcp.med.harvard.edu/ncs*), has also been developed (using innovations from the Munich version of the CIDI, the WHO CIDI, and the DIS-IV) for use with a new NCS cohort. The PTSD module of the NCS-R asks about exposure to 26 specific events (including violence against or sudden death of loved ones) and "any other" traumatic event. As with the WHO CIDI, after all events are queried, the respondent is asked to choose the "worst" event. In the NCS-R (as in the DIS but not the WHO CIDI), the worst event is identified by reading a short list of PTSD symptoms and asking the respondent to identify the specific event that was associated with the most symptoms. Additional information is then obtained about this "worst" event, including date of occurrence, duration, and details on the event. The respondent is then asked if he or she has had the specific PTSD symptoms that were either related to the event (e.g., memories) or that occurred during the time the event affected the subject the most (e.g., trouble sleeping). The NCS group has also developed an adolescent version of the NCS-R (the NCS-A) that contains a PTSD section similar to that of the adult version but with some modifications, such as the inclusion of a specific question about observation of domestic violence.

A common problem with these survey interviews involves their assessment of exposure. A large body of research demonstrates that asking more specific questions about PTEs elicits more reports of exposure than fewer, more general questions (cf. Weaver, 1998). For example, a meta-analysis of differences in women's self-reports of exposure to sexual abuse found that the key predictor across studies was the number of different questions asking about types of sexual assaults (Bolen & Scannapieco, 1999), with more specific questions producing higher exposure rates. Similarly, in a study of women with documented childhood sexual abuse (Williams, Siegel, & Pomeroy, 2000), four gate questions resulted in self-reports of abuse from 80% of those who had been abused, and eight questions resulted in reports from 90% of participants. In contrast, the DIS asks only one global sexual assault question ("being raped or sexually assaulted," although the item appears twice—for relatives and nonrelatives separately), and the CIDI versions ask about only two categories—rape and other sexual assault. The DISC asks just one very general question: "being forced to do something sexual that you did not want to do."

Some research has documented the reliability and validity of these survey assessments. Empirical examinations of the psychometric properties of the DIS have generally shown it to be reliable (e.g., Helzer et al., 1985) but have raised important questions about its validity. For example, Anthony et al. (1985) showed that for most disorders, diagnoses based on the DIS agreed poorly with diagnoses made by clinicians based on a semistructured clinical interview. Similarly, although the DIS-PTSD module was found in the NVVRS Preliminary Validation Study (Schlenger et al., 1992) to correspond reasonably well with diagnoses based on structured clinical interviews in a sample of Vietnam veterans undergoing treatment, Kulka et al. (1991) found it to have very poor sensitivity when used to assess a community sample of Vietnam veterans. Kilpatrick et al. (1994), however, used a modified version of the DIS designed to overcome the kinds of problems experienced in the NVVRS in the DSM-IV field trial and found better correspondence with PTSD diagnoses based on structured clinical interviews in a mixed clinical and community sample.

Kessler et al. (1995) compared PTSD diagnoses based on the UM-CIDI with diagnoses based on structured clinical interviews of 29 NCS participants who reported one or more PTEs in their UM-CIDI interviews. The UM-CIDI was found to underdiagnose PTSD relative to clinical assessment, but the kappa for correspondence was .75. Because only respondents who reported traumatic events in the UM-CIDI were reinterviewed by clinicians, however, these results do not reflect any validity problems resulting from underreporting of traumatic events, for example, underreporting associated with insufficiently detailed questions.

The Clinical Interview Approach

The clinical interview approach shares the survey interview approach's focus on specific symptoms but differs in at least two ways. First, the interview is conducted by an experienced clinician. Use of trained, experienced clinicians allows the integration of information gained through observation of the respondent during the interview rather than relying concretely on what the respondent said (e.g., the respondent denied experiencing "emotional numbing" but remained affectless throughout the interview, even when describing extreme combat events).

Second, the interview is semistructured—that is, it includes specific questions about all of the symptoms of interest, but the interviewer is encouraged to probe for more information where appropriate. Elicitation of additional information about symptoms through the use of follow-up probes (e.g., "Can you tell me more about that?"; "What was that like for you?") increases the validity of the symptom assessment. For example, in the NVVRS Preliminary Validation Study (Schlenger et al., 1992), we noticed that patients often responded affirmatively to symptom questions in survey interviews. When the patients were probed, however, the interviewers found that, although the experiences they described may have been psychiatric symptoms, they were often not the symptom described in the original question. Experiences such as these suggest that the constructs embodied in the symptoms that make up the DSM-IV definitions of psychiatric disorders may be difficult for many people to recognize on the basis of brief, survey interview questions. This problem underlines the importance of the role of clinical judgment in valid case identification.

The first semistructured clinical interview to support diagnosis of PTSD was the Structured Clinical Interview for DSM-III-R (SCID; Spitzer, Williams, Gibbon, & First, 1992). The PTSD module of the SCID was developed by the NVVRS research team and incorporated into Form NP-V of the SCID. Because it was developed for use in a study of combat-related PTSD, it focused largely on the kinds of extreme events that are associated with war-zone situations. All PTSD symptoms are assessed, including lifetime ("Have you ever had this symptom?") and current ("Do you have this symptom now?").

Subsequently, other clinical interview protocols have been developed. These include the Clinician-Administered PTSD Scale (CAPS; Blake et al., 1995) and the Structured Interview for PTSD (SI-PTSD; Davidson, Smith, & Kudler, 1989). The CAPS has the substantial advantage of including both frequency and severity ratings for each symptom (as opposed to the present–absent indicator of the SCID), and the SI-PTSD includes ratings of severity.

The Psychometric Approach

Both the survey-interview and clinical-interview approaches to case identification may be described as *rational* in that they are structured by the symptoms that make up the DSM definition of PTSD and impose DSM decision rules (e.g., at least one B criterion symptom, three or more C criterion symptoms, etc.) to identify cases. In other words, using these approaches, one decides whether an individual is a case by inquiring about the specific symptoms of PTSD and then applying the DSM definition of caseness to the symptom pattern reported.

The other two major approaches share a fundamentally different conceptualization of the problem of case identification, an approach that is better described as *empirical* than as *rational.* Both are based on the psychometric tradition of empirical validity, in which "scales" that measure specific "traits" (or "constructs") are derived by comparing the responses to sets of standardized stimuli ("items") of people who *have* the trait to the responses of those who *do not.* Items that discriminate between the known groups are incorporated into the test, and those that do not are not.

In what we refer to as the psychometric approach, stimuli—be they symptom descriptions, statements with which the participant is asked to agree or disagree, and so on—are presented to the participant, and his or her responses are recorded. Psychometric instruments are typically presented in a self-administered format (i.e., the participant reads the items and records responses without the intervention of an interviewer). An increasing body of evidence suggests that "sensitive" information is more likely to be revealed in self-report settings than in interview settings (e.g., Turner, Lessler, & Gfroerer, 1992; Turner et al., 1998), which may be an advantage for this method in assessing for PTSD.

Probably the best-known example of the psychometric approach to PTSD case identifications is the Mississippi Scale for Combat-Related PTSD (Keane, Caddell, & Taylor, 1988). The Mississippi Scale consists of 35 items with 5-point, Likert-style response categories. The scale was created from a pool of potential items developed by a group of clinicians experienced in treating Vietnam veterans with PTSD to represent broadly the kinds of complaints voiced by veterans with PTSD. From this pool, those items that were shown empirically to discriminate combat veterans with PTSD from those without were included in the scale. To reduce the potential impact of response set, 10 of the items are phrased in the negative direction (i.e., the low end of the scale is associated with PTSD). The Mississippi Scale has been shown to be reliable and strongly related to the clinical diagnosis of PTSD (Keane et al., 1988; Kulka et al., 1991). For the NVVRS, a "civilian" version of the Mississippi scale was created that appears to have promise for assessing noncombat PTSD (Vreven, Gudanowski, King, & King, 1995).

Another excellent example of the psychometric approach to PTSD case identification is the PTSD scale of the Minnesota Multiphasic Personality Inventory (MMPI; Keane, Malloy, & Fairbank, 1984). Using groups of combat veterans with and without PTSD, a set of 49 MMPI items was identified that significantly discriminated the groups. This scale has also been shown to be both reliable and strongly related to clinical diagnosis, and it has been carried into the new MMPI-2 (Butcher, Dahlstrom, Graham, Tellegen, & Kaemmer, 1989) as research scale PK. In addition, scale PS of the MMPI-2 represents an extension of the original scale and includes the original Keane et al. (1984) scale items that were cross-validated in the NVVRS sample, plus a number of new items that were found in the NVVRS to discriminate between Vietnam veterans with PTSD and those without.

Psychobiological Approaches

Psychobiological approaches are another step removed from the potential problems associated with relying on self-reports. These approaches involve identifying psychobiological correlates of PTSD—that is, reliable psychobiological differences between PTSD cases and noncases. If such differences exist, they would represent potentially a more "objective" method for identifying PTSD cases. Potential psychobiological correlates that have been studied to date have included both psychophysiological and neurobiological measures—psychophysiological reactivity in response to presentations of trauma-related stimuli (e.g., slides depicting combat scenes) and imagery, neuroimaging, and assessment of levels of cortisol and other stress-related neurochemicals.

Studies of physiological reactivity associated with trauma exposure have a long history, dating back as far as World War I, when veterans with "shell shock" were shown to demonstrate greater increases in heart rate and respiration than control participants in response to laboratory presentations of combat-related stimuli (Meakins & Wilson, 1918). Over the years, these findings have been extended to veterans of other wars as well (Blanchard, Kolb, Gerardi, Ryan, & Pallmeyer, 1986; Blanchard, Kolb, Pallmeyer, & Gerardi, 1982; McFall, Murburg, Roszell, & Veith, 1989; Malloy, Fairbank, & Keane, 1983; Pitman & Orr, 1993; Blanchard & Buckley, 1999; Orr & Kaloupek, 1997). Skin conductance, heart rate, electromyogram (EMG), and blood pressure measures have typically been found, either alone or in combination, to reliably discriminate PTSD cases from noncases among combat-exposed veterans.

Studies using these measures have revealed a consistent pattern of increased physiological reactivity to combat and military-related stimuli presentation in veterans with PTSD as compared with veterans who do not meet diagnosis for PTSD. Such challenge studies have used verbal imagery scripts (both general and idiosyncratic), audio stimuli, and audiovisual stimuli presentations. Tomarken (1995) has recently summarized important issues with respect to the psychometric properties of psychophysiological measures.

Findings from a related body of literature examining brain wave activity (including event-related potentials [ERPs], and general EEG activity) in veterans with PTSD offer insights into underlying mechanisms related to concentration difficulties and processing of emotional memories (McCaffrey, Lorig, Pendrey, McCutcheon, and Garrett, 1993; McFarlane, Weber, & Clark, 1993). Likewise, studies of startle response that have examined eyeblink EMG habituation to tones and magnitude of eyeblink response to intense auditory stimuli have also begun to elucidate types and patterns of responses displayed by PTSD versus non-PTSD cases.

Despite the promising results from these latter studies of cognitive processes and of startle response, reactivity to trauma-related stimuli remains the most well-studied symptom using psychophysiological techniques. In general, findings from studies of reactivity indicate that psychophysiological measures serve as a valid index of reactivity to trauma-related memories or stimuli (e.g., Blanchard & Buckley, 1999 Blanchard, Kolb, & Prins, 1991; Gerardi, Keane, Cahoon, & Klauminzer, 1994; Orr & Kaloupek, 1997; Pitman, Orr, Forgue, de Jong, & Claiborn, 1987; Shalev, Orr, Peri, Schreiber, & Pitman, 1992). Consequently, there have been efforts to utilize these measures as a marker for PTSD, and it has been suggested that consideration should be given to revising the diagnostic criteria to formalize the requirement of direct indicators of physiological reactivity into the diagnostic definition (Orr & Kaloupek, 1997).

Regardless of whether these measurement techniques will eventually be refined to sufficiently meet the standards as a "true" marker of the disorder, it is now widely recognized that state-of-the-art diagnostic assessment of PTSD should include a psychophysiological component (Fairbank et al., 2001; Litz, Penk, Gerardi, & Keane, 1992; Orr & Kaloupek, 1997). Among the recommended components of a multimethod assessment protocol (clinical interview, psychometric testing, psychophysiological assessment), psychophysiological assessment stands as the only data source not fully reliant on self-report. Although psychophysiological techniques have a certain appeal in that they offer more objective indicators of symptomatology, they are not error free and can be susceptible to "faking" (a common validity concern with more subjective self-report measures). Nonetheless, these techniques provide important convergent data to bolster diagnostic accuracy.

Although this considerable body of research indicates the significant potential of psychophysiological techniques for the assessment of PTSD, these studies have been conducted almost exclusively with war veterans who have had multiple exposures to traumatic events and chronic symptomatology. Recently, however, Shalev, Orr, and Pitman (1993) found that PTSD cases could be reliably discriminated from noncases among Israeli civilians exposed to noncombat trauma. These findings, if replicated, suggest that measuring psychophysiological responses to trauma-related imagery may be an effective assessment tool for PTSD related to a variety of traumatic exposures.

Although psychophysiological measures may seem difficult to "fake," is this, in fact, the case? This issue has not been intensively studied to date, but the results of a study conducted by Gerardi, Blanchard, and Kolb (1989) on the ability of veterans without PTSD to "fake" increased physiological reactivity in response to combat stimuli, serve as an important caveat. Findings indicated that, although the baseline levels of physiological reactivity of veterans with PTSD were significantly higher than those of veterans without PTSD, there were no differences in the responses to combat stimuli of veterans with and without PTSD who attempted to fake PTSD.

Finally, substantial issues surround the feasibility of using psychophysiological approaches, particularly in the context of community studies. The cost of equipment, the expertise necessary to conduct the assessment, and the requirements for a controlled environment would, in most cases, be prohibitive in such studies. Thus, although promising, the role of psychophysiological assessment in PTSD case identification in epidemiological studies is probably limited at present.

In addition, exciting technological advances in neuroimaging and developing research employing these technologies and other methodologies to examine neuroendocrinological and neurochemical factors are rendering dramatic findings that both shed light on the pathogenesis of PTSD and may suggest the development of new treatment techniques (Bremner, Southwick & Charney, 1999; Malizia & Nutt, 2000; Nutt, 2000; Pitman, Shin, Rauch, 2001; Yehuda, 2000). Converging data from studies examining the neurobiological underpinnings of PTSD are increasingly supportive of a model of biological dysregulation of the glutamatergic, noradrenergic, serotonergic, and neuroendocrine pathways in the development and maintenance of PTSD (Malizia & Nutt, 2000; Nutt, 2000; Yehuda, 2000).

Structural imaging studies have pointed to structural differences in the neuroanatomy of individuals with PTSD as compared with controls, including presence of nonspecific white matter lesions and reduced hippocampal volume (Pitman et al., 2001). With the advent of positron emission tomography (PET) and other functional neuroimaging techniques, researchers have been able to advance beyond the limitations of static measures of brain structure to conduct dynamic measurement of brain activity. One key finding from these studies is that the presentation of trauma-related stimuli to individuals with PTSD results in increased activity in areas of the brain thought to be involved in the processing of fear (amygdala and anterior paralimbic structures) and failure to activate areas of the brain thought to play an inhibitory role (cingulate cortex; Pitman et al., 2001). Although study results are not fully consistent, findings are suggestive that higher amygdala responsivity and underresponsive medial prefrontal cortex may play a role in the pathology of PTSD. Currently, there is considerable hope and enthusiasm that these evolving technologies and methodologies can further elucidate the underlying pathogenesis of PTSD and ultimately provide precise direction for the development of more targeted and effective treatment.

Studies have also begun to identify neurobiological correlates of PTSD that may ultimately prove useful in case identification. For example, Yehuda and her colleagues (Yehuda et al., 1990) found significantly lower mean 24-hour urinary cortisol levels in combat veterans with PTSD than in age-comparable, nonpsychiatric controls. Subsequently, Yehuda et al. (1995) found that Holocaust survivors with PTSD had lower mean 24-hour urinary cortisol levels than a comparison group of Holocaust survivors without PTSD and another comparison group of sociodemographically matched controls who were not exposed to the Holocaust. These latter findings strengthen the specificity of the relationship between urinary cortisol and PTSD, suggesting that this relationship may eventually be useful in PTSD case identification.

Research-Design-Based Approaches

Judicious selection of assessment techniques and instruments is not the only way to improve case identification in epidemiological studies. The ability to identify cases can be influenced by features of the research design as well. Traditionally, cohort studies are designed so that all participants undergo the same assessment procedure. When the disorder of interest is relatively rare, however—that is, when most people in the cohort *do not* have the disorder—alternative designs may be both more efficient and more effective.

For example, Kulka et al. (1991) note that the findings of seven major community epidemiological studies of the prevalence of PTSD among Vietnam veterans showed prevalence estimates ranging from 13 to 17%. In other words, more than 80% of the veterans who participated in these studies did *not* have PTSD. Comprehensive PTSD case identification, however, is resource intensive, and expending those resources on participants who probably do not have PTSD is inefficient.

One solution to this dilemma is the two-stage design (see Dohrenwend, 1989). In two-stage designs, all participants are first assessed with a brief screening instrument that has been shown to be related to the specific diagnosis being studied. This allows the investigators to divide the cohort into "likely cases" and "likely noncases." Then at the second stage, all of those who screen positive (i.e., the likely cases) and a subsample of the negatives (i.e., the likely noncases) are selected for a more comprehensive assessment.

By including in the second stage all of the apparent cases, the statistical power for risk factor and other analyses is increased, and a basis for estimating the sample-specific false-positive screening rate is established (i.e., what proportion of the "likely cases" identified by the screening are ultimately determined to be noncases?). Further, by including a subsample of the screen negatives, an empirical basis for estimating the sample-specific false-negative screening rate is also established (i.e., what proportion of the "likely non-cases" are ultimately determined to be PTSD cases?). Because the second-stage sample is a probability sample, second-stage findings can be weighted back to formulate unbiased prevalence estimates for the original cohort, corrected for the observed screening bias.

As an example of how this approach can be implemented, participants in the NVVRS (Kulka et al., 1990) were screened at the first stage with the Mississippi Scale. All veterans who scored over the specified cutoff of 89, which was selected to emphasize sensitivity over specificity (i.e., to increase the likelihood that all of the true PTSD cases in the sample screened positive and were therefore included in the second stage), were then included in the clinical examination sample, along with a subset of those who screened negative. Participants in the clinical examination underwent a comprehensive, multimeasure PTSD assessment, which served as the basis for the NVVRS composite PTSD diagnosis (details of this procedure are provided in Schlenger et al., 1992).

Thus a variety of ways exist to improve case identification in community epidemiological studies. Although opinions vary as to which method is "best," one fact is clear: No single existing method is "perfect"; that is, none provides a true "gold standard" for PTSD diagnosis. Spitzer (1983) recommends the LEAD standard (Longitudinal, Expert, and All Data), which emphasizes assessment by trained clinicians using multiple sources of information. The NVVRS research team (Schlenger et al., 1992) extended this to the Comprehensive Assessment of Multimethod–Multisource Information (CAMMI) standard. The CAMMI standard emphasizes the integration of information from multiple methods and multiple sources into case identification algorithms.

The point is that in the absence of a definitive biological marker that can be measured with near-absolute reliability, PTSD case identification must rely on less-than-perfect assessment measures. That is, although a number of "good" measures of PTSD exist, none is "perfect." Consequently, given the importance of valid case identification to internal validity, the use of multiple measures that employ varying methodologies and data sources is recommended. Relying on multiple measures and requiring multiple positive indications for an individual to be classified as a case are feasible, even in community studies, and increase confidence in the diagnosis.

ETHICAL CONSIDERATIONS

The fundamental principles of research ethics as defined in the *Belmont Report* (National Commission for the Protection of Human Subjects of Biomedical and Behavioral Research, 1979) are respect for persons, beneficence, and justice. As such, researchers must ensure that individuals have autonomy with regard to participating in research studies, that the possibility of harm is minimized and the possibility of benefit is maximized, and that the burdens and benefits associated with research are equitably distributed (i.e., studies must not be conducted so that certain populations or individuals take on most of the risks of research whereas others glean most of the benefits).

Although all of these principles must be considered in the design and conduct of any research study, the principles of respect and beneficence are particularly germane to studies of PTSD in community populations. Assessment of traumatic exposure and PTSD diagnosis involves focusing the attention of participants on experiences and symptoms that are likely to have been and may continue to be painful. This fact leads to concerns related to the protection of human participants: Do participants fully understand the nature of the research study in which they are being asked to participate? Do participants understand the potential risks and benefits of participation? Is participation in such assessments "harmful" to participants? What safeguards are prudent to guard against any potential negative consequences?

It can be argued that protection of human participants recruited for community epidemiological studies of PTSD begins as early as the design phase of a study (e.g., selection of specific assessment tools, determination of interviewer credentials required, development of training materials for interviewers, etc.). However, researchers are directly engaged in activities related to the protection of human participants during the informed consent process. That is, even before an individual has formally been defined as a research participant, the researcher is taking steps to certify the autonomy of that individual in making a decision to participate in a given research study.

For people to make autonomous decisions about participating in an epidemiological study, they must first be provided with information about the purpose of the study; study duration; study procedures, including any that are experimental; foreseeable risks or discomforts; benefits that may be expected; the extent to which confidentiality will be maintained; whom they may contact to answer questions about the study or their rights as a research participant; and the voluntary nature of participation in the study.[1] In the case of studies of trauma history and PTSD, "foreseeable risks and discomforts" include distress that may be experienced when participating in an assessment of traumatic events or psychological symptoms. Consequently, researchers must inform participants of the potential for such distress during the informed consent process.

Additionally, studies of trauma and ensuing psychological sequelae can involve gathering information that may necessitate mandatory reporting and therefore constitute a breach of confidentiality. For example, assessments of

[1] Additional elements must also be part of the informed consent process for studies that involve treatment of the participant, studies in which an investigator can terminate an individual's participation, studies of greater than minimal risk, studies involving pregnant women, studies in which findings from the study may influence a participant's willingness to continue participation, studies that involve additional costs to participants, and studies in which there are consequences to the participant for withdrawal.

abuse histories in children or adults who have perpetrated abuse could require that the researchers report certain information to the proper authorities in the state in which the study is conducted. The duty to report abuse is complicated by the fact that the mandatory reporting laws vary across states with regard to who must report; what must be reported, including the thresholds for mandatory reporters and for nonmandatory reporters; and to whom the report must be made. Likewise, assessments of psychological symptoms could lead to endorsement of suicidal or homicidal ideation or intent and may in some circumstances result in a required report of such information. Researchers must be informed about the laws of states in which they are conducting research, must utilize these laws to guide the development of a reporting protocol, and must inform potential research participants about the circumstances under which confidentiality will be broken and a report will be made.

An additional issue with regard to informed consent is the ability of a potential participant to act with autonomy in the immediate wake of a trauma. Although little empirical evidence speaks directly to this issue, DuMont and Stermac (1996) found that, among sexual assault survivors who had presented for treatment within 72 hours of the assault and signed a consent form to participate in a research study at that time, 14 out of 15 women in the study did not recall signing the consent form when contacted 39 months later. Although these findings are not definitive on the matter of ability to consent to or decline participation in a study during the hours immediately following a trauma, the participants' failure to remember the consent process and provision of consent in this situation is troubling.

Findings from a study (Ruzek & Zatzick, 2000) of hospitalized motor vehicle and assault victims who participated in a trauma-focused interview as part of a research study indicate that some individuals were not participating as informed participants (19% stated that they felt that they couldn't say no to the research, 2% did not understand the consent form, 6% did not feel free to skip questions, 3% did not think they could stop at any time). Although immediate posttrauma contact with individuals is relatively rare in community epidemiological studies, newer technologies (e.g., RDD surveys, Internet surveys) and more nimble funding mechanisms do make such contact more likely today than in the past. Consequently, when conducting studies with individuals who have experienced trauma within the previous few hours or days, researchers should proceed with particular care and take extra precautions to ensure that individuals are acting with autonomy in consenting to participate.

Once an individual has made an informed decision to participate in a study, the researcher has an obligation to conduct that study in ways that minimizes risk and maximizes potential for benefit. Obviously, to minimize risk, one must have an understanding of the potential harm that can ensue from participating in a research study. Until relatively recently, there has been little empirical study of the impact of participating in trauma-related research. However, a growing body of studies provides empirical findings to help guide trauma researchers in assessing risk and in taking action to minimize risk.

Newman, Walker and Gefland (1999) examined the ethical costs and benefits of conducting trauma research with 1,174 women enrolled in an HMO who participated in a trauma-related health survey. Specifically, these women were sent a mail survey that contained questions about childhood maltreatment (including sexual maltreatment) and experiencing symptoms of PTSD. A subsample of 252 women participated in a follow-up trauma-focused interview. Among the mail survey respondents, 10.5% stated that they experienced unexpected upset, but 77% stated that they had no regrets about having participated in the survey. Among the interview participants, 19% reported unexpected distress, but 86% stated that they had no regrets. These researchers examined the relationship of unexpected distress to regret and found, somewhat surprisingly, that among those who participated in the mail survey and were unexpectedly distressed, only 1.1% expressed regret at having participated in the study, and among those who reported unexpected distress to the interview, only one person expressed regret.

In a study of 641 Australian Vietnam veterans who participated in an epidemiological survey of PTSD, Parslow, Jorm, O'Toole, Marshall, and Grayson (2000) found that PTSD diagnosis was related to level of distress reported from participating in the study (75.3% of those with current PTSD reported distress from participating, 56.5% of those with past PTSD reported distress from participating, and 20.6% of those with no PTSD diagnosis reported distress from participating). However, distress was not related to whether or not they were willing to continue participating in the study.

Ruzek and Zatzick (2000) studied a more acutely traumatized population, 117 hospitalized motor vehicle accident or assault victims. Indivduals who agreed to participate were given a 1-hour interview that assessed traumatic life events, PTSD, depression, peritraumatic dissociation, and drug and alcohol use. Participants were also given 10 items from the Reactions to Research Questionnaire. In this more acutely traumatized population, a sizable minority reported indications of distress related to participating in the research (11% were more upset than expected; 32% stated it made them think about things they did not want to think about). However, over 95% of the participants reported that the benefits outweighed the costs and indicated that they would still agree to participate.

A recent study conducted by Griffin, Resick, Waldrop, and Mechanic (2003) offers additional data on the impact of participation in trauma research, specifically with regard to the duration of distress. In two samples of participants in trauma research, one assessed in the acute aftermath of a physical/sexual assault ($N = 170$) and the other assessed retrospectively following exposure to domestic violence ($N = 260$), these researchers found that, in general, participation in the trauma assessment was rated as minimally distressing by both samples. Additionally, most participants (95% of those assessed acutely and 98% of those assessed retrospectively) indicated that they would be willing to participate in this type of assessment again. The only part of the trauma assessment that was given moderately high distress ratings was participation in a trauma phase of a psychophysiological assessment protocol during which participants were asked to talk about their trauma. However, although the ratings of distress were higher during this section of the protocol, ratings of distress decreased after a final baseline phase that followed the trauma phase of the psychophysiological assessment, indicating that the increased distress was transient.

The findings of all of these studies taken together suggest that some percentage of participants will experience distress when participating in trauma-focused research; however, the available data indicate that this distress is not overwhelming and is transient in nature. Additionally, most participants in trauma-focused studies indicated that they obtained some benefit from participating in such studies and said that they would participate again. Further, these findings hold for both acute and nonacute populations and for those reporting high levels of PTSD symptomatology. Therefore, researchers conducting trauma research are provided some assurances that the level of risk for trauma-focused research studies is minimal and that, with the proper care and sensitivity in the conduct of these studies, participants will not be harmed.

In summary, researchers conducting community epidemiological studies of PTSD should (1) be aware that some participants may experience distress; (2) inform all potential participants in advance of that possibility; (3) train interviewers to manage emotional responsivity in participants and provide them support in doing so; and (4) arrange in advance a professional referral network for participants who request referral.

As an example of how these mandates can be implemented, even in the context of a national survey (Kulka et al., 1990), NVVRS survey interviews were conducted by experienced survey interviewers who were trained to administer the interview in a 10-day training session. In addition to covering the mechanics of the interview process, the training also focused on issues related to respecting the rights of research participants (e.g., voluntary participation, informed consent, confidentiality) and interviewer "sensitivity." In this component of the training, which was provided by a team of experienced clinicians expert in diagnosing and treating PTSD in combat veterans, trainers helped interviewers identify the parts of the interview that were most likely to evoke emotional responses. In addition, training focused on how to recognize cues that indicate emotional reactivity and how to *manage* such reactivity when it occurred. It is important to train survey interviewers to recognize and maintain appropriate role boundaries so that they do not make the error of attempting to provide "counseling" or other interventions that are beyond their professional competence.

In addition to this training, the NVVRS investigators established support networks for participants and/or interviewers. To support participants, interviewers always carried with them a list of local mental health treatment resources (e.g., veterans centers, community mental health centers) in the event that the participant requested information. In addition, interviewers were trained to report to the clinical training team anything "unusual" that occurred during their contacts with participants (e.g., during an interview, during a phone call in which the interviewer was trying to set up an interview). Clinicians would then discuss the facts of the case with the interviewer, and they would together decide on a course of action (e.g., the clinician might call the participant to make a referral). Furthermore, NVVRS participants were followed up by phone about a week after their interview and asked specifically about its impact on them, if any. During these calls, referral assistance was offered to all who requested it. In fact, the number of interviews in which participants were distressed was small, and no reactions were severe.

The NVVRS investigators also implemented a support network for interviewers in recognition of the fact that these interviews could be stressful both for participants and for interviewers. In addition to their special training, interviewers had access to clinical backup at all times (i.e., there was always a clinician whom they could call). In addition, we held periodic conference calls for small groups of interviewers with members of the clinical team to provide peer support, discuss specific problems, and allow interviewers to benefit from the experiences of their colleagues.

Safeguarding the privacy of the respondent during the assessment process is also a challenging aspect of community epidemiological research. Interviews in community studies are typically conducted in the participant's home, with family members and others also present. Precautions must be taken to protect the confidentiality of the participant's answers by conducting the interview out of the hearing range of others in the residence. Issues of privacy are particularly important for potentially vulnerable populations, such as children and adolescents, who could be placed at risk if their answers to sensitive questions (e.g., questions about substance use and abuse, sexual behavior) were overheard.

Several relatively recent technological advances in survey methods show considerable promise for enhancing the privacy of respondents in community studies of sensitive behaviors. Such advances include new computer technologies in which laptop computers "read" (prerecorded) interview questions to respondents wearing headphones and the interviewee responds by pressing the appropriate key on the computer's keyboard. This technology, referred to as audio-computer-assisted self-interviewing (A-CASI), has already been applied to several standardized assessment instruments and is likely soon to become the standard in community epidemiological studies of PTSD.

The even more recent technological advances that provide for collection of data via the Internet pose new ethical challenges for researchers. The Internet offers the opportunity to collect data from dispersed samples expeditiously and at a much lower cost than would be incurred using more conventional data collection methods. A report from a 1990 conference sponsored by the American Association for the Advancement of Science (Frankel & Siang, 1999) provides an overview of the ethical and legal challenges that face researchers conducting human-participants research on the Internet, including: the ability of researchers and participants to use pseudonym identities; complexities in obtaining informed consent; participants' expectations of privacy online; issues of public and private spaces in cyberspace; protection of confidentiality of data that is transmitted over the Internet; use of appropriate sampling techniques in Internet studies; and handling distressed participants. The federal Office for Human Research Protections (OHRP) has indicated that any institutional review board reviewing research that is to be conducted using the Internet must include, as a member or as a consultant, an individual with information technology credentials in order to appropriately evaluate that research and, therefore, to be in compliance with federal regulations. It follows, then, that researchers designing Internet studies must also either have such knowledge themselves or avail themselves of such knowledge via consultants in order to design a study that provides the appropriate human-participants protections. Because of the sensitive nature of trauma-focused studies and the potential for distress among some study participants, conducting trauma-focused research on the Internet poses a particular challenge. Developing procedures that ensure that the spirit of the current federal regulations included in Title 45 CFR Part 46 (Protection of Human Subjects) are met when conducting trauma-focused Internet research will require that researchers become informed about technology and are creative, flexible, and vigilant in their critique of their study methods.

SUMMARY

Community epidemiological studies of PTSD represent a vital cornerstone of our understanding of the phenomenology and etiology of the disorder and yield important clues with respect to how best to treat and prevent it. Because we do not randomize people to exposure to PTEs, however, it is critical that such studies be designed to include a variety of quasi-experimental comparisons that allow the ruling out of important alternative explanations of the findings and to assess multiple outcomes, some of which are selected for their ability to provide discriminant and construct validity information that can also help rule out alternative explanations.

Similarly, accurate assessment of exposure and case identification are two cornerstones of the internal validity of community epidemiological studies of PTSD. Inaccurate assessment of either can lead to unwarranted conclusions about PTSD incidence and prevalence, about its relationship to other disorders, and about its risk factors, all of which can detract from treatment and prevention efforts.

Assessment of exposure is complicated by the fact that there are many kinds of exposures that can lead to PTSD and that individuals can have multiple exposures of varying frequency and intensity. Most studies have assessed exposure via one-time survey interviews, although documented misclassifications associated with self-reports of exposure underscore the importance of independent corroboration. Although existing instruments have moved the field forward, it is clear that periodic assessment of exposure in the context of prospective, longitudinal studies represents an important advance and that independent corroboration should always be sought where feasible.

Because many PTEs strike without warning, rapid response is often mandatory. Newer approaches to survey interviewing help in this regard but are not without problems. Nonresponse is an important issue, although recent developments in the conceptualization of survey nonresponse are somewhat reassuring. Limited interview time forces use of brief assessments, which increases pressure for establishing the correspondence of the screening instruments with the underlying constructs (e.g., PTE exposure, PTSD diagnosis) in populations similar to those under study.

Case identification in community studies is complicated by the lack of a "presenting problem" to serve as a starting point for assessment. Instruments based on a variety of underlying approaches to diagnostic decision making have been developed that have acceptable psychometric properties. Nevertheless, none represents a true "gold standard." In the absence of such a standard, confidence in case identification can be improved by using multiple assessments that can provide an empirical basis for a "best estimate" diagnosis and through design features that focus assessment resources on people who are likely to have or to be at risk for PTSD.

Community epidemiological studies of PTSD involve some special ethical considerations. Investigators conducting such studies should train interviewers and other staff members in the details of human participants' protection, including voluntary participation, informed consent, and confidentiality. In addition, interviewers and others who have direct contact with research participants should be prepared in advance to identify and manage emotional reactivity on the part of some study participants. Investigators should plan for networks to support both participants and interviewers. Although recent empirical evidence with respect to the effects of participating in such studies is reassuring, safeguards remain important.

One implication of the preceding is that competent conduct of community epidemiological studies of PTSD requires skills from a variety of disciplines. Consequently, such studies are best conducted by multidisciplinary teams of investigators that can bring the full range of skills and expertise—psychological, sociological, anthropological, statistical, methodological, logistical, and ethical—to bear. Assembling such multidisciplinary teams and fielding the large-scale data collection efforts that these studies require are both expensive and time-consuming.

Finally, although the field has advanced rapidly since the official designation in 1980 of PTSD as a specific psychiatric disorder, many basic epidemiological questions remain unanswered. For PTSD related to some types of traumatic exposure (e.g., combat, rape), questions of prevalence and comorbidity have been relatively well studied, but for other exposures, basic questions remain. Across the board, however, important issues of etiology are still unresolved. Addressing these questions comprehensively will require large-scale, prospective cohort studies conducted by multidisciplinary teams of investigators using multiple measures of exposure and multiple case identification measures. In addition, they are likely to require rapid response and possibly multiple modes of assessment. These are important challenges, but the progress made over the past two decades in accumulating evidence about the epidemiology of PTSD provides good reason for optimism about future progress.

REFERENCES

American Psychiatric Association. (1980). *Diagnostic and statistical manual of mental disorders* (3rd ed.). Washington, DC: Author.

American Psychiatric Association. (1994). *Diagnostic and statistical manual of mental disorders* (4th ed.). Washington, DC: Author.

Anthony, J. C., Folstein, M., Romanoski, A. J., Von Korff, M. R., Nestadt, G. R., Chalal, R., et al. (1985). Comparison of the lay Diagnostic Interview Schedule and a standardized psychiatric diagnosis. *Archives of General Psychiatry, 42*, 667–676.

Blake, D. D., Weathers, F. W., Nagy, L. M., Kaloupek, D. G., Gusman, F. D., Charney, D. S., & Keane, T. M. (1995). The development of a clinician-administered PTSD scale. *Journal of Traumatic Stress, 8*, 75–90.

Blanchard, E. B., & Buckley, T. C. (1999). Psychophysiological assessment of posttraumatic stress disorder. In P. A. Saigh & J. D. Bremner (Eds.), *Posttraumatic stress disorder: A comprehensive text* (pp. 248–266). Boston: Allyn & Bacon.

Blanchard, E. B., Kolb, L. C., Gerardi, R. J., Ryan, P., & Pallmeyer, T. P. (1986). Cardiac response to relevant stimuli as an adjunctive tool for diagnosing posttraumatic stress disorder in Vietnam veterans. *Behavior Therapy, 17*, 592–606.

Blanchard, E. B., Kolb, L. C., Pallmeyer, T. P., & Gerardi, R. J. (1982). A psychophysiological study of posttraumatic stress disorder in Vietnam veterans. *Psychiatric Quarterly, 54*, 220–229.

Blanchard, E. B., Kolb, L. C., & Prins, A. (1991). Psychophysiological responses in the diagnosis of posttraumatic stress disorder in Vietnam veterans. *Journal of Nervous and Mental Disease, 179*, 99–103.

Bolen, R. B., & Scannapieco, M. (1999, September). Prevalence of child sexual abuse: A corrective meta-analysis. *Social Services Review*, 282–313.

Boudreaux, E., Kilpatrick, D. G., Resnick, H. S., Best, C. L., & Saunders, B.E. (1998). Criminal victimization, posttraumatic stress disorder, and comorbid psychopathology among a community sample of women. *Journal of Traumatic Stress, 11*, 665–678.

Bremner, J. D., Southwick, S. M., & Charney, D. S. (1999). The neurobiology of posttraumatic stress disorder: An integration of animal and human research. In P. A. Saigh & J. D. Bremner (Eds.), *Posttraumatic stress disorder: A comprehensive text* (pp 103–143). Boston: Allyn & Bacon.

Breslau, N., Davis, G. C., & Andreski, P. (1995). Risk factors for PTSD-related traumatic events: A prospective analysis. *American Journal of Psychiatry, 152*, 529–535.

Breslau, N., Davis, G. C., Andreski, P., & Peterson, E. (1991). Traumatic events and posttraumatic stress disorder in an urban population of young adults. *Archives of General Psychiatry, 48*, 216–222.

Breslau, N., Kessler, R. C., Chilcoat, H. D., Schultz, I. R., Davis, G. C., & Andreski, P. (1998). Trauma and posttraumatic stress disorder in the community: The 1996 Detroit Area Survey of Trauma. *Archives of General Psychiatry*, *55*, 626–632.

Bromet, E., & Dew, M. A. (1995). Review of psychiatric epidemiologic research on disasters. *Epidemiologic Reviews*, *17*, 113–119.

Butcher, J. N., Dahlstrom, W. G., Graham, J. R., Tellegen, A., & Kaemmer, B. (1989). *Minnesota Multiphasic Personality Inventory-2 (MMPI-2): Manual for administration and scoring*. Minneapolis: University of Minnesota Press.

Cook, T. D., & Campbell, D. T. (1979). *Quasi-experimentation*. Boston: Houghton Mifflin.

Costello, A. J., Edelbrock, C. S., Kalas, R., Kessler, M. D., & Klaric, S. H. (1982). *The National Institute of Mental Health Diagnostic Interview for Children (DISC)*. Rockville, MD: National Institute of Mental Health.

Davidson, H., Smith, R., & Kudler, H. (1989). Validity and reliability of the DSM-III criteria for posttraumatic stress disorder: Experience with a structured interview. *Journal of Nervous and Mental Disease*, *177*, 336–341.

Dohrenwend, B. P. (1989). The problem of validity in field studies of psychological disorders revisited. In L. N. Robins (Ed.), *Validity of psychiatric diagnosis*. New York: Raven Press.

DuMont, J., & Stermac, L. (1996). Research with women who have been sexually assaulted: Examining informed consent. *Canadian Journal of Human Sexuality*, *5*, 185–191.

Fairbank, J. A., Ebert, L., & Caddell, J. M. (2001). Posttraumatic stress disorder. In H. E. Adams & P. B. Sutker (Eds.), *Comprehensive handbook of psychopathology* (3rd ed.). New York: Kluwer Academic/Plenum.

Fairbank, J. A., Jordan, B. K., & Schlenger, W. E. (1996). Designing and implementing epidemiologic studies. In E. B. Carlson (Ed.), *Trauma research methodology*. Lutherville, MD: Sidran Press.

Fairbank, J. A., Schlenger, W. E., Caddell, J. M., & Woods, M. G. (1993). Posttraumatic stress disorder. In P. B. Sutker & H. E. Adams (Eds.), *Comprehensive handbook of psychopathology*. New York: Plenum Press.

Fairbank, J. A., Schlenger, W. E., Saigh, P. A., & Davidson, J. R. T. (1995). An epidemiologic profile of posttraumatic stress disorder: Prevalence, comorbidity, and risk factors. In M. J. Friedman, D. S. Charney, & A. Y. Deutch (Eds.), *Neurobiological and clinical consequences of stress: From normal adaptation to PTSD*. New York: Raven Press.

Frankel, M. S., & Siang, S. (1999). *Ethical and legal aspects of human subjects research on the Internet*. Washington, DC: American Association for the Advancement of Science. Retrieved from http://www.aaas.org/spp/dspp/sfrl/projects/intres/main.htm.

Galea, S., Ahern, J., Resnick, H., Kilpatrick, D., Bucuvalas, M., Gold, J., & Vlahov, D. (2002). Psychological sequelae of the September 11 terrorist attacks in New York City: *New England Journal of Medicine*, *346*, 982–987.

Gerardi, R. F., Blanchard, E. B., & Kolb, L. C. (1989). Ability of Vietnam veterans to dissimulate a psychophysiological assessment for posttraumatic stress disorder. *Behavior Therapy*, *20*, 229–243.

Gerardi, R. J., Keane, T. M., Cahoon, B. J., & Klauminzer, G. W. (1994). An in vivo assessment of physiological arousal in posttraumatic stress disorder. *Journal of Abnormal Psychology*, *103*, 825–827.

Graham, J. W., Hofer, S. M., & McKinnon, D. P. (1996). Maximizing the usefulness of data obtained with planned missing value patterns: An application of maximum likelihood procedures. *Multivariate Behavioral Research, 31*(2), 197–218.

Griffin, M. G., Resick, P. A., Waldrop, A. E., & Mechanic, M. B. (2003). Participation in trauma research: Is there evidence of harm? *Journal of Traumatic Stress, 16*, 221–227.

Helzer, J. E., Robins, L. N., McEvoy, L. T., Spitznagel, E. L., Stoltzman, R. K., Farmer, A., & Brockington, I. F. (1985). A comparison of clinical and Diagnostic Interview Schedule diagnoses. *Archives of General Psychiatry, 42*, 657–666.

Herman, J. J., Perry, J. C., & van der Kolk, B. A. (1989). Childhood trauma in borderline personality disorder. *American Journal of Psychiatry, 146*, 490–495.

Jordan, B. K., Schlenger, W. E., Caddell, J. M., & Fairbank, J. A. (1997). Etiologic factors in the development of borderline personality disorder in a sample of convicted women felons. In M. C. Zanarini (Ed.), *The role of sexual abuse in borderline personality disorder*. Washington, DC: American Psychiatric Press.

Keane, T. M., Caddell, J. M., & Taylor, K. L. (1988). Mississippi Scale for Combat-Related Posttraumatic Stress Disorder: Three studies in reliability and validity. *Journal of Consulting and Clinical Psychology, 56*, 85–90.

Keane, T. M., Malloy, P. F., & Fairbank, J. A. (1984). The empirical development of an MMPI subscale for the assessment of combat-related posttraumatic stress disorder. *Journal of Consulting and Clinical Psychology, 52*, 888–891.

Kessler, R. C., McGonagle, K. A., Zhao, S., Nelson, C. B., Hughes, M., Eshleman, S., et al. (1994). Lifetime and 12-month prevalence of DSM-IIIR psychiatric disorders in the United States. *Archives of General Psychiatry, 51*, 8–19.

Kessler, R. C., Sonnega, A., Bromet, E., Hughes, M., & Nelson, C. R. (1995). Posttraumatic stress disorder in the National Comorbidity Survey. *Archives of General Psychiatry, 52*, 1048–1060.

Kilpatrick, D. G., Resnick, H. S., & Freedy, J. R. (1991). *The Potential Stressful Events Interview*. Unpublished instrument, Medical University of South Carolina, Department of Psychiatry, Crime Victims Research and Treatment Center, Charleston, SC.

Kilpatrick, D. G., Resnick, H. S., Freedy, J. R., Pelcovitz, D., Resick, P., Roth, S., & van der Kolk, B. (1994). The posttraumatic stress disorder field trial: Emphasis on criterion A and overall PTSD diagnosis. In T. A. Widiger (Ed.), *DSM-IV source book* (Vol. 5). Washington, DC: American Psychiatric Press.

Kilpatrick, D. G., Saunders, B. E., Veronen, L. J., Best, C. L., & Von, J. M. (1987). Criminal victimization: Lifetime prevalence, reporting to police, and psychological impact. *Crime and Delinquency, 33*, 479–489.

Korn, E. L., & Graubard, B. I. (1999). Predictive margins for survey data. *Biometrics, 55*, 652–659.

Kubany, E. S., Haynes, S. N., Leisen, M. B., Owens, J. A., Kaplan, A. S., Watson, S. B., & Burns, K. (2000). Development and preliminary validation of a brief broad-spectrum measure of exposure to trauma: The Traumatic Life Events Questionnaire. *Psychological Assessment, 12*(2), 210–224.

Kulka, R. A., & Schlenger, W. E. (1993). Survey research and field designs for the study of posttraumatic stress disorder. In J. P. Wilson & B. Raphael (Eds.), *International handbook of traumatic stress syndromes*. New York: Plenum Press.

Kulka, R. A., Schlenger, W. E., Fairbank, J. A., Hough, R. L., Jordan, B. K., Marmar, C. R., & Weiss, D. S. (1990). *Trauma and the Vietnam War generation: Report of findings from the National Vietnam Veterans Readjustment Study*. New York: Brunner/Mazel.

Kulka, R. A., Schlenger, W. E., Fairbank, J. A., Hough, R. L., Jordan, B. K., Marmar, C. R., & Weiss, D. S. (1991). Assessment of posttraumatic stress disorder in the community: Prospects and pitfalls from recent studies of Vietnam veterans. *Psychological Assessment*, *3*, 547–560.

Little, R. J. A., & Rubin, D. B. (1987). *Statistical analysis with missing data*. New York: Wiley.

Litz, B. T., Penk, W. E., Gerardi, R. J., & Keane, T. M. (1992). Assessment of posttraumatic stress disorder. In P. A. Saigh (Ed.), *Posttraumatic stress disorder: A behavioral approach to assessment and treatment* (pp. 50–84). Needham Heights, MA: Allyn & Bacon.

Loftus, E. F., Garry, M., & Feldman, J. (1994). Forgetting sexual trauma: What does it mean when 38% forget? *Journal of Consulting and Clinical Psychology*, *62*, 1177–1181.

Malizia, A. L., & Nutt, D. J. (2000). Human brain imaging and post-traumatic stress disorder. In D. Nutt, J. R. Davidson, & J. Zohar (Eds.), *Post-traumatic stress disorder: Diagnosis, management and treatment* (pp. 41–51). London: Martin Dunitz.

Malloy, P. F., Fairbank, J. A., & Keane, T. M. (1983). Validation of a multimethod assessment of posttraumatic stress disorder. *Journal of Consulting and Clinical Psychology*, *51*, 488–494.

McCaffrey, R. J., Lorig, T. S., Pendrey, D. L., McCutcheon, N. B., & Garrett, J. C. (1993). Odor-induced EEG changes in PTSD Vietnam veterans. *Journal of Traumatic Stress*, *6*, 213–224.

McFall, M. E., Murburg, M., Roszell, D. K., & Veith, R. C. (1989). Psychophysiologic and neuroendocrine findings in posttraumatic stress disorder: A review of theory and research. *Journal of Anxiety Disorders*, *3*, 243–257.

McFarlane, A. C., Weber, D. L., & Clark, C. R. (1993). Abnormal stimulus processing in posttraumatic stress disorder. *Biological Psychiatry*, *34*, 311–320.

Meakins, J. C., & Wilson, R. M. (1918). The effect of certain sensory stimulations on respiratory and heart rate in cases of so-called "irritable heart." *Heart*, *7*, 17–22.

National Commission for the Protection of Human Subjects of Biomedical and Behavioral Research. (1979). *The Belmont Report: Ethical principles and guidelines for the protection of human subjects*. Washington, DC: National Institutes of Health, Office for Protection from Research Risks.

Neria, Y., & Bromet, E. J. (2000). Comorbidity of PTSD and depression. [Editorial]. *Biological Psychiatry*, *48*, 878–880.

Neria, Y., Bromet, E. J., & Marshall, R. (2002). The relationship between trauma exposure, posttraumatic stress disorder and depression [Letter to the editor]. *Psychological Medicine*, *32*, 1479–1480.

Newman, E., Walker, E., & Gefland, E. (1999). Assessing the ethical costs and benefits of trauma focused research. *General Hospital Psychiatry*, *21*, 187–196.

Norris, F. H. (1990). Screening for traumatic stress: A scale for use in the general population. *Journal of Applied Social Psychology*, *20*, 1704–1718.

Norris, F. H. (1992). Epidemiology of trauma: Frequency and impact of different potentially traumatic events on different demographic subgroups. *Journal of Consulting and Clinical Psychology*, *60*, 409–418.

Norris, F., Byrne, C., Diaz, E., & Kaniasty, K. (2002). *The range, magnitude, and du-*

ration of effects of natural and human-caused disasters: A review of the empirical literature. Boston, MA: National Center for PTSD. Retrieved June 26, 2002, from http://www.ncptsd.org/facts/disasters.

North, C. S., & Pfefferbaum, B. (2002). Research on the mental health effects of terrorism. *Journal of the American Medical Association, 288*, 633–636.

Nutt, D. J. (2000). The psychobiology of posttraumatic stress disorder. *Journal of Clinical Psychiatry, 61*(Suppl. 5), 24–29.

Orr, S. P., & Kaloupek, D. G. (1997). Psychophysiologic assessment of posttraumatic stress disorder. In J. P. Wilson & T. M. Keane (Eds.), *Assessing psychological trauma and PTSD* (pp. 69–97). New York: Guilford Press.

Parslow, R. A., Jorm, A. F., O'Toole, B. I., Marshall, R. P., & Grayson, D. A. (2000). Distress experienced by participants during an epidemiological survey of posttraumatic stress disorder. *Journal of Traumatic Stress, 13*, 465–471.

Pitman, R. K., & Orr, S. P. (1993). Psychophysiologic testing for posttraumatic stress disorder: Forensic psychiatric application. *Bulletin of the American Academy of Psychiatry and the Law, 21*, 37–52.

Pitman, R. K., Orr, S. P., Forgue, D. F., de Jong, J. B., & Claiborn, J. M. (1987). Psychophysiologic assessment of posttraumatic stress disorder imagery in Vietnam combat veterans. *Archives of General Psychiatry, 44*, 970–975.

Pitman, R. K., Shin, L. M., & Rauch, S. L. (2001). Investigating the pathogenesis of posttraumatic stress disorder with neuroimaging. *Journal of Clinical Psychiatry, 62*(Suppl. 17), 47–54.

Regier, D. A., Myers, J. K., Kramer, M., Robins, L. N., Blazer, D. G., Hough, R. L., et al. (1984). The NIMH Epidemiologic Catchment Area Program: Historical context, major objectives, and study population characteristics. *Archives of General Psychiatry, 41*, 934–941.

Resnick, H. S., Best, C. L., Freedy, J. R., Kilpatrick, D. C., & Falsetti, S. A. (1993). *Trauma assessment for adults*. Unpublished interview protocol, Medical University of South Carolina, Department of Psychiatry, Crime Victims Research and Treatment Center, Charleston, SC.

Resnick, H. S., Falsetti, S. A., Kilpatrick, D. C., & Freedy, J. R. (1996). Assessment of rape and other civilian trauma-related posttraumatic stress disorder: Emphasis on assessment of potentially traumatic events. In T. W. Miller (Ed.), *Stressful life events* (2nd ed.). New York: International Universities Press.

Resnick, H. S., Kilpatrick, D. C., Dansky, B. S., Saunders, B. E., & Best, C. L. (1993). Prevalence of civilian trauma and posttraumatic stress disorder in a representative national sample of women. *Journal of Consulting and Clinical Psychology, 61*, 984–991.

Robins, L. N., Helzer, J. E., Croughan, J., & Ratcliff, K. S. (1981). National Institute of Mental Health Diagnostic Interview Schedule: Its history, characteristics, and validity. *Archives of General Psychiatry, 38*, 381–389.

Robins, L. N., Wing, J., Wittchen, H. U., & Helzer, J. E. (1988). The Composite International Diagnostic Interview: An epidemiologic instrument suitable for use in conjunction with different diagnostic systems and in different cultures. *Archives of General Psychiatry, 45*, 1069–1077.

Rubin, D. B. (1976). Inference and missing data. *Biometrika, 63*, 581–592.

Ruzek, J. I., & Zatzick, D. F. (2000). Ethical considerations in research participation among acutely injured trauma survivors: An empirical investigation. *General Hospital Psychiatry, 22*, 27–36.

Saigh, P. A., & Bremner, J. D. (Eds.). (1999). *Posttraumatic stress disorder: A comprehensive text*. Boston: Allyn & Bacon.

Schafer, J. L. (1997). *Analysis of incomplete multivariate data*. Boca Raton, FL: Chapman & Hall/CRC.

Schafer, J. L., & Graham, J. W. (2002). Missing data: Our view of the state of the art. *Psychological Methods*, 7(2), 147–177.

Schlenger, W., Caddell, J., Ebert, L., Jordan, B. K., Rourke, K., Wilson, D. et al. (2002). Psychological reactions to terrorist attacks: Findings from the National Study of Americans' Reactions to September 11. *Journal of the American Medical Association*, *288*, 581–588.

Schlenger, W. E., Kulka, R. A., Fairbank, J. A., Hough, R. L., Jordan, B. K., Marmar, C. R., & Weiss, D. S. (1992). The prevalence of posttraumatic stress disorder in the Vietnam generation: A multimethod, multisource assessment of psychiatric disorder. *Journal of Traumatic Stress*, *5*, 333–363.

Schuster, M. A., Stein, B. D., Jaycox, L., Collins, R. L., Marshall, G. N., Elliott, M. N., et al. (2001). A national survey of stress reactions after the September 11, 2001 terrorist attacks. *New England Journal of Medicine*, *345*, 1507–1512.

Shaffer, D., Fisher, P., Lucas, C. P., Dulcan, M. K., & Schwab-Stone, M. E. (2000). NIMH Diagnostic Interview Schedule for Children—Version IV (NIMH DISC-IV): Description, differences from previous versions, and reliability of some common diagnoses. *Journal of the American Academy of Child and Adolescent Psychiatry*, *39*(1), 28–38

Shalev, A. Y., Orr, S. P., Peri, T., Schreiber, S., & Pitman, R. K. (1992). Physiologic responses to loud tones in Israeli patients with posttraumatic stress disorder. *Archives of General Psychiatry*, *49*, 870–875.

Shalev, A. Y., Orr, S. P., & Pitman, R. K. (1993). Psychophysiologic assessment of traumatic imagery in Israeli civilian patients with posttraumatic stress disorder. *American Journal of Psychiatry*, *150*, 620–624.

Shapiro, S., Skinner, E. A., Kessler, L. G., Von Korff, M., German, P. S., Tishler, G. L., et al. (1984). Utilization of health and mental health services: Three Epidemiologic Catchment Area sites. *Archives of General Psychiatry*, *41*, 971–978.

Silver, R., Holman, E., McIntosh, D., Poulin, M., & Gil-Rivas, V. (2002). Nationwide longitudinal study of psychological responses to September 11. *Journal of the American Medical Association*, *288*, 1235–1244.

Spitzer, R. L. (1983). Psychiatric diagnosis: Are clinicians still necessary? *Comprehensive Psychiatry*, *24*, 399–411.

Spitzer, R. L., Williams, J. B. W., Gibbon, M., & First, M. B. (1992). The Structured Clinical Interview for DSM-III-R (SCID): I. History, rationale, and description. *Archives of General Psychiatry*, *49*, 624–629.

Sudman, S., & Bradburn, N. (1973). Effects of time and memory factors on response in surveys. *Journal of the American Statistical Association*, *68*, 805–815.

Tomarken, A. J. (1995). A psychometric perspective on psychophysiological measures. *Psychological Assessment*, 7, 387–395.

Turner, C. F., Ku, L., Rogers, S. M., Lindberg, L. D., Pleck, J. H., & Sonenstein, F. L. (1998). Adolescent sexual behavior, drug use, and violence: Increased reporting with computer survey technology. *Science*, *280*, 867–873.

Turner, C. F., Lessler, J. T., & Gfroerer, J. C. (Eds.). (1992). *Survey measurement of drug use: Methodological studies*. Washington, DC: U.S. Government Printing Office.

Vreven, D. L., Gudanowski, D. M., King, L. A., & King, D. W. (1995). The civilian version of the Mississippi PTSD Scale: A psychometric evaluation. *Journal of Traumatic Stress, 8*, 91–109.

Weaver, T. L. (1998). Method variance and sensitivity of screening for traumatic stressors. *Journal of Traumatic Stress, 11*, 181–185.

Weiss, D. S., Marmar, C. R., Schlenger, W. E., Fairbank, J. A., Jordan, B. K., Hough, R. L., & Kulka, R. A. (1992). The prevalence of lifetime and partial posttraumatic stress disorder in Vietnam theater veterans. *Journal of Traumatic Stress, 5*, 364–376.

Williams, L. M. (1994a). Recall of childhood trauma: A prospective study of women's memories of child sexual abuse. *Journal of Consulting and Clinical Psychology, 62*, 1167–1176.

Williams, L. M. (1994b). What does it mean to forget child sexual abuse? A reply to Loftus, Garry, and Feldman. *Journal of Consulting and Clinical Psychology, 62*, 1182–1186.

Williams, L. M., Siegel, J. A., & Pomeroy, J. J. (2000). Validity of women's self-reports of documented child abuse. In A. Stone & J. S. Turkkan (Eds.), *The science of self-report: Implications for research and practice*. Mahwah, NJ: Erlbaum.

Wilson, J. P., & Raphael, B. (Eds.). (1993). *International handbook of traumatic stress syndromes*. New York: Plenum Press.

World Health Organization. (1992). *International statistical classification of diseases and related health problems* (rev. ed.). Geneva, Switzerland: Author.

Yehuda, R. (2000). Neuroendocrinology. In D. Nutt, J. R. Davidson, & J. Zohar (Eds.), *Post-traumatic stress disorder: Diagnosis, management and treatment* (pp. 53–68). London: Martin Dunitz.

Yehuda, R., Kahana, B., Binder-Byrnes, K., Southwick, S. M., Mason, J. W., & Giller, E. L. (1995). Low urinary cortisol excretion in Holocaust survivors with posttraumatic stress disorder. *American Journal of Psychiatry, 152*, 982–986.

Yehuda, R., Southwick, S. M., Nussbaum, G., Wahby, V., Giller, E. L., & Mason, J. W. (1990). Low urinary cortisol excretion in patients with posttraumatic stress disorder. *Journal of Nervous and Mental Disease, 178*, 366–369.

Zanarini, M. C., Gunderson, J. G., Marino, M. F., Schwartz, L. O., & Frankenburg, F. R. (1989). Childhood experiences of borderline patients. *Comprehensive Psychiatry, 30*, 18–25.

CHAPTER 10

The Assessment of Military-Related PTSD

TERENCE M. KEANE
AMY E. STREET
JANE STAFFORD

Since the diagnosis of posttraumatic stress disorder (PTSD) appeared in the third edition of the *Diagnostic and Statistical Manual of Mental Disorders* (DSM-III) of the American Psychiatric Association (1980), objective measurement of the psychological effects of combat and other military stressors has grown rapidly. Studies by Wilson (1979) and Egendorf, Kadushin, Laufer, Rothbart, and Sloan (1981) were among the first attempts to quantify the psychological effects of war when these investigators systematically examined the psychological status of American veterans of the Vietnam War. Since that time, the growth in the quantity and quality of instruments designed to assess exposure to potentially traumatic events and PTSD symptomatology has been extensive. Initially driven by the demand for instruments to be used in clinic settings, this development was maintained by studies funded in the public interest to estimate the prevalence of exposure to traumatic events and the development of PTSD in our society.

Our first goal in this chapter is to present the model for assessing and diagnosing PTSD that originated in our research program in Jackson, Mississippi (Keane, Fairbank, Caddell, Zimering, & Bender, 1985) and that was refined and enhanced in the National Center for PTSD in Boston. This method is premised upon the notion that all measures of a disorder are imperfectly related to the condition and that multiple measures from different domains improve diagnostic accuracy and confidence. This multimethod approach to assessment of PTSD is valuable clinically because it taps numerous domains of functioning and thus assists the clinician in identifying multiple targets for intervention. It is valuable in research because it increases the likelihood that patients classified as having PTSD for research purposes do indeed have PTSD.

A second purpose of this chapter is to review the extant literature on the development and evaluation of instruments that measure military-related trauma exposure and attendant PTSD. This is accomplished with an awareness of ongoing changes in the nature of military activities. As peacekeeping and humanitarian efforts increasingly become primary functions of military troops, members of the military are exposed to unique stressors. Efforts to quantify these experiences require a specific methodology that will permit the stable measurement of the complex life events for those serving in these roles. We offer one possible methodology for clinicians and researchers to employ when confronted with measuring stressor exposure in a unique environment and setting.

In addition to the ongoing changes in the types of activities to which members of the military are exposed, U.S. military forces themselves are becoming increasingly diverse. Racial and ethnic composition of the American military force is changing, and, with more minorities involved in military actions, assessment measures must be developed that are culturally sensitive and broadly based to permit accurate evaluations and comparisons across minority groups. Similarly, women are represented in the military in greater numbers, and their range of responsibilities and experiences has greatly expanded. Assessment instruments that are at once sensitive to different gender-based experiences in military assignments and also representative of women's unique responses to military stressors require special consideration. Thus we culminate this chapter with a discussion of strategies that will assist professionals in the successful development of instruments that meet these criteria.

MULTIMODAL ASSESSMENT

A comprehensive assessment of military-related PTSD requires a thorough evaluation of PTSD symptoms and stressors within a broad-based evaluation of general psychopathology (see Keane, Wolfe, & Taylor, 1987). Typical parameters for assessment include the individual's level of functioning within developmental, social, familial, educational, vocational, medical, cognitive, interpersonal, behavioral, and emotional domains across the time periods prior to, during, and subsequent to military service. Such an approach provides an adequate foundation on which to create accurate diagnostic and case formulations that account for the degree to which any pre- or post-war-zone experiences may contribute to the individual's current level of functioning.

Comprehensive PTSD assessment is best achieved through the use of multiple reliable and valid instruments, as every measure is associated with some degree of error (Keane et al., 1987). Therefore, a multimethod approach that combines data derived from self-report measures, structured clinical interviews, and, when possible, psychophysiological assessment is recommended

(Keane et al. 1985; Schnurr, Friedman, & Bernardy, 2002). Such multimodal assessment of PTSD combines each measure's relative strengths, minimizes the psychometric shortcomings of any one instrument, and maximizes correct diagnostic decisions (see Weathers, Keane, King, & King, 1997, for detailed information on psychometric theory).

In addition, the external validity of PTSD assessment can be enhanced by collecting information from multiple informants and available archives. Some individuals with PTSD may have difficulty specifying their symptoms, behaviors, and experiences due to denial, amnesia, avoidance, minimization, cognitive impairment, or motivational factors. Therefore, collateral reports from friends, family members, or health care workers can provide meaningful information to corroborate and clarify aspects of the individual's experiences. Any consistent patterns of discordance among informants can yield hypotheses about the individual's characteristic attributional style or the interpersonal consequences of the individual's behavior. Similarly, consultation of all relevant archives (e.g., medical, legal, military, and educational records) may provide corroborative data to support and amplify self-reports.

Although comprehensive assessments require measures and methods that assess more than military-related experiences and distress, a review of all potential measures that could be used in multidimensional assessment is beyond the scope of this chapter. Our review focuses on the most commonly used validated methods and measurement strategies applied specifically to the assessment of military-related PTSD, including measures of exposure, structured diagnostic and clinical interviews, self-report measures, and psychophysiological assessment. Given the chapter's emphasis on military-related PTSD, we give considerable weight to the assessment of exposure to potentially traumatic experiences that occur in the context of military duties. Several unpublished measures or measures that have not yet been validated are included in this review if they have noteworthy features or historical relevance. Unless otherwise specified, all measures of PTSD presented here assess PTSD symptoms using DSM-IV criteria for PTSD (American Psychiatric Association, 1994).

Evaluation of Exposure to Military-Related Potentially Traumatic Events

Deployment in a war zone does not by itself indicate that an individual has experienced a potentially traumatic event. Similarly, members of the military can be exposed to potentially traumatic events during military duty that do not involve service in a war zone. In order to assess whether or not an individual was exposed to a potentially traumatic event during his or her military service, detailed descriptions of military duties and experiences must be obtained. Although examination of military records may be a helpful adjunct to this assessment, overreliance on these records is ill advised, as there are often inaccuracies in these documents (e.g., Watson, Juba, & Anderson, 1989).

The assessment of PTSD symptomatology is scientifically more advanced than the assessment of stressor exposure in military and war settings. For example, few measures of war-zone stressor exposure are empirically validated, and only one study compared the relative performance of available combat exposure scales (Watson et al., 1989). The following brief review identifies the primary domains that must be considered when assessing exposure to military-related traumatic events and describes the most widely used measures within each of these domains. Table 10.1 provides a summary of the number of items, content areas covered, known internal consistency, and available convergent validity with measures of PTSD. Many measures of war-zone exposure focus exclusively on detailing the intensity, frequency, and duration of traditional combat experiences involving threat of danger, loss of life, or severe physical injury (Green, 1993). Such exposure has been documented as the key risk factor for the development of PTSD among veterans (e.g., Kulka et al., 1990). Although many exposure scales have been developed, few have been empirically validated. In the research literature, the most widely used measure to assess exposure to traditional combat experiences is the 7-item Combat Exposure Scale developed by Keane et al. (1989). This measure is primarily used in studies of Vietnam veterans (e.g., Keane et al., 1998), but has also been used in studies of veterans of the Korean conflict and World War II (McCranie & Hyer, 2000). Reports of combat exposure using the Combat Exposure Scale are consistent across two evaluation points separated by at least 4 years (Niles et al., 1998).

A second domain of military exposure that is related to PTSD symptoms includes those war-zone experiences that take place outside the realm of traditional combat (e.g., Grady, Woolfolk, & Budney, 1989; Green, Grace, Lindy, & Gleser, 1990; Yehuda, Southwick, & Giller, 1992). For example, in the context of combat-related activities, many soldiers are confronted with guerrilla warfare that includes exposure to grotesque death and mutilation and many forms of abusive violence (e.g., Laufer, Gallops, & Frey-Wouters, 1984). Both the 6-item Military Stress Scale (Watson, Kucula, Manifold, Vassar, & Juba, 1988) and the 7-item Combat Exposure Index (Janes, Goldberg, Eisen, & True, 1991) include an assessment of exposure to such experiences. A 24-item Graves Registration Duty Scale, developed to assess aspects of handling human remains (e.g., matching or identifying body parts, transporting body parts) was validated on a largely male sample of Operation Desert Storm troops (Sutker, Uddo, Brailey, Vasterling, & Errera, 1994). In addition, several psychometrically validated scales focus solely on the assessment of exposure to atrocities, such as the 6-item Atrocity Scale (Brett & Laufer, cited in Yehuda et al., 1992), and the 5-item Abusive Violence Scale (Hendrix & Schumm, 1990). A more recent assessment instrument, the 84-item War Events Scale, measures observation of atrocities, participation in atrocities, and current distress related to these events (Unger, Gould, & Babich, 1998).

TABLE 10.1. Self-Report Measures of Exposure to Military-Related Potentially Traumatic Events

Scale name	Authors	Type of exposure measured	Number of items	Alpha	Strength of the relationship with measures of PTSD
Abusive Violence Scale	Hendrix and Shumm (1990)	atrocities	5	.81	.28 (IES intrusion scale); .30 (IES avoidance scale)
Atrocity Scale	Brett and Laufer (cited in Yehuda, Southwick, and Giller, 1992)	atrocities	6	—	.70 (Mississippi Scale); .39 (Figley PTSD Scale)
Combat Exposure Index	Janes, Goldberg, Eisen, and True (1991)	guerrilla warfare	7	.84	—
Combat Exposure Scale	Keane et al. (1989)	traditional combat experiences	7	.85	.43 (Mississippi Scale)
Deployment Risk and Resiliency Inventory	King, King, and Vogt (2003)	10 different deployment/ war-zone factors	201[a]	.82–.94	.12–.52[b] (PTSD Checklist)
Graves Registration Duty Scale	Sutker, Uddo, Brailey, Vasterling, and Errera (1994)	handling human remains	24	.88	.27 (Number of SCID Criterion B symptoms)
Military Stress Scale	Watson, Kucala, Manifold, Vassar, and Juba (1988)	guerrilla warfare	6	—	.57 (PTSD Interview)
Sexual Experiences Questionnaire —DoD	Fitzgerald, Magley, Drasgow, and Waldo (1999)	sexual harassment and assault	22	.93–.94	—
VESI—Specific Stressor Subscale	Wilson and Krause (1980)	combat stress, environmental stress	46	.87–.95	.23–.57 (combat scale with symptom clusters); .25–.47 (environment scale with symptom clusters)

(continued)

TABLE 10.1. *(continued)*

Scale name	Authors	Type of exposure measured	Number of items	Alpha	Strength of the relationship with measures of PTSD
War Events Scale	Unger, Gould, and Babich (1998)	atrocities	84	.92–.95	—
War Zone Stress Index	King, King, Gudanowski, and Vreven (1995)	traditional combat experience; perceived threat; atrocities; malevolent environment	72	.83–.94	—

Note. —indicates not available.
[a] although individual factor measures may be administered separately.
[b] some correlations are in the negative direction, as would be predicted.

When assessing war-zone-related exposure to potentially traumatic events, another domain to consider is the many unpleasant general factors associated with service in a war zone (e.g., bad environmental conditions, adverse climate, problems with hygiene, lack of sleep, food and water deprivation, harassment on homecoming, etc.). In the 100-item NVVRS stressor measure (Kulka et al., 1990), several items assessed malevolent conditions related to deprivation and feeling removed from the world in addition to combat, grotesque death, and abusive violence (Schlenger et al., 1992). Accordingly, a 72-item measure of combat exposure, the War Zone Stress Index, was derived from the NVVRS stressor items that assessed perceived threat and malevolent environment in addition to traditional combat and exposure to atrocities (King, King, Gudanowski, & Vreven, 1995). Enduring such adversity was found to be a significant predictor of PTSD among male and female Vietnam veterans (King et al., 1995).

Similarly, Wilson and Krause (1980) designed a 46-item Specific Stressor in Vietnam subscale in the Vietnam Era Stress Inventory (VESI) that included many items regarding exposure to ongoing harsh daily circumstances. Despite the breadth and clinical acumen reflected in this scale, only three studies have examined its psychometric properties, and each was based on a modification of the measure (Green et al., 1990; McFall, Smith, Mackay, & Tarver, 1990; McFall, Smith, Roszell, Tarver, & Malais, 1990; Wilson, 1989).

In the past decade the experience of sexual harassment and sexual assault in the military has received considerable attention. Unfortunately, this type of victimization is quite common among those in the military, with high rates of victimization for both male and female personnel. The largest investigation of sexual trauma during military service, conducted by the Department of Defense (DoD) in 1995, reported annual rates for sexual harassment of 78% among women and 38% among men (43% overall) and rates for attempted or completed sexual assault of 6% for women and 1% for men (2% overall; Bastian, Lancaster, & Reyst, 1996). Sexual trauma in the military does not occur only during training or peacetime, and, in fact, the stress of war may be associated with increases in rates of sexual harassment and assault. Research with female Operation Desert Storm military personnel established that rates of sexual assault (7%), physical sexual harassment (33%), and verbal sexual harassment (66%) were higher than those typically found in peacetime military samples (Wolfe et al., 1998). The Sexual Experiences Questionnaire—DoD (Fitzgerald, Magley, Drasgow, & Waldo, 1999) is a military-specific version of the most widely used measure of sexual harassment. This instrument is the first measure of sexual harassment designed to meet traditional standards of reliability and validity. It is sensitive to the occurrence of sexual harassment and has been found to predict important psychological and organizational outcomes (Fitzgerald, Swan, & Magley, 1997). In addition, Wolfe, Brown, Furey, and Levin (1993) developed the Wartime Stressor Scale for Women to assess the social and environmental context of war-zone exposure specifically for women soldiers, including questions about sexual discrimination as well as sexual assault.

One recently developed measure, the Deployment Risk and Resilience Inventory (King, King, & Vogt, 2003), combines the assessment of traditional combat experiences with the assessment of a range of potentially traumatric war-zone and deployment experiences that occur outside of the realm of traditional combat. The 201-item inventory combines 14 measures that assess risk and resilience factors associated with possible militatry deployment stress reactions including two predeployment/prewar factors, 10 deployment/war-zone factors, and two postdeployment/postwar factors. The deployment/war-zone factors assessed are "sense of preparedness," "difficult living and working environment," "concerns about life and family disruptions," "deployment social support," "sexual harassment," "general harassment," "perceived threat," "combat experiences," "exposure to the aftermath of battle" and "self-reports of nuclear, biological, or chemical exposures." Any of the individual factor measures may be administered separately and the wording of all items is appropriate for contemporary military deployments. Initial psychometric evidence for this inventory is strong, suggesting that it holds great promise for reliably assessing a range of military-related potential traumatic events (King, King, Vogt, Knight, & Samper, 2004).

With the advent of DSM-IV (American Psychiatric Association, 1994), exposure to a traumatic event was defined both in terms of objective and subjective criteria. Criterion A of the PTSD diagnostic critieria specifies that a traumatic event must involve actual or threatened injury to oneself or others (criterion A1) and must engender concomitant feelings of fear, helplessness, or horror (criterion A2). Unfortunately, not one of the measures of military-related trauma exposure reviewed here includes assessment of the three specified emotional response domains indicated in criterion A2. However, two extensive structured interviews that assess lifetime exposure to all potentially traumatic events, including military-related experiences—the Potential Stressful Events Interview (Falsetti, Resnick, Kilpatrick, & Freedy, 1994; Resnick, Falsetti, Kilpatrick, & Freedy, 1996), and the Evaluation of Lifetime Stressors (Krinsley et al., 1994; Corcoran, Green, Goodman, & Krinsley, 2000)—include assessments of fear, helplessness, and horror. Similarly, many checklist measures of lifetime trauma exposure, including the widely used 24-item Traumatic Life Events Questionnaire (Kubany et al., 2000) assess emotional responses to a range of potentially traumatic events, including exposure to a war zone or combat.

Evaluation of PTSD Symptoms among Military Personnel

Structured Clinical Interviews

Several structured diagnostic interviews were developed for the assessment of PTSD as modules of comprehensive diagnostic tools or as independent PTSD measures. Modules offer expediency in diagnosis but have typically yielded only dichotomous symptom ratings. Interviews focused solely on PTSD diagnostic criteria often require more time investment, but many yield evaluation of symptoms on a continuum. We briefly present examples of each type of interview format that can be used to diagnose PTSD among military personnel.

PTSD modules are available in the Diagnostic Interview Schedule—IV (DIS-IV; Robins, Cottler, Bucholz, & Compton, 1997), the Structured Clinical Interview for DSM-IV (SCID; First, Spitzer, Williams, & Gibbon, 1997), and the Anxiety Disorders Interview Schedule—IV (ADIS-IV; Blanchard, Gerardi, Kolb, & Barlow, 1986; Di Nardo, Brown, & Barlow, 1994). Of all these measures, the SCID has demonstrated high interrater reliability and is strongly correlated to other measures of PTSD.

PTSD structured interviews used with veterans include the Clinician-Administered PTSD Scale (CAPS; Blake et al., 1990; Blake et al., 1995; Weathers, Keane, & Davidson, 2001), the PTSD Interview (PTSD-I; Watson, Juba, Manifold, Kucala, & Anderson, 1991), and the Structured Interview for PTSD (SI-PTSD; Davidson, Smith, & Kudler, 1989; Davidson, Malik, & Travers, 1997). Although all these measures performed well, the CAPS is noteworthy for the thorough analysis of its psychometric utility; its strengths include good psychometrics (e.g., alpha coefficient = .94; sensitivity = .84; specificity = .95; kappa coefficient = .78), clear behavioral anchors, a time frame concordant with that of DSM diagnostic criteria, and separate frequency and intensity ratings.

Self-Report Measures

Self-report checklists that provide information about PTSD symptomatology can be time- and cost-efficient tools in the multimethod assessment process. They can be combined to maximize efficiency, specificity, or sensitivity of the assessment battery. Many excellent self-report questionnaires are available to assess military-related PTSD; some solely assess diagnostic criteria, some correspond to the diagnostic criteria and their associated features, and other measures broadly sample the content of the disorder. We briefly review the measures that are commonly used in assessments of military personnel.

Several short scales have been developed that assess the 17 diagnostic symptoms of PTSD. Not surprisingly, they all have relatively comparable psychometric qualities, particularly internal consistency. The PTSD Checklist (PCL; Weathers, Litz, Herman, Huska, & Keane, 1993; Blanchard, Jones-Alexander, Buckley, & Forneris, 1996) has good sensitivity (.82) and specificity (.83) and is positively correlated with standard measures of PTSD (Mississippi Scale; $r = .93$; MMPI-2 PK Scale, $r = .77$; Impact of Event Scale, $r = .90$). The current version has excellent internal consistency (Cronbach alpha coefficient = .86), excellent specificity (.94 for both current and past PTSD), but weak sensitivity (current PTSD = .48, past PTSD = .48). The Purdue Post-Traumatic Stress Scale—Revised (PPTSD-R; Lauterbach & Vrana, 1996) is available in both military and civilian versions and has demonstrated good psychometric properties. However, the most recent version has yet to be validated with military populations.

Several validated self-report instruments exist that include PTSD symptoms and diagnosis and commonly associated features of the disorder. The Self-Rating Inventory for PTSD (SIP; Hovens, Bramsen, & van der Ploeg, 2002; Hovens et al., 1993; Hovens et al., 1994) consists of 22 items and was originally designed for use with Dutch World War II resistance fighters. It has extensive psychometric data and is available in both English and Dutch. The SIP includes trauma-related symptoms such as those classified under the proposed "diagnosis of extreme stress, not otherwise specified" classification (Herman, 1993). When compared with the CAPS as gold standard, the PTSD subscale of the SIP possesses excellent sensitivity (.92) and moderate specificity (.61) within a sample of civilian psychiatric outpatients and Dutch resistance fighters. The 43-item Los Angeles Symptom Checklist (LASC; King, King, Leskin, & Foy, 1995) also appears to be a psychometrically sound measure of PTSD symptoms among Vietnam veterans (alpha coefficient .91 for 17-item index and .94 for full index; test–retest reliability = .94 for the 17-item index and .90 for full index), although specificity and sensitivity data from military samples are still needed.

Several measures perform quite well in predicting PTSD diagnostic status that are not based directly on DSM diagnostic criteria. In fact, two of the primary self-report measures in the NVVRS, the Keane PTSD Scale of the MMPI (PK scale; Keane, Malloy, & Fairbank, 1984) and the Mississippi Scale for

Combat-Related PTSD (Keane, Caddell, & Taylor, 1988) were designed to measure broadly the construct of PTSD. The 49-item MMPI PK scale and the 46-item MMPI-2 PK have moderate or better psychometric performance, although the sensitivity and specificity of the PK scales have varied from study to study (e.g., Graham, 1993; Keane et al., 1984; Lyons & Keane, 1992; Query, Megran, & McDonald, 1986; Watson, 1990). In studies in which the diagnostic criterion is strongest (e.g., SCID or CAPS), the PK's performance is very good. When more questionable diagnostic criteria are employed (e.g., chart diagnosis), the PK has had more modest success. In addition, the MMPI-2 PK scale works as well when it is applied as a separate measure as it does when embedded within the full MMPI (Graham, 1993; Herman, Weathers, Litz, & Keane, 1996; Litz et al., 1991; Lyons & Scotti, 1994).

The 35-item Mississippi Scale for Combat-Related PTSD (Keane et al., 1988) is one of the most widely used PTSD measures among veteran populations (e.g., Kulka et al., 1990; McFall, Smith, Mackay, & Tarver, 1990; Perconte et al., 1993) and is available in numerous languages (e.g., Dutch, Spanish). Three abbreviated versions of the scale also show promising correlations (.90–.96) with the original scale (Fontana & Rosenheck, 1994; Hyer, Davis, Boudewyns, & Woods, 1991; Wolfe, Keane, Kaloupek, Mora, & Wine, 1993).

The 15-item Impact of Event Scale (IES; Horowitz, Wilner, & Alvarez, 1979; Zilberg, Weiss, & Horowitz, 1982; Weiss & Marmar, 1997), also used in the NVVRS preliminary validation trial (Kulka et al., 1991), was found to have less useful diagnostic utility than either the PK or Mississippi Scale, but nonetheless it performed as a good indicator of PTSD status (sensitivity = .92; specificity = .62; correct classification = 81.6%). The IES has been translated widely and used with many different national military forces (e.g., Kulka et al., 1990; Schwarzwald, Solomon, Weisenberg, & Mikulincer, 1987). Recent additions to the IES (i.e., IES—Revised; Weiss & Marmar, 1997) included the items associated with increased arousal and yield a more complete assessment of the PTSD diagnostic criteria.

Weathers and his colleagues (Weathers, Litz, Keane, Herman, Steinberg, Huska, & Kraemer, 1996) derived a 25-item War-Zone-Related PTSD subscale (WZ-PTSD) that is embedded in the Symptom Checklist 90—Revised (SCL-90-R; Derogatis, 1977). In two different samples, this scale demonstrated that the WZ-PTSD measure clearly outperforms the SCL-90-R Global Severity Index in identifying cases of PTSD.

Psychophysiological Assessment

Psychophysiological assessment can provide unique information on the extent of autonomic hyperarousal and startle responses in PTSD (Orr & Roth, 2000). In general, combat veterans with PTSD demonstrate significantly more psychophysiological reactivity to combat stimuli than do comparison groups, such as nonveterans with psychiatric disorders and combat veterans without psychiatric disorders (Keane et al., 1998; Prins, Kaloupek, & Keane, 1995). However, the specificity of psychophysiological assessment typically exceeds its sensitivity. A psychophysiological assessment of PTSD usually involves presenting an individual with standardized stimuli (e.g., combat photos, noises, odors) or personalized cues of traumatic life events (e.g., taped scripts of their traumatic experiences). Psychophysiological indices that can be assessed include heart rate, blood pressure, muscle tension, skin conductance level and response, and peripheral temperature (e.g., Blanchard, Kolb, Pallmeyer, & Gerardi, 1982; Orr et al., 1990; Pitman, Orr, Forgue, de Jong, & Claiborn, 1987; Shalev, Orr, & Pitman, 1992, 1993). Again, because no one psychophysiological index is error free, convergent measures of psychophysiology are recommended. Although psychophysiological assessment once required elaborate and expensive laboratory equipment, portable systems have made this technique more feasible than ever before. Orr, Metzger, Miller, and Kaloupek (Chapter 11, this volume) provide a more thorough discussion of the findings from studies of the psychophysiological assessment of PTSD. Findings in male and female veteran populations demonstrate the usefulness of this approach across genders (Peirce, Newton, Buckley, & Keane, 2002).

Interpretation of the Components of Multimodal Assessment

The ideal battery for the assessment of military-related PTSD incorporates data derived from the multiple methods described here. However, inconsistency across these domains is common in assessment and may result either from measurement artifacts or as manifestations of varying presentations of the disorder. Distinguishing noise from signal among these multiple measures is a complex task that relies on expertise in both clinical and empirical domains. Despite the wealth of psychometric data available regarding the performance of individual instruments, few studies are available that examine the relative contributions of particular instruments within a battery to the overall prediction of PTSD status. Two distinct strategies have evolved over time. In the NVVRS, a statistical algorithm was designed to approximate the process of clinical decision making and was used to reconcile cases in which disagreements occurred among various PTSD indicators (Kulka et al., 1991; Schlenger et al., 1992). This approach may be most useful in case determination for research and may provide data to inform clinical practice. Nonetheless, clinical judgment and expertise is also needed to interpret the qualitative contributions of particular measures and the manner in which individuals may minimize or distort their experiences. Thus a fundamental approach to interpretation incorporates a combination of good clinical skill and empirical knowledge about the relative psychometric qualities of each indicator. To facilitate the interpretation of multimodal data, Keane and his colleagues (1987) suggested the use of consensus among clinical team members who represent expertise in different arenas. This approach ensures that all data are considered, that bias is minimized, and that empirical and psychometric concerns are appropriately evaluated so that the most accurate interpretation of the data can be attained.

NEW CHALLENGES TO MEASURING MILITARY-RELATED PTSD

New Issues in Assessment of Military Trauma Exposure

In the current geopolitical climate, the types of missions in which military personnel will participate will be markedly different from the traditional conflicts of the past. In the coming years, it is likely that many of the more significant efforts of the U.S. Armed Forces will focus on multilateral peacekeeping, humanitarian relief, and peace enforcement operations with the goal of confronting regional instabilities that threaten world interests (Henshaw, 1993). Evidence of this type of military "humanitarianism" can be seen in recent missions, including "Operation Provide Comfort" in Kurdistan, the goal of which was to supply relief to refugees; "Operation Sea Angel" in Bangladesh, in which forces provided relief to victims of a flood; and "Operation Restore Hope," the purpose of which was to provide humanitarian aid and peacekeeping in Somalia (Moskos & Burk, 1994). Data on the psychological adjustment of participants in the peace enforcement mission in Somalia suggest that PTSD can develop as a result of the military-related stressors involved with this type of duty (Orsillo et al., 1994). In addition, recent military operations with a more traditional combat focus also provide exposure to a unique set of potentially traumatic events. For example, veterans of Operation Desert Storm and Operation Iraqi Freedom were confronted with the fear of weapons of mass destruction, including biological and chemical weapons (Norwood, Holloway, & Ursano, 2001; Knudson, 2001).

Although existing measures of military-related PTSD will most likely be appropriate for assessing symptom presentation, novel approaches to measuring exposure to potentially traumatic events must be developed to reflect the unique stressors that characterize these types of missions. Many factors suggest that, as the issues surrounding military missions change, so too does the direction mental health professionals need to take in assessing exposure to military-related traumatic events.

For instance, one challenge inherent in the assessment of trauma exposure among personnel engaged in these new military operations is the diverse nature and character of the missions. The actual role of participants in these experiences may vary widely. On the one extreme are conventional observer missions, in which forces serve as impartial observers of a truce between two or more formerly warring parties (Henshaw, 1993). In this situation, the goal of the mission is usually short term and quite clear, and the presence of troops is supported by all parties. However, modern military operations can range in levels of intervention to include missions that require a variety of activities that could potentially result in more direct exposure to potentially traumatic events, including the delivery of humanitarian assistance to starving people, disarmament of or preventative peacekeeping between potentially hostile forces, and activities involving conventional military capabilities (Eyre, Segal, & Segal, 1993; Henshaw, 1993) such as in Operation Enduring Freedom in Afghanistan or Operation Iraqi Freedom.

As mentioned, a multidimensional approach to the measurement of military-stressor exposure includes assessment of the general malevolence of the environment and the individual's subjective emotional response to traumatic events, in addition to an assessment of their participation in a wide range of military activities. Anecdotal reports from individuals who have served in peacemaking and peacekeeping operations suggest that a range of environmental stressors are often present (Grinfeld, 1993; Wilkinson, 1994). Findings from a preliminary survey of individuals serving in Somalia support the notion that these separate components of exposure are independently associated with the development of PTSD among peace enforcement participants (Orsillo et al., 1994). Thus it is important to consider these dimensions in the measurement of exposure within the new military missions as well.

Preliminary accounts also imply a wide range of subjective emotional responses among individuals who take part in these new types of military operations. Participants are often required to maintain the difficult balance of power with restraint in situations that could range in political climate from mildly confusing and disorganized to seriously and dangerously chaotic (Henshaw, 1993). Thus peacekeepers may feel overwhelmed with the boredom, isolation, and cultural deprivation that often accompanies the "observer" as compared to "intervener" role of their duties (Harris, Rothberg, Segal, & Segal, 1993), or they may become frustrated with the relatively inactive role they play in the peace process (Mortensen, 1990). Military personnel may also become disillusioned with their duties, as their role in the mission will not always result in an objectively defined success. Although the problems defined by the mission may be amenable to some degree of change, in many cases they may not always be resolvable (Henshaw, 1993).

Given the constantly evolving nature of modern military operations, multidimensional exposure scales may need to be tailored on a case-by-case basis to capture the full range of events included in each new military mission. In the next section, we delineate the steps one can take to develop a clinically sensitive measure of exposure that can be used in this rapidly changing military environment.

Suggestions for the Development of Military Stress Exposure Scales

The first step an assessor must take in developing a measure of exposure is initial item selection (content validity). Items for a test are most often generated and chosen on the basis of their face validity in relation to a theoretical understanding of the concept to be measured (Nunally, 1973). This pool of initial items can be developed in several ways. If one does not have direct contact with participants in the mission, there are at least two alternative methods of obtaining content information. One approach is to survey a panel of experts in the field of military-related PTSD who can use their clinical expertise in the determination of appropriate items for an exposure scale. Another option is to gather descriptive information presented in media accounts of anecdotal reports by participants on the mission. Although these approaches can result in the development of face-valid items, the best manner in which to collect content information is to directly sample participants.

Information for item development can be directly collected from participants in many ways. One approach is to construct a scale based on the techniques described here, and then to derive feedback regarding the items from individuals who have served, or who are currently serving, in the mission. Another method involves incorporating descriptive data obtained through clinical interviewing into the development of items. Although both these approaches can be easily implemented, a potentially more effective and rigorous technique that can be used to collect this type of qualitative data for item generation is the use of focus group interviewing.

Focus group interviewing is a technique by which information about a novel content area can be quickly and inexpensively obtained by observing participants interact with one another regarding a topic provided by the leader (Morgan, 1988). To use this methodology, an interested researcher would construct a focus group of participants who have been deployed to serve in the mission. Through directed group discussions about the nature of their duty, the unique stressors and conflicts that participants face should become readily apparent and can be incorporated into a measure of exposure. The selection of focus group members will inevitably vary according to the purpose of the assessment, but the group should typically include and consider the experiences of a wide variety of participants. For instance, different gender or ethnic groups may encounter very different stressors in the military, so it may be important to create groups that accurately reflect the demographics of the sample of interest. In addition, including participants of various branches and ranks of the military in a group or running subgroups of special individuals (e.g., a "front line" Marine focus group) may be fruitful. For instance, it has been theorized that members of elite combat units who are self-selected and subsequently trained and socialized in traditional combat activities may have a more difficult adjustment to the types of duties required in peacemaking (Segal & Segal, 1993). Finally, sampling groups widely across the time period of the mission will help to elicit data regarding the changing nature of the potentially traumatic events.

In addition to content, the method employed to format the questions that compose the scale needs attention (Golden, Sawicki, & Franzen, 1984). Items can either be open ended, allowing respondents to freely answer a question including any information they feel is relevant and pertinent, or restricted, such as a forced-choice (true/false) or multiple-choice item. Open-ended questions allow more personalized responses and may be helpful in providing detailed information about experiences in the war zone. However, these items are difficult to quantify and score. On the other hand, restricted items, although more standardized, are easier to interpret in a group or normative context. An assessment approach that includes both types of items and thus combines nomothetic and ideographic methodologies may be the most flexible in allowing clinicians to better understand exposure experiences.

Several surveys developed at the National Center for PTSD at the VA Boston Healthcare System successfully incorporated many of these methodological nuances into instrument development. For instance, Wolfe, Brown, and Kelley (1993) designed a survey to investigate the multidimensional components of exposure among individuals who served in Operation Desert Storm. Items were generated both from previously validated exposure measures and from feedback from Operation Desert Storm veterans, and the item format allowed for both fixed and open-ended responses.

In addition, Litz and his colleagues (Litz, Moscowitz, Friedman, & Ehlich, 1995) designed a survey to evaluate the long-term psychosocial sequelae that stem from participation in the peacekeeping mission in Somalia during Operation Restore Hope (ORH; later Operation Continue Hope, OCH). Items were generated based on anecdotal descriptions of events experienced by military personnel who were deployed to Somalia and qualitative information about the nature of the mission derived from debriefing groups. This survey also incorporated some open-ended questions to allow participants to report unique aspects of the stressors they faced. Each of these efforts serve as models for the future development of psychometrically sound measures of exposure.

Cultural Considerations in the Assessment of Military-Related PTSD

Another challenge to the assessment of military-related PTSD is the need to develop instruments that are culturally sensitive. Concurrent with changes in the function of the military, the demographic composition of the U.S. Armed Forces has also dramatically shifted. Over the past 20 years the proportion of women in the armed forces has grown from less than 2% to more than 15%, and the percentage of African Americans serving has doubled from 10 to 20% (Office of the Assistant Secretary of Defense, 2003). This change in the demographics of the armed forces necessitates that cultural and gender-based considerations be taken into account in stress assessment.

There are several clinical descriptions of responses to traumatic events that underscore the importance of culturally sensitive instrumentation. Racial conflicts, discrimination, bicultural struggles, and identification with the "enemy" have all been cited as stressors commonly experienced by minority veterans (Kraft, 1993; Loo, 1994; Parson, 1985). As well, differences in the level of exposure to war-zone related stressors and the severity of PTSD symptoms experienced between ethnic minority and Caucasian veterans have been empirically documented (e.g., Frueh, Brady, & Arellano, 1998; Green, Grace,

Lindy, & Leonard, 1990; Kulka et al., 1990). Although it is difficult to meaningfully interpret these group differences, some investigators have begun to identify possible mediators of the effect of ethnicity on the development of PTSD, such as discrimination and alienation (e.g., Ruef, Litz, & Schlenger, 2000). Unfortunately, much of the research in this area is limited by the use of assessment instruments that may not be optimal for all cultures present in the United States (Marsella, Friedman, & Spain, 1993).

Guidelines to Ethnocultural Assessment

In an effort to improve the research on ethnocultural aspects of psychopathology, several authors compiled guidelines for culturally sensitive assessment. First, an assessor should be clinically sensitive to ethnic issues and aware of his or her own prejudices and biases (Penk & Allen, 1991; Westermeyer, 1985). Second, researchers ought to go beyond comparing categories of ethnic groups as the sole means of understanding ethnocultural variability (Marsella et al., 1993: Penk & Allen, 1991). Moreover, the level of an individual's acculturation to the dominant culture must be assessed rather than assumed by their ethnic identity. Finally, it is key that instrumentation be developed that maintains equivalence across several different cultural groups.

Dimensions of Cultural Equivalence

Cultural equivalence in assessment is typically established within several different domains: content, semantic, technical, normative, and conceptual equivalence (Flaherty et al., 1988; Lonner, 1985; Marsella & Kameoka, 1988). First, it is important to ensure that the content being measured is relevant to the phenomena of each culture being studied. Next, semantic equivalence should be obtained to ensure, through translation and back translation by bilingual experts, that the meaning of each item is the same in each culture. Measures are determined to be technically equivalent when the method of assessment (e.g., self-report, interview) results in comparable comfort and familiarity between cultures. For instance, it is important to be aware, in developing a culturally sensitive assessment instrument, that a Likert-type scale may be meaningless to some ethnic groups (Flaskerud, 1988; Kinzie et al., 1982). Normative equivalence refers to the importance of using local norms to interpret findings. In many cases, because of cultural differences in definitions of problematic behavior, it may be inappropriate to use the criterion for caseness developed in one culture to determine the boundaries of pathology in another. Finally, it is crucial that conceptual equivalence be determined. This ensures that the instrument is measuring the same theoretical construct, such as shame or dependency, in each culture. Keane, Kaloupek, and Weathers (1996) provide a more thorough description of the process necessary for developing instruments necessary to appropriately and equivalently assess trauma across cultural and ethnic groups.

SUMMARY

Assessing traumatic life experiences and PTSD among veterans of military service is conceptually and practically challenging. Military service varies from one action to the next, and in the current era clinicians and researchers will need to modify and alter their approaches to assessment in accordance with the particular details of the military activities involved. Moreover, the demographic composition of the forces is continuing to vary, and instruments need to be developed that are sensitive to the cultural nuances of the cultures within our population. Efforts to ensure that women and ethnic minority populations are represented in all phases of instrument development are important to the ultimate usefulness of the assessment instruments, whether they be primarily for use in the clinic, in the field, or in laboratory research studies.

Today many instruments are available to assess military-related trauma exposure and associated PTSD. These instruments are responsible for the great expansion of our knowledge since 1980 on the psychological, social, and physical effects of traumatic events. Our ability to appropriately assess both trauma exposure and PTSD has led to widespread recognition and acceptance of the central role that these phenomena play in the lives of individuals in our society. Future research on military trauma exposure and PTSD will continue to figure prominently in the development of a humane and sensible public policy toward individuals who serve in the military. The development of assessment instruments and methods that are reliable and valid will assist immensely in that process.

REFERENCES

American Psychiatric Association. (1980). *Diagnostic and statistical manual of mental disorders.* Washington, DC: Author.

American Psychiatric Association. (1994). *Diagnostic and statistical manual of mental disorders* (4th ed.). Washington, DC: Author.

Bastian, L. D., Lancaster, A. R., & Reyst, H. E. (1996). *Department of Defense 1995 sexual harassment survey.* Arlington, VA: Defense Manpower Data Center.

Blake, D. D., Weathers, F. W., Nagy, L. N., Kaloupek, D. G., Gusman, F. D., Charney, D. S., & Keane, T. M. (1995). The development of a clinician-administered PTSD scale. *Journal of Traumatic Stress, 8,* 75–90.

Blake, D. D., Weathers, F. W., Nagy, L. N., Kaloupek, D. G., Klauminser, G., Charney, D. S., & Keane, T. M. (1990). A clinician rating scale for assessing current and lifetime PTSD: The CAPS-1, *Behavior Therapist, 18,* 187–188.

Blanchard, E. B., Gerardi, R. J., Kolb, L. C., & Barlow, D. H. (1986). The utility of the Anxiety Disorders Interview Schedule in the diagnosis of posttraumatic stress disorder (PTSD) in Vietnam veterans. *Behavior Research Therapy, 24,* 577–580.

Blanchard, E. B., Jones-Alexander, J., Buckley, T. C., & Forneris, C. A. (1996). Psychometric properties of the PTSD Checklist (PCL). *Behaviour Research and Therapy, 34,* 669–673.

Blanchard, E. B., Kolb, L. C, Pallmeyer, T. P., & Gerardi, R. (1982). A psychophysiological study of posttraumatic stress disorder in Vietnam veterans. *Psychiatric Quarterly*, *34*, 220–229.

Corcoran, C. B., Green, B. L., Goodman, B. L., & Krinsley, K. (2000). Conceptual and methodological issues in trauma history of assessment. In R. Shalev, R. Yehuda, & A. McFarlane (Eds.), *International handbook of human response to trauma* (pp. 223–232). New York: Kluwer/Plenum.

Davidson, J. R. T., Malik, M. A., & Travers, J. (1997). Structured Interview for PTSD (SIP): Psychometric validation for DSM-IV criteria. *Depression and Anxiety*, *5*, 127–129.

Davidson, J. R. T., Smith, R. D., & Kudler, H. S. (1989). Validity and reliability of the DSM-III criteria for posttraumatic stress disorder: Experience with a structured interview. *Journal of Nervous and Mental Disease*, *177*, 336–341.

Derogatis, L. R. (1977). *The SCL-90 manual: 1. Scoring, administration and procedures for the SCL-90*. Baltimore: John Hopkins University School of Medicine, Clinical Psychometrics Unit.

Di Nardo, P. A., Brown, T. A., & Barlow, D. H. (1994). *Anxiety Disorders Interview Schedule for DSM–IV: Lifetime Version (ADIS-IV-L)*. San Antonio, TX: Psychological Corporation.

Egendorf, A., Kadushin, C., Laufer, R. S., Rothbart, G., & Sloan, L. (1981). *Legacies of Vietnam: Comparative adjustment of veterans and their peers* (Vol. 3). New York: Center for Policy Research.

Eyre, D. P., Segal, D. R., & Segal, M. W. (1993). The social construction of peacekeeping. In D. R. Segal & M. W. Segal (Eds.), *Peacekeepers and their wives: American participation in the multinational force and observers* (pp. 42–55). Westport, CT: Greenwood Press.

Falsetti, S. A., Resnick, H. S., Kilpatrick, D. G., & Freedy, J. R. (1994). A review of the Potential Stressful Events Interview: A comprehensive assessment instrument of high and low magnitude stressors. *Behavior Therapist*, *17*, 66–67.

First, M. B., Spitzer, R. L., Williams, J. B. W., & Gibbon, M. (1997). *Structured Clinical Interview for DSM-IV (SCID)*. Washington, DC: American Psychiatric Association.

Fitzgerald, L. F., Magley, V. J., Drasgow, F., & Waldo, C. R. (1999). Measuring sexual harassment in the military: The SEQ-DoD. *Military Psychology*, *11*, 243–263.

Fitzgerald, L. F., Swan, S., & Magley, V. J. (1997). But was it really sexual harassment?: Legal, behavioral, and psychological definitions of the workplace victimization of women. In W. O'Donohue (Ed.), *Sexual harassment: Theory, research and treatment* (pp. 5–28). Boston: Allyn & Bacon.

Flaherty, J. A., Gaviria, F. M., Pathak, D., Mitchell, T., Wintrob, R., Richman, J. A., & Birz, S. (1988). Developing instruments for cross-cultural psychiatric research. *Journal of Nervous and Mental Disease*, *176*, 257–263.

Flaskerud, J. H. (1988). Is the Likert scale format culturally biased? *Nursing Research*, *37*, 185–186.

Fontana, A., & Rosenheck, R. (1994). A short form of the Mississippi Scale for measuring change in combat-related PTSD. *Journal of Traumatic Stress*, *7*, 407–414.

Frueh, B. C., Brady, K. L., & Arellano, M. A. (1998). Racial differences in combat-related PTSD: Empirical findings and conceptual issues. *Clinical Psychology Review*, 18, 287–305.

Golden, C. J., Sawicki, R. S., & Franzen, M. D. (1984). Test construction. In G.

Goldstein & M. Hersen (Eds.), *Handbook of psychological assessment* (pp. 19–37). New York: Pergamon Press.

Grady, D. A., Woolfolk, R. L., & Budney, A. J. (1989). Dimensions of war-zone stress: An empirical analysis. *Journal of Nervous and Mental Disease*, *177*, 347–350.

Graham, J. R. (1993). *MMPI-2: Assessing personality and psychopathology*. New York: Oxford University Press.

Green, B. L. (1993). Identifying survivors at risk: Trauma and stressors across events. In J. P. Wilson & B. Raphael (Eds.), *International handbook of traumatic stress syndromes* (pp. 135–144). New York: Plenum Press.

Green, B. L., Grace, M. C., Lindy, J. D., & Gleser, G. G. (1990). War stressors and symptom persistence in posttraumatic stress disorder. *Journal of Anxiety Disorders*, *4*, 31–39.

Green, B. L., Grace, M. C., Lindy, J. D., & Leonard, A. C. (1990). Race differences in response to combat stress. *Journal of Traumatic Stress*, *3*, 379–393.

Grinfeld, M. J. (1993, February). U.S. troops to the rescue again: Soldiers' mental health now a serious priority for military leadership. *Psychiatric Times*, *1*, 1–6.

Harris, J. J., Rothberg, J. M., Segal, D. R., & Segal, M. W. (1993). Paratroopers in the desert. In D. R. Segal & M. W. Segal (Eds.), *Peacekeepers and their wives: American participation in the multinational force and observers* (pp. 81–94). Westport, CT: Greenwood Press.

Hendrix, C., & Schumm, W. (1990). Reliability and validity of the Abusive Violence Scale. *Psychological Reports*, *66*, 1251–1258.

Henshaw, J. H. (1993). Forces for peacekeeping, peace enforcement and humanitarian missions. In B. M. Blechman, W. J. Durch, D. R. Graham, J. H. Henshaw, P. L. Reed, V. A. Utgoff, & S. A. Wolfe (Eds.), *The American military in the twenty-first century* (pp. 397–430). New York: St. Martins Press.

Herman, D. S., Weathers, F. W., Litz, B. T., & Keane, T. M. (1996). Psychometric properties of the embedded and stand-alone versions of the MMPI-2 Keane PTSD Scale. *Assessment*, *3*, 437–442.

Herman, J. L. (1993). Sequelae of prolonged and repeated trauma: Evidence for a complex posttraumatic stress disorder (DESNOS). In J. R. T. Davidson & E. B. Foa (Eds.), *Posttraumatic stress disorder: DSM-IV and beyond* (pp. 213–228).Washington, DC: American Psychiatric Press.

Horowitz, M. J., Wilner, N. R., & Alvarez, W. (1979). Impact of Event Scale: A measure of subjective distress. *Psychosomatic Medicine*, *41*, 208–218.

Hovens, J. E., Bramsen, I., & van der Ploeg, H. M. (2002). Self-Rating Inventory for Posttraumatic Stress Disorder: Review of the psychometric properties of a new brief Dutch screening instrument. *Perceptual and Motor Skills*, *94*, 996–1008.

Hovens, J. E., Falger, P. R. J., Op den Velde, W., Mweijer, P., de Grown, J. H. M., & van Duijn, H. (1993). A self-rating scale for the assessment of posttraumatic stress disorder in Dutch Resistance veterans of World War II. *Journal of Clinical Psychology*, *49*, 196–203.

Hovens, J. E., van der Ploeg, H. M., Bramsen, I., Klaarenbeek, M. T. A., Schreuder, J. N., & Rivero, V. V. (1994). The development of the Self-Rating Inventory for Posttraumatic Stress Disorder. *Acta Psychiatrica Scandinavica*, *90*, 172–183.

Hyer, L., Davis, H., Boudewyns, P., & Woods, M. G. (1991). A short form of the Mississippi Scale for Combat-Related PTSD. *Journal of Clinical Psychology*, *4*, 510–518.

Janes, G. R., Goldberg, J., Eisen, S. A., & True, W. R. (1991). Reliability and validity of a combat exposure index for Vietnam-era veterans. *Journal of Clinical Psychology*, *47*, 80–86.

Keane, T. M., Caddell, J. M., & Taylor, K. L. (1988). Mississippi Scale for Combat-Related Posttraumatic Stress Disorder: Three studies in reliability and validity. *Journal of Consulting and Clinical Psychology*, *56*, 85–90.

Keane, T. M., Fairbank, J. A., Caddell, J. M., Zimering, R. T., & Bender, M. (1985). A behavioral approach to assessing and treating PTSD in Vietnam veterans. In C. R. Figley (Ed.), *Trauma and its wake* (pp. 257–294). New York: Brunner/Mazel.

Keane, T. M., Fairbank, J. A., Caddell, J. M., Zimering, R. T., Taylor, K. L., & Mora, C. A. (1989). Clinical evaluation of a measure to assess combat exposure. *Psychological Assessment*, *1*, 53–55.

Keane, T. M., Kaloupek, D. G., & Weathers, F. W. (1996). Cross-cultural issues in the assessment of posttraumatic stress disorder. In A. J. Marsella, M. J. Friedman, E. Gerrity, & R. Scurfield (Eds.), *Ethnocultural aspects of posttraumatic stress disorder* (pp. 183–205). Washington DC: American Psychiatric Press.

Keane, T. M., Kolb, L. C., Kaloupek, D. G., Orr, S. P., Blanchard, E. B., Thomas, R. G., et al. (1998). Utility of psychophysiological measurement in the diagnosis of posttraumatic stress disorder: Results from a Department of Veterans Affairs cooperative study. *Journal of Consulting and Clinical Psychology*, *66*(6), 914–923.

Keane, T. M., Malloy, P. F., & Fairbank, J. A. (1984). Empirical development of an MMPI subscale for the assessment of combat-related posttraumatic stress disorder. *Journal of Consulting and Clinical Psychology*, *52*, 888–891.

Keane, T. M., Wolfe, J., & Taylor, K. L. (1987). Posttraumatic stress disorder: Evidence for diagnostic validity and methods of psychological assessment. *Journal of Clinical Psychology*, *43*, 32–43.

King, D. W., King, L. A., Gudanowski, D. M., & Vreven, D. L. (1995). Alternative representation of war zone stressors: Relationships to posttraumatic stress disorder in male and female Vietnam veterans. *Journal of Abnormal Psychology*, *104*, 184–196.

King, D. W., King, L. A., & Vogt, D. S. (2003). *Manual for the Deployment Risk and Resilience Inventory (DRRI): A collection of measures for studying deployment-related experiences in military veterans*. Boston, MA: National Center for PTSD.

King, L. A., King, D. W., Leskin, G., & Foy, D. W. (1995). The Los Angeles Symptom Checklist: A self-report measure of posttraumatic stress disorder. *Assessment*, *2*, 1–17.

King, L., King, D., Vogt, D., Knight, J., & Samper, R. (2004). *Development and psychometric properties of the Deployment Risk and Resilience Inventory*. Manuscript under review.

Kinzie, J. D., Manson, S. M., Vinh, D. T., Tolan, N. T., Anh, B., & Pho, T. N. (1982). Development and validation of a Vietnamese-language depression rating scale. *American Journal of Psychiatry*, *138*, 1276–1281.

Knudson, G. B. (2001). Nuclear, biological, and chemical training in the U.S. Army Reserves: Mitigating psychological consequences of weapons of mass destruction. *Military Medicine*, *166*, 63–65.

Kraft, S. (1993, January 30). Black like me: Troops in Somalia. *Los Angeles Times*, pp. 1, 13.

Krinsley, K., Weathers, F., Vielhauer, M., Newman, E., Walker, E., Young, L., & Kimerling, R. (1994). *Evaluation of Lifetime Stressors Questionnaire and Interview*. Unpublished manuscript.

Kubany, E. S., Haynes, S. N., Leisen, M. B., Owens, J. A., Kaplan, A. S., Watson, S. B., et al. (2000). Development and preliminary validation of a broad-spectrum measure of trauma exposure: The Traumatic Life Events Questionnaire (TLEQ). *Psychological Assessment, 12*, 428–444.

Kulka, R. A., Schlenger, W. E., Fairbank, J. A., Hough, R. L., Jordan, B. K., Marmar, C. R., & Weiss, D. S. (1990). *Trauma and the Vietnam war generation: Report of findings from the National Vietnam Veterans Readjustment Study*. New York: Brunner/Mazel.

Kulka, R. A., Schlenger, W. E., Fairbank, J. A., Jordan, B. K., Hough, R. L., Marmar, C. R., & Weiss, D. S. (1991). Assessment of posttraumatic stress disorder in the community: Prospects and pitfalls from recent studies of Vietnam veterans. *Psychological Assessment, 3*, 547–560.

Laufer, R. S., Gallops, M. S., & Frey-Wouters, E. (1984). War stress and trauma: The Vietnam veteran experience. *Journal of Health and Social Behavior, 25*, 65–85.

Lauterbach, D., & Vrana, S. R. (1996). Three studies on the reliability and validity of a self-report measure of posttraumatic stress disorder. *Assessment, 3*, 17–25.

Litz, B. T., Moscowitz, A., Friedman, M., & Ehlich, P. (1995). *Somalia Peacekeeping Survey*. Unpublished manuscript.

Litz, B. T., Penk, W., Walsh, S., Hyer, L., Blake, D. D., Marx, B., et al. (1991). Similarities and differences between Minnesota Multiphasic Personality Inventory (MMPI) and MMPI-2 applications to the assessment of posttraumatic stress disorder. *Journal of Personality Assessment, 51*, 238–254.

Lonner, W. J. (1985). Issues in testing and assessment in cross-cultural counseling. *Counseling Psvchologist, 13*, 599–614.

Loo, C. M. (1994). Race-related PTSD: The Asian American Vietnam veteran. *Journal of Traumatic Stress, 7*, 637–656.

Lyons, J. A., & Keane, T. M. (1992). Keane PTSD Scale: MMPI and MMPI-2 update. *Journal of Traumatic Stress, 5*, 111–117.

Lyons, J. A., & Scotti, J. R. (1994). Comparability of two administration formats of the Keane Posttraumatic Stress Disorder Scale. *Psychological Assessment*, 6, 209–211.

Marsella, A. J., Friedman, M. J., & Spain, E. H. (1993). Ethnocultural aspects of posttraumatic stress disorder. In J. M. Oldham, M. B. Riba, & A. Tasman (Eds.), *Review of Psychiatry* (Vol. 12, (pp. 157–181). Washington, DC: American Psychiatric Press.

Marsella, A. J., & Kameoka, V. A. (1988). Ethnocultural issues in the assessment of psychopathology. In S. Wetzler (Ed.), *Measuring mental illness: Psychometric assessment for clinicians* (pp. 231–256). Washington, DC: American Psychiatric Press.

McCranie, E. W., & Hyer, L. A. (2000). Posttraumatic stress disorder symptoms in Korean Conflict and World War II combat veterans seeking outpatient treatment. *Journal of Traumatic Stress, 13*(3), 427–439.

McFall, M. E., Smith, D. E., Mackay, P. W., & Tarver, D. J. (1990). Reliability and validity of Mississippi Scale for Combat-Related Posttraumatic Stress Disorder. *Psychological Assessment*, 2, 114–121.

McFall, M. E., Smith, D. E., Roszell, D. K., Tarver, D. J., & Malais, K. L. (1990). Convergent validity of measures of PTSD in Vietnam combat veterans. *American Journal of Psychiatry, 147*, 645–648.

Morgan, D. L. (1988). Focus groups as qualitative research. *Sage university paper series on qualitative research methods* (Vol. 16). Beverly Hills, CA: Sage.

Mortensen, M. S. (1990, August). *The UN peacekeeper: A new type of soldier? Preliminary studies of professional roles in military forces.* Paper presented to the American Sociological Association convention, Washington, DC.

Moskos, C. M., & Burk, J. (1994). The postmodern military. In J. Burk (Ed.), *The military in new times: Adapting armed forces to a turbulent world* (pp. 141–162). Boulder, CO: Westview Press.

Niles, B. L., Newman, E., Erwin, B. A., Fisher, L. M., Kaloupek, D. G., & Keane, T. M. (1998). Stability and fluctuation of Veterans' reports of combat exposure. In L. M. Williams & V. L. Banyard (Eds.), *Trauma and memory* (pp. 311–317). Thousand Oaks, CA: Sage.

Norwood, A. E., Holloway, H. C., & Ursano, R. J. (2001). Psychological effects of biological warfare. *Military Medicine, 166*(12 Suppl.), 27–28.

Nunally, J. (1973). *Psychometric theory.* New York: McGraw-Hill.

Office of the Assistant Secretary of Defense. (2003). *(Force Management Policy): Population representation in the military services, 2001.* Washington, DC: Author.

Orr, S., Claiborn, J. M., Altman, B., Forgue, D. F., de Jong, J. B., Pitman, R. K., & Herz, L. R. (1990). Psychometric profile of PTSD, anxious and healthy Vietnam veterans: Correlations with psychophysiological responses. *Journal of Consulting and Clinical Psychology, 58,* 329–335.

Orr, S. P., & Roth, W. T. (2000). Psychophysiological assessment: Clinical applications for PTSD. *Journal of Affective Disorders, 61,* 225–240.

Orsillo, S. M., Litz, B. T., Goebel, A. E., Friedman, M., Ehlich, P., & Bergman, E. D. (1994, November). *An investigation of the psychological sequelae associated with peacemaking in Somalia.* Paper presented at the annual meeting of the Association for Advancement of Behavior Therapy, San Diego, CA.

Parson, E. R. (1985). The intercultural setting: Encountering black Viet Nam. In S. M. Sonnenberg, A. S. Blank, & J. A. Talbott (Eds.), *The trauma of war: Stress and recovery in Viet Nam veterans* (pp. 359–388). Washington, DC: American Psychiatric Press.

Peirce, J. M., Newton, T. L., Buckley, T. C., & Keane, T. M. (2002). Gender and psychophysiology of PTSD. In R. Kimerling, P. C. Ouimette, & J. Wolfe (Eds.), *Gender and PTSD.* New York: Guilford Press.

Penk, W. E., & Allen, I. M. (1991). Clinical assessment of posttraumatic stress disorder (PTSD) among American minorities who served in Vietnam. *Journal of Traumatic Stress, 4,* 41–66.

Perconte, S., Wilson, A., Pontius, E., Dietrick, A., Kirsch, C., & Sparacino, C. (1993). Unit-based intervention for Gulf War soldiers surviving a SCUD missile attack: Program description and preliminary findings. *Journal of Traumatic Stress, 6,* 225–238.

Pitman, R. K., Orr, S. P., Forgue, D. F., de Jong, J. B., & Claiborn, J. M. (1987). Psychophysiologic assessment of posttraumatic stress disorder imagery in Vietnam combat veterans. *Archives of General Psychiatry, 44,* 970–975.

Prins, A., Kaloupek, D., & Keane, T. M. (1995). Psychophysiological evidence for autonomic arousal and startle in traumatized adult populations. In M. J. Friedman, D. Charney, & A. Deutch (Eds.), *Neurobiological and clinical consequences of stress: From normal adaptation to PTSD* (pp. 291–314). New York: Raven Press.

Query, W. T., Megran, J., & McDonald, G. (1986). Applying posttraumatic stress disorder MMPI subscale to World War II POW veterans. *Journal of Clinical Psychology, 42,* 315–317.

Resnick, H. S., Falsetti, S. A., Kilpatrick, D. G., & Freedy, J. R. (1996). Assessment of rape and other civilian trauma-related posttraumatic stress disorder: Emphasis on assessment of potentially traumatic events. In T. W. Miller (Ed.), *Stressful life events* (pp. 231–266). Madison, WI: International Universities Press.

Robins, L., Cottler, L., Bucholz, K., & Compton, W. (1997). *Diagnostic Interview Schedule for the DSM-IV (DIS-IV)*. St. Louis, MO: Washington University School of Medicine.

Ruef, A. M., Litz, B. T., & Schlenger, W. E. (2000). Hispanic ethnicity and risk for combat-related posttraumatic stress disorder. *Cultural Diversity and Ethnic Minority Psychology*, 6, 235–251.

Schlenger, W. E., Kulka, R. A., Fairbank, J. A., Hough, R. L., Jordan, B. K., Marmar, C. R., & Weiss, D. S. (1992). The prevalence of posttraumatic stress disorder in the Vietnam generation: A multimodal, multisource assessment of psychiatric disorder. *Journal of Traumatic Stress*, *5*, 333–363.

Schnurr, P. P., Friedman, M. J., & Bernardy, N. C. (2002). Research on posttraumatic stress disorder: Epidemiology, pathophysiology, and assessment. *Psychotherapy in Practice*, *58*(8), 877–889,

Schwarzwald, J., Solomon, Z., Weisenberg, M., & Mikulincer, M. (1987). Validation of the Impact of Event Scale for psychological sequelae of combat. *Journal of Consulting and Clinical Psychology*, *55*, 251–256.

Segal, D. R., & Segal, M. W. (1993). Research on soldiers of the Sinai multinational force and observers. In D. R. Segal & M. W. Segal (Eds.), *Peacekeepers and their wives: American participation in the multinational force and observers* (pp. 56–64). Westport, CT: Greenwood Press.

Shalev, A. Y., Orr, S. P., & Pitman, R. K. (1992). Psychophysiologic responses during script-driven imagery as an outcome measure in posttraumatic stress disorder. *Journal of Clinical Psychiatry*, *532*, 324–326.

Shalev, A. Y., Orr, S. P., & Pitman, R. K. (1993). Psychophysiologic assessment of traumatic imagery in Israeli civilian patients with posttraumatic stress disorder. *American Journal of Psychiatry*, *150*, 620–624.

Sutker, P. B., Uddo, M., Brailey, K., Vasterling, J. J., & Errera, P. (1994). Psychopathology in war-zone deployed and nondeployed Operation Desert Storm troops assigned graves registration duties. *Journal of Abnormal Psychology*, *103*, 383–390.

Unger, W. S., Gould, R. A., & Babich, M. (1998). The development of a scale to assess war-time atrocities: The War Events Scale. *Journal of Traumatic Stress*, 11, 375–383.

Watson, C. G. (1990). Psychometric posttraumatic stress disorder techniques: A review. *Psychological Assessment*, 2, 460–469.

Watson, C. G., Juba, M. P., & Anderson, P. E. D. (1989). Validities of five combat scales. *Psychological Assessment*, *1*, 98–102.

Watson, C. G., Juba, M. P., Manifold, V., Kucula, T., & Anderson, P. E. D. (1991). The PTSD interview: Rationale, descriptions, reliability, and concurrent validity of a DSM-III-based technique. *Journal of Clinical Psychology*, *47*, 179–188.

Watson, C. G., Kucula, T., Manifold, V., Vassar, P., & Juba, M. (1988). Differences between posttraumatic stress disorder patients with delayed and undelayed onsets. *Journal of Nervous and Mental Disease*, *176*, 568–572.

Weathers, F. W., Keane, T. M., & Davidson, J. R. T. (2001) The Clinician-Administered PTSD Scale: A review of the first ten years of research. *Depression and Anxiety*, *13*, 132–156.

Weathers, F. W., Keane, T. M., King, L. A., & King, D. W. (1997). Psychometric theory in the development of posttraumatic stress disorder assessment tools. In J. P. Wilson & T. M. Keane (Eds.), *Assessing psychological trauma and PTSD* (pp. 98–135). New York: Guilford Press.

Weathers, F. W., Litz, B. T., Herman, D. S., Huska, J. A., & Keane, T. M. (1993, October). *The PTSD checklist: Reliability, validity, and diagnostic utility.* Paper presented at the annual meeting of the International Society for Traumatic Stress Studies, San Antonio TX.

Weathers, F. W., Litz, B. T., Keane, T. M., Herman, D. S., Steinberg, H. R., Huska, J. A., & Kraemer, H. C. (1996). The utility of the SCL-90-R for the diagnosis of war-zone-related posttraumatic stress disorder. *Journal of Traumatic Stress, 9,* 111–128.

Weiss, D. S., & Marmar, C. R. (1997). The Impact of Event Scale–Revised. In J. P. Wilson & T. M. Keane (Eds.), *Assessing psychological trauma and PTSD* (pp. 399–411). New York: Guilford Press.

Westermeyer, J. (1985). Psychiatric diagnosis across cultural boundaries. *American Journal of Psychiatry, 142,* 798–805.

Wilkinson, T. (1994, October 21). GI suicides in Haiti alert army to the enemy within. *Los Angeles Times,* pp. 1, 8, 9.

Wilson, J. P. (1979). *The forgotten warrior project.* Cincinnati, OH: Disabled American Veterans.

Wilson, J. P. (Ed.) (1989). *Trauma transformation and healing.* New York: Brunner/Mazel.

Wilson, J. P., & Krause, G. E. (1980). *The Vietnam Era Stress Inventory.* Cleveland, OH: Cleveland State University.

Wolfe, J., Brown, P. J., Furey, J., & Levin, K. B. (1993). Development of a War-Time Stressor Scale for women. *Psychological Assessment, 5,* 330–335.

Wolfe, J., Brown, P. J., & Kelley, J. M. (1993). Reassessing war stress: Exposure and the Persian Gulf War. *Journal of Social Issues, 49,* 15–31.

Wolfe, J., Keane, T. M., Kaloupek, D. G., Mora, C. A., & Wine, P. (1993). Patterns of positive readjustment in Vietnam combat veterans. *Journal of Traumatic Stress, 6,* 179–193.

Wolfe, J., Sharkansky, E. J., Read, J., Dawson, R., Martin, J. A., & Ouimette, P. C. (1998). Sexual harassment and assault as predictors of PTSD symptomatology among U.S. Persian Gulf War personnel. *Journal of Interpersonal Violence, 13,* 40–57.

Yehuda, R., Southwick, S. M., & Giller, E. L. (1992). Exposure to atrocities and severity of chronic posttraumatic stress disorder in Vietnam combat veterans. *American Journal of Psychiatry, 149,* 333–336.

Zilberg, N. J., Weiss, D. S., & Horowitz, M. J. (1982). Impact of Event Scale: A cross-validation study and some empirical evidence supporting a conceptual model of stress responses syndromes. *Journal of Consulting and Clinical Psychology, 50,* 407–414.

PART III

Psychobiology

CHAPTER 11

Psychophysiological Assessment of PTSD

SCOTT P. ORR
LINDA J. METZGER
MARK W. MILLER
DANNY G. KALOUPEK

Over the past 20 years, and particularly within the past 10 years, research has provided the foundation for a psychobiological characterization of posttraumatic stress disorder (PTSD). Much of this work has used measures of peripheral autonomic and muscular activity to assess key features of the disorder as specified in the fourth edition of the *Diagnostic and Statistical Manual of Mental Disorders* (DSM-IV; American Psychiatric Association, 1994). More recently, there has been a notable increase in the use of measures of electrophysiological activity, specifically event-related potentials (ERPs), in the study of the disorder. Consistent with DSM criterion B5, the resulting findings have provided a relatively consistent picture of differential (e.g., greater) peripheral and central psychophysiological reactivity to stimuli related to an index traumatic event in individuals with PTSD that is not shown by individuals who experienced similar events but did not develop PTSD. Similarly, evidence from an array of psychophysiological studies supports the DSM-IV criterion D features of increased irritability or anger (D2), difficulty concentrating (D3), hypervigilance (D4), and exaggerated startle response (D5).

Research using psychophysiological measures also has examined the possibility that PTSD is characterized by persistently elevated levels of autonomic arousal. Other research has revealed psychophysiological characteristics that are not formally recognized as clinical or diagnostic features of PTSD but that are important to advancing our general understanding of the disorder. One of the most consistent findings of this type has been that of exaggerated heart rate (HR) responses to sudden, loud tones in individuals with PTSD. Such findings suggest that PTSD is characterized by a heightened sensitivity to aversive stimulation.

Despite successful application of psychophysiological methods to the study of posttraumatic adjustment, the practical aspects of using these measures and methods for the diagnosis, evaluation, and treatment of PTSD remain obscure to most clinicians. Although a few researchers have begun to discuss potential clinical application of psychophysiological assessment (Allen, 2002; Beuzeron-Mangina, 2000; Pitman & Orr, 1993), such discussions of the technology and methods for psychophysiological measurement are likely to appear intimidating to the nonexpert. At minimum, descriptions of technical matters can make for laborious reading. In the past, equipping and maintaining a state-of-the-art psychophysiological laboratory has been expensive and time-consuming. Fortunately, personal computers and integrated circuitry have reduced costs and eased the burden of psychophysiological data management and quantification. It is no longer necessary for an individual to have a high level of expertise in psychophysiological technology and methods and extensive resources in order to take advantage of the benefits offered by psychophysiological methods.

It is important to recognize that the PTSD diagnosis is presently based on subjective information that is not necessarily comparable to information recorded directly from physiological systems. Self-reported physiological activity and emotional experience often do not correlate well with measured physiological responses. General research on autonomic perception and response covariation (Eifert & Wilson, 1991; Spinhoven, Onstein, Sterk, & LeHaen-Versteijnen, 1993; Tyrer, Lee, & Alexander, 1980) makes it clear that self-reports of psychophysiological reactivity are not interchangeable with observations or recordings of such activity. With regard to fear, Lang (e.g., 1985) has long noted that self-report and concurrent psychophysiological arousal seldom have more than 10% shared variance. Limited convergence between self-reported emotion and physiological measures adds complexity to the assessment of PTSD, but it can be readily managed by a multimodal approach (e.g., Malloy, Fairbank, & Keane, 1983) that looks for convergence among diverse measures and considers measures that diverge from each other as a source of potentially valuable information for case conceptualization.

This chapter begins with a brief, nontechnical overview of psychophysiological methods and issues. We then summarize current findings related to individual DSM diagnostic criteria for PTSD before addressing both psychophysiological predictors of risk and remission and the use of psychophysiology to monitor treatment process and outcome. These clinically oriented topics are followed by coverage of relevant basic processes related to unconditioned or defensive responding, habituation, conditionability, and emotional–motivational states. Next, we outline threats to the validity of psychophysiological assessment and identify some potential conceptual aspects of PTSD that psychophysiology might address. Finally, we present a proposal for incorporating objective psychophysiological reactivity into the diagnostic criteria. Hopefully, both researchers and clinicians will be encouraged to seriously consider the potential value of this methodology in their respective contexts.

A BASIC PRIMER ON PSYCHOPHYSIOLOGICAL MEASURES AND METHODS

Use of psychophysiology measurement in research or clinical practice requires a conceptual grasp of the systems and methods, even if true technical understanding and mastery are not essential. Some knowledge of physiology, biomedical equipment, and computers is important. Expert consultation and assistance is necessary for someone new to these methods, regardless of whether they are at the stage of planning for, collecting, or interpreting psychophysiological data. Paradoxically, engaging a consultant tends to increase the need for knowledge about psychophysiology rather than diminishing it. This knowledge allows for the sharing of a common language and conceptual understanding, which increases the likelihood of successful communication and collaboration.

This section provides a brief overview of some of the common measurement and interpretational issues related to the use of psychophysiological methods. An edited volume by Cacioppo, Tassinary, and Berntson (2000) provides a comprehensive and up-to-date discussion of psychophysiological theory, methodology, and analysis. This handbook is recommended as a resource for anyone, expert or novice, interested in psychophysiology.

Four Key Physiological Systems

Cardiovascular

Heart rate (HR) and blood pressure (BP) are the most commonly used cardiovascular measures. Heart rate can be obtained manually by palpating and counting the number of beats, or it can be obtained more reliably and with greater temporal resolution by recording the electrocardiogram (ECG) and either counting R-waves or measuring the time between them directly or by means of a cardiotachometer that translates time intervals to beats-per-minute equivalent values. Blood pressure can be recorded manually by the auscultatory (i.e., cuff and stethoscope) method used in routine physical examinations or by means of similar automated methods involving an inflatable cuff placed on an arm. Whether manual or automated, these methods produce intermittent readings. A recent innovation in psychophysiological recording allows for continuous recording of blood pressure and HR from a finger cuff.

Heart rate is typically expressed in beats per minute, whereas interbeat interval or heart period is expressed in milliseconds. Blood pressure is expressed in millimeters of mercury pressure (Hg). The rate of sampling and level of precision required for obtaining HR and blood pressure data will be determined by the manner in which the signals are recorded, as well as by the issues addressed by the measures. For example, if one is interested in assessing resting level, samples might be obtained a few times per minute over an extended period of time, from several minutes to hours. However, if the objective is to evaluate responsivity to a brief stimulus, the recording interval should be relatively short. For HR, it would be desirable to capture each successive beat during the stimulus presentation, as well as for a short period immediately before and after the stimulus is presented. Although some HR responses to a stimulus may occur quickly, within 1–2 seconds, other responses may evolve more slowly, perhaps requiring 20–30 seconds to reach their peak.

Electrodermal

Sweat gland activity is perhaps the most widely studied response system, including measures of skin conductance (SC), resistance, and potential. Even though sweating serves a thermoregulatory function and is influenced by such factors as ambient temperature and humidity, when these factors are controlled there is a high correlation between output from the sympathetic nervous system (SNS) and SC responses (Wallin, 1981). In fact, Lang, Bradley, and Cuthbert (1990) have stated that "conductance change is a near-direct measure of general sympathetic nervous system activity" (p. 383). This specificity makes SC especially useful for assessing emotional arousal that is presumed to have a strong SNS component. Skin conductance is recorded by maintaining a very small constant voltage between two electrodes and measuring the variations in current that result from sweat gland activity in the underlying area. Conductance increases when the sweat ducts fill, membrane permeability changes, and sweat diffuses into the skin (Edelberg, 1972). Skin conductance is typically recorded from the fingers or palm of the nondominant hand through metal or silver/silver chloride electrodes. The contact area between the skin and electrode paste, as well as the distance between the two recording electrodes, will influence the value of SC level. For high-quality measurement, it is important to use an isotonic paste that approximates the salinity of sweat (see guidelines provided by Fowles et al., 1981) and not an electrolytic paste such as that used for ECG and other types of biological signal recording that is formulated to progressively reduce skin resistance (impedance) as it remains in contact with the skin.

Electromyographic

Muscle activity can be recorded through small surface electrodes placed over the muscle(s) of interest. Accurate location of the electrodes is very important so as to maximize detection of activity of the muscle group of interest and minimize that associated with nearby muscles. A discussion of the technical aspects of electromyogram (EMG) recording and description of where to position electrodes for specific muscle groups of the face and body can be found in Cacioppo, Tassinary, and Fridlund (1990). Careful consideration should be given to selection of muscle sites and adherence to recommended procedures for electrode placement. For example, measuring frontalis EMG by locating electrodes over each eye (Andreassi, 1980), a common practice in biofeedback applications, is highly susceptible to nonselective muscle activity and is unsuitable for most nonbiofeedback applications. Recording EMG activity requires equipment that can amplify the microvolt signals and provide filtering of the raw signal so as to include the primary frequencies associated with muscle activity. It is usually desirable to rectify (make positive) and integrate (smooth) the raw EMG so that the signal more clearly reflects meaningful changes and is less sensitive to momentary fluctuations. Proper abrading of the recording site and use of an electrolytic paste are two important steps for reducing resistance in the skin and achieving high-quality EMG recordings.

Electrocortical

Electrocortical activity recorded in electroencephalograhic (EEG) and event-related potential (ERP) studies is measured by placing electrodes on the scalp at specific locations, and then amplifying and filtering the microvolt signals so that they are discriminated from background noise and reflect the process of interest (e.g., attention). Electrodes are commonly fitted inside an elasticized cap, much like a bathing cap, which positions and holds them at the correct locations on the head according to the standardized 10–20 international system (Jasper, 1958). The number of electrodes may range from as few as 10 to more than 100 depending on the particular application. Electrodes also are placed near the eyes so that vertical and horizontal eye movements can be detected. Muscle activity associated with movement of the eyes, as well as the head or neck, can introduce artifact into the EEG recording. Data from trials that include significant movement are usually eliminated from analyses or corrected using mathematical algorithms.

EEG studies of brain asymmetry and emotion typically involve continuous recording of electrocortical activity from opposing sites on each side of midline (e.g., F3 and F4, T3 and T4 of the 10–20 international system) under baseline or emotionally evocative conditions. Studies have focused almost exclusively on alpha activity (8–13 Hz) because this power band is assumed to be inversely related to general brain activation. Alpha power is derived using a fast Fourier transform, and values often are log-transformed to normalize the distribution. Most commonly, asymmetry index scores are calculated by subtracting alpha power recorded at the left electrode site from that recorded at the right site. Positive scores indicate greater alpha power at the right than the left electrode site, which is assumed to reflect greater left- than right-sided brain activation.

Methodologies for measuring ERP components involve averaging the EEG signal over many trials to improve signal-to-noise ratio, because most ERP components are relatively small compared with the background EEG activity. This is accomplished by repeated presentations of either one stimulus or one type of stimulus (e.g., a tone of a specific intensity and frequency or a set of words related to a traumatic event) and averaging the recorded epochs for trials of the same type. Signal recording is typically initiated prior to stimulus onset in order to establish a baseline that can be used as a point of reference for each recorded epoch. Adjustment relative to baseline involves centering the voltage on a mean of zero over the prestimulus sampling period and is accomplished by subtracting the average baseline voltage from each measurement point in the poststimulus sampling epoch. Like EEG studies, the electrical signals are digitally filtered, and trials free of excessive eye-movement artifact are retained for signal averaging. Peak ERP component amplitudes (i.e., the maximal voltage deflection identified in a designated latency range) and their corresponding latencies are then scored for each stimulus type. An ERP waveform consists of a series of positive and negative voltages that are characteristically labeled with "P" or "N," to denote whether they are positive or negative, along with a number to indicate the latency of the component's peak or their ordinal position in the waveform. For example, "P300" or "P3" is a positive-going component that occurs approximately 300 milliseconds, and is the third positive component, after stimulus onset. It is worth noting that the convention for visual display of these waveforms has positive components going downward and vice versa.

Personal computers have revolutionized EEG and ERP research because they can be programmed to handle nearly all of the otherwise time-intensive data management and scoring tasks. As computers become more powerful, new methods of assessing and depicting brain activity are becoming available, including topographical maps that produce pictures to concisely represent a composite of brain electrical activity. Despite these advances, anyone considering this type of measurement should be aware that the technology remains rather intricate, data scoring and management still can be time-consuming, and many of the scoring and interpretational issues are complex.

Two Key Measurement Issues

Measuring Resting and Prestimulus Levels

Most psychophysiological investigations assess resting levels at the beginning of the procedure as a reference point for comparison with subsequent values. It also is common to obtain additional baseline values from rest periods at points throughout the procedure as a means of tracking shifts in tonic arousal. A decision must be made regarding the optimal amount of time for stabilization and collection of initial resting-level data. A review of studies that collected resting HR levels by Hastrup (1986) noted a negative correlation between subsequent HR level and duration of the rest period, indicating that shorter rest periods yield higher HR levels. In general, it appears that 15 minutes may be optimal for initial stabilization before assessing basal HR level, although decisions about baseline length are best viewed as application specific. Considerations that influence the decision include the fact that overly long rest periods may result in boredom, restlessness, and even sleep, whereas overly brief rest periods will not allow sufficient time for physiological stabilization, especially if participants have been physically active prior to the rest (e.g., coming directly into the lab from outside activities).

Periodic sampling of resting baseline values throughout a recording session is important for determining general physiological trends or to provide reference values for calculating the magnitude of responses (e.g., to trauma-relevant stimuli). Because physiological levels can change over time, especially when a variety of stimuli or tasks are being presented, it often is desirable to obtain baseline or nontask comparison values that precede and are proximal to the target of interest (e.g., prior to presentation of a particular stimulus). Suitable reference levels may be obtained from relatively brief periods of recording if the individual is sitting quietly and is not extremely anxious. For example, in the studies of trauma-related imagery (e.g., Orr, Pitman, Lasko, & Herz, 1993), baseline data were collected for 30 seconds prior to each script and 1–3 minutes were between trials. In ERP research, electrocortical recording commonly begins 100 milliseconds or so prior to each stimulus presentation. The mean level during this baseline interval is subtracted from values during the remainder of the recording interval to provide baseline correction for each trial. Intervals between trials can be as short as 2 seconds for procedures that use ERP measures. Depending on the protocol and type of stimuli being used, as well as the particular measure(s) being recorded, more or less time between stimulus presentations may be needed to allow for stabilization.

Deciding How Many Measures to Record

The most frequently used indices of emotional arousal in psychophysiological studies of PTSD have been measures of peripheral autonomic activity (i.e., HR, SC, and BP). A number of studies also have used facial EMG to assess emotional reactivity, whereas relatively fewer studies have recorded cortical ERPs in order to evaluate cognitive processing in PTSD. The selection of measures generally is determined by the conceptual and theoretical issues to be addressed, but there are practical considerations as well. These include such issues as previous use and popularity, amount of technical expertise required for data collection and interpretation, availability of instrumentation, and expense.

There is ample evidence that measures are differentially sensitive to emotional and psychological states and behaviors. It is important to recognize that one measure cannot simply be substituted for another. Fowles (1980) in particular has explored some of the differential value of HR and SC as psychophysiological indicators. His model proposes that HR will better index responding associated with active avoidance behavior, whereas SC will better index active inhibition. Although HR and SC can provide useful indices of general arousal, they are not necessarily informative about its valence (i.e., whether it is positive or negative). In contrast, measures of facial EMG activity may not index intensity very well, but they are particularly good at providing information about the valence of the emotional arousal (Fridlund & Izard, 1983). For example, an increase in zygomaticus major activity (the muscle group involved in smiling) is characteristic of a pleasant emotional experience, whereas increased corrugator activity (the muscle group involved in frowning) has been found to accompany a depressed mood (Sirota & Schwartz, 1982). Corrugator EMG is especially useful for discriminating between positively and negatively valenced emotions.

Finally, it is important to recognize that there often are differences between individuals in the relative degree to which responses appear in one system versus another (Stern & Sison, 1990). For example, exposure to a generic stressor such as mental arithmetic may produce an increase in HR and SC levels for some individuals, whereas other individuals will show change in one system but not the other, and still others may show small or no changes at all. Measurement of only a single system greatly increases the likelihood that reactivity will be underestimated or missed completely in individuals who happen to be more responsive in another system.

OVERVIEW OF PSYCHOPHYSIOLOGICAL EVIDENCE IN RELATION TO TRAUMA AND PTSD

Reactivity to Trauma-Related Cues: Criterion B5

Theoretically, the critical element in physiological response to trauma-related cues is activation of the memory network in which a traumatic event is encoded. Once such a memory is activated, emotions that are associatively linked with it also become activated, along with their accompanying physiological responses. Interestingly, physiological reactivity to trauma-related cues was moved from the category of arousal symptoms (criterion D6) as it appeared in DSM-III-R to the category of reexperiencing symptoms (criterion B5) in DSM-IV. This change is of conceptual significance because it recognizes physiological reactivity as a measure of the degree to which an event is emotionally reexperienced rather than as a pathological symptom indicative of generally heightened arousal. The revision also is supported by findings, discussed later, that demonstrate that increased physiological reactivity is relatively specific to trauma-related stimuli and does not appear to generalize to other (i.e., non-trauma-related) stressful or emotionally negative stimuli (Casada, Amdur, Larsen, & Liberzon, 1998; Orr et al., 1993; Pitman et al., 1990; Pitman, Orr, Forgue, de Jong, & Claiborn, 1987).

The Standardized Audiovisual Method of Assessment

The standardized approach involves presentation of a fixed set of stimuli, such as light flashes, combat sounds (mortar explosions or gunfire), and pictures of combat situations, while psychophysiological responses are recorded (e.g., Blanchard, Kolb, Gerardi, Ryan, & Pallmeyer, 1986; Dobbs & Wilson, 1960; Malloy et al., 1983; McFall, Murburg, Ko, & Veith, 1990). The intensity level of the auditory stimuli may be varied within the procedure, beginning at a low level of sound or trauma-relevant content and increasing to progressively higher levels. Responses to standardized neutral stimuli that are not related to the trauma (e.g., music or slides depicting outdoor scenes) provide a comparison for physiological reactivity specific to trauma-relevant content.

Reactivity to any stimulus format can be calculated as difference scores between periods with contrasting content. For example, if trauma-related auditory stimuli are interspersed with neutral stimuli (e.g., music), a response score can be computed by subtracting the physiological level during the neutral presentation of the neutral stimulus from that recorded during the trauma-related presentation. This difference score represents the individual's relative reactivity to the two stimuli, with a positive value indicating greater trauma-related reactivity. Conceptually, scores of this sort reflect excess (i.e., trauma-specific) reactivity by taking account of both individual differences in physiological characteristics (e.g., responsivity or baseline levels) and reactivity to the task itself (e.g., listening to sounds) that are extraneous to the quantity of interest.

The use of standardized stimuli to assess psychophysiological reactivity allows maximal control over the selection and presentation of the stimuli. Furthermore, each individual's reactivity is measured to the same set of cues. Thus differences in physiological reactivity are more readily attributable to individual differences in the emotional relevance of the stimuli. A limitation of the use of standardized stimuli, especially in studies of emotion, is that the selected stimuli may not match a particular individual's unique experience(s). This can result in less than optimal activation of the target emotion(s).

The Script-Driven Imagery Method of Assessment

The imagery-based approach is derived from procedures developed by Peter Lang and his colleagues for the study of fear and phobias (Cook, Melamed, Cuthbert, McNeil, & Lang, 1988; Lang, Levin, Miller, & Kozak, 1983; McNeil, Vrana, Melamed, Cuthbert, & Lang, 1993). Details of the methodology as applied to trauma-exposed individuals can be found in Pitman et al. (1987) and Orr et al. (1993). Briefly, the procedure involves preparing various scripts that portray actual or hypothetical experiences of the person being assessed, including the two most stressful trauma-related experiences they can recall. Other experiences may include stressful lifetime experiences not related to the trauma, positive experiences, or neutral experiences, depending on the most relevant comparison for the question at hand. A written description of each personal experience is reviewed and edited to produce a script of about 30-second duration, composed in the second person, present tense. Standard scripts portraying various hypothetical experiences also are included and provide a means for comparing responses to stimuli that are the same for all individuals within or between studies. Scripts are recorded in a neutral voice for playback in the laboratory while psychophysiological activity is measured. Individuals are instructed to listen carefully during the playing of each script and to imagine them as vividly as possible. The reading and imagining of each script is followed by a period for relaxation, after which several self-reports are made on Likert-type scales. A response score is calculated for each physiological dependent variable, separately for each script, by subtracting the preceding baseline period value from the value during imagery.

An important feature of the script-driven-imagery method is its flexibility. Scripts can be tailored to capture an individual's unique experience of a traumatic event and can also be used to assess emotional reactivity to most any traumatic event. For example, a Vietnam veteran whose job was handling dead bodies in a morgue might be unresponsive to standard combat-related sights and sounds but prove highly reactive to a script describing the personally relevant experience of working in a morgue. The potential limitations of this method include its reliance on participants' ability to recall the events in question and their willingness to comply with instructions to vividly imagine the experiences. Failure in either regard can result in an underestimate of an individual's emotional reactivity.

Summary of Evidence for Trauma-Specific Responding

One of the most consistent findings is that psychophysiological reactivity to cues reminiscent of the traumatic event is heightened in individuals diagnosed with PTSD but not in trauma-exposed individuals who fail to meet PTSD diagnostic criteria (for reviews, see McFall, Murburg, Roszell, & Veith, 1989; Orr, Metzger, & Pitman, 2002; Prins, Kaloupek, & Keane, 1995; Shalev & Rogel-Fuchs, 1993). Studies that have examined psychophysiological reactivity to trauma-related cues are summarized in Table 11.1. A number of studies have presented standardized audiovisual cues to combat veterans. Typically, combat sounds, such as mortar explosions or gunfire, and pictures of combat situations both have produced larger responses in HR, BP, electrodermal activity, and forehead EMG in veterans with PTSD than in those without PTSD (Blanchard et al., 1986; Blanchard, Kolb, Pallmeyer, & Gerardi, 1982; Blanchard, Kolb, Taylor, & Wittrock, 1989; Casada et al., 1998; Dobbs & Wilson, 1960; Malloy et al., 1983; McFall et al., 1990; Pallmeyer, Blanchard, & Kolb, 1986). Standardized combat-related words also have produced larger SC responses in combat veterans with PTSD than in combat veterans with other psychiatric disorders (McNally et al., 1987). Although the majority of

TABLE 11.1. Studies That Have Examined Psychophysiological Reactivity to Trauma-Related Stimuli in Individuals with and without PTSD

Study	Sample gender and trauma type	Sample size	Measures on which PTSD > non-PTSD	Trauma cue format
Blanchard, Hickling, Buckley, Taylor, Vollmer, & Loos (1996)	MVA	PTSD = 38 TC = 32 NC = 54	HR*, F-EMG, SBP, DBP	SDI, videotape
Blanchard, Hickling, Taylor, Loos, & Gerardi (1994)	Combat	PTSD = 23 TC = 17 NC = 40	SC, HR*, F-EMG, SBP, DBP	SDI, videotape
Blanchard, Kolb, Gerardi, Ryan, & Pallmeyer (1986)	Combat	PTSD = 57 TC = 34	HR*	Combat sounds
Blanchard, Kolb, Pallmeyer, & Gerardi (1982)	Combat	PTSD = 11 NC = 11	SC, HR*, F-EMG*, SBP*, DBP	Combat sounds
Blanchard, Kolb, Taylor, & Wittrock (1989)	Combat	PTSD = 59 TC = 12	HR*	Combat sounds
Carson et al. (2000)	Women exposed to war zone trauma	PTSD = 17 TC = 21	SC*, HR*, LF-EMG*, C-EMG	SDI
Casada, Amdur, Larsen, & Liberzon (1998)	Combat	PTSD = 15 TC = 10 NC = 11	SC, HR*, F-EMG†	Combat sounds
Davis, Adams, Uddo, Vasterling, & Sutker (1996)	Combat	PTSD = 10 TC = 18	SC, HR, LF-EMG	SDI
Gerardi, Blanchard, & Kolb (1989)	Combat	PTSD = 18 TC = 18	SR*, HR*, F-EMG*, SBP, DBP	Combat sounds
Keane et al. (1998)	Combat	PTSD = 631+ TC = 319+	SC*, HR*, LF-EMG*, SBP, DBP*	SDI, audiovisual
Kinzie et al. (1998)	Combat, refugees	PTSD = 38 TC =22 NC = 22	HR	Audiovisual
Lanius et al. (2001)	Mixed trauma	PTSD = 9 TC = 9	HR*	SDI
Malloy, Fairbank, & Keane (1983)	Combat	PTSD = 10 TC = 10	SR, HR*	Audiovisual

(continued)

TABLE 11.1 *(continued)*

Study	Sample gender and trauma type	Sample size	Measures on which PTSD > non-PTSD	Trauma cue format
McDonagh-Coyle et al. (2001)[a]	♀ Sexual abuse	*N* = 371	SC, HR*, LF-EMG†	SDI
McFall, Murburg, Ko, & Veith (1990)	♂ Combat	PTSD = 10 TC/NC = 11	HR*, SBP, DBP*	Audiovisual
McNally et al. (1987)	♂ Combat	PTSD = 10 TC = 10	SC*	Words
Orr, Lasko, et al. (1998)	♀ Sexual abuse	PTSD = 29 TC = 18	SC, HR*, LF-EMG, C-EMG*	SDI
Orr, Pitman, Lasko, & Herz (1993)	♂ Combat	PTSD = 8 TC = 12	SC*, HR*, LF-EMG, C-EMG	SDI
Pallmeyer, Blanchard, & Kolb (1986)	♂ Combat	PTSD = 12 TC = 10 NC =5	HR*, SC*, F-EMG, SBP*, DBP*	Combat sounds
Pitman et al. (2001)	♀ Breast cancer	PTSD = 5 TC = 25	SC*, HR*, LF-EMG, C-EMG*	SDI
Pitman et al. (1990)	♂ Combat	PTSD = 7 TC = 7	SC*, HR, LF-EMG*	SDI
Pitman et al. (1987)	♂ Combat	PTSD = 18 TC = 15	SC*, HR, LF-EMG*	SDI
Shalev, Orr, & Pitman (1993)	♂ ♀ Mixed trauma	PTSD = 13 TC = 13	SC, HR*, LF-EMG*	SDI
Wolfe et al. (2000)	♀ Women exposed to war zone trauma	PTSD = 8 TC = 20	SC*, HR, SBP*, DBP	Audiovisual

Note. SR, skin resistance; SC, skin conductance; HR, heart rate; F-EMG, forehead EMG; LF-EMG, lateral frontalis EMG; C-EMG, corrugator EMG; TC, trauma-exposed control group; NC, normal (non-trauma-exposed) control group; MVA, motor vehicle accident; SDI, script-driven imagery; SBP, systolic blood pressure; DBP, diastolic blood pressure.

[a]A correlational approach was used in this study.

* $p < .05$; † $p < .10$.

studies using standardized audiovisual cues have involved male military veterans, recent research also has demonstrated heightened psychophysiological reactivity in female veterans and in veterans' service organization volunteers with PTSD related to their experiences during the Vietnam War (Wolfe et al., 2000). Only one published study did not find larger responses to videotaped scenes of the Vietnam War in veterans with than without PTSD (Kinzie et al., 1998). However, even this study found a larger HR response to videotaped scenes of a Cambodian refugee camp in Cambodians with PTSD than in those without PTSD. Overall, the pattern of findings is extremely consistent.

Studies that have used individually tailored imagery scripts as the means for cue presentation also have found larger SC, HR, and/or facial EMG (lateral frontalis) responses during recollection of trauma-related experiences in individuals with PTSD than in those without PTSD. This trauma-specific reactivity has been found with male Vietnam, World War II, and Korean combat veterans (Orr et al., 1993; Pitman et al., 1990; Pitman et al., 1987), adult females with a history of childhood sexual abuse (McDonagh-Coyle et al., 2001; Orr, Lasko, et al., 1998), female nurse veterans who witnessed injury or death during military service in Vietnam (Carson et al., 2000), and breast cancer survivors (Pitman et al., 2001), as well individuals exposed to other civilian traumatic events (Blanchard et al., 1996; Blanchard, Hickling, Taylor, Loos, & Gerardi, 1994; Shalev, Orr, & Pitman, 1993). The findings for Vietnam veteran nurses and breast cancer survivors are of particular interest as evidence consistent with the position taken in DSM-IV concerning the ability of "witnessing a traumatic event" and "being diagnosed with a life-threatening illness" to act as potential causes for PTSD. Finally, a large multisite study involving more than 1,300 male Vietnam veterans applied both standardized audiovisual and script-driven imagery procedures in an examination of combat-related PTSD (Keane et al., 1998). Results of this study replicated findings of heightened physiological reactivity in combat veterans with PTSD, although the magnitude of the effect is somewhat smaller than that obtained in smaller studies.

Findings from two studies stand in contrast to those demonstrating the relative specificity of heightened psychophysiological reactivity to trauma-related cues in individuals with PTSD. A study by Beckham and colleagues (Beckham et al., 2002) observed larger systolic blood pressure and a trend toward larger HR responses in Vietnam combat veterans during recollection of a past experience of anger than in veterans without PTSD. This finding is not surprising in light of previous evidence for greater anger and hostility shown by individuals with PTSD (e.g., Beckham, Moore, & Reynolds, 2000). In a second study, male and female Cambodian refugees with PTSD from prolonged and intense trauma showed elevated HR responses, relative to controls without trauma, to videotaped scenes of a Cambodian refugee camp but also to scenes of an auto accident, domestic violence, the Vietnam War, and a hurricane (Kinzie et al., 1998). The reason for generalized reactivity in the Cambodians with PTSD is not clear, but one possible explanation is the use of a finger pulse plethysmograph to measure HR. This instrument can be susceptible to artifact produced by muscle movement. Consistent with this possibility, behavioral observations indicated that the Cambodian refugees with PTSD reacted more strongly across scenes.

This body of evidence supports the idea that physiological responses can provide an index of the emotional experience associated with reactivation of memory for a traumatic event. An extension of this idea is that the presence of clinical pathology can be inferred from reactivity to trauma-related cues. Several investigators (e.g., Blanchard, Kolb, & Prins, 1991; Malloy et al., 1983; Orr et al., 1998; Pitman et al., 1987; Shalev et al., 1993) have attempted to use one or more indices of psychophysiological reactivity as a marker for PTSD. These diagnostic applications have produced sensitivity values in the range of 60–90% and specificity values of 80–100%.

Reactivity to Generic Stressors

Although individuals with PTSD respond with increased reactivity to trauma cues, they appear to show relatively normal levels of responding to generic stressors unrelated to trauma. For example, studies measuring autonomic responses while performing mental arithmetic have reported comparably large (Blanchard et al., 1986; Orr, Meyerhoff, Edwards, & Pitman, 1998) and even somewhat smaller (Keane et al., 1998; McDonagh-Coyle et al., 2001) responses in individuals with PTSD than in those without. A purely physical stressor, orthostatic challenge, also produced comparably large increases in HR and BP in groups with and without PTSD (Orr, Meyerhoff, et al., 1998). However, individuals with PTSD are more physiologically reactive to aversive stimuli, such as loud sounds or mild electric shock (e.g., Casada et al., 1998). Increased reactivity to aversive unconditioned stimuli such as loud noises or shock could represent a heightened sensitivity of the nervous system, of which sensitization of the amygdala may play a central role (see Pitman, Shalev, & Orr, 1999).

Use of Neuroimaging Methods

Recently, challenge studies have begun to employ more sophisticated measures of brain activation, such as positron emission tomography (PET) and functional magnetic resonance imaging (fMRI) to identify the neural circuitry associated with increased responsiveness to trauma cues. Some of these studies have incorporated peripheral psychophysiological measures, including HR, SC, and facial EMG, to provide concurrent validation of emotional responding to the challenge task. Similar to findings described previously, these studies have reported increased HR responding during traumatic stimulation in individuals with PTSD compared with individuals without PTSD (Lanius et al., 2001; Shin et al., 1999) or with baseline-neutral conditions (Pissiota et al., 2002; Rauch et al., 1996). The integration of neuroimaging and psychophysiological assessment is an important direction for future research, as the simultaneous measurement of regions of brain activation and psychophysiological responding should ultimately improve our understanding at both levels.

Numbing of General Responsiveness: Criteria C4–6

Despite clear evidence for heightened physiological reactivity to trauma reminders, many individuals with PTSD also report a diminished ability to experience emotions. This complaint is reflected in the DSM-IV criteria for PTSD that address symptoms of disinterest (C4), detachment (C5), and restricted range of affect (C6). Theorists have hypothesized that the hyperarousal and numbing symptoms of PTSD are inversely related and are characterized by alternating periods of intense reexperiencing and negative arousal followed by intervals of dampened affective responsivity (Herman, 1992; Horowitz, 1986; van der Kolk, 1987; van der Kolk, Greenberg, Boyd, & Krystal, 1985).

Litz (1992) also proposed that emotional numbing in PTSD is phasic but conceptualized the phenomenon as a transient depletion or reduction in the capacity for *positive* emotion that follows and is tied to episodes of intense reexperiencing and trauma-related arousal. In other words, Litz's model posits that affective abnormalities in PTSD are: (1) secondary to either acute or sustained activation of trauma-related emotional responses and (2) reflected in hyporeactivity to stimuli that normally evoke a positive or appetitive hedonic response. Litz also proposed that (3) exposure to trauma-related cues primes the psychobiological systems underlying aversive emotional states, resulting in facilitation of subsequent defensive responses and reactivity to unpleasant stimuli. Preliminary support for the first two of these propositions has been provided by evidence that self-reports of emotional numbing symptoms are most strongly predicted by hyperarousal symptoms (Litz et al., 1997; Flack, Litz, Hsieh, Kaloupek, & Keane, 2000) and by laboratory data showing that activation of a trauma-related emotional response produced phasic reductions in the expression of positive affect in individuals with PTSD (Litz, Orsillo, Kaloupek, & Weathers, 2000).

In the Litz et al. (2000) study, combat veterans with and without PTSD viewed emotionally evocative pictures before and after exposure to a combat-related audiovisual presentation while their self-report and physiological responses, including facial EMG, were recorded. Results revealed that the two groups exhibited equivalent patterns of affective response prior to the trauma-related challenge, yet after that manipulation, participants with PTSD exhibited suppressed zygomaticus EMG (i.e., smile) responses during viewing of pleasant images relative to controls. A follow-up study by Miller and Litz (in press) replicated the equivalent patterns of psychophysiological response under baseline conditions in veterans with and without PTSD. However, in this study, individuals with PTSD showed facilitation of negative emotional responses after exposure to trauma-related cues without evidence of change in indicators of positive emotion. Although the results of the two studies diverge with regard to the acute consequences of activating trauma-related emotions, they are broadly consistent with models that emphasize the phasic nature of affective disturbance in individuals with PTSD.

Sleep Disturbance: Criterion D1

Although there is extensive research and clinical literature regarding psychophysiological assessment of sleep and sleep problems (see Pivik, 2000), PTSD-related work of this type is only now beginning to emerge. For example, Woodward, Murberg, and Bliwise (2000) measured EEG during sleep and noted a trend toward reduced low-frequency power during non-rapid-eye-movement sleep in veterans with combat-related PTSD compared with controls without PTSD. A difference also was noted for the ratio of rapid eye movement (REM) to non-REM beta-band EEG between individuals with and without PTSD. A recent study of the effects of cognitive behavioral therapy noted a reduction in heart rate variability (HRV) during REM sleep in 5 patients who improved with therapy compared with an increase in HRV in the single patient who did not improve (Nishith et al., 2003). These pilot findings suggest that improvement in PTSD symptoms may be associated with a reduction in HRV. The application of psychophysiological measures and methods to PTSD-related sleep disturbances is a promising direction for future research.

Irritability or Anger: Criterion D2

Findings from a number of studies using self-report measures (Beckham, Feldman, et al., 2000; Butterfield, Forneris, Feldman, & Beckham, 2000; Lasko, Gurvits, Kuhne, Orr, & Pitman, 1994) support the DSM criterion regarding heightened anger and hostility as a feature of PTSD. One noteworthy study recently examined whether individuals with PTSD also show increased psychophysiological reactivity during recollection and reliving of a past personal anger-provoking situation. Beckham et al. (2002) measured HR and BP in combat veterans with and without PTSD when cued to relive a memory in which they felt angry, frustrated, or upset with another person. Veterans with PTSD were quicker to indicate the onset of anger and produced larger HR and diastolic BP responses while reliving their anger situations. These findings raise the possibility that at least some subpopulations with PTSD may be characterized by heightened physiological reactivity to stimuli associated with anger, in addition to stimuli related to the index traumatic event.

Difficulty Concentrating: Criterion D3

Several studies have reported abnormalities in an ERP component linked to attentional processing in PTSD, thereby providing electrophysiological evidence for the DSM-IV symptom of disturbed concentration. Specifically, researchers have used the auditory oddball procedure to examine P3 responses in individuals with PTSD. The auditory oddball is the most common procedure for eliciting the P3 response and has been widely used in the study of attention in clinical disorders (Polich & Herbst, 2000). In this procedure, individuals listen to a series of infrequently presented "target" tones that are interspersed among highly frequent "common" tones and infrequent "distractor" tones. The tones differ in pitch, with the target tone often having the highest (e.g., 2000 Hz), the distractor tone having the lowest (e.g., 500 Hz), and the common tone having an intermediate (e.g., 500 Hz) pitch. Participants are instructed to sit quietly with their eyes open and to press a button (or keep a mental count) in response to target tones, while ignoring all other tones. During performance of this task, the individual's ERPs are recorded during a 1-second interval starting 100 milliseconds prior to tone onset. The P3 response is scored as the most positive point of electrical activity in the time window between approximately 300 and 500 milliseconds following tone onset. In normal individuals, the P3 response to the target stimulus at the midline parietal (Pz) recording site is larger relative to the P3 response to common stimuli and is often larger than the response to distractor stimuli. The relative amplitude of the P3 response reflects task relevancy (i.e., importance) and infrequency (i.e., low probability) of the target stimulus and is widely presumed to index the amount of attentional resources directed at the eliciting stimulus. In line with findings reported for several other clinical disorders, samples of men and women with PTSD have produced smaller P3 response amplitudes to target stimuli than have their respective comparison groups, suggesting that they have increased difficulty concentrating (Charles et al., 1995; Felmingham, Bryant, Kendall, & Gordon, 2002; Galletly, Clark, McFarlane, & Weber, 2001; McFarlane, Weber, & Clark, 1993; Metzger, Orr, Lasko, Berry, & Pitman, 1997; Metzger, Orr, Lasko, & Pitman, 1997).

It is noteworthy that this ERP indicator has not been found in PTSD samples containing individuals on psychoactive medications (Kimble, Kaloupek, Kaufman, & Deldin, 2000; Metzger, Orr, Lasko, & Pitman, 1997), as might be expected if one effect of medication is to improve attention and concentration. Neylan et al. (2003) did not find smaller P3 response amplitudes to auditory and visual targets in a sample of male Vietnam veterans that included a mixture of medicated and unmedicated individuals, nor were there differences in P3 between medicated and unmedicated participants. Interpretation of these findings is complicated by a strikingly small mean P3 response for the group without PTSD, compared with previously published P3 means for control groups. Finally, a recent study of unmedicated female veterans who had served as military nurses in Vietnam demonstrated significantly *larger* P3 amplitudes to target stimuli in those with PTSD than in those without the disorder (Metzger et al., 2002). This is a curious finding and difficult to reconcile given that P3 amplitude abnormalities in clinical populations are typically associated with reduced responses. One possible explanation is that the larger P3 responses in the nurse veterans with PTSD represent increased attention and concentration used to compensate for limitations associated with having PTSD.

Hypervigilance: Criterion D4

Psychophysiological support for the DSM-IV symptom of hypervigilance recently has been provided by studies using both peripheral and central measures. Two studies of conditionability in PTSD (Orr et al., 2000; Peri, Ben-Shakhar, Orr, & Shalev, 2000) found that individuals with PTSD showed larger SC-orienting responses to initial presentations of the to-be-conditioned neutral stimulus (i.e., slides of colored circles), suggesting increased vigilance toward novel stimuli. A study of motor vehicle accident victims found that those with PTSD showed a greater number of SC-orienting responses to both neutral and threatening words, supporting the possibility of a generally heightened orienting response among these individuals (Bryant, Harvey, Gordon, & Barry, 1995).

Support for increased orienting responses in women with PTSD also is provided by an ERP study in which they showed a larger negative-going deflection when a novel stimulus is presented within a repeated stimulus chain (so-called mismatch negativity; Morgan & Grillon, 1999). Likewise, a relatively increased frontal P3 response amplitude to novel distractor stimuli has been reported for male Vietnam combat veterans (Kimble et al., 2000). Such enhanced cortical responses to novel stimuli may index the clinical symptoms of hypervigilance. However, a recent study that compared frontal P3 responses to both novel auditory and visual stimuli between male Vietnam combat veterans with and without PTSD did not find evidence supporting increased orienting in PTSD (Neylan et al., 2003).

Tendency to suppress or reduce an early positive ERP response (i.e., P50) to the second of two stimuli presented in close temporal proximity can be interpreted as an indicator of vigilance. Four studies have examined this effect, indexed as the ratio of P50 responses to a series of paired clicks in individuals with PTSD. In normal individuals, the amplitude of the P50 response to the second click of a pair is appreciably smaller than the response amplitude to the first click. This reduction presumably is the result of a central inhibitory function or sensory gating response at the neuronal level. Both male Vietnam combat veterans (Gillette et al., 1997; Neylan et al., 1999) and female rape victims (Skinner et al., 1999) with PTSD have failed to show a reduction in P50 response amplitude to the second of the paired clicks, resulting in abnormally large P50 ratios. One study of female military nurses who were veterans of war in Vietnam (Metzger et al., 2002) failed to find support for sensory gating abnormalities specific to PTSD, although this study did find that P50 ratios were related to measures of general psychopathology. This finding is consistent with evidence that P50 ratios are abnormally increased in several other clinical disorders, particularly schizophrenia.

Finally, researchers have measured ERP P3 responses to combat-related words (Stanford, Vasterling, Mathias, Constans, & Houston, 2001) and pictures (Attias, Bleich, Furman, & Zinger, 1996; Attias, Bleich, & Gilat, 1996; Bleich, Attias, & Furman, 1996) in the context of an emotional oddball paradigm. Modeled after the three-tone oddball procedure, this procedure used trauma-related pictures or words as infrequent, to-be-ignored "distractors" that were interspersed among common (e.g., home furnishings) and target (e.g., domestic animals) stimuli. In each study, combat veterans with PTSD produced larger P3 waveform components to the trauma-related stimuli than did veterans without PTSD. In similar studies of normal individuals, the P3 has been shown to be sensitive to the intrinsic emotional or informational value of a stimulus and is presumed to provide an index of the attentional resources devoted to processing the stimulus. Importantly, combat veterans with PTSD do not show larger P3 response amplitudes to social threat words (Stanford et al., 2001), suggesting that the involuntary attentional bias is specific to trauma-related cues, perhaps due to their increased emotional significance, and does not generalize across all negative emotional cues.

The P3 response to trauma-related stimuli recorded at the parietal site has been found to correctly classify 90% of Israeli combat veterans with PTSD and 85% of the veterans without PTSD (Attias, Bleich, & Gilat, 1996). This is consistent with the sensitivity and specificity values obtained for autonomic measures and supports the potential diagnostic utility of ERP measures. To date, only one published study has not found evidence of larger P3 amplitude responses to trauma-related words in PTSD. In this instance, a mixed trauma group with PTSD showed smaller P3 amplitudes across neutral, positive, and trauma-related words presented in the context of an emotional Stroop color-naming task (Metzger, Orr, Lasko, McNally, & Pitman, 1997). The smaller P3 amplitudes are suggestive of attentional difficulties (e.g., concentration difficulties, as discussed previously) and might reflect poorer performance due to the more difficult than usual format of the Stroop task in this study, which entailed indicating the color of words (via button press) while ignoring word meaning. Importantly, although participants with PTSD did not show selective differences in P3 amplitudes to trauma-related words, behaviorally they did take longer to indicate the color of trauma-related words, consistent with the presence of a cognitive bias for trauma-related information. Because participants are asked to ignore all nontarget stimuli in each of these tasks, both larger P3 amplitudes and longer color-naming reaction times appear to reflect an automatic, involuntary cognitive response. Therefore, these findings suggest that PTSD is characterized by "selective cognitive sensitivity" to stimuli reminiscent of the traumatic event (Stanford et al., 2001), which might be a component of a more general hypervigilant state.

Exaggerated Startle Response: Criterion D5

Exaggerated startle responding has been recognized as a core subjective symptom of posttrauma reactions since the earliest descriptions of combat soldiers suffering adverse effects of exposure to the stress of combat (Cambell, 1918; Grinker & Spiegel, 1945; Southard, 1919). Kardiner (1941), one of the first to systematically describe the syndrome, considered exaggerated startle to be a central element of the disorder which he related to the hyperarousal symptoms. Recent empirical studies have confirmed the association between self-reports of exaggerated startle, PTSD, and the hyperarousal symptoms. Indeed, startle may be one of the most reliably reported symptoms of the disorder. For example, Davidson, Hughes, Blazer, and George (1991) found that exaggerated startle was endorsed by 88% of participants with a diagnosis of PTSD, making it the second most commonly reported symptom following reexperiencing of the trauma. Similarly, Pynoos et al. (1993) examined the strength of the association between each PTSD symptom and diagnostic status using discriminant function analysis and found that self-report of exaggerated startle accounted for the second largest proportion of variance in diagnostic status, preceded only by intrusive thoughts. Likewise, Meltzer-Brody, Churchill, and Davidson (1999) found that exaggerated startle was the PTSD symptom that best differentiated individuals who met full diagnostic criteria from those who did not.

There also is evidence based on self-reports suggesting that exaggerated startle is one of the first symptoms to emerge following trauma exposure. Among survivors of an industrial disaster, Weisaeth (1989) found that intense startle was the most commonly reported PTSD symptom within 1 week of the disaster, being endorsed by 80% and 86% of participants with moderate and high levels of exposure to the accident, respectively. Similarly, Southwick and colleagues (Southwick et al., 1993; Southwick et al., 1995) examined the development of PTSD symptoms over time in two units of Gulf War veterans and found that increased startle was the most frequently reported PTSD symptom at 1 month, the third most common symptom at 6 months, and the second most frequently endorsed symptom 2 years after returning from the war.

From a psychophysiological perspective, the startle response is a constellation of defensive reflexive motor movements, phasic autonomic responses, and voluntary orienting movements that occur (in that temporal order) in response to any sudden, intense change in stimulus intensity. The reflexive component of the reaction begins with an eyeblink between 20 and 50 milliseconds after onset of a startle-eliciting stimulus and spreads distally to produce upper-limb, truncal, and lower-limb flexion. The reflex follows a similar, though not identical, pattern between individuals and is distinguished from the subsequent autonomic nervous system responses (e.g., phasic heart rate acceleration and deceleration; SC increases) and voluntary motor movements (i.e., postural adjustments and orienting toward a stimulus source) that have a longer latency and are characterized by greater interindividual variation in form and duration (Howard & Ford, 1992).

Generating and measuring the human startle response is relatively simple. It is usually accomplished by exposing individuals to stimuli that have an appropriate combination of (high) intensity and (sudden) onset and then quantifying the magnitude of muscular or autonomic reactivity they produce. Acoustic stimuli, either brief bursts of white noise or pure tones, with intensities ranging from 85 to 116 dB, are commonly used for generating startle responses in the laboratory. In humans, the startle reflex is typically measured from EMG recordings of the contraction of the orbicularis oculi muscle that subserves eyeblink response, an index that is considered the most reliable and persistent component of the startle complex (Landis & Hunt, 1939). Eyeblink responses are typically elicited by an acoustic stimulus (e.g., a brief burst of loud white noise presented over headphones), although visual (e.g., light flashes) and tactile stimuli (e.g., air puffs) can also be used. The orbicularis oculi EMG signal typically is scored off-line using mathematical algorithms or visual inspection to determine the onset latency and magnitude, in microvolts, of the muscle contraction.

In contrast to clear and consistent evidence regarding subjective startle as a core feature of PTSD, laboratory evidence for exaggerated startle is equivocal. As summarized in Table 11.2, 19 published laboratory studies have compared the acoustic eyeblink startle reflex in individuals with and without PTSD. Data analyses in all of these studies have focused on indices of baseline or overall startle amplitude. Some also examined group differences in habituation of the startle response or included more complex manipulations (prepulse inhibition, e.g., Grillon, Morgan, Southwick, Davis, & Charney, 1996; fear potentiation of startle, e.g., Grillon, Ameli, Goddard, Woods, & Davis, 1994). Overall, 11 out of the 19 studies have reported significant blink-amplitude differences between individuals with and without PTSD. This trend suggests that heightened EMG-indexed startle is associated with PTSD but also that there may be one or more important moderating or mediating factors that have not been consistently addressed by procedures used in past startle studies.

What might account for the discrepancy between findings from self-report versus psychophysiological studies of startle? One theoretically and biologically substantive possibility is that exaggerated startle in PTSD is a context- or state-dependent phenomenon related to anxiety (Grillon & Morgan, 1999; Grillon, Morgan, Davis, & Southwick, 1998b). This hypothesis follows from research by Davis and colleagues (e.g., Davis, Walker, & Lee, 1997, 1999) on the neurobiology of fear, anxiety, and startle. The evidence shows that, although amplitude of the startle response is potentiated by both exposure to contextual threat (i.e., anxiety, as in returning to the location of previous aversive conditioning) and explicit threat (i.e., fear, as in exposure to a conditioned stimulus signaling imminent shock), these responses are mediated by different neurobiological systems. Specifically, the response conditional to contextual threat is mediated by the corticotropin-releasing hormone (CRH) system of the bed nucleus of the stria terminalis, whereas the response conditional to explicit threat cues is mediated by the central nucleus of the amygdala.

The body of findings based on humans suggests that exaggerated startle in PTSD is an anxiety-based or context-dependent phenomenon. It appears that differences between groups with and without PTSD are most reliably observed under test conditions involving distal anticipation of an aversive stimulus and are not observed under conditions involving proximal threat. As shown in Table 11.2, all 4 studies involving contextual anxiety cues (e.g., an-

TABLE 11.2. Studies That Have Examined Exaggerated Startle, As Measured from the Eyeblink Response, in Individuals with and without PTSD

Study	Sample gender and trauma type	Sample size	Startle amplitude for PTSD > non-PTSD	Procedures create aversive context
Butler et al. (1990)	Combat	PTSD = 20 Non = 18	Yes	No
Cuthbert et al. (2003)	Assorted traumas	PTSD = 22 Non = 108	No	No
Grillon & Morgan (1999)	Combat	PTSD = 13 Non = 14	Yes	Yes
Grillon, Morgan, Davis, & Southwick (1998a)	Combat	PTSD = 19 Non = 13	Yes	No
Grillon, Morgan, Davis, & Southwick (1998b)	Combat	PTSD = 34 Non = 31	Yes	Yes
Grillon, Morgan, Southwick, Davis, & Charney (1996)	Combat	PTSD = 21 Non = 27	No	No
Ladwig et al. (2002)	Cardiac survivors	PTSD = 11 Non = 19	Yes	No
Medina, Mejia, Schell, Dawson, & Margolin (2001)	Domestic abuse	PTSD = 7 Non = 39	No	No
Metzger et al. (1999)	Childhood sexual abuse	PTSD = 21 Non = 13	No	No
Morgan, Grillon, Southwick, Nagy, et al. (1995)	Combat	PTSD = 18 Non = 11	Yes	Yes
Morgan, Grillon, Southwick, Davis, & Charney (1995)	Combat	PTSD = 9 Non = 10	Yes	Yes
Morgan, Grillon, Southwick, Davis, & Charney (1996)	Combat	PTSD = 10 Non = 22	Yes	No
Morgan, Grillon, Lubin, & Southwick (1997)	Sexual assault	PTSD = 13 Non = 16	Yes	No
Orr, Lasko, Shalev, & Pitman (1995)	Combat	PTSD = 37 Non = 19	Yes	No
Shalev, Peri, Orr, Bonne, & Pitman (1997)	Assorted traumas	PTSD = 30 Non = 28	Yes	No
Orr, Solomon, et al. (1997)	Combat	PTSD = 19 Non = 74	No	No

(continued)

TABLE 11.2. *(continued)*

Study	Sample gender and trauma type	Sample size	Startle amplitude for PTSD > non-PTSD	Procedures create aversive context
Ross et al. (1989)	Combat	PTSD = 9 Non = 9	No	No
Shalev et al. (2000)	Assorted traumas; mainly MVA	PTSD = 36 Non = 182	No	No
Shalev, Orr, Peri, Schreiber, & Pitman (1992)	Unspecified trauma	PTSD = 14 Non = 34	No	No

ticipation of a threatened shock or needle stick) found significant group differences in baseline startle amplitude, whereas only 7 of 14 studies that lack explicit anticipation of aversive stimulation found such differences. More direct evidence has been provided by Grillon et al. (1998b), who examined startle responses in veterans with and without PTSD during an initial laboratory session that involved no aversive manipulation, followed several days later by startle testing during an aversive conditioning procedure that involved anticipation of a mild shock. Significant group differences in baseline startle amplitude were observed only during session 2, suggesting that group effects were linked to the anxiogenic context in which the shock conditioning took place. No group differences in the fear response to presentation of conditioned threat cues (i.e., a CS+) were found, consistent with the possibility that exaggerated startle in PTSD is linked exclusively to the neurobiological system underlying contextual anxiety and not to the system underlying fear.

A recent study by Pole, Neylan, Best, Orr, and Marmar (2003) found that PTSD symptom severity was positively related to SC response magnitude under low and moderate but not high (i.e., imminent) threat conditions. Eyeblink EMG response magnitude was positively related to symptom severity only under the moderate threat condition. When the physiological responses measured under low threat were added to a regression model predicting PTSD symptom severity, they explained an additional 22% of the variance beyond the 11% explained by self-reported startle alone. This finding is especially interesting because it suggests that self-reported startle and physiological measures of startle may be tapping different aspects of PTSD symptom severity.

Persistent Autonomic Arousal

A chronic stress-related disorder such as PTSD has potential to produce long-term dysregulation of sympathetic activity that would be manifested as, for example, persistent elevations in BP, HR, and SC levels. Some of these alterations are recognized as precursors to serious health consequences, including hypertension and cardiovascular disease (Blanchard, 1990). In fact, a recent study showed evidence of increased atrioventricular conduction deficits, non-specific ECG abnormalities, and infarctions in a group of 54 Vietnam veterans with combat-related PTSD (Boscarino & Chang, 1999). The presence of these cardiovascular abnormalities appeared unrelated to comorbid depression and other anxiety disorders, alcohol consumption, smoking, demographic variables, body mass, and so forth.

Questions about elevated psychophysiological levels in PTSD typically have been addressed through second-order analyses applied to data collected during challenge studies involving trauma-related or threat (i.e., electric shock) tasks. Physiological levels are recorded while subjects sit quietly prior to exposure to the primary study stimuli or tasks. Some studies have reported elevated HR, BP, and SC levels at rest in participants with PTSD compared with controls (Blanchard, 1990; Casada et al., 1998; Kinzie et al., 1998; Orr et al., 2000), whereas a number of other studies have not (Blanchard et al., 1994; Blanchard et al., 1986; McFall et al., 1990; Orr et al., 1993; Pitman et al., 1990; Shalev et al., 1993). Relative elevations in HR and BP levels, recorded manually by a triage nurse, also have been found in a retrospective examination of the medical records of Vietnam combat veterans with PTSD who were seeking medical or psychiatric help at a VA hospital, compared with similar help-seeking Vietnam-era veterans without PTSD (Gerardi, Keane, Cahoon, & Klauminzer, 1994).

It is problematic to draw conclusions regarding basal physiological state based on data collected prior to a challenge procedure or medical appointment because, as noted elsewhere (Buckley & Kaloupek, 2001; Gerardi et al., 1994; Prins et al., 1995), higher readings for individuals with PTSD may be the result of entering a psychologically threatening situation rather than reflecting a biologically stable elevation in autonomic activation. Thus anxiety generated by anticipation of the trauma-related stimuli may explain the observed elevations in resting psychophysiological levels. One way to address this possibility is to collect physiological data during a laboratory session when participants know that they will not discuss or be exposed to trauma-related material. Very few studies of PTSD have assessed basal psychophysiological levels outside of a context that includes exposure to trauma-related cues. One strategy for circumventing anticipatory arousal is to collect basal readings during a time when individuals are not expecting to confront reminders of their traumatic experience. Two studies that took this approach (McFall, Veith, & Murberg, 1992; Orr, Meyerhoff, et al., 1998) found comparable physiological levels at rest for combat veterans with and without PTSD.

Another approach to assessing tonic physiological levels is to measure activity outside of a laboratory or medical setting. This procedure has the advantage of obtaining measures under relatively natural conditions that may provide a more accurate representation of individual physiological activity in relation to life activities and stressors. One study has reported higher ambulatory HR levels in a small sample of Vietnam combat veterans with PTSD (Muraoka, Carlson, & Chemtob, 1998). However, two other studies found comparable mean ambulatory (Beckham, Feldman, et al., 2000) or resting (Orr, Meyerhoff, et al., 1998) HR levels in Vietnam combat veterans with and without PTSD. A study that examined HR during sleep also found comparable HR levels in male, inpatient Vietnam veterans with PTSD and normal controls (Woodward et al., 2000).

Buckley and Kaloupek (2001) conducted a meta-analysis of 34 studies that measured baseline or ambulatory cardiovascular activity, including most of those described previously, with the aim of determining whether the research literature as a whole indicates tonic elevations in physiological activity associated with PTSD. The average effect sizes computed across challenge, acoustic startle, and nonchallenge studies indicated higher basal levels for HR and, to a lesser degree, BP shown by individuals with PTSD. Basal HR was highest among studies involving individuals with chronic PTSD, consistent with the hypothesis that elevated basal cardiovascular activity develops over many years, perhaps as the result of adaptation to repeated stress response.

Studies addressing the question of whether PTSD is characterized by persistent arousal have relied on measures of sympathetic nervous system activity, only recently beginning to examine possible parasympathetic contributions. Three studies by Cohen and colleagues (2000; 1998; 1997) have applied spectral analysis to HR data to quantify variability and tease apart the roles of parasympathetic and sympathetic influences with respect to elevated basal HR. These studies involved individuals with PTSD caused by a variety of trauma exposure types. Results show higher resting HR in participants with PTSD relative to controls. This HR difference is accompanied by lower high-frequency (HF) and higher low-frequency (LF) spectral components, indicating that PTSD is characterized by both increased sympathetic tone (LF component) and decreased parasympathetic tone (HF component) under resting conditions. In contrast, Sahar, Shalev, and Porges (2001) reported normal resting parasympathetic tone in PTSD. They found that trauma-exposed individuals with and without PTSD did not differ on measures of respiratory sinus arrhythmia, which is presumed to index vagal (i.e., parasympathetic) regulation of heart rate.

Whether or not PTSD is associated with long-term alterations of sympathetic and/or parasympathetic activity remains unclear; the findings are mixed, even from studies that did not involve exposure to trauma-related materials. If such alterations exist, they seem to develop over time as PTSD becomes chronic and unremitting. A longitudinal study of trauma victims found that the individuals who eventually developed PTSD showed elevated HR resting levels in the emergency room and 1 week later, but the HR levels were no longer elevated and were comparable to those of individuals who did not develop PTSD at 1- and 4-month follow-ups (Shalev et al., 1998). Thus the initial HR level differences had disappeared even as PTSD became evident and diagnosable. A key question is whether HR levels will again become elevated over time in the subset of individuals who show unremitting PTSD.

The issue of whether there is a long-term alteration of sympathetic activity associated with PTSD is unlikely to be answered by the continued collection of data from small convenience samples in cross-sectional studies primarily designed to test other questions. A stronger scientific strategy is to follow acutely trauma-exposed individuals over an extended period of several years to determine when sympathetic and/or parasympathetic alterations become evident, if at all, and what factors mediate or moderate these changes.

CLINICAL APPLICATIONS OF PSYCHOPHYSIOLOGICAL METHODS

The clinical applicability of psychophysiological findings covered thus far has been primarily in relation to diagnosis. Two other domains of clinical application also have been evident in the literature: prediction of adjustment following trauma exposure and assessment of treatment-related responding.

Predicting Risk and Remission in PTSD

Findings from prospective studies offer some indication that early posttrauma alterations in basal HR may predict the development of PTSD. Resting HR and BP have been measured in studies of miscellaneous trauma survivors (Shalev et al., 1998) and motor vehicle victims (Bryant, Harvey, Guthrie, & Moulds, 2000) during immediate postincident emergency room (ER) or hospital treatment. Both studies found that trauma victims who went on to develop PTSD had significantly higher posttrauma resting HR, but not BP, compared with those who did not develop PTSD. Bryant and Harvey (2002) further reported that five of the original motor vehicle victims who had delayed-onset PTSD (i.e., met diagnostic criteria for PTSD 2 years, but not 6 months, following the traumatic event) also had elevated resting HR levels at the initial posttrauma hospital assessment. Furthermore, Shalev et al. (1998) found comparable resting HR levels between groups with and without PTSD at 1- and 4-month follow-ups, suggesting that only the initial elevation in HR was associated with PTSD risk.

In contrast to findings suggesting that elevated HR shortly after a traumatic event can predict risk of developing PTSD, a study by Blanchard, Hickling, Galovski, and Veazey (2002) found that motor vehicle accident victims with elevated HR levels in the ER were *less* likely to meet criteria for PTSD 13 months after their accidents. The reason for this opposite finding may be due to important methodological differences. In particular, the

Blanchard et al. study recruited individuals seeking treatment for psychological problems related to their accidents approximately 13 months after they occurred, with HR and BP readings obtained retrospectively from ER documents. Selection bias introduced by self-initiated help-seeking may have resulted in a sample that differed in important ways from samples studied by Shalev et al. (1998) and Bryant et al. (2000), which were not limited to individuals who initiated psychological treatment seeking. The Blanchard et al. (2002) study applied an additional restriction that only individuals who were currently symptomatic could be enrolled. Thus sample differences are a credible explanation for the discrepant findings.

Breslau and Davis (1992) conducted a large-scale study of young adults who experienced a traumatic event. They observed that those with chronic PTSD (i.e., lasting 1 year or longer) were more likely to report experiencing psychological and physiological overreactivity to stimuli that symbolized the traumatic event than were individuals who had PTSD that remitted within 1 year. Supporting psychophysiological evidence for this difference in subjective experience comes from a longitudinal study by Blanchard et al. (1996) that examined psychophysiological reactivity in acute trauma victims. In this study, Blanchard and colleagues measured HR and BP responses during trauma-related imagery in individuals who had experienced a recent motor vehicle accident within the previous 1–4 months and then reassessed them 1 year later. Two important findings emerged. First, accident victims with acute PTSD showed greater HR reactivity during trauma-related imagery than those without PTSD, as has been demonstrated consistently in individuals with chronic PTSD. Second, the investigators found that individuals who had PTSD that did not remit within 1 year of the accident produced significantly larger HR responses to the initial trauma-related imagery assessment than individuals who had PTSD that did remit. This latter finding is of substantial importance, because it demonstrates the potential value of early assessment of psychophysiological reactivity for identifying individuals at increased risk for developing chronic PTSD.

Finally, psychophysiology also may have value as a predictor of the clinical course of PTSD. An early study by Meakins and Wilson (1918) exposed soldiers diagnosed with "irritable heart" (probably PTSD) to bright flashes and blank pistol discharges while pulse rate and respiration were monitored. Individuals who showed the larger physiological responses were the ones who were subsequently unable to return to duty.

Assessing Treatment Process and Outcome

The application of psychophysiological methods to treatment-related issues in PTSD remains in its infancy, with only a handful of published studies and case reports. Existing work has focused on two general uses of psychophysiology: tracking of treatment process and demonstration of treatment outcome. Any of the methods discussed earlier could potentially be used to assess whether or not therapy produces measurable changes in physiological reactivity. Very simply, reactivity to trauma-related cues or startle responses could be assessed prior to, and then following, an intervention to determine the degree of changes associated with treatment. The choice of index would be dictated by the nature of the process of interest (i.e., emotion or attention).

Treatment Process Indicators

Exposure-based therapeutic techniques (e.g., imaginal flooding or desensitization) are particularly well suited to process measurement because of a model of efficacy formulated by Foa and Kozak (1986) that identifies three key markers of therapeutic process: initial response to cue exposure, within-session habituation, and between-session habituation. These markers often are assessed by simply asking a client to provide periodic ratings of subjective distress. In addition to, or instead of, self-reported distress, it is possible to continuously monitor physiological arousal for the same purpose. Accordingly, change in physiological arousal might be used by a therapist to determine how best to proceed in a particular session or between sessions. Particularly during exposure-based treatment, a gradual decrease in physiological arousal might be taken as an indication that specific cues are becoming less distressing for the client. Alternatively, a precipitous decrease in arousal might indicate that the client has disengaged from the task, perhaps because it has become overwhelming (Rachman & Whittal, 1989). In contrast, a gradual increase in physiological arousal could indicate that a client is becoming emotionally engaged in the therapeutic task or, if sustained, it might suggest that the particular therapeutic approach was not having the desired effect.

A few studies have examined the use of psychophysiological measures as indicators of emotional arousal during treatment. Most notably, Pitman and colleagues recorded HR, SC, and facial EMG during imaginal flooding treatment (Pitman, Orr, Altman, Longpre, Poire, Macklin, et al., 1996). Strong trends were observed for relationships between both within-session HR habituation ($r = .51, p < .05$) and between-session HR habituation ($r = .46, p < .05$) and reduction in number of daily intrusion symptoms. In contrast, a study that examined treatment of combat-related PTSD using eye movement desensitization and reprocessing (EMDR) therapy did not show these relationships between process indicators and outcome (Pitman, Orr, Altman, Longpre, Poire, & Macklin, 1996). The reason for the difference in findings is not clear, but a recent direct comparison of prolonged exposure and EMDR found that prolonged exposure was more effective in reducing reexperiencing (which includes intrusive recollections of the traumatic event) and avoidance symptoms than EMDR (Taylor et al., 2003). Such evidence raises the intriguing possibility that physiological indicators of therapy process have unique information value in relation to therapeutic process.

Treatment Outcome Indicators

Change in physiological reactivity to trauma-related cues from before treatment to after treatment may provide a useful index of clinical improvement both for group comparisons and individual cases. For example, it can be used to compare the efficacy of one therapy relative to another, or it might be used to determine whether or not a therapy has had the desired effect for a given client. Whatever its potential, use of psychophysiological methods to assess treatment outcome remains a relatively unexplored area in the PTSD literature, with only a few published reports to date. An early case report of combat-related PTSD treated with imaginal flooding by Keane and Kaloupek (1982) demonstrated that improvement was associated with a reduction in HR response magnitude during subsequent recollection of the trauma. Shalev, Orr, and Pitman (1992) found psychophysiological responses during trauma-related imagery to be sensitive to psychiatric improvement following a systematic desensitization procedure. Similarly, Boudewyns and Hyer (1990) reported that decrease in SC response to trauma-related imagery following treatment was associated with a higher "adjustment" score at 3 months posttreatment.

The measurement of HR variability before and after a 4-month course of treatment with the medication fluoxetine was used by Cohen and colleagues (Cohen, Kotler, Matar, & Kaplan, 2000) to assess change in sympathetic and parasympathetic tone and to examine the relationship of such change to improvement in PTSD-related symptoms. An uncontrolled trial by Tucker et al. (2000) found that 10 weeks of treatment with a similar medication, fluvoxamine, produced subjective symptom improvement and showed reduced physiological reactivity to trauma-related imagery by the PTSD patients. Although suggestive, this positive finding must be interpreted with caution, because there is clear evidence that reactivity to trauma-related cues is decreased on a second testing occasion, even when there is no intervening treatment (Blanchard et al., 1996; Keane et al., 1998). Nonetheless, evidence suggests the utility of psychophysiological reactivity as an index of treatment outcome.

There is preliminary evidence suggesting that change in P3 amplitude may provide a useful gauge of a patient's response to treatment with psychotropic medication. Although no studies have directly examined the effects of psychotropic medications on P3 amplitudes in PTSD, one study has reported normal P3 amplitudes in medicated, but not unmedicated, patients with PTSD (Metzger, Orr, Lasko, & Pitman, 1997). Such normalizing effects of medications on P3 amplitude have been reported for other clinical disorders, including depression and attention-deficit/hyperactivity disorder (ADHD). Additionally, increases in P3 amplitude following methylphenidate treatment were found to successfully predict the long-term benefits in children with ADHD (Young, Perros, Price, & Sadler, 1995). Thus assessment of P3 response amplitude appears to hold promise for both predicting and evaluating the efficacy of psychotropic intervention in various clinical disorders (Polich & Herbst, 2000), including PTSD.

APPLICATION OF PSYCHOPHYSIOLOGICAL METHODS TO BASIC PROCESSES

Unconditioned or Defensive Response and Habituation

Autonomic Measures

Similar to startle, a second approach to studying psychophysiological reactivity involves administration of multiple presentations of the same high intensity stimulus, most often a 95-decibel, 500-millisecond, pure tone with 0-millisecond rise and fall times (Orr, Lasko, Shalev, & Pitman, 1995; Shalev, Orr, Peri, Schreiber, & Pitman, 1992). Heart rate and SC responses to the stimulus presentations have been measured, along with eyeblink EMG, to provide indices of autonomic reactivity to the high intensity stimuli. It is important to note that these studies have used stimuli with longer durations than have studies focusing exclusively on EMG startle (e.g., Butler et al., 1990), because longer duration may produce a particular type of physiological reaction termed a defensive response (e.g., Graham, Anthony, & Zeigler, 1983, p. 392) in addition to startle, whereas shorter duration stimuli (< 500 milliseconds) may not produce the defensive component. Response scores for each trial are computed by subtracting the mean level immediately preceding tone onset from the maximum increase in level within a prespecified window following the tone. Because there are differences in the latencies of response onsets, the window is longer for autonomic (1–4 seconds) than for eyeblink (20–200 milliseconds) responses.

An advantage of using a single intensity level is that it allows for examination of decline in response magnitude across trials. This habituation of responding reflects the ability to learn *not* to respond to repetitive stimuli, essentially learning to ignore irrelevant information. Habituation is commonly measured in two ways: absolute and relative. Absolute habituation measures the number of trials required to reach a prespecified criterion for nonresponse, such as two successive trials for which there is no response (or an extremely small one). Relative habituation, on the other hand, measures the rate of decline (i.e., steepness of the slope) in response magnitude across a given set of trials.

The magnitudes of autonomic responses to repeated presentations of intense (i.e. loud) auditory stimuli have been found to be greater in individuals with PTSD. Specifically, they produce larger HR responses and/or show a slower rate of decline of SC response magnitude than individuals without PTSD (Metzger et al., 1999; Orr, Lasko, Metzger, & Pitman, 1997; Orr et al., 1995; Orr, Solomon, Peri, Pitman, & Shalev, 1997; Paige, Reid, Allen, & Newton, 1990; Rothbaum, Kozak, Foa, & Whitaker, 2001; Shalev et al.,

1992; Shalev et al., 2000; Shalev, Peri, Orr, Bonne, & Pitman, 1997). To date, only two studies have failed to find evidence for larger HR responses to loud tones in individuals with PTSD (Rothbaum et al., 2001; Shalev et al., 1997). However, both of these studies did show slower absolute SC response habituation in individuals with PTSD.

Findings in identical twins indicate that that there are strong genetic determinants of responsivity and habituation for both HR (Boomsma & Gabrielli, 1985; Carroll, Hewitt, Last, Turner, & Sims, 1995; Ditto, 1993; Kotchoubei, 1987) and SC (Lykken, Iacono, Haroian, McGue, & Bouchard, 1988). The possibility that the greater HR reactivity and slower decline of SC responses observed in individuals with PTSD may reflect a constitutional risk factor rather than a consequence of trauma was addressed in a recent twin study of Vietnam combat veterans and their identical twin brothers who did not serve in Vietnam. The findings from this study clearly demonstrate that, whereas veterans with combat-related PTSD showed elevated HR responding to startle-producing tones, their genetically identical twin brothers did not (Orr et al., 2003). In addition, a prospective study (Shalev et al., 2000) found that, although trauma victims who went on to develop PTSD showed elevated HR responses to startle-producing tones at 1- and 4-month posttrauma assessments, they did not show these elevated responses at a 1-week posttrauma assessment. Together, these findings provide compelling support for the position that larger HR responses to sudden, loud tones in individuals with PTSD represent an acquired, rather than a preexisting, condition. In contrast to the acquired nature of larger HR responses, the Orr et al. (2003) study also provided suggestive evidence that slower relative SC response habituation reflects a pretrauma vulnerability factor for PTSD. More specifically, both veterans with PTSD and their brothers showed a tendency toward slower SC habituation compared with that shown by the veterans without PTSD and their brothers.

It is important to note that heightened psychophysiological reactivity to intense auditory stimuli is not unique to PTSD; individuals with other types of anxiety disorders show increased reactivity as well. For example, studies of generalized anxiety disorder (GAD), agoraphobia, social phobia (Lader, 1967; Lader & Wing, 1964), and panic disorder (Roth, Ehlers, Taylor, Margraf, & Agras, 1990) have observed a slower decline in SC responses to repeated presentations of intense auditory stimuli for the groups with anxiety disorder.

Electrocortical Measures

Responses to high-intensity stimuli also have been studied by measuring cortical activity, particularly P2 response amplitude, to tones of varying intensity levels. In this work, cortical activity is typically recorded from the central midline (Cz) site while participants passively listen to the random presentations of 74-, 84-, 94-, and 104-decibel tones having rise and fall times of 25 milliseconds (Metzger et al., 2002; Paige et al., 1990). EEG is recorded beginning 100 milliseconds prior to tone onset and ending 500 milliseconds after tone onset. The EEG data from each trial are averaged separately for each tone intensity level, and the P2 response peak (the most positive point between approximately 140 and 230 millisecond posttone onset) is determined for the averaged waveform for each stimulus intensity level. Slope for the P2 response is then calculated from the regression line of the P2 response peaks across tones of increasing intensity.

Studies of electrocortical responses to intense stimuli provide additional evidence consistent with heightened defensive responses in individuals with PTSD. Two ERP studies (Lewine et al., 2002; Paige et al., 1990) found that, when exposed to tones of increasing intensity, male combat veterans with PTSD produced decreased P2 amplitudes to higher intensity tones (i.e., a decreased P2 slope or so-called "reducing" response). This pattern differed from that observed in combat veterans without PTSD and other normal participants, a pattern that reflects the typical "augmenting" whereby P2 amplitudes get progressively larger to louder tones. Paige et al. (1990) interpret the propensity to show diminishing P2 response amplitudes in PTSD as a state of protective inhibition. In other words, the nervous system is thought to have heightened sensitivity to stimulation, to which it adapts in self-protective fashion by dampening the impact of the increasingly loud tones.

Two studies contrast with the electrocortical "reducing" findings. A study of female veterans who served as nurses in Vietnam used a procedure nearly identical to that employed by Paige et al. (1990) but found increasing, rather than decreasing, P2 response amplitudes to tones of increasing intensities for participants with PTSD (Metzger et al., 2002). Finally, children with PTSD resulting from physical and/or sexual abuse also were found to produce increased P2 response amplitudes to progressively louder tones compared with abused children without PTSD (McPherson, Newton, Ackerman, Oglesby, & Dykman, 1997). Interpretation of this finding is complicated by the fact that the paradigm used with children deviated substantially from the passive-listening paradigm used in studies with adults in that the children were required to make a button-press response to all tones and were provided with feedback and a monetary award for responding quickly and without blinking.

Conditionability

Conditionability refers to the tendency to acquire and resist extinction of conditioned responses. Individual differences in this characteristic have been offered as one explanation for the fact that only some of the individuals who are exposed to a traumatic event go on to develop PTSD. In a test of this model, Orr and colleagues (Orr et al., 2000) randomly presented participants with two different-colored circles on a computer monitor. One of the colored circles (CS+) was paired with a highly annoying, but not painful, 500-millisecond electric shock (unconditioned stimulus; UCS), whereas the other colored circle (CS-) was not. Individuals with PTSD resulting from various traumas demonstrated larger HR, SC, and facial EMG responses to CS+ compared with CS- trials during the acquisition phase when only the CS+ was paired with the UCS. They also demonstrated larger differential SC responses during an extinction phase in which participants were told they would no longer receive the electric shocks. These findings suggest that individuals with PTSD acquire a larger and more persistent conditioned autonomic response to an aversive stimulus.

Two other studies failed to find evidence for increased conditionability among individuals with PTSD. In one, Gulf War veterans with PTSD actually were slower than those without PTSD in acquiring a conditioned response to a CS+ paired with a mild electric shock UCS (Grillon & Morgan, 1999). This study used eyeblink response to a startle probe presented in the context of CS+ and CS- rather than autonomic measures to assess conditioned response strength. It is noteworthy that veterans with PTSD demonstrated increased eyeblink during both CS- and CS+ training trials, suggesting a generalized fear response. A second study of mixed trauma victims used a loud noise as the UCS and recorded both SC and HR responses to CS+ and CS- presentations (colored slides) to assess CR strength. Individuals with PTSD produced larger SC responses during the extinction phase to both CS+ and CS- trials, but they did not show a larger differential fear response (Peri et al., 2000). The explanation for these discrepant findings is not clear, but it may well be related to differences in both experimental methods and dependent measures.

Assessing Emotional and Clinical States

Emotional and motivational states have been studied in both clinical and normal populations using electrophysiological measures of cortical arousal. This research is based on neuropsychological models relating different patterns of brain activity to psychologically significant states. In their simplest form (Davidson, 1984; Heller, 1990), these models contend that greater activation of the left than the right frontal hemisphere is associated with positive emotional states and approach-related motivational tendencies, whereas relatively greater activation of the right frontal hemisphere is associated with negative emotional states and withdrawal-related tendencies. Although findings from a number of studies support this positive-left/negative-right link, a subset of studies report inconsistent, and even contradictory, results. Of special note are recent studies showing that greater left-sided frontal activation is associated with negative emotional states, specifically anger (Harmon-Jones & Allen, 1998; Harmon-Jones & Sigelman, 2001) and anxiety (Heller, Nitschke, Etienne, & Miller, 1997). Such findings have led researchers to revise original asymmetry models in favor of more complex ones. For example, Heller and colleagues (Heller et al., 1997) have proposed that negative emotional states, including anxiety subtypes, are associated with unique patterns of regional brain activation. Specifically, "anxious apprehension" (i.e., rumination and worry) is associated with greater left-sided frontal activity, whereas "anxious arousal" (i.e., physiological arousal and hyperreactivity) is associated with greater right-sided activity, particularly in tempoparietal regions.

To date, two studies have examined the relative activation of the left versus the right hemisphere in individuals with PTSD. In a study of male Vietnam combat veterans, those with PTSD and no comorbid major depression showed greater left-sided frontal activation than veterans without PTSD (Metzger et al., 1998). Although greater left-sided frontal activation has been found to be associated with anger and, therefore, might represent increased irritability and anger in PTSD (criterion D2), this pattern also can be viewed as consistent with anxious apprehension in PTSD. A second study examined the relationship between PTSD symptom severity and patterns of regional (frontal, temporal, and parietal) brain asymmetry in female Vietnam nurse veterans with current, lifetime, or no PTSD (Metzger et al., in press). In contrast to the findings for male combat veterans, measures of PTSD symptom severity were not related to frontal asymmetry. However, severity of PTSD-related arousal symptoms was associated with increased right-sided parietal activation. Although different, the findings from both studies support the contention that particular patterns of asymmetrical brain activation are associated with negative states of emotion or arousal and encourage further application of this electrophysiological approach to the study of PTSD.

POTENTIAL INFLUENCES ON THE QUALITY AND VALIDITY OF ASSESSMENT

Appropriateness of Trauma Cue Presentations

A critical factor potentially accounting for part of the imperfect association between psychophysiological reactivity and PTSD diagnosis (e.g., Keane et al., 1998) is cue adequacy. A question that must be addressed each time a trauma-related psychophysiological challenge is administered concerns how well the stimulus material matches the individual's traumatic event. In this respect, there may be an advantage to idiographic approaches to trauma cue selection. Although standardized presentations benefit from uniformity and their potential for allowing tight experimental control, they suffer the disadvantage of variable correspondence with individual experience. Idiographic presentations may be designed to closely approximate the internal (memory) representations of the traumatic experience and thereby improve the validity of assessment.

Compliance with Protocol Demands

Any psychophysiological protocol requires that participants understand and adhere to a particular set of demands. The complexity of these demands will be determined by the nature of the protocol and the physiological measures being obtained. Validity and interpretability of the psychophysiological data will be significantly influenced by the degree of compliance. Even simple tasks, such as listening to a series of tones, require that individuals sit quietly and keep their eyes open. Although these may appear to be modest requirements, they can be challenging for an individual who is, for example, very anxious. More complex tasks may make significant demands on the physical and cognitive abilities of even well-functioning individuals, including the need to understand and remember a detailed set of instructions, concentrating and focusing attention for a sustained period, discriminating among several different types of stimuli, and staying motivated to perform a task despite the fact that it is repeated for tens or hundreds of trials. Of particular importance to trauma-related assessment are the emotional demands of the task. It may be very difficult for individuals to remain engaged in a procedure that produces significant emotional discomfort, as when they are exposed to reminders of a traumatic event. Individuals may try to reduce distress by averting their gaze from a visual stimulus or by distracting themselves when they are supposed to be vividly recalling an upsetting experience. Emotional distress may cause an increase in motor activity, such as fidgeting, that can artificially elevate physiological activity.

Occasional deviations from a protocol are inevitable; therefore, it is routine to plan ways to identify them and assess their impact. It is important to have some means for monitoring an individual as he or she goes through the assessment protocol. A closed-circuit video system can be used to observe gross body movements or to verify that an individual is generally complying with task demands. A former research participant decided to use the initial baseline-recording period of a study as an opportunity to clean out his wallet, even though he had been previously instructed to sit quietly. A glance at the closed-circuit TV monitor made it clear why the physiological measures had suddenly become erratic. Emotional provocation or challenge testing also offer unique opportunities for observing an individual during exposure to trauma-related cues, offering another reason that it is advantageous to have some means by which the individual can be unobtrusively observed. Although individuals' failure to comply with task demands, such as viewing or vividly recalling trauma-related materials, may reduce the interpretability of psychophysiological data, it also may be clinically informative as a form of behavior relevant to their PTSD.

Dissociation

It is possible that some psychological traits or response dispositions serve to decouple the relationship between subjective emotional experiences and psychophysiological reactivity. For example, individuals with dissociative tendencies may show reduced physiological reactivity to trauma-related stimuli, even though they report a high level of PTSD-related symptoms. The tendency to dissociate could partially explain the roughly 40% of individuals who meet full DSM criteria for PTSD despite being physiologically nonreactive. In a demonstration of this point, Griffin, Resick, and Mechanic (1997) assessed physiological reactivity in women who had developed PTSD following sexual assault and found that women who retrospectively reported greater peritraumatic dissociation (depersonalization) at the time of the rape were less physiologically reactive while describing the experience in detail compared to women who reported less dissociation. However, the negative relationship between self-reported peritraumatic dissociation and psychophysiological reactivity in the laboratory was not replicated in a recent study by Kaufman et al. (2002). This work was based on secondary analysis applied to the very large data set available for the multisite study in which Keane et al. (1998) conducted challenge testing with male Vietnam combat veterans. One potentially important difference between this study and the one by Griffin and colleagues is the chronic nature of PTSD in the veteran sample and the contrasting acute nature of PTSD among the assault victims.

More broadly, chronic depersonalization disorder has been found to be associated with smaller SC reactivity to unpleasant pictures (Sierra et al., 2002). And, in contrast to the findings of decreased physiological reactivity, results from a study of individuals who had previously suffered a serious cardiac event suggest that reactivity may be increased in individuals who report high peritraumatic dissociation (Ladwig et al., 2002). Individuals who retrospectively reported high dissociation were found to produce larger SC and eyeblink EMG responses to startling tones than individuals who reported little or no peritraumatic dissociation. Within the group that reported high peritraumatic dissociation, comparisons between individuals with full or partial PTSD and those without PTSD yielded significantly larger EMG, but not SC, responses to the loud tones in the PTSD subgroup.

Dissimulation

Available evidence is limited on the issue of faking in the context of PTSD-related psychophysiological assessment. A study by Gerardi, Blanchard, and Kolb (1989) showed that veterans with PTSD were unable to significantly alter their responses when instructed to do so, whereas veterans without PTSD were able to increase their physiological reactivity so as not to differ from those with PTSD on several measures. On the other hand, a high level of correct classification regarding true PTSD status was obtained when a previously used HR cutoff score was combined with baseline HR level as predictors. Similarly, Orr and Pitman (1993) instructed a group of veterans without PTSD to try to increase their reactivity during trauma-related imagery so as to appear as though they had PTSD. A discriminant function based on SC and corrugator EMG responses accurately classified 16 of 16 veterans when they were not trying to simulate PTSD and 12 of the 16 veterans when they were attempting to simulate PTSD, this despite the fact that during simulation these veterans were able to produce HR responses as large as those of individuals with PTSD.

A study of PTSD related to the missile attacks on Israel during the Gulf War of 1991 (Laor et al., 1998) examined HR, BP, and forehead EMG responses to audiotape presentations of various experiences, including a set of stimuli associated with a missile attack (e.g., alert siren, emergency code words, and missile explosion). Participants were asked to try to "fake" their physiological responses by either increasing them (non-PTSD group) or preventing them from increasing (PTSD group) during a second presentation of the missile-attack audiotape. Contrary to the findings of Gerardi et al. (1989), the non-PTSD group was unable to significantly increase their physiological responses during the simulation, whereas individuals with PTSD were able to significantly decrease their responses when instructed to do so. Taken together, these findings suggest some potential for dissimulation but indicate that it is difficult for individuals without PTSD, as a group, to reliably simulate the pattern of physiological responses of individuals with PTSD.

Individual Biological Influences

A variety of factors that can influence psychophysiological reactivity arise from characteristics such as age, sex, skin pigmentation, continental race, menstrual cycle phase, and physical fitness level. Although relationships to autonomic activity have been established in the general psychophysiological literature, there are few examples from the trauma literature that directly examine the impact of these factors. One study by Shalev et al. (1993) did find that female participants with PTSD demonstrated 33% (albeit nonsignificantly) greater physiological responding to their trauma script than males with PTSD. This example raises the question of whether such differences are sex related per se or the result of covarying influences such as differences in types of trauma exposure between men and women. More work like this can be expected as the literature on the psychophysiology of trauma develops.

Pharmacological Agents

Central and peripheral physiological levels and responses can be strongly influenced by a variety of substances, including prescribed and nonprescribed medications, alcohol, caffeine, and nicotine. For example, beta-blocking agents that are commonly prescribed for hypertension can reduce cardiovascular activity level and attenuate reactivity (Fredrikson et al., 1985). The anticholinergic drugs that are commonly used to treat depression can produce a substantial elevation in resting HR level. As noted previously, psychotropic medications have been found to normalize ERP components, particularly P3 amplitude, in clinical samples (Metzger, Orr, Lasko, & Pitman, 1997). Unfortunately, little is known about the impact of many of the medications on psychophysiological responding, making it difficult to estimate their impact.

Although it is not often possible to perform clinical psychophysiological testing on individuals in a medication-free state, on occasion such testing may be coordinated with a change in medication and may take place prior to beginning a new regimen. This assumes that the biological half-life of the discontinued medication is relatively short. In some instances, it may be possible to use physiological measures that are not influenced by a particular medication. For example, Fredrikson et al. (1985) found that measures of cardiovascular activity and reactivity were influenced by a beta blocker but that SC level and reactivity were not. In research it may be possible to obtain a subgroup of medication-free individuals who can be compared with those taking medications, as well as with the control group(s). Such subgroup comparisons can provide effect size estimates to guide determinations of whether medications are having a substantive effect on the measures of interest. Medication use by patients or participants should be noted as a matter of course, so that this information is available for subsequent consideration (e.g., to account for anomalies in responding).

Nicotine, caffeine, and alcohol are commonly used substances that also can influence physiological systems. Unfortunately, they do not have uniform impact across physiological systems, and the effect of withdrawal can be as problematic as that of consumption (Hughes, 1993; Lane & Williams, 1985; Lyvers & Miyata, 1993; Perkins, Epstein, Jennings, & Stiller, 1986; Ratliff-Crain, O'Keeffe, & Baum, 1989). For example, it is a common practice to ask individuals to abstain from using nicotine or caffeine for a period of time (often 30 minutes or more) prior to testing. However, some individuals may find that even brief abstinence produces discomfort, and it is difficult to know how this will influence test results. Despite uncertainty about how to adjust for their effects, it is typically a good idea to obtain estimates of an individual's daily consumption of nicotine, caffeine (coffee and soda), and alcohol prior to testing.

POTENTIAL CONCEPTUAL INSIGHTS

Relationshiop between PTSD and Other Disorders

Much of the preceding discussion has focused on psychophysiological methods applied to questions of clinical interest. In addition, psychophysiological data can provide evidence for conceptual models concerning the nature of PTSD. For example, it may be noteworthy that the heightened physiological reactivity to trauma-related stimuli observed in PTSD is similar to that observed when phobia-related cues are presented to individuals with simple phobia (Cook et al., 1988; McNeil et al., 1993). Simple phobics show larger HR and SC responses during imagery of their phobic objects than do other anxious groups who have less specific fears, such as agoraphobics. In fact, individuals with agoraphobia have been found to be physiologically unresponsive during imagery of their fear-related contexts (Cook et al., 1988; Zander &

McNally, 1988). An important factor in determining or modulating physiological reactivity across various anxiety disorders appears to be the specificity of the fear. In terms of Lang's (1985) bioinformational theory of emotion, the memory networks associated with specific fears may be more readily or strongly activated than less specific fears because the external cues used to trigger the fear are more closely matched with its internal representation. Thus both PTSD and simple phobia would appear to have fear networks that are highly specific and thereby easily activated.

Whereas the specificity of responses to trauma-related cues suggests a similarity with simple phobia, the findings of slower habituation of SC responses to intense auditory stimuli (Orr et al., 1995; Shalev et al., 1992) suggest a similarity with disorders characterized by more diffuse forms of anxiety. Interestingly, one study (Lader, 1967) that included a group of individuals with simple phobia reported that they did not differ from nonanxious individuals in their rate of SC habituation. Also, as noted earlier, both PTSD and panic disorder have been found to be associated with an elevated eyeblink startle response. Increased P50 ratio (Gillette et al., 1997) and reduced P3 amplitude (McFarlane et al., 1993) observed in PTSD also have been observed for other disorders, including schizophrenia and depression. Polich and Herbst (2000) described the P3 component of ERP as a general, but nonetheless utilitarian, measure of "cognitive efficiency that reflects how well an individual's CNS can process and incorporate incoming information" (p. 6). The nonspecificity of these findings suggests that various clinical disorders may share similar sensory and cognitive impairments. Taken together, these psychophysiological studies provide information that may be important in shaping the conceptualization of PTSD as an anxiety disorder, as well as identifying features that it shares with other disorders outside the anxiety spectrum.

Underlying Biological and Psychological Mechanisms of PTSD

The possibility that exaggerated startle in PTSD is a context-dependent phenomenon reflecting activation of the corticotropin-releasing hormone (CRH) system of the bed nucleus of the stria terminalis is consistent with evidence suggesting that patients with PTSD show elevated levels of CRH in the cerebrospinal fluid (Baker et al., 1999; Bremner et al., 1997) coupled with low basal levels of cortisol, a hormone that inhibits the production of CRH (Yehuda, 2002). Considered in conjunction with evidence that CRH potentiates startle (Lee & Davis, 1997; Swerdlow, Britton, & Koob, 1989) and that hydrocortisone administration attenuates startle (Buchanan, Brechtel, Sollers, & Lovallo, 2001), these findings point to a possible link between the symptom of exaggerated startle and hypothalamic–pituitary–adrenal-axis abnormalities in PTSD.

A second potentially fruitful avenue for research might be to examine whether the laboratory-based demonstration that baseline startle amplitude is context dependent can be validated by the "real world" experience of patients with PTSD. That is, does exaggerated startle occur primarily in specific situations or contexts, and, if so, what defines them? To do so, it may be necessary to conduct ambulatory assessment of startle responding and develop instruments for assessing self-reported startle with increased temporal resolution. Research along these lines has the potential to clarify the discrepancy between findings from self-report versus psychophysiological studies of exaggerated startle and to shed light on the mechanisms underlying this symptom.

Finally, decreased P3 response amplitude is popularly interpreted as indicative of attention-related difficulties. Yet Felmingham et al. (2002) found that reduced P3 response amplitudes were associated with increased numbing symptoms in their study of assault and accident victims. It is possible that reduced P3 response amplitude in PTSD reflects disinterest or lack of emotional engagement with a task, rather than a primary disturbance in attention. The fact that female Vietnam nurse veterans with PTSD showed larger, rather than smaller, P3 response amplitudes (Metzger et al., 2002) additionally brings into question the primary psychological mechanism related to this cortical response abnormality. However, it is possible that the modulation of the P3 response in the nurse veterans was related to increased, as opposed to decreased, emotional engagement. The authors speculate that the larger P3 amplitude responses shown by this high-functioning PTSD sample might represent an effortful "overcompensation" of attention resources to ensure successful performance of the task (Metzger et al., 2002). It will be important for future research to address alternative psychological factors that potentially mediate this cortical response abnormality in PTSD.

A RECOMMENDATION FOR RESEARCH AND CLINICAL PRACTICE

Reliance on interview-based self-report as the means for establishing a formal PTSD diagnosis (e.g., according to DSM-IV criteria) is standard for mental disorders and is practical in terms of applicability. On the other hand, PTSD is relatively unique among the diagnostic categories for mental disorders in requiring specification of the experience that is presumed to have caused symptoms to develop. Although this requirement can be cumbersome and can precipitate diagnostic ambiguities, it also can be viewed as a positive reflection of the knowledge base on which the diagnostic criteria for PTSD have developed. Which is to say, if we knew the experiences that cause depression or schizophrenia, this information would likely be included as part of the diagnostic criteria for these disorders, too. In order to further extend PTSD as a model diagnostic entity, it may be time to consider refining the criteria to make them less dependent on subjective evidence. In particular, we propose that the accumulated findings from studies using trauma-relevant challenge tasks are substantial enough to justify a greater role for direct psychophysiological evidence in the diagnostic determination.

Relocation of the DSM symptom concerned with physiological reactivity to trauma cues from the arousal category (D) to the reexperiencing category (B) was a first step in this direction. However, although it captures the emphasis on evocation of emotion-related physiological reactions, it still allows the evidence to remain subjective. This latitude seems unnecessary given the accumulation of psychophysiological findings and, as we have noted earlier, the increased availability of relatively inexpensive and easy-to-use physiological recording devices. Furthermore, there is already a subjective symptom option in category B referenced to "intense psychological distress" upon exposure to trauma cues (B4), which potentially overlaps with the content of symptom B5. Given the fact that only one B symptom is required for the PTSD diagnosis, these symptoms appear to be redundant as subjective complaints.

An alternative approach might be to separate the inherently subjective symptoms in category B (B1–4) from symptoms that can be demonstrated by objective physiological reactivity (B5). Consistency with the current diagnostic standard could be maintained by requiring one symptom from the B1–4 group *or* concrete psychophysiological evidence consistent with B5. Among the advantages of this approach is that it preserves the possibility that some individuals who may have difficulty reporting on their subjective state (e.g., young children; certain stroke victims) would still have a means for providing evidence of reexperiencing.

This call for a limited application of psychophysiological methods to document physiological arousal to trauma reminders does not add a new requirement for the presence of physiological reactivity to confer the diagnosis of PTSD. It can, however, serve as a starting point for refinement of the diagnostic standard for PTSD and can stimulate new avenues of empirical study that may lead to such a development. Exaggerated startle response (D5) is another symptom that may eventually warrant consideration of formal physiological documentation, but the current evidentiary base for this change is not as well developed as that for physiological reactivity. It should be added that this proposal is not intended as an endorsement of the taxonomic approach to PTSD diagnosis; it merely recognizes the important role that DSM plays in providing standardization for the study and treatment of the disorder, given the limits of our knowledge about the enduring impact of traumatic stress.

CONCLUSION

Psychophysiological assessment sometimes has an exaggerated image as a truly objective means for detecting an individual's psychological or emotional state. Although psychophysiological measures and methods can provide unique information, they are not inherently more valid or objective than typical assessment methods involving self-report or interviews. It is usually necessary to interpret psychophysiological information in the context of evidence collected via these other assessment methods. Because it is not uncommon for psychophysiological assessments to provide ambiguous evidence about diagnostic status or psychological state just as other methods do, there is often no choice but to rely on convergence from multiple sources of evidence. Even so, divergence between different sources of information can be highly informative and can provide clinical guidance. For example, an individual who reports that he or she is not bothered by reminders of a previous traumatic event yet who shows heightened physiological reactivity in the laboratory when recalling the event may be unaware of or denying the impact that this event is having on his or her emotional well-being. On the other hand, an individual who shows a generalized pattern of high distress reporting (e.g., one of the so-called "overreporters") may be more easily engaged in constructive clinical dialogue about his or her reporting style when presented with evidence that his or her physiological reactivity is not consistent with his or her subjective experience.

To date, most PTSD-related psychophysiological research has focused on demonstrating differences between groups of individuals with and without PTSD. Although this work has contributed substantially to the conceptual understanding of the disorder, the evidence for group differences rarely has direct value for the clinician and individual patient. This disjunction between laboratory and clinic reflects the fact that little effort has been devoted to the translation of research findings into clinically useful applications. For example, although a number of studies have demonstrated greater physiological responses to trauma-related stimuli, larger eyeblink startle, and reduced P3 responses in groups of individuals with PTSD, they provide little guidance for determining whether the physiological responses of a given individual are "heightened," represent an "exaggerated" startle response, or reflect "disturbed" attention. Perhaps future diagnostic criteria will offer standards for determining whether a particular response represents a clinically meaningful elevation or diminution. The research that is required in order for this to happen fits with a major challenge facing health care in the United States and worldwide concerning the need for increased efforts to translate laboratory and preclinical research into clinical advances (Fontanarosa & DeAngelis, 2003; Sung et al, 2003). It is encouraging that the blossoming of evidence regarding psychophysiology and PTSD over the past 10 years may now have reached the point at which it can provide a suitable base from which to pursue this translational goal in the trauma field.

REFERENCES

Allen, J. J. (2002). The role of psychophysiology in clinical assessment: ERPs in the evaluation of memory. *Psychophysiology*, *39*(3), 261–280.

American Psychiatric Association. (1994). *Diagnostic and statistical manual of mental disorders* (4th ed.). Washington, DC: Author.

Andreassi, J. L. (1980). *Psychophysiology: Human behavior and physiological response.* New York: Oxford University Press.

Attias, J., Bleich, A., Furman, V., & Zinger, Y. (1996). Event-related potentials in posttraumatic stress disorder of combat origin. *Biological Psychiatry, 40*(5), 373–381.

Attias, J., Bleich, A., & Gilat, S. (1996). Classification of veterans with posttraumatic stress disorder using visual brain-evoked P3s to traumatic stimuli. *British Journal of Psychiatry, 168*, 110–116.

Baker, D. G., West, S. A., Nicholson, W. E., Ekhator, N. N., Kasckow, J. W., Hill, K. K., et al. (1999). Serial CSF corticotropin-releasing hormone levels and adrenocortical activity in combat veterans with posttraumatic stress disorder. *American Journal of Psychiatry, 156*(4), 585–588.

Beckham, J. C., Feldman, M. E., Barefoot, J. C., Fairbank, J. A., Helms, M. J., Haney, T. L., et al. (2000). Ambulatory cardiovascular activity in Vietnam combat veterans with and without posttraumatic stress disorder. *Journal of Consulting and Clinical Psychology, 68*(2), 269–276.

Beckham, J. C., Moore, S. D., & Reynolds, V. (2000). Interpersonal hostility and violence in Vietnam combat veterans with chronic posttraumatic stress disorder: A review of theoretical models and empirical evidence. *Aggression and Violent Behavior, 5*, 451–466.

Beckham, J. C., Vrana, S. R., Barefoot, J. C., Feldman, M. E., Fairbank, J., & Moore, S. D. (2002). Magnitude and duration of cardiovascular responses to anger in Vietnam veterans with and without posttraumatic stress disorder. *Journal of Consulting and Clinical Psychology, 70*(1), 228–234.

Beuzeron-Mangina, J. H. (2000). Clinical psychophysiology in neurological, neurosurgical and psychiatric diseases. *International Journal of Psychophysiology, 37*, 1–2.

Blanchard, E. B. (1990). Elevated basal levels of cardiovascular responses in Vietnam veterans with PTSD: A health problem in the making? *Journal of Anxiety Disorders, 4*, 233–237.

Blanchard, E. B., Hickling, E. J., Buckley, T. C., Taylor, A. E., Vollmer, A., & Loos, W. R. (1996). Psychophysiology of posttraumatic stress disorder related to motor vehicle accidents: Replication and extension. *Journal of Consulting and Clinical Psychology, 64*(4), 742–751.

Blanchard, E. B., Hickling, E. J., Galovski, T., & Veazey, C. (2002). Emergency room vital signs and PTSD in a treatment seeking sample of motor vehicle accident survivors. *Journal of Traumatic Stress, 15*(3), 199–204.

Blanchard, E. B., Hickling, E. J., Taylor, A. E., Loos, W. R., & Gerardi, R. J. (1994). Psychological morbidity associated with motor vehicle accidents. *Behaviour Research and Therapy, 32*(3), 283–290.

Blanchard, E. B., Kolb, L. C., Gerardi, R. J., Ryan, P., & Pallmeyer, T. P. (1986). Cardiac response to relevant stimuli as an adjunctive tool for diagnosing posttraumatic stress disorder in Vietnam veterans. *Behavior Therapy, 17*, 592–606.

Blanchard, E. B., Kolb, L. C., Pallmeyer, T. P., & Gerardi, R. J. (1982). A psychophysiological study of posttraumatic stress disorder in Vietnam veterans. *Psychiatric Quarterly, 54*(4), 220–229.

Blanchard, E. B., Kolb, L. C., & Prins, A. (1991). Psychophysiological responses in the diagnosis of posttraumatic stress disorder in Vietnam veterans. *Journal of Nervous and Mental Disease*, *179*(2), 97–101.

Blanchard, E. B., Kolb, L. C., Taylor, A. E., & Wittrock, D. A. (1989). Cardiac responses to relevant stimuli as an adjunct in diagnosing posttraumatic stress disorder: Replication and extension. *Behavior Therapy*, *20*, 535–543.

Bleich, A. V., Attias, J., & Furman, V. (1996). Effect of repeated visual traumatic stimuli on the event-related P3 brain potential in posttraumatic stress disorder. *International Journal of Neuroscience*, *85*(1–2), 45–55.

Boomsma, D. I., & Gabrielli, W. F., Jr. (1985). Behavioral genetic approaches to psychophysiological data. *Psychophysiology*, *22*(3), 249–260.

Boscarino, J. A., & Chang, J. (1999). Electrocardiogram abnormalities among men with stress-related psychiatric disorders: Implications for coronary heart disease and clinical research. *Annals of Behavioral Medicine*, *21*(3), 227–234.

Boudewyns, P., & Hyer, L. (1990). Physiological response to combat memories and preliminary treatment outcome in Vietnam veteran PTSD patients with direct therapeutic exposure. *Behavior Therapy*, *21*, 63–87.

Bremner, J. D., Licinio, J., Darnell, A., Krystal, J. H., Owens, M. J., Southwick, S. M., et al. (1997). Elevated CSF corticotropin-releasing factor concentrations in posttraumatic stress disorder. *American Journal of Psychiatry*, *154*(5), 624–629.

Breslau, N., & Davis, G. C. (1992). Posttraumatic stress disorder in an urban population of young adults: Risk factors for chronicity. *American Journal of Psychiatry*, *149*(5), 671–675.

Bryant, R. A., & Harvey, A. G. (2002). Delayed-onset posttraumatic stress disorder: A prospective evaluation. *Australian and New Zealand Journal of Psychiatry*, *36*(2), 205–209.

Bryant, R. A., Harvey, A. G., Gordon, E., & Barry, R. J. (1995). Eye movement and electrodermal responses to threat stimuli in posttraumatic stress disorder. *International Journal of Psychophysiology*, *20*(3), 209–213.

Bryant, R. A., Harvey, A. G., Guthrie, R. M., & Moulds, M. L. (2000). A prospective study of psychophysiological arousal, acute stress disorder, and posttraumatic stress disorder. *Journal of Abnormal Psychology*, *109*(2), 341–344.

Buchanan, T. W., Brechtel, A., Sollers, J. J., & Lovallo, W. R. (2001). Exogenous cortisol exerts effects on the startle reflex independent of emotional modulation. *Pharmacology, Biochemistry, and Behavior*, *68*(2), 203–210.

Buckley, T. C., & Kaloupek, D. G. (2001). A meta-analytic examination of basal cardiovascular activity in posttraumatic stress disorder. *Psychosomatic Medicine*, *63*(4), 585–594.

Butler, R. W., Braff, D. L., Rausch, J. L., Jenkins, M. A., Sprock, J., & Geyer, M. A. (1990). Physiological evidence of exaggerated startle response in a subgroup of Vietnam veterans with combat-related PTSD. *American Journal of Psychiatry*, *147*(10), 1308–1312.

Butterfield, M. I., Forneris, C. A., Feldman, M. E., & Beckham, J. C. (2000). Hostility and functional health status in women veterans with and without posttraumatic stress disorder: A preliminary study. *Journal of Traumatic Stress*, *13*(4), 735–741.

Cacioppo, J. T., Tassinary, L. G., & Berntson, G. G. (Eds.). (2000). *Handbook of psychophysiology* (2nd ed.). Cambridge, UK: Cambridge University Press.

Cacioppo, J. T., Tassinary, L. G., & Fridlund, A. J. (1990). The skeletomotor system. In J. T. Cacioppo & L. G. Tassinary (Eds.), *Principles of psychophysiology: Phys-*

ical, social, and inferential elements (pp. 325–384). New York: Cambridge University Press.

Cambell, C. M. (1918). The role of instinct, emotion and personality disorders of the heart. *Journal of the American Medical Association, 71*, 1621–1626.

Carroll, D., Hewitt, J. K., Last, K. A., Turner, J. R., & Sims, J. (1995). A twin study of cardiac reactivity and its relationship to parental blood pressure. *Physiology and Behavior, 34*, 103–106.

Carson, M. A., Paulus, L. A., Lasko, N. B., Metzger, L. J., Wolfe, J., Orr, S. P., et al. (2000). Psychophysiologic assessment of posttraumatic stress disorder in Vietnam nurse veterans who witnessed injury or death. *Journal of Consulting and Clinical Psychology, 68*(5), 890–897.

Casada, J. H., Amdur, R., Larsen, R., & Liberzon, I. (1998). Psychophysiologic responsivity in posttraumatic stress disorder: Generalized hyperresponsiveness versus trauma specificity. *Biological Psychiatry, 44*(10), 1037–1044.

Charles, G., Hansenne, M., Ansseau, M., Pitchot, W., Machowski, R., Schittecatte, M., et al. (1995). P300 in posttraumatic stress disorder. *Neuropsychobiology, 32*(2), 72–74.

Cohen, H., Benjamin, J., Geva, A. B., Matar, M. A., Kaplan, Z., & Kotler, M. (2000). Autonomic dysregulation in panic disorder and in posttraumatic stress disorder: Application of power spectrum analysis of heart rate variability at rest and in response to recollection of trauma or panic attacks. *Psychiatry Research, 96*(1), 1–13.

Cohen, H., Kotler, M., Matar, M., & Kaplan, Z. (2000). Normalization of heart rate variability in posttraumatic stress disorder patients following fluoxetine treatment: Preliminary results. *Israel Medical Association Journal, 2*(4), 296–301.

Cohen, H., Kotler, M., Matar, M. A., Kaplan, Z., Loewenthal, U., Miodownik, H., et al. (1998). Analysis of heart rate variability in posttraumatic stress disorder patients in response to a trauma-related reminder. *Biological Psychiatry, 44*(10), 1054–1059.

Cohen, H., Kotler, M., Matar, M. A., Kaplan, Z., Miodownik, H., & Cassuto, Y. (1997). Power spectral analysis of heart rate variability in posttraumatic stress disorder patients. *Biological Psychiatry, 41*(5), 627–629.

Cook, E. W., III, Melamed, B. G., Cuthbert, B. N., McNeil, D. W., & Lang, P. J. (1988). Emotional imagery and the differential diagnosis of anxiety. *Journal of Consulting and Clinical Psychology, 56*(5), 734–740.

Cuthbert, B. N., Lang, P. J., Strauss, C., Drobes, D., Patrick, C. J., & Bradley, M. M. (2003). The psychophysiology of anxiety disorder: Fear memory imagery. *Psychophysiology, 40*, 407–422.

Davidson, J. R., Hughes, D., Blazer, D. G., & George, L. K. (1991). Posttraumatic stress in the community: An epidemiological study. *Psychological Medicine, 21*, 713–721.

Davidson, R. J. (1984). Hemispheric asymmetry and emotion. In K. Schere & P. Ekman (Eds.), *Approaches to emotion* (pp. 39–57). Hillsdale, NJ: Erlbaum.

Davis, J. M., Adams, H. E., Uddo, M., Vasterling, J. J., & Sutker, P. B. (1996). Physiological arousal and attention in veterans with posttraumatic stress disorder. *Journal of Psychopathology and Behavioral Assessment, 18*, 1–20.

Davis, M., Walker, D. L., & Lee, Y. (1997). Roles of the amygdala and bed nucleus of the stria terminalis in fear and anxiety measured with the acoustic startle reflex:

Possible relevance to PTSD. *Annals of the New York Academy of Sciences*, *821*, 305–331.

Davis, M., Walker, D. L., & Lee, Y. (1999). Neurophysiology and neuropharmacology of startle and its affective modulation. In M. E. Dawson, A. M. Schell, & A. H. Bohmelt (Eds.), *Startle modification: Implications for neuroscience, cognitive science, and clinical science*. Cambridge, UK: Cambridge University Press.

Ditto, B. (1993). Familial influences on heart rate, blood pressure, and self-report anxiety responses to stress: Results from 100 twin pairs. *Psychophysiology*, *30*(6), 635–645.

Dobbs, D., & Wilson, W. P. (1960). Observations on the persistence of war neurosis. *Diseases of the Nervous System*, *21*, 686–691.

Edelberg, R. (1972). Electrical activity of the skin: Its measurement and uses in psychophysiology. In N. S. Greenfield & R. A. Sternbach (Eds.), *Handbook of psychophysiology* (pp. 367–418). New York: Holt, Rinehart, & Winston.

Eifert, G. H., & Wilson, P. H. (1991). The triple response approach to assessment: A conceptual and methodological reappraisal. *Behaviour Research and Therapy*, *29*(3), 283–292.

Felmingham, K. L., Bryant, R. A., Kendall, C., & Gordon, E. (2002). Event-related potential dysfunction in posttraumatic stress disorder: The role of numbing. *Psychiatry Research*, *109*(2), 171–179.

Flack, W. F., Litz, B. T., Hsieh, F. Y., Kaloupek, D. G., & Keane, T. M. (2000). Predictors of emotional numbing, revisited: A replication and extension. *Journal of Traumatic Stress*, *13*, 611–618.

Foa, E. B., & Kozak, M. J. (1986). Emotional processing of fear: Exposure to corrective information. *Psychological Bulletin*, *99*, 20–35.

Fontanarosa, P. B., & DeAngelis, C.D. (2003). Translational medical research. *Journal of the American Medical Association*, *289*, 2133.

Fowles, D. C. (1980). The three-arousal model: Implications of Gray's two-factor learning theory for heart rate, electrodermal activity, and psychopathy. *Psychophysiology*, *17*(2), 87–104.

Fowles, D. C., Christie, M. J., Edelberg, R., Grings, W. W., Lykken, D. T., & Venables, P. H. (1981). Publication recommendations for electrodermal measurements. *Psychophysiology*, *18*(3), 232–239.

Fredrikson, M., Danielssons, T., Engel, B. T., Frisk-Holmberg, M., Strom, G., & Sundin, O. (1985). Autonomic nervous system function and essential hypertension: Individual response specificity with and without beta-adrenergic blockade. *Psychophysiology*, 22(2), 167–174.

Fridlund, A. J., & Izard, C. E. (1983). Electromyographic studies of facial expressions of emotion and patterns of emotions. In J. T. Cacioppo & R. E. Petty (Eds.), *Social psychophysiology: A sourcebook* (pp. 243–286). New York: Guilford Press.

Galletly, C., Clark, C. R., McFarlane, A. C., & Weber, D. L. (2001). Working memory in posttraumatic stress disorder: An event-related potential study. *Journal of Traumatic Stress*, *14*(2), 295–309.

Gerardi, R. J., Blanchard, E. B., & Kolb, L. C. (1989). Ability of Vietnam veterans to dissimulate a psychophysiologic assessment for posttraumatic stress disorder. *Behavior Therapy*, *20*, 229–243.

Gerardi, R. J., Keane, T. M., Cahoon, B. J., & Klauminzer, G. W. (1994). An in vivo assessment of physiological arousal in posttraumatic stress disorder. *Journal of Abnormal Psychology*, *103*(4), 825–827.

Gillette, G. M., Skinner, R. D., Rasco, L. M., Fielstein, E. M., Davis, D. H., Pawelak, J. E., et al. (1997). Combat veterans with posttraumatic stress disorder exhibit decreased habituation of the P1 midlatency auditory evoked potential. *Life Sciences, 61*(14), 1421–1434.
Graham, F. K., Anthony, B. J., & Zeigler, B. L. (1983). The orienting response and developmental processes. In D. Siddle (Ed.), *Orienting and habituation: Perspectives in human research* (pp. 371–417). New York: Wiley.
Griffin, M. G., Resick, P. A., & Mechanic, M. B. (1997). Objective assessment of peritraumatic dissociation: Psychophysiological indicators. *American Journal of Psychiatry, 154*, 1081–1088.
Grillon, C., Ameli, R., Goddard, A., Woods, S. W., & Davis, M. (1994). Baseline and fear-potentiated startle in panic disorder patients. *Biological Psychiatry, 35*(7), 431–439.
Grillon, C., & Morgan, C. A., III. (1999). Fear-potentiated startle conditioning to explicit and contextual cues in Gulf War veterans with posttraumatic stress disorder. *Journal of Abnormal Psychology, 108*(1), 134–142.
Grillon, C., Morgan, C. A., III, Davis, M., & Southwick, S. M. (1998a). Effect of darkness on acoustic startle in Vietnam veterans with PTSD. *American Journal of Psychiatry, 155*(6), 812–817.
Grillon, C., Morgan, C. A., III, Davis, M., & Southwick, S. M. (1998b). Effects of experimental context and explicit threat cues on acoustic startle in Vietnam veterans with posttraumatic stress disorder. *Biological Psychiatry, 44*(10), 1027–1036.
Grillon, C., Morgan, C. A., Southwick, S. M., Davis, M., & Charney, D. S. (1996). Baseline startle amplitude and prepulse inhibition in Vietnam veterans with posttraumatic stress disorder. *Psychiatry Research, 64*(3), 169–178.
Grinker, R. R., & Spiegel, J. P. (1945). *War neuroses*. Philadelphia: Blakiston.
Harmon-Jones, E., & Allen, J. J. (1998). Anger and frontal brain activity: EEG asymmetry consistent with approach motivation despite negative affective valence. *Journal of Personality and Social Psychology, 74*(5), 1310–1316.
Harmon-Jones, E., & Sigelman, J. (2001). State anger and prefrontal brain activity: Evidence that insult-related relative left-prefrontal activation is associated with experienced anger and aggression. *Journal of Personality and Social Psychology, 80*, 797–803.
Hastrup, J. L. (1986). Duration of initial heart rate assessment in psychophysiology: Current practices and implications. *Psychophysiology, 23*(1), 15–18.
Heller, W. (1990). The neuropsychology of emotion: Developmental patterns and implications for psychopathology. In N. Stein, B. L. Leventhal, & T. Trabasso (Eds.), *Psychological and biological approaches to emotion* (pp. 167–211). Hillsdale, NJ: Erlbaum.
Heller, W., Nitschke, J. B., Etienne, M. A., & Miller, G. A. (1997). Patterns of regional brain activity differentiate types of anxiety. *Journal of Abnormal Psychology, 106*(3), 376–385.
Herman, J. L. (1992). *Trauma and recovery*. New York: Basic Books.
Horowitz, M. (1986). *Stress response syndromes* (2nd ed.). Northvale, NJ: Aronson.
Howard, R., & Ford, R. (1992). From the jumping Frenchmen of Maine to posttraumatic stress disorder: The startle response in neuropsychiatry. *Psychological Medicine, 22*(3), 695–707.
Hughes, J. R. (1993). Possible effects of smoke-free inpatient units on psychiatric diagnosis and treatment. *Journal of Clinical Psychiatry, 54*, 109–114.

Jasper, H. H. (1958). The ten-twenty electrode system of the International Federation. *Electroencephalography and Clinical Neurophysiology*, *10*, 371–375.

Kardiner, A. (1941). *The traumatic neuroses of war*. New York: Hober.

Kaufman, M. L., Kimble, M. O., Kaloupek, D. G., McTeague, L. M., Bachrach, P., Forti, A. M., & Keane, T. M. (2002). Peritraumatic dissociation and physiological response to trauma-relevant stimuli in Vietnam combat veterans with posttraumatic stress disorder. *Journal of Nervous and Mental Disease*, *190*, 167–174.

Keane, T. M., & Kaloupek, D. G. (1982). Imaginal flooding in the treatment of a posttraumatic stress disorder. *Journal of Consulting and Clinical Psychology*, *50*(1), 138–140.

Keane, T. M., Kolb, L. C., Kaloupek, D. G., Orr, S. P., Blanchard, E. B., Thomas, R. G., et al. (1998). Utility of psychophysiological measurement in the diagnosis of posttraumatic stress disorder: Results from a Department of Veterans Affairs Cooperative Study. *Journal of Consulting and Clinical Psychology*, *66*(6), 914–923.

Kimble, M., Kaloupek, D., Kaufman, M., & Deldin, P. (2000). Stimulus novelty differentially affects attentional allocation in PTSD. *Biological Psychiatry*, *47*(10), 880–890.

Kinzie, J. D., Denney, D., Riley, C., Boehnlein, J., McFarland, B., & Leung, P. (1998). A cross-cultural study of reactivation of posttraumatic stress disorder symptoms: American and Cambodian psychophysiological response to viewing traumatic video scenes. *Journal of Nervous and Mental Disease*, *186*(11), 670–676.

Kotchoubei, B. I. (1987). Human orienting reaction: The role of genetic and environmental factors in the variability of evoked potentials and autonomic components. *Activitas Nervosa Superior (Praha)*, *29*(2), 103–108.

Lader, M. H. (1967). Palmar skin conductance measures in anxiety and phobic states. *Journal of Psychosomatic Research*, *11*, 271–281.

Lader, M. H., & Wing, L. (1964). Habituation of the psycho-galvanic reflex in patients with anxiety states and in normal subjects. *Journal of Neurology, Neurosurgery, and Psychiatry*, *27*, 210.

Ladwig, K. H., Marten-Mittag, B., Deisenhofer, I., Hofmann, B., Schapperer, J., Weyerbrock, S., et al. (2002). Psychophysiological correlates of peritraumatic dissociative responses in survivors of life-threatening cardiac events. *Psychopathology*, *35*(4), 241–248.

Landis, C., & Hunt, W. A. (1939). *The startle pattern*. New York: Farrar & Rinehart.

Lane, J. D., & Williams, R. B., Jr. (1985). Caffeine affects cardiovascular responses to stress. *Psychophysiology*, *22*(6), 648–655.

Lang, P. J. (1985). The cognitive psychophysiology of emotion: Fear and anxiety. In A. Tuma & J. Maser (Eds.), *Anxiety and anxiety disorders* (pp. 131–170). Hillsdale, NJ: Erlbaum.

Lang, P. J., Bradley, M. M., & Cuthbert, B. N. (1990). Emotion, attention, and the startle reflex. *Psychological Review*, *97*(3), 377–395.

Lang, P. J., Levin, D. N., Miller, G. A., & Kozak, M. J. (1983). Fear behavior, fear imagery, and the psychophysiology of emotion: The problem of affective response integration. *Journal of Abnormal Psychology*, *92*(3), 276–306.

Lanius, R. A., Williamson, P. C., Densmore, M., Boksman, K., Math, K. B., Gupta, M. A., Madhulika, A., et al. (2001). Neural correlates of traumatic memories in posttraumatic stress disorder: A functional MRI investigation. *American Journal of Psychiatry*, *158*(11), 1920–1922.

Laor, N., Wolmer, L., Wiener, Z., Reiss, A., Muller, U., Weizman, R., et al. (1998). The function of image control in the psychophysiology of posttraumatic stress disorder. *Journal of Traumatic Stress, 11*, 679–695.

Lasko, N. B., Gurvits, T. V., Kuhne, A. A., Orr, S. P., & Pitman, R. K. (1994). Aggression and its correlates in Vietnam veterans with and without chronic posttraumatic stress disorder. *Comprehensive Psychiatry, 35*(5), 373–381.

Lee, Y., & Davis, M. (1997). Role of the hippocampus, the bed nucleus of the stria terminalis, and the amygdala in the excitatory effect of corticotropin-releasing hormone on the acoustic startle reflex. *Journal of Neuroscience, 17*(16), 6434–6446.

Lewine, J. D., Thoma, R. J., Provencal, S. L., Edgar, C., Miller, G. A., & Canive, J. M. (2002). Abnormal stimulus-response intensity functions in posttraumatic stress disorder: An electrophysiological investigation. *American Journal of Psychiatry, 159*(10), 1689–1695.

Litz, B. T. (1992). Emotional numbing in combat-related posttraumatic stress disorder: A critical review and reformulation. *Clinical Psychology Review, 12*, 417–432.

Litz, B. T., Orsillo, S. M., Kaloupek, D., & Weathers, F. (2000). Emotional processing in posttraumatic stress disorder. *Journal of Abnormal Psychology, 109*(1), 26–39.

Litz, B. T., Schlenger, W. E., Weathers, F. W., Caddell, J. M., Fairbank, J. A., & LaVange, L. M. (1997). Predictors of emotional numbing in posttraumatic stress disorder. *Journal of Traumatic Stress, 10*, 607–617.

Lykken, D. T., Iacono, W. G., Haroian, K., McGue, M., & Bouchard, T. J., Jr. (1988). Habituation of the skin conductance response to strong stimuli: A twin study. *Psychophysiology, 25*(1), 4–15.

Lyvers, M., & Miyata, Y. (1993). Effects of cigarette smoking on electrodermal orienting reflexes to stimulus change and stimulus significance. *Psychophysiology, 30*(3), 231–236.

Malloy, P. F., Fairbank, J. A., & Keane, T. M. (1983). Validation of a multimethod assessment of posttraumatic stress disorders in Vietnam veterans. *Journal of Consulting and Clinical Psychology, 51*(4), 488–494.

McDonagh-Coyle, A., McHugo, G. J., Friedman, M. J., Schnurr, P. P., Zayfert, C., & Descamps, M. (2001). Psychophysiological reactivity in female sexual abuse survivors. *Journal of Traumatic Stress, 14*(4), 667–683.

McFall, M. E., Murburg, M. M., Ko, G. N., & Veith, R. C. (1990). Autonomic responses to stress in Vietnam combat veterans with posttraumatic stress disorder. *Biological Psychiatry, 27*(10), 1165–1175.

McFall, M. E., Murburg, M. M., Roszell, D. K., & Veith, R. C. (1989). Psychophysiologic and neuroendocrine findings in posttraumatic stress disorder: A review of theory and research. *Journal of Anxiety Disorders, 3*, 243–257.

McFall, M. E., Veith, R. C., & Murburg, M. M. (1992). Basal sympathoadrenal function in posttraumatic distress disorder. *Biological Psychiatry, 31*(10), 1050–1056.

McFarlane, A. C., Weber, D. L., & Clark, C. R. (1993). Abnormal stimulus processing in posttraumatic stress disorder. *Biological Psychiatry, 34*(5), 311–320.

McNally, R. J., Luedke, D. L., Besyner, J. K., Peterson, R. A., Bohm, K., & Lips, O. J. (1987). Sensitivity to stress-relevant stimuli in posttraumatic stress disorder. *Journal of Anxiety Disorders, 1*, 105–116.

McNeil, D. W., Vrana, S. R., Melamed, B. G., Cuthbert, B. N., & Lang, P. J. (1993). Emotional imagery in simple and social phobia: Fear versus anxiety. *Journal of Abnormal Psychology, 102*(2), 212–225.

McPherson, W. B., Newton, J. E., Ackerman, P., Oglesby, D. M., & Dykman, R. A. (1997). An event-related brain potential investigation of PTSD and PTSD symptoms in abused children. *Integrative Physiological and Behavioral Science*, *32*(1), 31–42.

Meakins, J. C., & Wilson, R. M. (1918). The effect of certain sensory stimulations on respiratory and heart rate in cases of so-called "irritable heart." *Heart: A Journal for the Study of the Circulation*, 7, 17–22.

Medina, A. M., Mejia, V. Y., Schell, A. M., Dawson, M. E., & Margolin, G. (2001). Startle reactivity and PTSD symptoms in a community sample of women. *Psychiatry Research*, *101*(2), 157–169.

Meltzer-Brody, S., Churchill, E., & Davidson, J. R. (1999). Derivation of the SPAN, a brief diagnostic screening test for posttraumatic stress disorder. *Psychiatry Research*, *88*(1), 63–70.

Metzger, L. J., Carson, M. A., Paulus, L. A., Lasko, N. B., Paige, S. R., Pitman, R. K., et al. (2002). Event-related potentials to auditory stimuli in female Vietnam nurse veterans with posttraumatic stress disorder. *Psychophysiology*, *39*(1), 49–63.

Metzger, L. J., Orr, S. P., Berry, N. J., Ahern, C. E., Lasko, N. B., & Pitman, R. K. (1999). Physiologic reactivity to startling tones in women with posttraumatic stress disorder. *Journal of Abnormal Psychology*, *108*(2), 347–352.

Metzger, L. J., Orr, S. P., Lasko, N. B., Berry, N. J., & Pitman, R. K. (1997). Evidence for diminished P3 amplitudes in PTSD. *Annals of the New York Academy of Sciences*, *821*, 499–503.

Metzger, L. J., Orr, S. P., Lasko, N. B., McNally, R. J., & Pitman, R. K. (1997). Seeking the source of emotional Stroop interference effects in PTSD: A study of P3s to traumatic words. *Integrative Physiological and Behavioral Science*, *32*(1), 43–51.

Metzger, L. J., Orr, S. P., Lasko, N. B., & Pitman, R. K. (1997). Auditory event-related potentials to tone stimuli in combat-related posttraumatic stress disorder. *Biological Psychiatry*, *42*(11), 1006–1015.

Metzger, L. J., Paige, S. R., Carson, M. A., Lasko, N. B., Paulus, L. A., Pitman, R. K., & Orr, S. P. (in press). Opposite patterns of parietal EEG asymmetry associated with PTSD arousal vs. depressive symptoms. *Journal of Abnormal Psychology*.

Metzger, L. J., Paige, S. R., Lasko, M. V., Tomarken, A. J., Orr, S. P., & Pitman, R. K. (1998). *Resting frontal brain asymmetry in combat-related PTSD*. Paper presented at the annual neeting of the International Society for Traumatic Stress Studies, Washington, DC.

Miller, M.W, & Litz, B. T. (in press). Emotional processing in posttraumatic stress disorder: II. Startle reflex modulation during picture processing. *Journal of Abnormal Psychology*.

Morgan, C. A., III, & Grillon, C. (1999). Abnormal mismatch negativity in women with sexual assault-related posttraumatic stress disorder. *Biological Psychiatry*, *45*(7), 827–832.

Morgan, C. A., III, Grillon, C., Lubin, H., & Southwick, S. M. (1997). Startle reflex abnormalities in women with sexual assault-related posttraumatic stress disorder. *American Journal of Psychiatry*, *154*(8), 1076–1080.

Morgan, C. A., III, Grillon, C., Southwick, S. M., Davis, M., & Charney, D. S. (1995). Fear-potentiated startle in posttraumatic stress disorder. *Biological Psychiatry*, *38*(6), 378–385.

Morgan, C. A., III, Grillon, C., Southwick, S. M., Davis, M., & Charney, D. S. (1996).

Exaggerated acoustic startle reflex in Gulf War veterans with posttraumatic stress disorder. *American Journal of Psychiatry*, *153*(1), 64–68.

Morgan, C. A., III, Grillon, C., Southwick, S. M., Nagy, L. M., Davis, M., Krystal, J. H., et al. (1995). Yohimbine-facilitated acoustic startle in combat veterans with posttraumatic stress disorder. *Psychopharmacology (Berl)*, *117*(4), 466–471.

Muraoka, M. Y., Carlson, J. G., & Chemtob, C. M. (1998). Twenty-four-hour ambulatory blood pressure and heart rate monitoring in combat-related posttraumatic stress disorder. *Journal of Traumatic Stress*, *11*(3), 473–484.

Neylan, T. C., Fletcher, D. J., Lenoci, M., McCallin, K., Weiss, D. S., Schoenfeld, F. B., et al. (1999). Sensory gating in chronic posttraumatic stress disorder: Reduced auditory P50 suppression in combat veterans. *Biological Psychiatry*, *46*(12), 1656–1664.

Neylan, T. C., Jasiukaitis, P. A., Lenoci, M., Scott, J. C., Metzler, T. J., Weiss, D. S., et al. (2003). Temporal instability of auditory and visual event-related potentials in posttraumatic stress disorder. *Biological Psychiatry*, *53*(3), 216–225.

Nishith, P., Duntley, S. P., Domitrovich, P. P., Uhles, M. L., Cook, B. J., & Stein, P. K. (2003). Effect of cognitive behavioral therapy on heart rate variability during REM sleep in female rape victims with PTSD. *Journal of Traumatic Stress*, *16*(3), 247–250.

Orr, S. P., Lasko, N. B., Metzger, L. J., Berry, N. J., Ahern, C. E., & Pitman, R. K. (1998). Psychophysiologic assessment of women with posttraumatic stress disorder resulting from childhood sexual abuse. *Journal of Consulting and Clinical Psychology*, *66*(6), 906–913.

Orr, S. P., Lasko, N. B., Metzger, L. J., & Pitman, R. K. (1997). Physiologic responses to non-startling tones in Vietnam veterans with posttraumatic stress disorder. *Psychiatry Research*, *73*(1–2), 103–107.

Orr, S. P., Lasko, N. B., Shalev, A. Y., & Pitman, R. K. (1995). Physiologic responses to loud tones in Vietnam veterans with posttraumatic stress disorder. *Journal of Abnormal Psychology*, *104*(1), 75–82.

Orr, S. P., Metzger, L. J., Lasko, N. B., Macklin, M. L., Hu, F. B., Shalev, A. Y., et al. (2003). Physiologic responses to sudden, loud tones in monozygotic twins discordant for combat exposure: Association with posttraumatic stress disorder. *Archives of General Psychiatry*, *60*(3), 283–288.

Orr, S. P., Metzger, L. J., Lasko, N. B., Macklin, M. L., Peri, T., & Pitman, R. K. (2000). De novo conditioning in trauma-exposed individuals with and without posttraumatic stress disorder. *Journal of Abnormal Psychology*, *109*(2), 290–298.

Orr, S. P., Metzger, L. J., & Pitman, R. K. (2002). Psychophysiology of posttraumatic stress disorder. *Psychiatric Clinics of North America*, *25*(2), 271–293.

Orr, S. P., Meyerhoff, J. L., Edwards, J. V., & Pitman, R. K. (1998). Heart rate and blood pressure resting levels and responses to generic stressors in Vietnam veterans with posttraumatic stress disorder. *Journal of Traumatic Stress*, *11*(1), 155–164.

Orr, S. P., & Pitman, R. K. (1993). Psychophysiologic assessment of attempts to simulate posttraumatic stress disorder. *Biological Psychiatry*, *33*(2), 127–129.

Orr, S. P., Pitman, R. K., Lasko, N. B., & Herz, L. R. (1993). Psychophysiological assessment of posttraumatic stress disorder imagery in World War II and Korean combat veterans. *Journal of Abnormal Psychology*, *102*(1), 152–159.

Orr, S. P., Solomon, Z., Peri, T., Pitman, R. K., & Shalev, A. Y. (1997). Physiologic responses to loud tones in Israeli veterans of the 1973 Yom Kippur War. *Biological Psychiatry*, *41*(3), 319–326.

Paige, S. R., Reid, G. M., Allen, M. G., & Newton, J. E. (1990). Psychophysiological correlates of posttraumatic stress disorder in Vietnam veterans. *Biological Psychiatry*, *27*(4), 419–430.

Pallmeyer, T. P., Blanchard, E. B., & Kolb, L. C. (1986). The psychophysiology of combat-induced posttraumatic stress disorder in Vietnam veterans. *Behaviour Research and Therapy*, *24*(6), 645–652.

Peri, T., Ben-Shakhar, G., Orr, S. P., & Shalev, A. Y. (2000). Psychophysiologic assessment of aversive conditioning in posttraumatic stress disorder. *Biological Psychiatry*, *47*(6), 512–519.

Perkins, K. A., Epstein, L. H., Jennings, J. R., & Stiller, R. (1986). The cardiovascular effects of nicotine during stress. *Psychopharmacology (Berl)*, *90*(3), 373–378.

Pissiota, A., Frans, O., Fernandez, M., von Knorring, L., Fischer, H., & Fredrikson, M. (2002). Neurofunctional correlates of posttraumatic stress disorder: A PET symptom provocation study. *European Archives of Psychiatry and Clinical Neuroscience*, *252*(2), 68–75.

Pitman, R. K., Lanes, D. M., Williston, S. K., Guillaume, J. L., Metzger, L. J., Gehr, G. M., et al. (2001). Psychophysiologic assessment of posttraumatic stress disorder in breast cancer patients. *Psychosomatics*, *42*(2), 133–140.

Pitman, R. K., & Orr, S. P. (1993). Psychophysiologic testing for posttraumatic stress disorder: Forensic psychiatric application. *Bulletin of the American Academy of Psychiatry and Law*, *21*(1), 37–52.

Pitman, R. K., Orr, S. P., Altman, B., Longpre, R. E., Poire, R. E., & Macklin, M. L. (1996). Emotional processing during eye movement desensitization and reprocessing therapy of Vietnam veterans with chronic posttraumatic stress disorder. *Comprehensive Psychiatry*, *37*(6), 419–429.

Pitman, R. K., Orr, S. P., Altman, B., Longpre, R. E., Poire, R. E., Macklin, M. L., et al. (1996). Emotional processing and outcome of imaginal flooding therapy in Vietnam veterans with chronic posttraumatic stress disorder. *Comprehensive Psychiatry*, *37*(6), 409–418.

Pitman, R. K., Orr, S. P., Forgue, D. F., Altman, B., de Jong, J. B., & Herz, L. R. (1990). Psychophysiologic responses to combat imagery of Vietnam veterans with posttraumatic stress disorder versus other anxiety disorders. *Journal of Abnormal Psychology*, *99*(1), 49–54.

Pitman, R. K., Orr, S. P., Forgue, D. F., de Jong, J. B., & Claiborn, J. M. (1987). Psychophysiologic assessment of posttraumatic stress disorder imagery in Vietnam combat veterans. *Archives of General Psychiatry*, *44*(11), 970–975.

Pitman, R. K., Shalev, A. Y., & Orr, S. P. (1999). Posttraumatic stress disorder: Emotion, conditioning, and memory. In M. S. Gazzaniga (Ed.), *The cognitive neurosciences* (pp. 1137–1147). Cambridge, MA: MIT Press.

Pivik, R. T. (2000). Sleep and dreaming. In J. T. Cacioppo, L. G. Tassinary, & G. G. Bernston (Eds.), *Handbook of psychophysiology* (2nd ed., pp. 687–716). Cambridge, UK: Cambridge University Press.

Pole, N., Neylan, T. C., Best, S. R., Orr, S. P., & Marmar, C. R. (2003). Fear-potentiated startle and posttraumatic stress symptoms in urban police officers. *Journal of Traumatic Stress*, *16*, 471–479.

Polich, J., & Herbst, K. L. (2000). P300 as a clinical assay: Rationale, evaluation, and findings. *International Journal of Psychophysiology, 38*(1), 3–19.

Prins, A., Kaloupek, D. G., & Keane, T. M. (1995). Psychophysiological evidence for autonomic arousal and startle in traumatized adult populations. In M. J. Friedman, D. Charney, & A. Deutch (Eds.), *Neurobiological and clinical consequences of stress: From normal adaption to PTSD* (pp. 291–314). New York: Raven Press.

Pynoos, R. S., Goenjiam, A., Tashjian, M., Karakashian, M., Manjikian, R., Manoukian, G., et al. (1993). Posttraumatic stress reactions in children after the 1988 Armenian earthquake. *British Journal of Psychiatry, 163*, 239–247.

Rachman, S., & Whittal, M. (1989). Fast, slow and sudden reductions in fear. *Behaviour Research and Therapy, 27*(6), 613–620.

Ratliff-Crain, J., O'Keeffe, M. K., & Baum, A. (1989). Cardiovascular reactivity, mood, and task performance in deprived and nondeprived coffee drinkers. *Health Psychology, 8*(4), 427–447.

Rauch, S. L., van der Kolk, B. A., Fisler, R. E., Alpert, N. M., Orr, S. P., Savage, C. R., et al. (1996). A symptom provocation study of posttraumatic stress disorder using positron emission tomography and script-driven imagery. *Archives of General Psychiatry, 53*, 380–387.

Ross, R. J., Ball, W. A., Cohen, M. E., Silver, S. M., Morrison, A. R., & Dinges, D. F. (1989). Habituation of the startle reflex. *Journal of Neuropsychiatry, 1*, 305–307.

Roth, W. T., Ehlers, A., Taylor, C. B., Margraf, J., & Agras, W. S. (1990). Skin conductance habituation in panic disorder patients. *Biological Psychiatry, 27*, 1231–1243.

Rothbaum, B. O., Kozak, M. J., Foa, E. B., & Whitaker, D. J. (2001). Posttraumatic stress disorder in rape victims: Autonomic habituation to auditory stimuli. *Journal of Traumatic Stress, 14*(2), 283–293.

Sahar, T., Shalev, A. Y., & Porges, S. W. (2001). Vagal modulation of responses to mental challenge in posttraumatic stress disorder. *Biological Psychiatry, 49*(7), 637–643.

Shalev, A. Y., Orr, S. P., Peri, T., Schreiber, S., & Pitman, R. K. (1992). Physiologic responses to loud tones in Israeli patients with posttraumatic stress disorder. *Archives of General Psychiatry, 49*(11), 870–875.

Shalev, A. Y., Orr, S. P., & Pitman, R. K. (1992). Psychophysiologic response during script-driven imagery as an outcome measure in posttraumatic stress disorder. *Journal of Clinical Psychiatry, 53*(9), 324–326.

Shalev, A. Y., Orr, S. P., & Pitman, R. K. (1993). Psychophysiologic assessment of traumatic imagery in Israeli civilian patients with posttraumatic stress disorder. *American Journal of Psychiatry, 150*(4), 620–624.

Shalev, A. Y., Peri, T., Brandes, D., Freedman, S., Orr, S. P., & Pitman, R. K. (2000). Auditory startle response in trauma survivors with posttraumatic stress disorder: A prospective study. *American Journal of Psychiatry, 157*(2), 255–261.

Shalev, A. Y., Peri, T., Orr, S. P., Bonne, O., & Pitman, R. K. (1997). Auditory startle responses in help-seeking trauma survivors. *Psychiatry Research, 69*(1), 1–7.

Shalev, A. Y., & Rogel-Fuchs, Y. (1993). Psychophysiology of the posttraumatic stress disorder: From sulfur fumes to behavioral genetics. *Psychosomatic Medicine, 55*(5), 413–423.

Shalev, A. Y., Sahar, T., Freedman, S., Peri, T., Glick, N., Brandes, D., et al. (1998). A prospective study of heart rate response following trauma and the subsequent development of posttraumatic stress disorder. *Archives of General Psychiatry, 55*(6), 553–559.

Shin, L. M., McNally, R. J., Kosslyn, S. M., Thompson, W. L., Rauch, S. L., Alpert, N. M., et al. (1999). Regional cerebral blood flow during script-driven imagery in childhood sexual abuse-related PTSD: A PET investigation. *American Journal of Psychiatry, 156*(4), 575–584.

Sierra, M., Senior, C., Dalton, J., McDonough, M., Bond, A., Phillips, M. L., et al. (2002). Autonomic response in depersonalization disorder. *Archives of General Psychiatry, 59*, 833–838.

Sirota, A. D., & Schwartz, G. E. (1982). Facial muscle patterning lateralization during elation and depression imagery. *Journal of Abnormal Psychology, 91*(1), 25–34.

Skinner, R. D., Rasco, L. M., Fitzgerald, J., Karson, C. N., Matthew, M., Williams, D. K., et al. (1999). Reduced sensory gating of the P1 potential in rape victims and combat veterans with posttraumatic stress disorder. *Depression and Anxiety, 9*(3), 122–130.

Southard, E. E. (1919). *Shell shock and other neuropsychiatric problems presented in 589 case histories from the war literature 1914–1918*. Boston: Leonard.

Southwick, S. M., Krystal, J. H., Morgan, C. A., Johnson, D., Nagy, L. M., Nicolaou, A., et al. (1993). Abnormal noradrenergic function in posttraumatic stress disorder. *Archives of General Psychiatry, 50*(4), 266–274.

Southwick, S. M., Morgan, C. A., Darnell, A., Bremner, J. D., Nicolaou, A. L., Nagy, L. M., et al. (1995). Trauma-related symptoms in veterans of Operation Desert Storm: A 2-year follow-up. *American Journal of Psychiatry, 152*, 1150–1155.

Spinhoven, P., Onstein, E. J., Sterk, P. J., & LeHaen-Versteijnen, D. (1993). Discordance between symptom and physiological criteria for the hyperventilation syndrome. *Journal of Psychosomatic Research, 37*, 281–289.

Stanford, M. S., Vasterling, J. J., Mathias, C. W., Constans, J. I., & Houston, R. J. (2001). Impact of threat relevance on P3 event-related potentials in combat-related posttraumatic stress disorder. *Psychiatry Research, 102*, 125–137.

Stern, R. M., & Sison, C. E. (1990). Response patterning. In J. T. Cacioppo & L. G. Tassinary (Eds.), *Principles of psychophysiology: Physical, social, and inferential elements* (pp. 193–215). New York: Cambridge University Press.

Sung, N. S., Crowley, W. F., Genel, M., Salber, P., Sandy, L., Sherwood, L. M., et al. (2003). Central challenges facing the national clinical research enterprise. *Journal of the American Medical Association, 289*, 1278–1287.

Swerdlow, N. R., Britton, K. T., & Koob, G. F. (1989). Potentiation of acoustic startle by corticotropin-releasing factor (CRF) and by fear are both reversed by alpha-helical CRF (9–41). *Neuropsychopharmacology, 2*(4), 285–292.

Taylor, S., Thordarson, D. S., Maxfield, L., Fedoroff, I. C., Lovell, K. & Ogrodniczuk, J. (2003). Comparative efficacy, speed, and adverse effects of three PTSD treatments: Exposure therapy, EMDR, and relaxation. *Journal of Consulting and Clinical Psychology, 71*, 330–338.

Tucker, P., Smith, K. L., Marx, B., Jones, D., Miranda, R., & Lensgraf, J. (2000). Fluvoxamine reduces physiologic reactivity to trauma scripts in posttraumatic stress disorder. *Journal of Clinical Psychopharmacology, 20*(3), 367–372.

Tyrer, P., Lee, I., & Alexander, J. (1980). Awareness of cardiac function in anxious, phobic and hypochondriacal patients. *Psychological Medicine, 10*(1), 171–174.

Van der Kolk, B. (1987). *Psychological trauma.* Washington, DC: American Psychiatric Press.

Van der Kolk, B., Greenberg, M., Boyd, H., & Krystal, J. (1985). Inescapable shock, neurotransmitters, and addiction to trauma: Toward a psychobiology of posttraumatic stress. *Biological Psychiatry, 20,* 314–325.

Wallin, B. G. (1981). Sympathetic nerve activity underlying electrodermal and cardiovascular reactions in man. *Psychophysiology, 18*(4), 470–476.

Weisaeth, L. (1989). The stressors and the posttraumatic stress syndrome after an industrial disaster. *Acta Psychiatrica Scandinavica, 80*(Suppl. 355), 25–37.

Wolfe, J., Chrestman, K. R., Ouimette, P. C., Kaloupek, D., Harley, R. M., & Bucsela, M. (2000). Trauma-related psychophysiological reactivity in women exposed to war-zone stress. *Journal of Clinical Psychology, 56*(10), 1371–1379.

Woodward, S. H., Murburg, M. M., & Bliwise, D. L. (2000). PTSD-related hyperarousal assessed during sleep. *Physiology and Behavior, 70*(1–2), 197–203.

Yehuda, R. (2002). Current status of cortisol findings in posttraumatic stress disorder. *Psychiatric Clinics of North America, 25*(2), 341–368, vii.

Young, E. S., Perros, P., Price, G. W., & Sadler, T. (1995). Acute challenge ERP as a prognostic of stimulant therapy outcome in attention-deficit hyperactivity disorder. *Biological Psychiatry, 37*(1), 25–33.

Zander, J. R., & McNally, R. J. (1988). Bio-informational processing in agoraphobia. *Behaviour Research and Therapy, 26*(5), 421–429.

CHAPTER 12

Assessing Neuropsychological Concomitants of Trauma and PTSD

JEFFREY A. KNIGHT
CASEY T. TAFT

During the past decade, empirical studies increasingly focused on examining brain-based correlates of clinical symptoms from a broader range of psychiatric conditions, including posttraumatic stress disorder (PTSD). Having a better understanding of these correlates will prove essential for developing more effective behavioral and pharmacological treatment protocols for PTSD, as well as for devising strategies geared toward preventing the development of PTSD symptoms after exposure to trauma. However, the process of studying these correlates is complicated, because, as with psychiatric disorders in general, PTSD does not present with the types of structural lesions that would be diagnostic in classic neurological disorders. Unlike a tumor, stroke, aneurysm, or multiple sclerosis, psychiatric disorders often have few or no corresponding neuroanatomical correlates that are pathognomonic and identifiable via autopsy, computed tomography (CT) scan, or magnetic resonance imaging (MRI) scan (Raz, 1989). When structural findings are present, they may not reliably correlate with the level of functional deficits or symptom severity (Devous, 1989, p. 219). The presence of comorbid conditions with PTSD further complicates interpretations of structure–function relationships. Nonetheless, advances in the behavioral neurosciences, electrophysiological measurement (quantitative electroencephalogram [EEG], evoked potential responding), and functional neuroimaging techniques (positron emission tomography [PET], single photon emission computerized tomography [SPECT], functional MRI) have shown promise for investigating the pathogenesis of

PTSD via volumetric studies and cognitive activation paradigms (Pitman, Shin, & Rauch, 2001; Segalowitz, Lawson, & Berge, 1993), and for developing nonpsychological models of functional disorders (Andreasen, 1989; McGuire, Shah, & Murray, 1993; Orsillo & McCaffrey, 1992). Neuropsychological assessment has also been employed as a noninvasive approach to studying the relationship between PTSD and brain functioning, as well as the effects of trauma on neurocognitive abilities (Knight, 1997). Neuropsychological tests designed to measure brain–behavior associations are often used to determine whether corresponding functional deficits exist when abnormal findings are detected from imaging protocols. Although there are clear challenges for researchers and clinicians who study brain–behavior correlates of trauma and PTSD, the literature highlights trends toward examining the interaction of brain-based factors and trauma variables using multimethod assessment protocols designed to measure the relevant comorbid effects.

The increased interest in understanding how brain functioning relates to PTSD is a natural progression in the growth of the comparatively young literature on mechanisms of trauma-related disorders. Early in the PTSD literature, the major emphases centered around defining the set of primary PTSD criteria and associated features, debating the validity of its status as a unique anxiety disorder, and creating reliable diagnostic interviews and psychological methods for measuring PTSD. Having stable PTSD diagnostic criteria and standardized assessment methods for classifying cases in clinical and research protocols has facilitated examinations into the causes and effects of trauma-related problems. Studying the structure and function of brain systems to search for etiologies and mechanisms that produce PTSD and traumatic dysfunction is a logical next step. Protocols that measure neurobiological and neurobehavioral factors will be required, although the neurobiological protocols can be complicated to conduct and the necessary technical resources might not be readily available. The clinical–behavioral effects of trauma may be more amenable to study than the neurobiological causal factors, and as a result they have predominated in the literature to date. However, to continue advancing the field regarding brain-related correlates of trauma, more research should be conducted and more interventions designed from a clinical neuroscience perspective, which assumes that alterations in brain functioning underlie observed clinical changes. This may require a shift in viewpoint for the clinician or clinical researcher from one that is purely psychological or psychiatric to one that is more neuropsychiatric.

At an abstract level, few would disagree with the notion that alterations in the brain's functional status play a significant role in generating the clinical presentations observed in patients with PTSD. However, many different points of view would be expressed in a debate regarding the degree of emphasis brain-related factors should receive in planning studies, clinical assessments, and treatment interventions. In essence, when attempting to account for the incidence and severity of PTSD symptoms, the variety of symptom patterns, and the overall dysfunction associated with PTSD, how much weight should be given to brain-related variables? The question reflects professional worldviews, training, and the available data. Even with the recent growth of studies related to this question, it cannot easily be answered due to the array of PTSD presentations and outcomes that must be explained, the complexity introduced by multiple coexisting disorders and problems, and the variability in exposure to models and investigational methods of PTSD and brain-based comorbidities across researchers and clinicians. Relative to training for other disorders, comparatively few clinical neuroscientists, neuropsychologists, and neuropsychiatrists have trauma-focused training. Similarly, few traumatologists are formally trained to assess and study brain–behavior relationships. Acquiring knowledge of methods and models from both the trauma and neurosciences areas is important for assessing, treating, and researching the effects of trauma on brain functioning and for understanding the role of brain functioning on PTSD development, maintenance, alteration, and resolution. An integrated approach is particularly relevant for assessing and treating individuals with known neuropsychological comorbidities (Merskey, 1992).

To assist in the process of conceptualizing the role of brain-related factors in trauma research and clinical work, this chapter focuses on issues surrounding the evaluation of common neurocognitive concomitants observed in populations with trauma and PTSD. The primary aims are to provide information to practitioners and clinical researchers regarding conditions that can produce comorbid neuropsychological problems, to consider specific problems that can arise when conducting neuropsychological evaluations with populations with trauma, and to discuss topics to be addressed in future research that investigates the interaction of PTSD and neurocognitive factors. Individual sections of the chapter also identify common sources of neuropsychogenic trauma, review the current literature on the neuropsychological evaluation of PTSD and trauma in combat and noncombat populations, and discuss process issues for testing male and female adults with trauma histories. The chapter is also intended to increase awareness among neuropsychologists of PTSD-specific factors that are not ordinarily considered or addressed during neuropsychological evaluations and to highlight for trauma clinicians and researchers relevant neuropsychological variables that should be considered in their work.

CONCEPTUALIZING THE NEUROPSYCHOLOGICAL COMORBIDITIES OF PTSD

The range of comorbid medical and psychiatric problems in chronic PTSD populations can be extensive and can produce significant impact across multiple domains of everyday functioning. When neuropsychological comorbidities are found or suspected from the medical history or behavioral observations, case formulations become more complex and the assessment process more complicated. Depending on the population of interest, the assessment context, and the goals for the assessment, the current literature may or may not be useful for clinicians and researchers as a guide for developing clinical hypotheses and structuring their diagnostic process. Findings are often mixed for portions of the literature that focus on acquired or developmental neurological injuries as causal factors for the development of PTSD. Other aspects of the literature that mainly address the coexistence of neurological conditions and PTSD need more empirical research.

When specific studies of brain-based factors cannot be used as a guide to assessment or treatment planning, consulting general models can often be helpful. Current explanatory models of hypothetical brain-based contributions to PTSD symptom development are either fairly systemic (e.g., *changes at synaptic levels of cortical neurons from protracted and excessive sensitizing stimulation*, Kolb, 1989; *beta-adrenergic activation and memory for emotional events*, Cahill, Prins, Weber, & McGaugh, 1994; altered *functioning of brainstem catecholaminergic systems in childhood PTSD*, Perry, 1994), linked to a brain structure or cortical area (e.g., *reduced right hippocampal volume*, Bremner et al., 1995; *anterior cingulate cortex*, Hamner, Lorberbaum, & George, 1999; *left frontal, temporal, or anterior regions*, Ito, Teicher, Glod, & Harper, 1993; *hippocampus, parietal lobes and orbital frontal complex*, Semple, Goyers, McCormick, & Morris, 1993; *locus coeruleus and amygdala*, Watson, Hoffman, & Wilson, 1988; *limbic system, septal–hippocampal–amygdalar complex*, Vasterling et al., 2002), or are specific to a neurocognitive deficit (e.g., *memory problems*, Elzinga & Bremner, 2002; Vasterling, Brailey, Constans, & Sutker, 1998; Yehuda & Harvey, 1997). These models might help to guide one's conceptual understanding, but their components may not be specific enough for use with individual cases. As a result, individual evaluations will frequently require a process of constructing and testing clinical hypotheses. Clinical researchers may need to employ similar processes for group designs. The separate main effects of trauma-related and neuropsychological factors, as well as their synergistic effects, will need to be addressed. Traumatologists should consider the possibility that events capable of producing psychological and physical trauma could also cause neurological damage, and neuropsychologists should consider the potential for significant reciprocal influences between psychological trauma and neurocognitive sequelae. The final analysis will weigh information about hypothesized neurobiological systems, logical inferences from other related clinical disorders, and patterns among clinical symptoms to address the relationship between the traumatic experiences, PTSD development, observed neurocognitive impairments, and possible brain functions associated with the patterns of cognitive symptoms that manifest clinically. One clear component of this analytic process is an awareness of neurological conditions that could combine with trauma-related variables to produce neurocognitive problems. We discuss these factors subsequently.

Multivariate approaches that account for complex PTSD presentations should resonate with anyone who has worked with chronic PTSD populations because of the multiple psychiatric and medical conditions that often coexist with PTSD symptoms (Sierles, Chen, McFarland, & Taylor, 1983). However, whereas dual diagnostic formulations have been modeled for other psychiatric disorders and behavioral medicine models have been applied to the interaction of psychological and medical disorders (e.g., chronic pain and PTSD), our models for understanding the neuropsychological comorbidities for PTSD are comparatively less well developed. The relative absence of developed models is somewhat puzzling, as it is evident that many of the events known to cause psychological and physical trauma to the body have an equally high potential to produce brain injuries that affect neurocognitive functioning. High-impact mechanical accidents can injure multiple body systems that directly and indirectly affect brain functioning. The nature of military activities, modes of military ground and air transportation, and proximity to lethal weaponry possess a high potential for neurological injury. Physical beatings typically involve repeated blows to the face and head, with either hands, fists, feet, or hard objects, which can be severe enough to produce episodes of unconsciousness or sequelae reflecting minor head injury even in the absence of lost consciousness. Suicide attempts involving strangulation, suffocation, carbon monoxide poisoning, and near drownings can produce hypoxic or anoxic episodes, with residual brain damage from periods of restricted or lost oxygenation of brain tissue. As is discussed further in later sections, the context for these events can be civilian, military, occupational, nonoccupational, interpersonal, social, intentional, incidental, or accidental and can be experienced by males and females across the lifespan. Although certain types of traumatic experiences may be more prevalent in children, adults, males, or females—the events that cause neurological injuries can occur in most populations. The process of studying the neuropsychological concomitants of PTSD is complicated further by the number of prior traumatogenic events the survivors have experienced and by the parameters of their responses to these events. A person's trauma history can also interact with other demographic factors, such as gender, age at the time of traumatic injury, education, general medical health status, and familial history of heritable disorders, to influence the severity of neurocognitive problems.

In summary, even though our understanding of the neuropsychological factors in trauma contexts is evolving, rationally based formulations can now be developed using existing knowledge about the individual trauma and neuropsychological conditions. The joint effects of the many possible comorbid combinations will often be untested. The first step in the analysis is to identify the types of conditions having the potential to cause neurocognitive problems that might interact with traumatic experiences.

Identifying Neuropsychogenic Events and Concomitants

By definition, PTSD is an acquired disorder that is dependent on exposure to a traumatic event. Neurological conditions can be either developmental or acquired. Thus neurological conditions that coexist with PTSD can precede the traumatic event, codevelop with the traumatic event, or occur at some interval after the traumatic event. When both types of disorders are present, a complete assessment should evaluate clinical and historical information about all relevant developmental and acquired neuropsychogenic factors. PTSD interviews or checklists assess the manifestations of psychological trauma. These interviews are not designed to address neurocognitive problems. Neuropsychological evaluations will gather information about medical conditions and factors that could produce neurocognitive impairments (e.g., strokes, tumors, head injuries, dementias, developmental problems, substance abuse, toxic exposures, familial disorders), but sampling of trauma variables is limited. Formal neuropsychological testing contributes performance information about the direct and indirect effects of both neurological and psychological conditions. In combination, these sources of clinical and historical data should form the basis for profiling the effects of comorbidity on trauma survivors' clinical presentations.

PTSD and Developmental Neurological Conditions

Combinations of conditions in this category can be found across the lifespan and develop independently of acquired disorders. They can create vulnerabilities that could facilitate the onset of PTSD following traumatic exposure, limit cognitive capacities that a person could marshal to cope with acute symptoms of PTSD, or cause a decline in neurocognitive functioning that makes previously manageable PTSD symptoms unmanageable. The age at which the conditions manifest, as well as the pattern and degree of neurocognitive deficits, will vary across developmental conditions. Thus the point at which the trauma or traumas occur during the lifespan will interact with the developmental condition and stage of cognitive maturation.

Learning disabilities and attention-deficit disorder (ADD) are developmental conditions found in adults and children. Adults with developmental disorders often present with a set of behavioral and learning problems in verbal and nonverbal modalities that can predate traumatic experiences (Gaddes, 1985; Rourke, 1985; Spreen, 1988). Learning disabilities and attention-deficit disorder may occur separately or in conjunction with each other and concurrently with anxiety and depression (Biederman, Newcorn, & Sprich, 1991; Bigler, 1990). Features of PTSD and ADD that behaviorally resemble each other may stem from different roots. Although clinical correlations have been observed, the contributions of learning disabilities and attention-deficit disorder to the development and maintenance of PTSD also need more empirical study. Establishing the existence of these conditions as part of the clinical history in patients undergoing psychiatric evaluations is important, though, for differential diagnosis, for appraising potential interaction effects between conditions, and for interpreting neuropsychological test findings. An example of a potential interaction is hypervigilance and ADD. Hypervigilant individuals scan the environment for sources of imagined or real threat. This behavior preoccupies them and can produce fatigue from the sustained effort. For patients with ADD, their focus of attention is involuntarily shifted to salient and often irrelevant stimuli in the surrounding environment. Shifting attention from one salient stimulus to another can overtly resemble hypervigilant scanning. It is also possible that the distractibility and reduced capacity to concentrate that accompanies ADD intensifies PTSD-related hypervigilance because of the difficulty the individual has inhibiting reactions to stimuli in the surrounding environment. Both conditions interfere with attention and concentration abilities, which in turn affects encoding and storage processes necessary for good memory. Neuropsychological testing can assist with the clinical differentiation of these behaviors by examining patterns of attentional problems under low-distraction conditions.

Neurocognitive Factors That Increase Risk for Experiencing Traumatic Events

Various neurological conditions can produce impairments in areas of higher cognitive processing involved in learning and memory, attention, planning, reasoning, judgment, monitoring of the environment, awareness of consequences, volition, sequencing abilities, controlling impulsivity, integration of complex information, and self-regulation (Brooks, 1989; Lezak, 1989). The impact of impairments in these areas can increase the risk of incurring a trauma (Cuffe, McCullough, & Pumariega, 1994; Famularo, Kinscherff, & Fenton, 1992). Alterations in judgment and decreased appreciation of behavioral consequences may lead to psychological trauma from various kinds of accidents, beatings, or assaults. Brain damage that reduces the capacity to attend to the most relevant aspects of the environment, to process and appraise information quickly, and to recognize danger will increase risk for experiencing a trauma. Individuals presenting with neurocognitive deficits in these domains should be assessed for past trauma exposure.

PTSD Emergence or Exacerbation Following the Onset of a Neurological Condition

Individuals in this category present with increased PTSD symptoms following the gradual development of a neurological disorder or the onset of an acute neurological condition. The exacerbation may result from (1) the extra demand on cognitive and emotional resources produced by adding a neurological condition to existing trauma symptoms, (2) precipitation of traumatic distress that is directly related to the new neurological condition, or (3) triggering hyperarousal related to themes of fear and helplessness because the new neurological disorder is a threat to health. Chemtob and Herriott (1994) described a case of PTSD as a sequela of severe Guillain–Barré syndrome in a 24-year-old female. Cassidy and Lyons (1992) reported on the case of a 63-

year-old World War II male combat veteran who experienced increased dissociative episodes of hand-to-hand combat, intrusive recall of traumatic memories, and avoidance of reminders of the war after surviving a cerebral vascular accident (CVA). These case examples illustrate conditions that cause a change in symptom status. In one case, the PTSD is secondary to the neurological condition, and in the other, PTSD symptoms increase after the neurological event. A reduced capacity to inhibit or modulate PTSD symptoms is common to both examples.

PTSD and Acquired Neurological Conditions

Together with trauma-related variables, clinical and research protocols should include assessments of acquired conditions capable of producing neuropsychological deficits, such as neurotoxic exposures, hypoxic/anoxia episodes, chronic alcohol abuse, dementias, and traumatic head injuries. Ignoring the impact of these conditions—which could have been acquired before, during, or after the traumatic event—increases the risk of misattributing the sources of observed clinical problems and impaired neuropsychological test performances.

Neurotoxic Exposure

Neurotoxic exposure can occur during military combat, industrial accidents, environmental accidents, suicide attempts, and intentional or accidental poisonings. It can be the primary traumatic event or an associated aspect of a psychological trauma. The negative effects of toxin exposure on neurocognitive abilities, affect, and personality have been well described (Hartman, 1988, 1992; Levy, 1988; White, Feldman, & Proctor, 1992). Schottenfeld and Cullen (1985) reported that PTSD frequently developed in workers who were acutely or chronically exposed to toxins. Toxin-exposed individuals may be immediately aware that the exposure occurred, may experience fear for their health or their lives during the exposure, and may immediately develop acute stress disorder that later progresses to PTSD. Others may experience chronic exposure or may not be aware of an acute exposure, becoming aware of it only after the fact. The onset of PTSD symptoms may be linked to the moment when they become aware of the past threat to their health. Reexperiencing and hyperarousal symptoms can subsequently be triggered when strong chemical smells are encountered in the ambient environment, even if the odor is different from the one involved in the original toxin exposure. Extreme patterns of avoidance behavior may develop as a strategy to prevent repeated exposure to the chemicals attributed to be the cause of current emotional, medical, and neuropsychological problems. These avoidance behaviors may closely resemble in form and severity those that are often associated with phobias and obsessive–compulsive disorder. In conceptualizing individual cases, the comorbid effects of neurotoxic exposure and PTSD will need to be differentiated from general psychological distress, neurocognitive sequelae, and other anxiety disorders with overlapping symptoms.

Hypoxic/Anoxia Episodes

Psychologically traumatic events involving suicide attempts via carbon monoxide poisoning; respiratory-suppressing drug overdoses; near drownings; fires; or other near-death experiences from stabbings, shootings, strangulation, suffocation, chest wounds that affect circulation (e.g., crush injuries), toxic spills, and electrocution (Cooper & Milroy, 1994; Daniel, Haben, Hutcherson, Botter, & Long, 1985; Hopewell, 1983; Mellen, Weedn, & Kao, 1992; Miller, 1993) can produce neurological damage from reduced flows of oxygen to the brain. An acute or chronic impact on cognitive abilities can result. A variety of neuropsychological deficits have been noted to occur from the nonspecific neuropathological changes following anoxia, including dysfunctional memory attributed to reductions in hippocampal volume (Hopkins, Weaver, & Kesner, 1994; Hopkins et al., 1995). Recovery from anoxic episodes will be affected by the age and health of the person. Little is known at this time about the clinical interactions of trauma-related symptoms and hypoxia/anoxia. However, residual tissue damage following hypoxic and anoxic episodes can be diffuse, potentially affecting many brain cortical and subcortical systems. Damage that impairs the efficiency of these brain systems may reduce emotion regulation capacities, making psychological distress and PTSD symptoms more difficult to manage.

Chronic Alcohol Abuse in PTSD

Chronic alcohol abuse can also produce damage to multiple brain regions involved in the regulation of behavior, cognition, and emotion. Harper, Kril, and Daly (1987) reported neuropathological findings showing reduced brain weights and increased pericerebral space that was attributed to loss of white matter, particularly neuronal cell death and axonal degeneration in the anterior frontal lobe. This radiological evidence of cortical atrophy in chronic alcoholics and in heavy social drinkers correlated with clinical and neuropsychological deficits. Alcohol use can increase the risk of acquiring a brain injury. Hillbom and Holm (1986) reported a strong association between substance abuse problems and motor vehicle accidents, and Gill and Sparadeo (1988) noted that 50–70% of all patients who received head injuries in motor vehicle accidents had been drinking. The presence of alcohol in the body can exacerbate the acute effects of head injury and can delay or complicate recovery. Edna (1982) reported that injured patients having alcohol in the bloodstream presented with lower levels of consciousness when admitted to the hospital and had longer durations of coma that were not accounted for by factors such as skull fractures and hematomas.

Individuals with PTSD frequently abuse alcohol as an agent for regulating physiological arousal, promoting sleep, decreasing pain, and numbing responsiveness (Keane & Wolfe, 1990). Although alcohol may have some effectiveness in the short term for symptom management, chronic use can lead to persistent behavioral dysregulation, drug tolerance, and a separate substance abuse dependence that parallels the PTSD condition. The disinhibitory effects of acute alcohol intoxication can also add to the problems patients with PTSD have in controlling their negative emotions, exhibiting good judgment, and containing behavioral reactions. Given the high comorbidity between the two disorders, the neuropsychological effects of chronic alcohol use are also particularly salient for patients with PTSD. Parsons (1987) found that neuropsychological deficits were predicted by number of drinking occasions and the maximum quantity consumed each time. As the chronicity of drinking increased, neuropsychological impairment approached that of brain-damaged patients.

The interactions of neurocognitive deficits, chronic alcohol abuse, and PTSD are complex. Although PTSD or chronic alcohol abuse symptoms could be viewed as the main problem needing to be addressed for any given case, the impact of neurocognitive impairments needs to be equally considered. Screening for neurocognitive problems in a clinical assessment can be difficult in clinical patients who have long-standing PTSD and alcohol abuse, if their memory for autobiographical details is absent or unreliable. To facilitate recall, time lines should be collected to refine the details of alcohol use; potential head injury events from motor vehicle accidents, fights or beatings, falls and work accidents; PTSD symptoms; and neurocognitive problems. This interviewing method is helpful, and formal neuropsychological testing will complement the history information to further define areas of neurocognitive impairment. The assessment information from all of these sources will be needed to characterize the clinical problems resulting from the many possible combinations of comorbid symptoms.

Dementias

Dementia has been defined as an acquired, persistent impairment of intellectual functioning with compromise in at least three of the following spheres of mental activity: language, memory and visuospatial skills, emotion or personality, and higher cognitive abilities (Cummings & Benson, 1992). PTSD could coexist with dementia as a separate disorder caused by traumatic events occurring earlier in life or ones experienced in later life. If only subclinical levels of PTSD symptoms were present premorbidly, the onset of dementia could precipitate the emergence of the full PTSD criteria by exacerbating these symptoms, or, secondary to marked cognitive decline, new psychological traumas could have a greater impact because needed cognitive resources are no longer available to manage the distress that is experienced. For instance, problems with response inhibition can increase the difficulty for the patient with dementia in containing emotional reactions that are triggered by trauma-related cues. If PTSD-related factors are not assessed as part of the evaluation process, the emotional dysregulation, anxiety, irritability, impaired attention/distraction, and depressed mood might be completely attributed to symptoms of dementia. Although these clinical symptoms are common to both PTSD and dementia, they might respond uniquely to interventions that target the disorders separately. Alternatively, the interaction of the two disorders might produce distinct effects that do not respond well unless treated in combination. More empirical study is needed that focuses on dementias and PTSD.

Traumatic Head Injury

Although they commonly co-occur, the comorbid effects of PTSD and traumatic head injury are generally underevaluated by traumatologists and neuropsychologists. Many military and civilian events can cause neurological and psychological trauma. The following sources of traumatic psychological stress should be considered for their concomitant head injury potential: natural disasters, intimate relationship violence or violence by family members (Glod, 1993; Kiser, Heston, Millsap, & Pruitt, 1991; Stein, Kennedy, & Twamley, 2002), stranger violence (Shepard, Quercohi, & Preston, 1990), injuries during torture (*violence*, Jacobs & Iacopino, 2001; Rassmussen, 1990; Weinstein, Fucetola, & Mollica, 2001; *nutritional deprivation/starvation by captors*, Gurvit, 1993; Sutker, Allain, & Winstead, 1987; Sutker, Galina, West, & Allain, 1990; Thygesen, Hermann, & Willanger,1970), rape and other sexual trauma with physical injury to the head (Jenkins, 2000; Jenkins, Langlais, Delis, & Cohen, 1998; Reeves, Beltzman, & Killu, 2000), high-risk sports (Downs & Abwender, 2002; Matser, Kessels, Lezak, & Troost, 2001; Roberts, Allsop, & Barton, 1990), transportation accidents as a driver, passenger, or pedestrian (Kuch, Evans, & Watson, 1991), military-related combat and noncombat injuries (Trudeau et al., 1998), and industrial/occupational accidents.

When the index traumatic event falls into one of the preceding categories, neuropsychologists should ask additional questions about possible PTSD symptoms, and traumatologists should ask questions about prior head injuries and any consequent physical or cognitive problems that resulted. Surveying the preceding categories of potential traumatic brain injury (TBI) events as part of clinical history taking will often elicit additional traumatic experiences. Routinely employing a structured interview process helps to address one of the factors that limits spontaneous reporting of possible head injury events by patients; that is, that events without loss of consciousness or with short intervals of lost consciousness may not be remembered as an injury. Emerging from a short interval of lost consciousness may be perceived by patients as awakening from a form of sleep. In addition, many potential head injuries can occur during activities that could be regarded by the patient as occupational hazards and thus are not remembered as significant. For example, in the military, head injuries can occur in battle from stabbings, low- and high-velocity missile wounds, explosions of land mines, hand grenades, bombs, rockets, mortars, large-scale artillery weapons, or falls from training equipment, helicopters, trees, buildings, and moving armored vehicles. The loss of consciousness and the concussions that may have resulted from these combat events may be blended generally into the context of the psychological trauma or may be considered of minor importance compared to surviving combat.

The preceding examples illustrate the main types of traumatic brain injury that can coexist with psychological trauma: penetrating head injury (PHI) and major, minor, or mild closed head injury (CHI). PHIs constitute 2–6% of all head injuries and can include open head wounds from knives or sharp or blunt objects, skull fractures associated with falls, beatings, and crush injuries, and missile wounds from gunshots, shrapnel, and other projectiles. Military combat, crime episodes, and miscellaneous accidents are the most common sources of PHI (Kampen & Grafman, 1989). The amount of damage depends on the velocity of the penetrating object and the cavitation surrounding the track of the object. Hemorrhaging occurs locally and throughout the brain. High-velocity wounds are frequently fatal, whereas low-velocity wounds (e.g., stabbings) produce local damage. Changes in behavior, affect, and cognition are a product of the tissue damage and the resulting alteration in regional brain metabolism. PHI will always be obvious and reportable by the patient. In contrast, CHI events may not always be remarkable when only momentary loss of consciousness or transient symptoms accompanied the event.

CHI events vary in severity and can produce sequelae ranging from frank neurocognitive deficits to various emotional and behavioral disturbances that could be attributed to psychiatric origins. In severe CHI, gross acceleration–deceleration movements of the brain within the skull produce widespread diffuse damage due to axonal shearing and concussive damage to the surface of the cortex in orbitofrontal, anterior, and inferior temporal regions of the brain (Davidoff, Kessler, Laibstain, & Mark, 1988; McAllister, 1992). For minor head injuries, movement effects are less pronounced and result in more circumscribed deficits related to abilities mediated by the anterior cortex, such as memory, attention and concentration, judgment, and abstract reasoning (Barth et. al., 1983; Bigler & Snyder, 1995; Kwentus, Hart, Peck & Kornstein, 1985). Even in cases of common whiplash injuries, in which no head contact or loss of consciousness is reported, complex attentional processing can be impaired (Radanov, Stefano, Schnidrig, Sturzenegger, & Augustiny, 1993). Segalowitz et al. (1993) reported an incident rate of 30% for head injuries among a large community sample of 3,961 people. Presence of head injury was significantly related to reports of hyperactivity, sleep disturbance, depression, and problems with social functioning. Neurobehavioral effects of CHI can overlap with symptoms of anxiety, depression, manic behavior, and personality disorder (McAllister, 1992).

The combined effects of CHI and PTSD can produce difficulties with inhibiting behavior, regulating emotional reactivity, and suppressing trauma-related intrusive memories. The presence of a CHI can increase levels of hypervigilance, flashbacks, intrusive memories, and physiological hyperarousal or panic and can decrease ability to control negative emotions and expressions of anger or to shut down physical reactions that persist after being startled. Depending on the location of the head injury, other problems may exist, including poor concentration, increased cognitive rigidity, perseveration on ideas or plans, misperception of social cues, reduced verbal abstract reasoning, and distorted interpretations of nonverbal information. These problems can worsen under conditions of increased and persistent physiological arousal and can potentially limit the benefits derived from psychotherapy. Levin (1985) noted that in some patients with minor CHI, residual deficits might be manifested only under conditions of stress.

The TBI–PTSD Controversy

An active debate is ongoing in the current literature surrounding two main questions related to whether TBI and PTSD are mutually exclusive: (1) Can PTSD coexist with TBI? and (2) can PTSD develop following a traumatic head injury when the survivor cannot recall the details of the event due to neurogenic amnesia? Both questions are important for theoretical and practical reasons. Theoretically, they speak to the potential neurobiological mechanisms for PTSD. Practically, the answers to these questions have medicolegal implications for injury-related lawsuits and workers' compensation claims, as the causal linkage is important for assigning fault and awarding payment for damages. Psychologists and neuropsychologists who provide expert testimony to the courts might be called on to address these questions in their evaluations.

These questions have become controversial (Bontke, 1996; Bryant, 2001; Levy, 1996; Stephen & Masterson, 1999), in part because opposite, empirically supported conclusions have been reached by different researchers. Findings from some studies in the literature support the argument against the development of PTSD following TBI (Mayou, Bryant, & Duthie, 1993; Sbordone, 1991, 1999; Sbordone & Liter, 1995; Ursano et al., 1999; Warden et al., 1997), whereas other case studies and group-design studies have reported that PTSD can develop following mild to severe TBIs (incidence rates of 17–56%; Bryant, 1996; Bryant & Harvey, 1995, 1998, 1999a,b, 2002; Bryant, Marosszeky, Crooks, & Gurka, 2000; Bryant, Marosszeky, Crooks, Baguley, & Gurka, 2001; Feinstein, Hershkop, Ouchterlony, Jardine & McCullagh, 2002; Grisgsby & Kaye, 1993; Harvey & Bryant, 2000, 2001; Hibbard, Uysal, Keple, Bogdany, & Silver, 1998; Hickling, Gillen, Blanchard, Buckley, & Taylor, 1998; Horton, 1993; Layton & Wardi-Zonna, 1995; Mayou, Black, & Bryant, 2000; McMillan, 1991, 1996; Middleboe, Andersen, Birket-Smith, & Frist, 1992; Ohry, Rattok, & Solomon, 1996; Parker, 1998; Rattok & Ross, 1993; Williams, Evans, Wilson, & Needham, 2002; Wright & Telford, 1996).

The argument against the development of PTSD following TBI states that trauma-related symptoms are not likely to develop when consciousness is lost and amnesia exists for details of the head injury event. In the absence of conscious recall for the event, it is assumed that psychological distress, feelings of being threatened or endangered, intrusions, flashbacks, nightmares, and reactivity should not develop. Consequently, patterns of avoidance should also not develop, and hypervigilance should be unnecessary. Implicit in the logic behind this argument is the assumption that the psychological effects of amnesia for a traumatic event are the same as if one had never experienced the event. That is, without a traumatic experience, PTSD symptoms should not develop. This logic makes amnesia the causal factor that determines PTSD symptom development. When low incidences of PTSD following TBI have been observed, some researchers (Klein, Caspi, & Gil, 2003; O'Brien & Nutt, 1998) have interpreted this finding to mean that sustaining a TBI may even serve a protective function against the development of traumatic stress reactions. The memory loss that is secondary to the TBI supposedly protects against PTSD by preventing the formation of distressing memories. However, the presence of amnesia and the absence of PTSD reexperiencing symptoms may be correlated in time but not causally related, and they might reflect different outcomes resulting from damage sustained to multiple brain regions during the same TBI event. Considering that PTSD symptoms develop in portions of TBI survivors and also when psychogenic amnesia is present, the absence of recall of the traumatic event is not sufficient to account for all the patterns in the data. More complete explanations for these empirical observations need to proposed and evaluated.

One possible hypothesis accounts for the discordant findings in the literature by postulating that subgroups of TBI survivors encode the head injury event differently. In the subgroup that lost consciousness during the event, that is now completely amnestic for the details of the event, and that does not manifest current PTSD symptoms, the traumatic content and associated emotional distress cannot be accessed because they were not stored in memory in any form. In the other subgroups that developed PTSD following TBI, two alternative explanations are possible. The first possibility is that autobiographical recall for details of the head injury is completely intact because consciousness was not lost and the event was fully encoded in memory or that partial memory exists because some encoding occurred during fleeting moments of consciousness. These "islands of memory" could develop in the presence of fluctuating levels of consciousness (Forrester, Encel, & Geffen, 1994; Gronwall & Wrightson, 1980; King, 1997; McMillan, 1996; McNeil & Greenwood, 1996). Memory for the head injury event in either of these two instances would be linked to moments of conscious processing, with PTSD reexperiencing, avoidance, and hyperarousal symptoms developing around the discontinuous fragments of memory. The second possibility is that aspects of the traumatic/TBI event were encoded as memories under state-dependent conditions and are most susceptible to being triggered when similar stimulus conditions reoccur. Thus PTSD symptoms would be less likely to form around the narrative memory of the TBI event. Brewin, Dalgleish, and Joseph (1996) discussed this possibility in their dual-representation theory of PTSD, which accounts for symptom development under these conditions by making a distinction between conscious memories of a traumatic event, which are verbally accessible, and fear-conditioned avoidance/arousal symptoms, which are situationally accessible. Conscious attention during the traumatic event is required in this model in order for verbally accessible information to be sufficiently organized, encoded, and stored for later recall. States of unconsciousness secondary to a traumatic brain injury would interfere with or prevent conscious information processing. In contrast, the situationally accessible information would be encoded and stored within a distributed perceptual system in the brain and automatically retrieved when elicited by trauma-related cues. The situationally accessible information stored in memory would include conditioned components of fear, anxiety, and distress. When cued, they would be reexperienced as psychological and physiological reactivity to which patterns of avoidance behaviors could develop. Consistent with this model, studies have found patients with moderate to severe TBI who met only partial PTSD criteria, manifesting as avoidance and hyperarousal in the absence of reexperiencing (Warden et al., 1997; Bryant & Harvey, 1996). Baggaley and Rose (1990) observed PTSD without symptoms of intrusive recall but with nightmares characterized by unretrievable content and with phobic avoidance to trauma-specific cues. Watson (1990) reported examples of trauma reexperiencing that took the form of specific pain and other physical symptoms. The preceding formulations rely on fluctuations in consciousness during the TBI and in variability in post-TBI recall to reconcile the discrepant findings in the literature regarding PTSD development. Other methodological factors might shape interpretations of the findings in the literature.

Approaches to assessing traumatic experiences will determine incidence rates of PTSD, and poor autobiographical memory will set upper limits on the availability of historical information for this diagnostic process. The inability to recall the details of a traumatic experience could reflect psychogenic amnesia, neurogenic amnesia, a drug-induced blackout episode secondary to severe chronic alcohol abuse, or a combination of all three, as might be the case with a chronic alcohol abuser who sustains a closed head injury with a momentary loss of consciousness during a motor vehicle accident and reports a history of dissociating in response to stress and blacking out from intoxication while driving. In this example, it would be difficult to determine the cause for any presenting amnestic disturbance using currently available diagnostic methods. However, at the time that diagnostic information is being collected, determining the cause of the amnesia may be a lower priority, as all three conditions functionally interfere with or prevent retrieval of information. The potential for recall at some later time, however, could vary across the different sources. Obtaining valid self-appraisals of the degree of consciousness maintained during the traumatic event will likewise be confounded by limited recall. The ambiguity about level of consciousness throughout the event makes it equally difficult to predict whether some post-TBI cued reactivity might develop and, if so, in what form. Moreover, for individuals with past histories of multiple trauma who present with PTSD symptoms after a recent TBI, amnesia for the most recent TBI event may actually be unrelated to the PTSD symptoms that present clinically. Thus proper interpretation of information from diagnostic interviews requires that symptom ratings be correctly linked, to the extent that it is possible, to their corresponding traumatic event. Interpretive schemas might also require some modification in order to account for atypical but valid patterns of PTSD symptoms associated with TBI.

The methods employed for assessing criterion A will also affect the rates of PTSD reported after a TBI. In order for a PTSD diagnosis to be assigned using DSM-IV, individual PTSD symptom criteria must be associated with a traumatic event that meets the PTSD A_1 and A_2 criteria. However, if interviews are used to establish the PTSD diagnosis, and if the traumatic event and reactions to the event cannot be recalled by the TBI survivor, then PTSD criterion A cannot be established by self-report. The DSM-IV PTSD diagnosis technically cannot be conferred in the absence of criterion A. From a diagnostic perspective, the nature of the events that produced the brain injury clearly meet the DSM-IV A_1 criterion definition of *exposure to a traumatic event* in which the individual experiences or is confronted with actual or threatened death or serious injury or threat to physical integrity of self or others. The A_2 criterion, which reflects psychological distress experienced about the event, further requires that the person must also have reacted with fear, horror, or helplessness or, in the case of children, with agitated or disorganized behavior. If the TBI survivor had even momentary awareness of the injury, fear was probably elicited. Although it may be implicit in the diagnostic criteria that the person remembers having reactions of fear or helplessness, recall of these reactions is not explicitly required for the PTSD diagnosis. If others observed these reactions in the person, they could report these observations during a collateral interview. Thus criterion A_1 will be met by virtue of surviving a life-threatening head injury, and the more subjective A_2 criterion might need to be corroborated by observers of the person in the acute phase of injury. In cases in which PTSD B, C, and D criteria symptoms are present but autobiographical memory for the traumatic event is absent, rates of diagnosis of no PTSD will be higher.

Various self-report interview and questionnaire methods, discussed in more detail in other chapters in this volume, are used to measure the construct of PTSD or the 17 PTSD symptoms directly. Some methods primarily rate presence or absence of each symptom, whereas others additionally assess frequency, intensity, or severity. With methods that measure all of the DSM-IV PTSD symptoms, thousands of possible combinations of the 17 PTSD symptoms would meet criteria for the PTSD diagnosis. For example, some individuals might just meet the minimum PTSD symptom requirements (i.e., 1 B criterion, 3 C criterion, and 2 D criterion symptoms), whereas others might present with most of the 17 PTSD symptoms. However, regardless of the number and pattern of symptoms, after crossing the DSM-IV diagnostic threshold, all individuals receive the PTSD diagnosis, and they all could be included in the PTSD group for research studies. Yet, compared with the person with many PTSD symptoms, much less demand on cognitive resources will be experienced by an individual with the minimum required number of PTSD symptoms.

The preceding discussion underscores the fact that PTSD is not a unitary construct, and the incidence of PTSD following TBI will vary depending on the diagnostic scheme and the thresholds employed to establish caseness. The criterion A determination process will affect PTSD prevalence rates by defining whether a qualifying event occurred to which PTSD symptoms could form. The diagnostic thresholds set for the 17 individual PTSD symptoms will limit the sensitivity for detecting psychopathology. TBI survivors could potentially be excluded from the PTSD diagnosis if they miss the diagnostic cutoff by one individual symptom in one of the B, C, or D criterion groups. Future studies should examine the impact of diagnostic decisions and analyze PTSD symptoms as a continuous variable, as well as a dichotomous diagnostic variable. A continuous variable may offer more sensitivity to the range of clinical presentations that could manifest. For research that compares the functioning of patients with PTSD with other external neurocognitive criteria, the variability in the test performances should also be examined as a function of different symptom patterns among the members of the PTSD group.

Time of measurement is also important when defining the rates of PTSD following TBI. The point in time at which the diagnostic determination is made can influence conclusions about the effect of TBI on the development of PTSD. Bryant and Harvey (1998) observed that, among survivors with mild TBI, 24% met PTSD criteria in the first month postinjury. Among patients with mild TBI who were initially diagnosed with acute stress disorder, 24% developed PTSD at 6 months postinjury. Prospective data from a separate study (Harvey & Bryant, 2000) found that 80% of survivors with mild TBI who were diagnosed with acute stress disorder following a motor vehicle accident met criteria for PTSD 2 years after injury. Over the course of time, intrusive memories have been found to decrease in patients with TBI and to increase in survivors with TBI (Bryant & Harvey, 1995; Bryant & Harvey, 2001). In cases of initial amnesia for the event, memory functioning may show a general improvement over time (Harvey & Bryant, 2001), and this improvement may be accompanied by a corresponding increase in details recalled. PTSD symptoms might increase as more details are remembered. These data suggest the possibility that the emergence of PTSD may parallel the TBI recovery process or that having a TBI increases the risk of developing delayed PTSD reactions.

In conclusion, the existing literature shows that PTSD and TBI can clearly coexist; however, the issue of PTSD development following a TBI remains open. The presence of amnesia for details of the TBI event drives the argument against PTSD development and is viewed by some as a protective factor that prevents distress. Alternatively, moments of conscious processing during the TBI event may explain why PTSD develops in some people but not in others. Additional variables related to how PTSD is diagnosed and when PTSD is assessed post-TBI could also account for some patterns among the existing findings. To advance the literature, it might be more fruitful in the future to shift the emphasis of the comorbidity debate from the current question to questions with more clinical relevance. For example, under what conditions does amnesia not only block access to details of the TBI event but also cause a reduction in general psychological problems and trauma-specific symptoms? Is amnesia for the event a separate process or secondary to the global neurogenic memory loss, and could exposure treatment methods elicit recall of the event?

The theoretical and medicolegal aspects of the comorbidity debate are academic compared with the tangible clinical needs of survivors of TBI who have PTSD. They are academic in that case examples of a single TBI and a newly emergent PTSD condition in someone who is free from premorbid neurological problems and psychopathology will represent only a small portion of the clinical population likely to present for evaluation and treatment. Whether the PTSD symptoms are related to the present TBI, to other TBIs, or to other traumas is mostly irrelevant when the clinical goal is to understand and treat whatever functional problems present. Survivors of TBI with trauma from childhood abuse and combat veterans with PTSD who sustained CHIs during the service or after discharge as civilians populate mental health clinics.

The impact of TBI for patients with PTSD is usually not subtle, especially if frontal brain systems are involved. These patients will regularly identify the TBI as the factor responsible for the reduction in their capacity to inhibit behavioral and emotional responding to the trauma-related intrusive memories and flashbacks and to manage general hyperarousal. They report that before the CHI occurred they had been able to push intrusion away, were not as quickly angered, recovered from startle sooner, and had much better concentration. The problems resulting from PTSD and TBI are unequivocal in the clinical presentations of these patients. It would be extremely unfortunate if the difficulties resulting from PTSD–TBI comorbidity were underdiagnosed or invalidated because the literature suggests that the two disorders cannot coexist.

Related to the validity of TBI–PTSD coexistence is the notion that a TBI functions as a protective factor. The term "protective" implies that receiving a brain injury is somehow a positive life event. In a circumscribed way, although the absence of some reexperiencing criteria may prevent the PTSD diagnosis from being assigned, the effects of moderate to severe TBIs on brain functioning are not positive. The use of the term "protective" should be reconsidered in light of the existing assessment and rehabilitation literature on the negative impact of TBI. Calling TBIs protective could mislead caregivers and evaluators into discounting the legitimacy of the presence of PTSD after

TBI and the severity of potential functional consequences for survivors of TBI. Clinical case conceptualizations, treatment plans, or opinions advanced in court cases could also be affected.

To guard against the development of biases that could have unintentional negative effects for patients, much more needs to be known about causes for the low rates of PTSD observed in some TBI survivors and whether the conclusions based on the limited number of existing TBI–PTSD studies would generalize to other age groups and individuals who had experienced multiple closed head injuries. The evolving literature will benefit from more empirically supported conclusions about TBI comorbidity based on a wider sampling of TBI survivors who have experienced a broader range of traumas.

REVIEW OF THE EXISTING LITERATURE

The published studies examining neuropsychological test performances from patients with PTSD to date are relatively few and vary in format, from single clinical case studies to large-sample group designs. A range of populations with PTSD have been examined. At this point, no consensus neuropsychological test battery has evolved for evaluating PTSD, although the neurocognitive domains of attention, concentration, executive functioning, and memory are commonly assessed. The following sections divide available studies into combat-trauma and non-combat-trauma groups, and the main findings are reviewed. A general discussion follows at the end of this section, addressing issues that are common to these studies.

Studies with Combat Veteran Populations

Findings of neuropsychological impairment among combat veteran populations have been mixed due to several factors, including variability in the degree to which comorbid and preexisting pathology have been taken into account, a lack of control groups in some studies, failure to match comparison groups on key variables, differences in type of sample examined (e.g., clinical versus population-based), differences in PTSD severity across studies, and variations in sample size and statistical power to detect differences.

Several studies appearing early in the literature failed to document an association between PTSD and neuropsychological impairment among samples of combat veterans. In a study of 36 POW survivors of the Bataan Death March during World War II, Moses and Maruish (1988) found scores on the Luria–Nebraska Neuropsychological Battery (LNNB) to fall within the normal range compared with the normative sample. However, although several of the participants were noted to exhibit a variant of PTSD, no diagnostic information was given. Similarly, Dalton, Pederson, and Ryan (1989) found few deficit performances on neuropsychological testing among a sample of PTSD-positive Vietnam veteran inpatients. Only the Trail Making Test-Part B, the

Benton Visual Retention Test, and the Stroop Color–Word Naming Test showed slightly reduced group performances, and these findings were interpreted as reflecting mild anxiety effects, as would be expected in psychiatric inpatient samples. Gurvits et al. (1993) found few differences between groups of Vietnam combat veterans with and without PTSD on neuropsychological testing, though the group with PTSD showed more neuropsychological soft signs on neurological examination. In a more recent study, Golier and colleagues (1997) did not find differences on a sustained-attention task between a group of Vietnam combat veterans with PTSD and a PTSD-negative control group.

In contrast to the studies that failed to find neuropsychological deficits among combat veterans with PTSD, a growing literature documents clinical impairments on tests of *memory* (Bremner, Southwick, Johnson, Yehuda, & Charney, 1993; Bremner, Scott, et al., 1993; Gilbertson, Gurvits, Lasko, Orr, & Pitman, 2001; Sutker, Allain, & Johnson, 1993; Sutker, Winstead, Galina, & Allain, 1991; Uddo, Vasterling, Brailey, & Sutker, 1993), *attention* (Uddo et al., 1993; Vasterling et al., 2002), *executive functioning* (Beckham, Crawford, & Feldman, 1998), and *global intellectual functioning* (Gil, Calev, Greenberg, Kugelmass, & Lerer, 1990; McNally & Shin, 1995; Sutker et al., 1991; Vasterling et al., 2002). In a few studies of veterans with combat-related PTSD, short-term memory impairment has shown some association with reduced volume in the hippocampus, a structure considered critical for new learning and memory (see Bremner, 1999, for a review). Some researchers have concluded that the accumulating evidence demonstrates the presence of frontal-limbic-system dysfunction among combat veterans with PTSD (e.g., Vasterling et al., 2002).

Perhaps the most salient confound in the examination of the relationship between PTSD and neuropsychological deficits among combat veterans is the issue of comorbidity. Studies differ substantially regarding the degree to which comorbid psychiatric and neurological conditions are systematically considered when designing studies and interpreting data. As previously discussed, combat veterans with PTSD typically present with multiple comorbidities, many of which impair cognitive functioning to differing degrees. Some studies have attempted to account for comorbidity by comparing groups with PTSD only to those with PTSD and other comorbid problems. For example, Barrett, Green, Morris, Giles, and Croft (1996) compared the neuropsychological functioning of four groups of Vietnam veterans: those with a lifetime history of PTSD and a current diagnosis of anxiety, depression, or substance abuse; those with PTSD diagnoses only; those with diagnoses of anxiety, depression, or substance abuse only; and normal controls with no psychiatric diagnoses. Interestingly, these researchers found no neuropsychological impairment among the group with PTSD only. In contrast, the group with PTSD and comorbid diagnoses displayed the most impairment on all measures of cognitive functioning. This group generated impaired performances on tests of concept formation, problem solving, verbal memory, and visual organization. The authors concluded that PTSD, in isolation, did not appear to be associated with cognitive impairment.

It has been argued (Gilbertson et al., 2001; Knight, 1997) that the very high rates of comorbidity among veterans with PTSD greatly hinders attempts to obtain a "pure PTSD" group in comparative studies and that such a sample may not adequately reflect the patterns of symptomatology typically observed in the population with PTSD. Attempts to match groups with PTSD and control groups on comorbid problems may lead to overly pathological control groups and to groups with PTSD who have relatively low levels of symptoms, which could mask differences between groups. As these authors discuss, it may be more fruitful to examine the interrelationships among comorbid problems and their unique effects on neuropsychological functioning. These researchers found attention and memory deficits among a group of combat veterans with PTSD, relative to combat veterans without PTSD. In addition, associations between PTSD and these two neuropsychological variables were independent of trauma exposure severity, IQ, depression, alcohol use history, and history of developmental learning problems.

Whether neuropsychological sequelae manifest differently for PTSD than for other psychiatric conditions remains an open question and has been the focus of studies that compared veterans with PTSD to those with other psychiatric problems. In this regard, Gil et al. (1990) evaluated the neuropsychological test performances among a group of men with PTSD only, matched psychiatric controls, and normal controls. Across a full battery of tests, the patients with PTSD showed significant impairment relative to normal controls but levels of impairment similar to the matched psychiatric controls. The authors interpreted the findings as supporting the presence of a general cognitive dysfunction, rather than a PTSD-specific dysfunction. Among a large population-based sample (n = 723) of Vietnam-era veterans, Zalewski, Thompson, and Gottesman (1994) compared neuropsychological testing performances among a group of those with PTSD, a group of individuals with generalized anxiety disorder, and a group with no lifetime history of psychiatric disorder. In this study, there were no differences between the two psychiatric groups on neuropsychological testing, and these two groups also did not differ from the nonpsychiatric control group. Similar findings were obtained in a reanalysis of a smaller subsample of this larger data set, in a comparison of veterans with PTSD who were in distress at the time of evaluation, veterans with PTSD who were not in distress at the time of evaluation, veterans diagnosed with a psychiatric disorder other than PTSD, and a matched control group (Crowell, Kieffer, Siders, & Vanderploeg, 2002).

Another question that has received relatively little attention is whether neuropsychological deficits are the precursors or the sequelae of trauma. Vasterling et al. (2002) reviewed several studies demonstrating associations between PTSD and indirect, pretrauma estimates of intellectual functioning. In their comparison of veterans with PTSD and a group of veterans with no mental disorders on a neuropsychological test battery, these researchers attempted to account for pretrauma deficits by controlling for estimated premorbid intelligence. In addition, and in contrast to many prior studies, considerable efforts were made to account for comorbid problems. Veterans were excluded if they had a positive history of head injury, central nervous system disease, alcohol or substance abuse disorder, lifetime history of bipolar or psychotic disorders, or subthreshold PTSD. As previous researchers had found, estimated premorbid intelligence was associated with PTSD severity, and a diagnosis of PTSD was associated with impairments on tasks of sustained attention, working memory, and initial learning. These associations remained even after controlling for premorbid intelligence. It was concluded that, although pretrauma cognitive functioning may be a risk factor, PTSD appears to be associated with neuropsychological deficits that are independent of the effects of premorbid functioning.

Some researchers have examined the associations between specific events encountered during combat and later neuropsychological functioning. For example, Trudeau et al. (1998) demonstrated that combat veterans with PTSD and a history of blast concussion performed more poorly on a test of attention than those with PTSD and no history of blast concussion. Levy (1988) compared the neuropsychological functioning of a group of Vietnam combat veterans exposed to Agent Orange with a nonexposed group. He found that the exposed group performed relatively poorer on the Wechsler Adult Intelligence Scale (WAIS) Vocabulary subtest, the Rey Auditory Verbal Test, the Symbol Digit Modalities Test, and the Word Fluency Test. Agent Orange exposure was also associated with the presence of PTSD, and combat exposure could not account for this association. PTSD accounted for the observed differences on neuropsychological testing.

Finally, as some have argued (e.g., Crowell et al., 2002), failures to find universal neuropsychological deficits among combat veterans with PTSD may stem from a lack of ecological validity among such studies. That is, typical neuropsychological paradigms may not necessarily capture the manner in which PTSD symptoms cause problems for combat veterans in the real world. Symptoms of PTSD typically are triggered by trauma-related cues in the environment. This is not captured by most neuropsychological testings, in which distractions are minimized as much as possible. One study (Yehuda, Keefe, Harvey, & Levengood, 1995) has found veterans with PTSD to exhibit a specific impairment in their retention of a word list following exposure to an intervening word list and normal performances on tests of initial attention, immediate memory, cumulative learning, and active interference from previous learning. The authors suggest that memory impairment among these individuals may stem from a reduced ability to inhibit attending to reexperiencing symptoms that occur in the form of intrusive memories or flashbacks. Another study (Zeitlin & McNally, 1991) has found combat veterans with PTSD to exhibit relatively heightened recall for combat-related words in implicit and explicit memory paradigms, suggesting a processing bias for trauma-specific stimuli.

Studies with Noncombat Trauma Populations

Relative to studies of combat veterans with PTSD, the examination of the neuropsychological functioning of noncombat populations with PTSD has received very little attention. The majority of these studies have examined samples of children or adolescents who have experienced different forms of child abuse or adult victims of various forms of violence (e.g., physical abuse, sexual abuse). With regard to the former, Tarter, Hegedus, Winsten, and Alterman (1984) found court-referred delinquent adolescents to exhibit primary difficulties in verbal or linguistic processing realms on neuropsychiatric testing. Dinklage and Grodzinsky (1993) showed that relative to matched psychiatric controls, a group of abused children had higher levels of inattentiveness, poorer impulse control, and below-average verbal memory. The group differences were not apparent on standard IQ measures. Moradi, Doost, Taghavi, Yule, and Dalgleish (1999) examined the memory function of a sample of 40 children and adolescents, 18 of whom were diagnosed with PTSD due to recent interpersonal violence or traffic accidents. On a test of everyday memory problems, children in the PTSD group scored lower than the control group and the normative sample on general memory, and these differences were independent of comorbid depression and reading ability. Using a more comprehensive neuropsychological test battery, Beers and De Bellis (2002) compared the cognitive functioning of a group of pediatric outpatients with PTSD from sexual abuse or from witnessing or experiencing physical abuse with that of a group of sociodemographically similar children without histories of PTSD or maltreatment on measures of language, attention, abstract reasoning/executive function, learning and memory, visual–spatial processing, and psychomotor function. Findings revealed deficits on tests of attention and abstract reasoning/executive function among those in the PTSD group. These researchers did not replicate the findings of general memory deficits obtained by Moradi et al. (1999), though results suggested deficits in verbal long-term memory.

Similar to the literature on combat veterans with PTSD, results from examinations into the neuropsychological functioning of adult female trauma victims have been mixed. Jenkins et al. (1998) examined learning and memory function among three groups: treatment-seeking rape survivors with PTSD, treatment-seeking rape survivors without PTSD, and nontraumatized controls. The group with PTSD scored significantly lower than the other two groups on the delayed-free-recall index of the California Verbal Learning Test (CVLT; Delis, Kramer, Kaplan, & Ober, 1987), with one-third of this group falling at least two standard deviations below the normative mean. A similar pattern of impaired performances was observed for the group with PTSD in sustained and divided attention. These differences were not accounted for by group differences in depression, comorbid anxiety disorders, or alcohol use. A trend was also reported for short-term memory deficits for the PTSD group relative to the other two groups. In contrast to this study, Stein, Kennedy, and Twamley (2002) recently found no differences on CVLT or Wechsler Memory Scale-III (WMS-III) verbal learning and memory scores between victims of intimate partner violence who had PTSD, victims of intimate partner violence who did not have PTSD, and nontraumatized controls. The PTSD group did, however, evidence lower scores on the Trail Making Test-Part B compared with the other two groups, with scores falling approximately two standard deviations below the normative group, consistent with some work demonstrating executive function deficits among combat veterans (Beckham et al., 1998). In addition, the two traumatized groups performed more poorly than controls on measures of visuoconstruction, visual memory, sustained attention, and auditory working memory. The authors concluded that deficits in neuropsychological test performances among abused women may be better explained by the experience of trauma or preexisting differences than the presence of PTSD.

Few neuropsychological studies have been conducted among older victims of noncombat trauma. An exception to this pattern was a recent study by Golier and colleagues (2002), who examined implicit and explicit memory function among a sample of Holocaust survivors. Holocaust survivors with PTSD were found to exhibit poorer explicit memory than Holocaust survivors without the disorder and healthy controls, independent of major depression. These findings, combined with a lack of differences between groups on implicit memory, suggested a relative deficit among these individuals on hippocampal-dependent memory function. The PTSD group also reported lower educational attainment and performed more poorly on the WAIS-R than the other two groups. Interestingly, significantly stronger inverse relationships were found between age and memory for the group with PTSD than for the other groups, raising the possibility of accelerated memory decline among Holocaust survivors with PTSD.

Overall, the findings in the preceding sets of studies are mixed regarding the presence and extent of neuropsychological impairments in PTSD and trauma-related disorders. At issue is the challenge of replicating, under structured neuropsychological testing conditions, the degree of neurocognitive impairments reported by patients in clinical contexts. When trauma patients describe the information-processing problems that they experience, a clear disruption in normal thought processes is evident, and the descriptions often resemble problems reported by neurological patients with known brain damage. However, under formal testing conditions, some investigators obtain normal or near normal mean test performances from PTSD groups. When impaired performances are found, the levels of impairment may approximate psychiatric comparison groups. In contrast, other investigators find significant impairment in the expected cognitive domains. Absence of neuropsychological deficits has been interpreted to mean that psychological distress, not PTSD, causes the information-processing problems reported clinically or that these problems are not static but arise mainly when PTSD reexperiencing symptoms are active.

Drawing general conclusions from the group of studies is difficult, however, because many of the study parameters are dissimilar. Populations varied, and sample sizes ranged from small to large. Reporting on basic study information was inconsistent for variables such as PTSD and neurological diagnostic procedures, trauma history evaluation methods, inclusion/exclusion criteria, matching variables employed for the control groups, and the neuropsychological testing protocol employed. Trauma factors that might account for variance in the findings (e.g., magnitude of the stressors, the presence of multiple traumas, or symptom chronicity and severity) were not standardly available. None of the studies we reviewed for this chapter reported on methods to account for potential reactivity to the neuropsychological testing process. For some of the studies reviewed, it is possible that test performances were influenced by altered engagement with the tasks. As we discussed in more detail later in this chapter, deficits in attention and memory functioning can result from the presence of trauma-related intrusions and physiological reactivity during testing.

Basic knowledge of neuropsychological performances from adults and children with PTSD is slowly accumulating. However, initial research and cross-validation studies at all ages across the lifespan are needed. It is unclear at this point in time which test instruments might be the most sensitive or whether traditional clinical neuropsychological measures are best suited for assessing the cognitive problems accompanying PTSD. Clinical neuropsychological tasks that are useful for examining cognitive functioning in neurological populations may prove too prone to ceiling effects in traumatized patients. In order to choose sensitive and specific neuropsychological tests, the most relevant cognitive domains must first be selected. PTSD, uncomplicated by CVA or other comorbid neurological disorders involving the dominant cerebral hemisphere, will typically produce few speech problems. Symptom complaints from patients with PTSD usually include attention/concentration, memory, and some executive dysfunction. In a recent review of studies on neuropsychological functioning in PTSD, Horner & Hamner (2002) found that 16 of 19 studies reported impairments in attention/concentration, immediate memory, or both. Using tests with established literatures is a reasonable starting strategy, but if future studies that are better controlled should find few deficits, then the overall composition of test batteries will need to be reconsidered. Finally, research studies that examine neurocognitive problems in PTSD patients with neurological disorders should examine incremental deficits linked to PTSD that are above the level of impairment known to result from the neurological condition alone.

CONSIDERATIONS FOR INTERPRETING NEUROPSYCHOLOGICAL TEST PERFORMANCES FROM TRAUMA POPULATIONS

The preceding sections focused on the nature of PTSD and comorbid neuropsychological conditions to raise awareness of the complexity created by co-existing disorders and of the importance of systematically evaluating these combinations. The next section discusses issues that are central to interpreting neuropsychological test performances from trauma populations. Patients with PTSD can present unique test administration and interpretation challenges. Most of the issues to be discussed have not been adequately accounted for by studies in the literature and, in all likelihood, have contributed to the mixed findings regarding the neuropsychological deficits that exist in groups with PTSD.

Preinterpretation Factors

Some general concerns, commonly understood to be important for neuropsychological test interpretation, have added significance when testing patients with PTSD in clinical settings and should be routinely reviewed in order to assess whether the examinee was able to commit all facets of attention and remain engaged throughout the testing process.

1. *Recent sleep quality and sleep patterns should be assessed.* Chronic sleep problems are often present in patients with PTSD (Woodward, 1993), including sleep apnea (Boza, Trujillo, Millares, & Liggett, 1984) and REM-sleep behavior disorder (Lapierre & Montplaisir, 1992). Neuropsychological deficits resulting from hypoxia secondary to sleep apnea range from global, diffuse cognitive dysfunction to isolated memory problems (Greenberg, Watson, & Deptual, 1987; Martzke & Steenhuis, 1993). Other sleep problems stem from increased sleep onset latencies and midsleep awakenings caused by regularly occurring PTSD-related nightmares. In some patients, the emotional aftereffects of the trauma-related nightmare during the previous night persist into the next day and may produce sustained increases in hyperarousal, hypervigilance, and more frequent or intense flashbacks. Short daytime naps may be the only sleep obtained to compensate for lost nighttime sleep. Circadian rhythms could be affected, and the patient could become fatigued more easily during the testing process.

2. *Residual effects of peripheral physical damage resulting from the traumatic experience should be systematically evaluated for their potential to produce impaired test performances.* Examples include damage to ears, eyes, and fingers among torture survivors or damage from explosions, booby traps, and exposure to neurotoxins among combat veterans. Some types of damage may not be reported by the examinee, and, if not evident from clinical observa-

tions, this damage could confound interpretations of impaired performances that might otherwise suggest cortical dysfunction.

3. *Medication and psychoactive substance use should be assessed, including pattern of usage and any recent changes.* Fluctuations in usage patterns may parallel phasic changes in PTSD symptoms (e.g., increases in alcohol and drugs consumed to induce sleep) or may be related to anticipatory anxiety about the testing process. For some, the increased use of medication or psychoactive substances may facilitate performances by reducing anxiety. In others, it may be excessive and detract from test performances.

4. *The role of compensation seeking, litigation, and secondary gain should be considered.* PTSD is a compensable disorder in the VA system, in workers' compensation claims, and in lawsuits. Recent controversies over PTSD in the courtroom and false memory syndrome in childhood sexual abuse cases could increase interest in forensic cases on contextual aspects of the neuropsychological assessment findings. Due to concerns related to maintaining compensation, test takers may worry that testing may yield signs that show clinical improvement, as these findings might threaten their compensation status. Including neuropsychological measures of effort in the test battery will assist in evaluating suspected, intentionally manipulated performances.

5. *Particular emphasis should be given to evaluating attentional problems.* Systematic investigation of attentional functions is generally required to establish the patient's ability to engage the tests. Intact attentional abilities are the foundation for higher cognitive information-processing abilities, including memory and language (Mirsky, Fantie, & Tatman, 1995). As attention is not a unitary construct, specific measures of multiple modes of attention should be included in test batteries. This recommendation is of particular importance when testing patients with PTSD who experience hypervigilance, intrusive recollections, hyperarousal, and dissociation that may disrupt engagement with the testing process when they occur during the session.

In addition to the standard data analysis and test interpretation process, the neuropsychological evaluation should ultimately address the following fundamental questions.

1. *Do any deficits exist?* This can be addressed by comparing the test performances with age- and education-matched normative values when available.

2. *When deficits are present, what is the pattern?* The pattern of deficits can first be described as lateralized, localized, or diffuse relative to normative population values. Qualitative performance features can be characterized in a similar manner and, when available, evaluated against normative values. Once performance levels for each test are established, levels within and across tests can be compared for patterns of relative strengths and weaknesses in the neurocognitive domains sampled.

3. *Is the pattern of deficits similar to those of other disorders, and is this*

pattern typical of PTSD populations? Obtained patterns of deficits can be analyzed against those of other known disorders. However, given the high incidence of observed comorbidity, this exercise may have less utility in chronic PTSD samples. Without a suitable set of comorbid comparison groups, determining whether the pattern is typical of PTSD will be more complicated. Based on an absence of consensus findings from the review of the literature in the previous section, the question of the best variables or test patterns to use is open to debate.

4. *Was the clinical testing process free from the effects of unintended affective priming? If present, did the priming produce a main effect across tests or interact with various components of the test battery to produce differential responding?* A previous investigation by Zimering, Caddell, Fairbank, and Keane (1993) demonstrated the effects of affective priming on task performance using an experimental paradigm. Exposure to auditory combat sounds produced subsequent decrements in performance on a motor steadiness task and letter vigilance during a continuous performance task. Corresponding increases in frightening and violent intrusive thoughts were also reported during the postprime intervals.

5. *When present, do cognitive problems at the time of testing represent an exacerbation of existing symptoms typical of the phasic variation of PTSD or a stable level of symptoms? Do the observed cognitive problems covary with general level of distress and symptom severity, or is there an interaction pattern among subsets of symptoms, with some deficits remaining relatively stable and others showing variations correlated with PTSD reexperiencing symptoms?* Answering these questions requires knowledge of the history of symptom fluctuations. The pattern of symptom variations serves as the context for referencing test findings and for generating clinical recommendations. For example, combat veterans with PTSD can experience cyclical variation in symptoms related to seasons of the year, anniversary reactions, and national holidays. Thus the level of test performances for any given administration could represent cyclical variation in PTSD symptoms that may regress toward the mean on retesting or influences due to changes in cognitive functioning from a variety of factors. Neither may be reported spontaneously by the patient.

PTSD Status and Reactivity to the Testing Process

One of the underlying assumptions for validity of neuropsychological test interpretations is that maximal performances were obtained during data collection. Methods for determining the role of confounding factors that attenuate performance must be systematically included in the testing process. Standardizing the test administration procedures, creating a conducive testing environment, and minimizing error due to non-test-related factors are some methods commonly incorporated for optimizing validity of the data collected. For neurological disorders and syndromes in which the lesion is static or progressive, variations in the pattern of test performances are assumed to be attributable to the underlying lesion. In psychiatric samples with distorted reality testing, skewed information-processing tendencies, and disturbances of mood, neuropsychological test performances can more proportionately reflect transient psychiatric status. For patients with PTSD, the neuropsychological testing process can interact with their trauma histories, resulting in performance impairments that inaccurately reflect neurocognitive functioning. This occurs because PTSD reexperiencing symptoms are cued by triggers in the environment. These triggers can elicit reactivity during the testing process. Studies in the literature to date have not adequately accounted for the range of reactivity to the testing process that can exist when assessing patients with PTSD.

Interaction of Trauma Histories and Administrator Characteristics

When traumatic events occur within an interpersonal context (e.g., physical violence, rape, or threat to life by another person), patients will remember both general and specific characteristics of the perpetrator or assailant. These details and general descriptions constitute cues that function to evoke physiological arousal and memories of the trauma when encountered in the everyday environment. The interpersonal context for testing is often a small office where the patient meets with the test administrator, who by virtue of gender or race alone may be a triggering stimulus for recall of traumatic experiences (e.g., an Asian person for Vietnam veterans).

Beyond general characteristics, trauma survivors may remember small details about the perpetrator that have become associated with threat or that may have served as warning signals cuing escape or avoidance in the past. For instance, incest survivors who were abused when the perpetrator was intoxicated may have learned the connection between the bloodshot eyes associated with drinking and an increased probability of molestation. Should the test examiner's eyes resemble the perpetrator's bloodshot eyes for other reasons, such as allergies or contact lenses, intrusive memories or dissociative episodes may be unintentionally triggered. Smells and odors can also function as powerful memory retrieval cues for trauma survivors. What would under usual circumstances be regarded as benign characteristics of the examiner can become significant in the testing process. Without knowledge of the examinee's trauma history, the test administrator may be unaware of stimulus characteristics that could elicit reactivity during testing. The reactivity may go unreported, and the examinee manages it by disengaging. Disengagement with the testing process by the examinee may be as subtle as a focused stare at the test stimuli or increased response latencies during the task.

Interaction of Trauma Histories and Testing Environment

A number of other features in the testing environment may combine to produce a disruption in the examinee's level of task engagement. For example, if a trauma involved being in a confined space (e.g., holding cells for prisoners), the combination of a small testing room and features of the test administrator may elicit intrusions, panic reactions, or flashbacks during testing. If the room is not sound isolated, noise in the hallway or adjoining rooms may repeatedly draw the attention of the hypervigilant patient away from the testing. Spurious outside noise problems are often managed by masking them with white noise generators or small fan devices in the room. Although they are successful in blocking other noises, the constant low-level din emitted from the masking device can resemble the characteristics of background noise from past traumas and may trigger memories for patients who were in chaotic combat, accidents, or natural disasters. Combat veterans exposed to the concussive effects of artillery explosions and torture survivors may have chronic tinnitus that is compounded by the masking devices (Graessner, 1993).

Patients with chronic PTSD who have developed a pattern of attending to stimuli around them and then escaping cognitively from triggered intrusive images may automatically engage in these monitoring processes and employ dissociative escape strategies during testing without reporting them. Effects on test performances could include slower reaction times, longer times to completion, interference with storage during memory tasks, incomplete processing of instructions for the task, inconsistent responding across tests, or premature discontinuation of some tasks, which appears as if the examinee simply "gave up." Examiners should try to be aware of these possibilities, as they often go undetected if not reported freely by the test taker.

For a portion of trauma survivors, a conditioned emotional response may be elicited by moments of silence during testing. Combat veterans who waited in silence while setting an ambush or ones who noticed the silence before being ambushed on patrol may become more agitated in sound-reduced testing rooms. Victims of incest and crime who hid in silence may have similar reactions. Silence is also an environmental condition that offers nothing for the PTSD patient to monitor, and without a stimulus present to capture attention, unwanted thoughts of the trauma may intrude. To prevent silences, patients may talk at fairly continuous rates and provide overly detailed answers to free-response sections of tests.

Interaction of Trauma Histories with Test Features and Task Requirements

In patients with PTSD, a generalization gradient may develop over time from a specific trauma event cue or set of cues to broader classes of stimuli. The neuropsychological test examiner may encounter unexpected reactions to the test materials that are associated with traumatic experiences. Patients with dementias, CVAs, or neoplasms but without PTSD are not likely to have cued emotional reactions to features of the test stimuli or the task. Frustration and some catastrophic reactions can be observed when these patients notice poor performances, but idiosyncratic associations are more rare. A case example of a military combat veteran illustrates how test characteristics can interact with an examinee's history.

A veteran whose trauma involved a near-death experience from artillery fire showed a series of responses during neuropsychological testing that culminated in discontinuation of the testing process because of his level of distraction. Shortly after the start of a computerized administration of the Continuous Performance Test—a task that requires sustained monitoring for the appearance of an *X* in one condition and an *X* preceded by an *A* in another condition—he developed heightened levels of physiological arousal because the colored-letter stimuli presented during the task seemed to him to "explode" onto the screen. His vigilance became heightened, and memories of the shelling he experienced were evoked. Once he was primed by these memories, subsequent tests were affected. During the Visual Span task from the Wechsler Memory Scale—Revised, he again experienced intrusive recollections of his traumatic experience. This test required the patient to observe and reproduce a sequence that is finger-tapped by the administrator on small, red-colored squares printed on a stimulus card. The process of reproducing the tapped sequence on the red squares reminded him of incoming small arms and artillery fire from the enemy. During motor speed testing with the Finger Tapping test, he associated tapping with past experiences of squeezing the trigger to fire a machine gun while on guard duty. During this association, he raised his head, looked out the window, and experienced a momentary flashback of the landscape around his guard post. The effects of these experiences lingered and manifested during the Sensory–Perceptual Examination, producing sensory errors that were inconsistent ipsilaterally and contralaterally. Subsequent retesting of his sensory–perceptual functions on another day produced a within-normal-limits performance. Had he not provided information on the distraction he experienced from the intrusions, the inconsistency in his performance could have been misconstrued as possible motivational problems or malingering.

Computerized tasks such as the Continuous Performance Test that present stimuli at short repeating intervals may elicit dissociation in patients who are prone to dissociating under stress. Although the precise explanations for this reaction are unclear, this response during testing is an acute, reactive state that limits the potential of examinees to generate their optimal performance. It may be that when targets are presented on the screen at a rapid rate, the examinee may feel unable to process the information, which produces feelings of failure, inadequacy, and helplessness associated with past trauma. Alternatively, the dissociative experience may be a manifestation of a photosensitive seizure or a reflex epilepsy. Photosensitive seizures can result from the presentation of synchronized visual stimuli such as flickering light in specific frequency ranges. Monochromatic red light has been shown to be more potent than other colors (Engel, 1989). Complex reflex epilepsies are elicited by very specific stimuli or stimulus conditions that frequently involve some level of cognitive or emotional appreciation of the stimulus (Forster, 1977).

The previous discussion illustrates how the presentation of visually oriented test stimuli can elicit reactions. Procedures that limit sight can be equally distressing. For example, neuropsychological tests that require wearing a blindfold (e.g., Tactual Performance Test) may be problematic for survivors of nighttime physical or sexual assault or for veterans with combat experiences such as being tortured, ambushed in the dark, or temporarily blinded by explosions. More generally, wearing a blindfold increases feelings of vulnerability by reducing one's ability to be vigilant of the environment, and these feelings in turn may exacerbate PTSD symptoms during testing.

Thematic Associations Cued by Testing

The testing process may activate a variety of themes associated with traumatic experiences in patients with PTSD. Abstract themes involving the absence of prediction and control may be aroused during testing and may manifest as overt discomfort and agitation when faced with ambiguity. Anxious anticipation during testing can prompt a search for information that may increase distractibility and confound performances on initial tests within the neuropsychological battery. Performance anxiety can also induce physiological arousal and intrusions during testing. During traumatic events, physiological reactions can be a very prominent aspect of the experience (e.g., feeling or hearing one's own heartbeat may have been paired with the silence of sitting still and keeping quiet while hiding from a sexual abuse perpetrator).

Poor test performance can activate cognitive schemas surrounding feelings of guilt associated with responsibility for the consequences of underperforming in the past (e.g., when negative consequences happened to others or when lives were at stake). If the examinees notice that their performance is flagging, feelings of "failure" may cue intrusive memories of the trauma. Feelings of low self-esteem and low self-worth may interact with intrusive memories to further depress or interrupt test performances. If survival in the past was linked to an error-free performance, defined as either exhibiting or inhibiting a response at the right time, the similarity of task requirements during neuropsychological testing may activate this schema. The possibility of this activation should be considered for tasks that require demonstration or suppression of specific responses (e.g., motor Go/No-Go tests), and for procedures in which direct feedback in the form of "correct" or "incorrect" is standardly given during the task (e.g., the Wisconsin Card Sorting Test, the Categories Test).

Single words may be sufficient to cue a theme. Previous findings using the Stroop paradigm (Litz & Herman, 1993; McNally, Kaspi, Riemann, & Zeitlin, 1990) have shown increased latencies for color naming of trauma-relevant words in combat veterans. Tests that assess language may inadvertently trigger associations. For example, during the Controlled Oral Word Association procedure, which measures verbal fluency by asking patients to generate as many words as possible starting with a target letter, traumatized patients may generate words directly related to their trauma that then function to prime affect and cue intrusive recollections (e.g., words beginning with "S" for combat veterans: shrapnel, shelling, sharpshooter, sniping).

Other idiosyncratic responses to neuropsychological tests have been observed in combat veterans. Items in subtests IV, V, and VI of the Categories Test include configurations that resemble defensive physical perimeters of compounds as viewed from aerial maps. Establishing defensive perimeters and planning missions that targeted enemy positions often involved detection of pattern configurations. To some, Mesulum's (1985) Letter and Shape Cancellation task resembles a schematic of a minefield. The recall trials of the Rey–Osterrieth Complex Figure and the Visual Reproduction subscale of the Wechsler Memory Scale can remind some of diagrammatic renderings of enemy compounds. Spatial associations linked to visual memory may rapidly induce intrusive recollections.

Veterans with PTSD may report that receiving instructions for completing neuropsychological tests feels like being briefed for an upcoming mission. As they listen to the instructions from the examiner, their attentional focus narrows so that the objectives would be clear. In some, this narrowing of focus leads to an intense, successful engagement with the task that produces enhanced performance. For others, if instructions are closely linked to a trauma experience, it may be distracting. Using the computerized Continuous Performance Test (visual *X/A – X* version) again as an example, a veteran reported that listening to instructions elicited a "mission mode" in him as he prepared to engage the task. Testing requirements that required him to respond to target letters as quickly as possible on the screen paralleled mission requirements to quickly spot an enemy soldier in the bushes or jungle and to shoot before being shot ("This test was like shooting at something coming out of the dark"). Pressing the computer key to respond on this task was analogous to pulling the trigger. Assuming a mission mentality can produce responses that are either facilitated or impaired by this narrow focus of attention. Short-latency commission errors can increase because the examinee responds too rapidly to any on-screen stimulus change (the "shoot-first" strategy); whereas omissions, defined as "missed targets," can distressingly resemble being symbolically shot by the enemy because of poor vigilance.

For trauma survivors whose traumatic events involved violations of interpersonal trust or who have become highly distrustful subsequent to the trauma, the testing process may evoke emotional reactions. Abused children may distrust adults, and adult trauma survivors may distrust authority figures, the government, institutions, hospitals, and staff affiliated with medical centers. Impersonal treatment, which can be part of the patient experience in large institutions, often inflames existing agitations. Military veterans are known to express feelings of being experimented on, and some have documentation of their military mistreatment (e.g., radiation exposure from being placed in open trenches during nuclear bomb testing). Even the word *testing* can elicit reactions because it seems like a direct challenge or something that must be endured. General negative associations with testing may be present for many patients who had poor academic histories, past aversive experiences taking tests in school, or learning disabilities. Developing good examiner–patient rapport is central to reducing the potential arousal that accompanies feelings of vulnerability from these factors.

Accounting for Potential Process Confounds

The degree to which the aforementioned parameters alter neuropsychological test results should receive stronger consideration in clinical case examinations and in research protocols. Neuropsychological testing with populations with PTSD for clinical or research purposes needs to include mechanisms for addressing the presence of altered states of engagement with the testing. The test administrator should be aware of the general range of potential reactions exhibited by traumatized populations. Individual testing sessions may need to be tailored based on clinical knowledge of the examinee's trauma history. For example, whereas some patients with PTSD need a clear view of the exits in order to feel less hypervigilant, others may need to have the furniture configured so that they could exit easily if necessary.

During testing, levels of arousal should be carefully observed as signs that attention may be shifting internally to intrusions or externally due to an increase in hypervigilance. Self-reporting of attentional shifts may not occur spontaneously. Patients with PTSD avoid stimuli and circumstances that arouse memories and physiological reactivity. They may be uncomfortable with self-observation and discussion of their reactions, especially if increased anxiety results from disclosure. Encouraging them to report attentional shifts that occur during testing increases the likelihood of detecting such shifts. Preparation for testing by the referral source, thorough explanation of each upcoming procedure, and efforts by the test administrator to build rapport will help to reduce anxiety and facilitate the disclosure process. To further ensure the validity of test interpretations, process checks should be included with data collection so that patterns of deficits can be correctly attributed to reactivity when present rather than to underlying lesions. Structured process recording forms should be available for recording observations during testing, and examiners should be trained in observing the many diverse reactions demonstrated by patients with PTSD.

For the groups of patients with more chronic PTSD and with greater symptom severity, the cognitive demand of sustained, focused mental activity may produce fatigue, accompanied by increased hypervigilance and vulnerability to intrusive recollections as their cognitive capacity to inhibit these reactions wanes. Thus patients with PTSD may not be able to tolerate a lengthy battery of tests and should be monitored for fatigue. Veteran populations have been described as "commonly reporting fatigue, concentration difficulties, somatic distress, and other complaints that impair capacity to endure lengthy testing sessions" (Dalton et al., 1989). To minimize fatigue for clinical evaluations, long batteries can be divided into shorter sessions. Although this assists in maintaining peak performance for each session, it also complicates the correlation of test findings across sessions because the patient is open to experiences between testings that may exacerbate symptoms and alter mood states. In controlled settings, acute shifts in clinical presentation primarily result from sleep disturbance, nightmares, flashbacks, increased intrusions, carryover effects of therapy groups, and interactions with visitors. For outpatients, similar experiences are possible, with the added potential of substance abuse and increased use of prescription medication to control symptom escalation.

Blind interpretation of testing data from PTSD protocols can be confounded because transient alterations in attention from intrusions or dissociations are difficult to rule in or rule out by examining the pattern among test performances. Attentional measures within the neuropsychological test battery are often examined to make a judgment about the examinee's ability to concentrate, and if they fall within expected ranges, a generalized assumption of adequate attention across all tests in the battery may be inferred. However, the transient nature of PTSD-related alterations in attention from cuing during portions of the testing process makes this practice potentially problematic for establishing the validity of the whole test battery.

CONCLUSIONS

The primary focus of this chapter was the interaction of trauma and neurological conditions. Common comorbid combinations were identified, along with processes for conceptualizing and evaluating their impacts on clinical presentations. Salient confounds that could affect the interpretation of test results, diagnostic decisions, and formulations of treatment plans were presented. The importance of considering the time of onset for neurological disorders was highlighted, given that these disorders might occur as a function of development or might be acquired before, during, or after a traumatic event. Any particular clinical presentation could reflect the influences of multiple traumas and multiple neurological conditions. Examples were reviewed that illustrated how neurological conditions can exacerbate PTSD symptoms and how PTSD might increase the risk of acquiring a neurological condition. Specific test administration issues and their potential impact on the interpretation of neuropsychological test results were delineated, and examples illustrated how PTSD symptoms interacted with the testing process. Finally, strategies for minimizing potential barriers to testing were discussed.

The primary intent of this chapter was to present issues related to comorbidity that are important for traumatologists and neuropsychologists to consider for research and clinical evaluations. The literature examining the basic mechanisms underlying the development and maintenance of PTSD from a neuroscience perspective continues to grow, and this new knowledge will inform clinical practice. Clinical models developed from practical knowledge of comorbidity patterns could help to structure hypotheses regarding brain-based determinants of PTSD. For individual cases, considering the role of neuropsychological concomitants should assist in assessing and treating complex PTSD presentations.

REFERENCES

Andreasen, N. C. (1989). *Brain imaging applications in psychiatry*. Washington, DC: American Psychiatric Press.

Baggaley, M. R., & Rose, J. (1990). Post-traumatic stress disorder [Letter to the editor]. *British Journal of Psychiatry*, *156*, 911.

Barrett, D. H., Green, M. L., Morris, R., Giles, W. H., & Croft, J. B. (1996). Cognitive functioning and posttraumatic stress disorder. *American Journal of Psychiatry*, *153*(11), 1492–1494.

Barth, J., Macciocchi, S., Giordani, B., Rimel, R., Jane, J., & Boll, T. (1983). Neuropsychological sequelae of minor head injury. *Neurosurgery*, *13*, 529–533.

Beckham, J. C., Crawford, A. L., & Feldman, M. E. (1998). Trail Making Test performance in Vietnam combat veterans with and without posttraumatic stress disorder. *Journal of Traumatic Stress*, *11*, 811–819.

Beers, S. R., & De Bellis, M. D. (2002). Neuropsychological function in children with maltreatment-related posttraumatic stress disorder. *American Journal of Psychiatry*, *159*, 483–486.

Biederman, J., Newcorn, J., & Sprich, S. (1991). Comorbidity of attention deficit hyperactivity disorder, with conduct, depressive, anxiety and other disorders. *American Journal of Psychiatry*, *148*, 564–577.

Bigler, E. D. (1990). The neurobiology and neuropsychology of adult learning disorders. *Journal of Learning Disabilities*, *25*, 488–506.

Bigler, E. D., & Snyder, J. L. (1995). Neuropsychological outcome and quantitative neuroimaging in mild head injury. *Archives of Clinical Neuropsychology*, *10*, 159–174.

Bontke, C. (1996). Do patients with mild brain injuries have posttraumatic stress disorder too? *Journal of Head Trauma Rehabilitation*, *11*, 95–102.

Boza, R. A., Trujillo, M., Millares, S., & Liggett, S. B. (1984, August). Sleep apnea and associated neuropsychiatric symptoms. *VA Practitioner*, 43–45.

Bremner, J. D. (1999). Does stress damage the brain? *Society of Biological Psychiatry*, *45*, 797–805.

Bremner, J. D., Randall, R., Scott, T. M., Bronen, R. A., Seibyl, J. P., Southwick, S. M., et al. (1995). MRI-based measurement of hippocampal volume in patients with combat-related posttraumatic stress disorder. *American Journal of Psychiatry*, *152*, 973–981.

Bremner, J. D., Scott, T. M., Delaney, R. C., Southwick, S. W. Mason, J. W., Johnson, D. R., et al. (1993). Deficits in short-term memory in posttraumatic stress disorder. *American Journal of Psychiatry*, *150*, 1015–1019.

Bremner, J. D., Southwick, S. M., Johnson, D. R., Yehuda, R., & Charney, D. S. (1993). Childhood physical abuse and combat-related posttraumatic stress disorder in Vietnam veterans. *American Journal of Psychiatry*, *150*, 235–239.

Brewin, C. R., Dalgleish, T., & Joseph, S. (1996). A dual representation theory of posttraumatic stress disorder. *Psychological Review*, *103*, 670–686.

Brooks, N. (1989). Closed head trauma: Assessing the common cognitive problems. In M. D. Lezak (Ed.), *Assessment of the behavioral consequences of head trauma*. New York: Liss.

Bryant, R. A. (1996). Posttraumatic stress disorder, flashbacks, and pseudomemories in closed head injury. *Journal of Head Trauma Rehabilitation*, *9*, 621–629.

Bryant, R. A. (2001). Posttraumatic stress disorder and mild brain injury: Controversies, causes, and consequences. *Journal of Clinical and Experimental Neuropsychology*, *23*(6), 718–728.

Bryant, R. A., & Harvey, A. G. (1995). Acute stress response: A comparison of head-injured and non-head-injured patients. *Psychological Medicine*, *25*, 869–873.

Bryant, R. A., & Harvey, A. G. (1996). Initial posttraumatic stress response following motor vehicle accidents. *Journal of Head Trauma Rehabilitation*, *9*, 223–234.

Bryant, R. A., & Harvey, A. G. (1998). Relationship of acute stress disorder and posttraumatic stress disorder following mild traumatic brain injury. *American Journal of Psychiatry*, *155*, 625–629.

Bryant, R. A., & Harvey, A. G. (1999a). Postconcussive symptoms and posttraumatic stress disorder after mild traumatic brain injury. *Journal of Nervous and Mental Disease*, *187*(5), 302–305.

Bryant, R. A., & Harvey, A. G. (1999b). The influence of traumatic brain injury on acute stress disorder and posttraumatic stress disorder following motor vehicle accidents. *Brain Injury*, *13*(1), 15–22.

Bryant, R. A., & Harvey, A. G. (2001). Reconstructing trauma memories: A prospective study of "amnesic" trauma survivors. *Journal of Traumatic Stress*, *14*(2), 277–282.

Bryant, R. A., & Harvey, A. G. (2002). Delayed-onset posttraumatic stress disorder: A prospective evaluation. *Australian and New Zealand Journal of Psychiatry*, *36*(2), 205–209.

Bryant, R. A., Marosszeky, J. E., Crooks, J., Baguley, I. J., & Gurka, J. A. (2001). Posttraumatic stress disorder and psychosocial functioning after severe traumatic brain injury. *Journal of Nervous and Mental Disease*, *189*(2), 109–113.

Bryant, R. A., Marosszeky, J. E., Crooks, J., & Gurka, J. A. (2000). Posttraumatic stress disorder after severe traumatic brain injury. *American Journal of Psychiatry*, *157*, 629–631.

Cahill, L., Prins, B., Weber, M., & McGaugh, J. L. (1994). Beta-adrenergic activation and memory for emotional events. *Nature*, *371*, 702–704.

Cassidy, K. L., & Lyons, J. A. (1992). Recall of traumatic memories following cerebral vascular accident. *Journal of Traumatic Stress*, *5*, 627–631.

Chemtob, C. M., & Herriott, M. G. (1994). Posttraumatic stress disorder as a sequela of Guillain-Barré syndrome. *Journal of Traumatic Stress*, *7*, 705–711.

Cooper, P. N., & Milroy, C. M. (1994). Violent suicide in South Yorkshire, England. *Journal of Forensic Sciences*, *39*, 657–667.

Crowell, T. A., Kieffer, K. M., Siders, C. A., & Vanderploeg, R. D. (2002). Neuropsychological findings in combat-related posttraumatic stress disorder. *Clinical Neuropsychologist*, *16*, 310–321.

Cuffe, S. P., McCullough, E. L., & Pumariega, A. J. (1994). Comorbidity of attention-deficit hyperactivity disorder and posttraumatic stress disorder. *Journal of Child and Family Studies*, *3*, 327–336.

Cummings, J. L., & Benson, D. F. (1992). *Dementia: A clinical approach*. Boston: Butterworth-Heinemann.
Dalton, J. E., Pederson, S. L., & Ryan J. J. (1989). Effects of posttraumatic stress disorder on neuropsychological test performances. *International Journal of Clinical Neuropsychology, 11*, 121–124.
Daniel, M., Haban, G. F., Hutcherson, W. L., Botter, J., & Long, C. (1985). Neuropsychological and emotional consequences of accidental, high-voltage shock. *International Journal of Clinical Neuropsychology, 7*, 102–106.
Davidoff, D. A., Kessler, H. R., Laibstain, D. F., & Mark, V. H. (1988). Neurobehavioral consequence of minor head injury: A consideration of postconcussive versus posttraumatic stress disorder. *Cognitive Rehabilitation, 6*, 8–13.
Delis, D. C., Kramer, J. H., Kaplan, E., & Ober, B. A. (1987). *The California Verbal Learning Test*. New York: Psychological Corporation.
Devous, M. D. (1989). Imaging brain function by single-photon emission computer tomography. In N. C. Andreasen (Ed.), *Brain imaging applications in psychiatry* (pp. 216–232). Washington, DC: American Psychiatric Press.
Dinklage, D., & Grodzinsky, G. M. (1993, February). *Neuropsychological deficits in severely sexually abused children*. Paper presented at the annual meeting of the International Neuropsychological Society, Galveston, TX.
Downs, D. S., & Abwender, D. (2002). Neuropsychological impairment in soccer athletes. *Journal of Sports Medicine and Physical Fitness, 42*(1), 103–107.
Edna, T. (1982). Alcohol influence and head injury. *Acta Chirurgica Scandinavia, 148*, 209–212.
Elzinga, B. M., & Bremner, J. D. (2002). Are the neural substrates of memory the final common pathway in posttraumatic stress disorder (PTSD)? *Journal of Affective Disorders, 70*(1), 1–17.
Engel, J. (1989). *Seizures and epilepsy*. Philadelphia: Davis.
Famularo, R., Kinscherff, R., & Fenton, T. (1992). Psychiatric diagnoses of maltreated children: Preliminary findings. *Journal of the American Academy of Child and Adolescent Psychiatry, 31*, 863–867.
Feinstein, A., Hershkop, S., Ouchterlony, D., Jardine, A., & McCullagh, S. (2002). Posttraumatic amnesia and recall of a traumatic event following traumatic brain injury. *Journal of Neuropsychiatry and Clinical Neurosciences, 14*(1), 25–30.
Forrester, G., Encel, J., & Geffen, G. (1994). Measuring posttraumatic amnesia (PTA): An historical review. *Brain Injury, 8*, 175–184.
Forster, F. M. (1977). *Reflex epilepsy, behavioral therapy and conditioned reflexes*. Springfield, IL: Thomas.
Gaddes, W. H. (1985). *Learning disabilities and brain function: A neuropsychological approach* (2nd ed.). New York: Springer-Verlag.
Gil, T., Calev, A., Greenberg, D., Kugelmass, S., & Lerer, B. (1990). Cognitive functioning in posttraumatic stress disorder. *Journal of Traumatic Stress, 3*, 29–45.
Gilbertson, M. W., Gurvits, T. V., Lasko, N. B., Orr, S. R., & Pitman, R. K. (2001). Multivariate assessment of explicit memory function in combat veterans with posttraumatic stress disorder. *Journal of Traumatic Stress, 14*, 413–432.
Gill, D., & Sparadeo, F. (1988, August). *Neurobehavioral complications from alcohol use prior to head injury*. Paper presented at the meeting of the American Psychological Association, Atlanta, GA.
Glod, C. A. (1993). Long-term consequences of childhood physical and sexual abuse. *Archives of Psychiatric Nursing, 7*, 163–173.

Golier, J., Yehuda, R., Cornblatt, B., Harvey, P., Gerber, D., & Levengood, R. (1997). Sustained attention in combat-related posttraumatic stress disorder. *Integrative Physiological and Behavioral Science*, *32*, 52–61.

Golier, J., Yehuda, R., Lupien, S. J., Harvey, P. D., Grossman, R., & Elkin, A. (2002). Memory performance in Holocaust survivors with posttraumatic stress disorder. *American Journal of Psychiatry*, *159*, 1682–1688.

Graessner, S. (1993). Tinnitus in torture survivors. *Torture*, *3*, 47.

Greenberg, G. D., Watson, R. K., & Deptual, D. (1987). Neuropsychological dysfunction in sleep apnea. *Sleep*, *10*, 254–262.

Grisgsby, J., & Kaye, K. (1993). Incidence and correlates of depersonalization following head trauma. *Brain Injury*, *7*, 507–513.

Gronwall, D., & Wrightson, P. (1980). Duration of posttraumatic amnesia after mild head injury. *Journal of Clinical Neuropsychology*, *2*, 51–60.

Gurvit, I. H. (1993). Neurological complications of repeated hunger strikes. *Torture*, *3*, 47.

Gurvits, T. V., Lasko, N. B., Schachter, S. C., Kutine, A. A., Orr, S. P., & Pitman, R. K. (1993). Neurological status of Vietnam veterans with chronic posttraumatic stress disorder. *Journal of Neuropsychiatry and Clinical Neurosciences*, *5*, 183–188.

Hamner, M. B., Lorberbaum, M. D., & George, M. S. (1999). Potential role of the anterior cingulate cortex in PTSD: Review and hypothesis. *Depression and Anxiety*, *9*, 1–14.

Harper, C., Kril, J., & Daly, J. (1987). Are we drinking our neurons away? *British Medical Journal*, *294*, 534–536.

Hartman, D. E. (1988). *Neuropsychological toxicology: Identification and assessment of human neurotoxic syndromes*. Oxford, UK: Pergamon Press.

Hartman, D. E. (1992). Neuropsychological toxicology. In A. E. Puente, R. J. McCaffrey III (Eds.), *Handbook of neuropsychological assessment: A biopsychosocial perspective*. New York: Plenum Press.

Harvey, A. G., & Bryant, R. A. (2000). A two-year prospective evaluation of the relationship between acute stress disorder and posttraumatic stress disorder following mild traumatic brain injury. *American Journal of Psychiatry*, *157*, 626–628.

Harvey, A. G., & Bryant, R. A. (2001). Reconstructing trauma memories: A prospective study of "amnesic" trauma survivors. *Journal of Traumatic Stress*, *14*(2), 277–282.

Hibbard, M., Uysal, S., Keple, K., Bogdany, J., & Silver, J. (1998). Axis I psychopathology in individuals with traumatic brain injury. *Journal of Head Trauma Rehabilitation*, *13*(4), 24–39.

Hickling, E. J., Gillen, R., Blanchard, E. B., Buckley, T., & Taylor, A. (1998). Traumatic brain injury and posttraumatic stress disorder: A preliminary investigation of neuropsychological test results in PTSD secondary to motor vehicle accidents. *Brain Injury*, *12*, 265–274.

Hillbom, M., & Holm, L. (1986). Contributions of traumatic head injuries to neuropsychological deficits in alcoholics. *Journal of Neurology, Neurosurgery, and Psychiatry*, *49*, 1348–1353.

Hopewell, C. A. (1983). Serial neuropsychological assessment in a case of reversible electrocution encephalopathy. *Clinical Neuropsychology*, *5*, 61–65.

Hopkins, R. O., Gale, S. D., Johnson, S. C., Anderson, C. V., Bigler, E. D., Blatter, D. D., & Weaver, L. K. (1995). Severe anoxia with and without concomitant brain atrophy and neuropsychological impairments. *Journal of the International Neuropsychological Society, 1*, 501–509.

Hopkins, R. O., Weaver, L. K., & Kesner, R. P. (1994, May). *Qualitative MRI analysis of the hippocampus corresponds with persistent memory impairments in carbon monoxide poisoned subjects.* Paper presented at the Theoretical and Experimental Neuropsychology meeting, Montreal, Quebec, Canada.

Horner, M. D., & Hamner, M. B. (2002). Neurocognitive functioning in posttraumatic stress disorder. *Neuropsychology Review, 12*(1), 15–30.

Horton, A. M. (1993). Posttraumatic stress disorder and mild head trauma: Follow-up of a case study. *Perceptual and Motor Skills, 76*, 243–246.

Ito, Y., Teicher, M. H., Glod, C. A., & Harper, D. (1993). Increased prevalence of electrophysiological abnormalities in children with psychological, physical, and sexual abuse. *Journal of Neuropsychiatry and Clinical Neurosciences, 5*, 401–408.

Jacobs, U., & Iacopino, V. (2001). Torture and its consequences: A challenge to clinical neuropsychology. *Professional Psychology: Research and Practice, 32*, 458–464.

Jenkins, M. A. (2000). Attentional dysfunction associated with posttraumatic stress disorder among rape survivors. *Clinical Neuropsychologist, 14*(1), 7–12.

Jenkins, M. A., Langlais, P. J., Delis, D., & Cohen, R. (1998). Learning and memory in rape victims with posttraumatic stress disorder. *American Journal of Psychiatry, 155*, 278–279.

Kampen, D. L., & Grafman, J. (1989). Neuropsychological evaluation of penetrating head injury. In M. D. Lezak (Ed.), *Assessment of the behavioral consequences of head trauma* (pp. 183–201). New York: Liss.

Keane, T. M., & Wolfe, J. (1990). Comorbidity in posttraumatic stress disorder: An analysis of community and clinical studies. *Journal of Applied Social Psychology, 20*, 1776–1788.

King, N. S. (1997). Posttraumatic stress disorder and head injury as a dual diagnosis: "Islands" of memory as a mechanism. *Journal of Neurology, Neurosurgery, and Psychiatry, 62*, 82–84.

Kiser, L. J., Heston, J., Millsap, P. A., & Pruitt, D. B. (1991). Physical and sexual abuse in childhood: Relationship with posttraumatic stress disorder. *Journal of the American Academy of Child and Adolescent Psychiatry, 30*, 776–783.

Klein, E., Caspi, Y., & Gil, S. (2003). The relation between memory of the traumatic event and PTSD: Evidence from studies of traumatic brain injury. *Canadian Journal of Psychiatry, 48*(1), 28–32.

Knight, J. A. (1997). Neuropsychological assessment in posttraumatic stress disorder. In J. P. Wilson & T. M. Keane (Eds.), *Assessing psychological trauma and PTSD* (pp. 448–492). New York: Guilford Press.

Kolb, L. C. (1989). Chronic posttraumatic stress disorder: Implications of recent epidemiological and neuropsychological studies. *Psychological Medicine, 19*, 821–824.

Kuch, K., Evans, R., & Watson, C. P. N. (1991). Accidents and chronic myofascial pain. *Pain Clinic, 4*, 79–86.

Kwentus, J., Hart, R., Peck, E., & Kornstein, S. (1985). Psychiatric complications of closed head trauma. *Psychosomatics, 26*, 8–17.

Lapierre, O., & Montplaisir, J. (1992). Polysomnographic features of REM sleep behavior disorder: Development of a scoring method. *Neurology, 42*(7), 1371–1374.

Layton, B. S., & Wardi-Zonna, K. (1995). Posttraumatic stress disorder with neurogenic amnesia for the traumatic event. *Clinical Neuropsychologist, 9*, 2–10.

Levin, H. (1985). Neurobehavioral recovery. In D. P. Becker & J. T. Povlishock (Eds.), *Central nervous system status report* (pp. 281–299). Washington, DC: NINCDS/NIH.

Levy, A. (1996, June). *PTSD and brain injury: The impossible coexistence.* Paper presented at the World Conference of the International Society for Traumatic Stress Studies, Jerusalem.

Levy, C. J. (1988). Agent Orange exposure and posttraumatic stress disorder. *Journal of Nervous and Mental Disease, 176*, 242–245.

Lezak, M. D. (1989). Assessment of psychosocial dysfunctions resulting from head trauma. In M. D. Lezak (Ed.), *Assessment of the behavioral consequences of head trauma* (pp. 113–144). New York: Liss.

Litz, B. T., & Herman, D. S. (1993, October). The parameters of selective attention in combat-related PTSD. In P. Resnick (Chair), *The role of cognition in PTSD.* Symposium presented at the meeting of the International Society for Traumatic Stress Studies, San Antonio, TX.

Martzke, J. S., & Steenhuis, R. E. (1993). *Isolated memory disturbance in the absence of global dysfunction in patients with sleep apnea.* Paper presented at the annual meeting of the International Neuropsychological Society, Galveston, TX.

Matser, J. T., Kessels, A. G. H., Lezak, M. D., & Troost, J. (2001). A dose–response relations of headers and concussions with cognitive impairment in professional soccer players. *Journal of Clinical and Experimental Neuropsychology, 23*(6), 770–774.

Mayou, R. A., Black, J., & Bryant, B. M. (2000). Unconsciousness, amnesia, and psychiatric symptoms following road traffic accidents. *British Journal of Psychiatry, 177*, 540–545.

Mayou, R. A., Bryant, B. M., & Duthie, R. (1993). Psychiatric consequences of road traffic accidents. *British Medical Journal, 307*, 647–651.

McAllister, T. W. (1992). Neuropsychiatric sequelae of head injuries. *Psychiatric Clinics of North America, 15*, 395–413.

McGuire, P. K., Shah, G. M. S., & Murray, R. M. (1993). Increased blood flow in Broca's area during auditory hallucinations in schizophrenia. *Lancet, 342*, 703–706.

McMillan, T. M. (1991). Posttraumatic stress disorder and severe head injury. *British Journal of Psychiatry, 159*, 431–433.

McMillan, T. M. (1996). Posttraumatic stress disorder following minor and severe head injury: 10 single cases. *Brain Injury, 10*, 749–758.

McNally, R. J., Kaspi, S. P., Riemann, B. C., & Zeitlin, S. B. (1990). Selective processing of threat cues in posttraumatic stress disorder. *Journal of Abnormal Psychology, 99*, 398–402.

McNally, R. J., & Shin, L. M. (1995). Association of intelligence with severity of posttraumatic stress disorder symptoms in Vietnam combat veterans. *American Journal of Psychiatry, 152*(6), 936–938.

McNeil, J., & Greenwood, R. (1996). Can PTSD occur with amnesia for the precipitating event? *Cognitive Neuropsychiatry, 1*, 239–246.

Mellen, P. F., Weedn, V. W., & Kao, G. (1992). Electrocution: A review of 155 cases with emphasis on human factors. *Journal of Forensic Sciences, 37*, 1016–1022.

Merskey, H. (1992). Psychiatric aspects of the neurology of trauma. *Neurology Clinics, 10*(4), 895–905.

Mesulam, M. M. (1985). *Principles of behavioral neurology*. Philadelphia: F. A. Davis.

Middleboe, T., Andersen, H. S., Birket-Smith, M., & Friis, M. L. (1992). Psychiatric sequelae of minor head injury: A prospective follow-up study. *European Psychiatry, 7*, 183–189.

Miller, L. (1993). Toxic tests: Clinical, neuropsychological, and forensic aspects of clinical and electrical injuries. *Journal of Cognitive Rehabilitation, 11*, 6–18.

Mirsky, A. F., Fantie, B. D., & Tatman, J. E. (1995). Assessment of attention across the lifespan. In R. L. Mapou & J. Spector (Eds.), *Clinical neuropsychological assessment: A cognitive approach*. New York: Plenum Press.

Moradi, A. R., Doost, H. T. N., Taghavi, M. R., Yule, W., & Dalgleish, T. (1999). Everyday memory deficits in children and adolescents with PTSD: Performance on the Rivermead Behavioural Memory Test. *Journal of Child Psychology and Psychiatry, 40*, 357–361.

Moses, J. A., & Maruish, M. E. (1988). A critical review of the Luria-Nebraska neuropsychological battery literature: V. Cognitive deficit in miscellaneous psychiatric disorders. *International Journal of Clinical Neuropsychology, 60*(2), 63–73.

O'Brien, M., & Nutt, D. (1998). Loss of consciousness and posttraumatic stress disorder. *British Journal of Psychiatry, 173*, 102–104.

Ohry, A., Rattok, J., & Solomon, Z. (1996). Posttraumatic stress disorder in brain injury patients. *Brain Injury, 10*, 687–695.

Orsillo, S. M., & McCaffrey, R. J. (1992). Anxiety disorders. In A. E. Puente & R. J. McCaffrey (Eds.), *Handbook of neuropsychological assessment: A biological perspective* (pp. 215–261). New York: Plenum Press.

Parker, R. S. (1998). The spectrum of emotional distress and personality changes after minor head injury incurred in a motor vehicle accident. *Brain Injury, 10*, 287–302.

Parsons, O. A. (1987). Neuropsychological consequences of alcohol abuse: Many questions—some answers. In O. A. Parsons, N. Butlers, & P. E. Nathan (Eds.), *Neuropsychology of alcoholism: Implications for diagnosis and treatment* (pp. 153–175). New York: Guilford Press.

Perry, B. D. (1994). Neurobiological sequelae of childhood trauma: PTSD in children. In M. M. Murburg (Ed.), *Catecholamine function in posttraumatic stress disorder: Emerging concepts* (pp. 233–255). Washington, DC: American Psychiatric Press.

Pitman, R. K., Shin, L. M., & Rauch, S. L. (2001). Investigating the pathogenesis of posttraumatic stress disorder with neuroimaging. *Journal of Clinical Psychiatry, 62*(Suppl. 17), 47–54.

Radanov, B. P., Stefano, G. D.., Schnidrig, A., Sturzenegger, M., & Augustiny, K. F. (1993). Cognitive functioning after whiplash. *Archives of Neurology, 50*, 87–91.

Rassmussen, O. V. (1990). Medical aspects of torture. *Danish Bulletin of Medicine, 33*, 1–88.

Rattok, J., & Ross, B. P. (1993, June). *Posttraumatic stress disorder in the traumatically head injured.* Paper presented at the 15th European Conference of the International Neuropsychological Society, Funchal, Madeira, Portugal.

Raz, S. (1989). Structural brain abnormalities in the major psychoses. In E. D. Bigler, R. A. Yeo, & E. Turkheimer (Eds.), *Neuropsychological function and brain imaging* (pp. 245–267). New York: Plenum Press.

Reeves, R. H., Beltzman, D., & Killu, K. (2000). Implications of traumatic brain injury for survivors of sexual abuse: A preliminary report of findings. *Rehabilitation Psychology, 45*, 205–211.

Roberts, G. W., Allsop, D., & Barton, C. J. (1990). The occult aftermath of boxing. *Journal of Neurology, Neurosurgery, and Psychiatry, 53*, 373–378.

Rourke, B. P. (1985). Overview of learning disability subtypes. In B. P. Rourke (Ed.), *Neuropsychology of learning disabilities* (pp. 3–14). New York: Guilford Press.

Rowan, A. B., & Foy, D. W. (1993). Posttraumatic stress disorder in child sexual abuse survivors: A literature review. *Journal of Traumatic Stress, 6*, 3–20.

Sbordone, R. J. (1991). *Neuropsychology for the attorney*. Orlando, Fl.: Deutsch Press.

Sbordone, R. J. (1999). Posttraumatic stress disorder: An overview and its relationship to closed head injury. *Neurorehabilitation, 13*, 69–78.

Sbordone, R. J., & Liter, J. C. (1995). Mild traumatic brain injury does not produce posttraumatic stress disorder. *Brain Injury, 9*, 405–412.

Schottenfeld, R. S., & Cullen, M. R. (1985). Occupation-induced posttraumatic stress disorders. *American Journal of Psychiatry, 142*(2), 198–202.

Segalowitz, S. J., Lawson, S. M., & Berge, B. E. (1993, February). *Unreported head injury in the general population: Subtle residual effects.* Paper presented at the annual meeting of the International Neuropsychological Society, Galveston, TX.

Semple, W. E., Goyers, P., McCormick, R., & Morris, E. (1993). Preliminary report: Brain blood flow using PET in patients with posttraumatic stress disorder and substance abuse histories. *Biological Psychiatry, 34*, 115–118.

Shepard, J. P., Quercohi, R., & Preston, M. S. (1990). Psychological distress after assaults and accidents. *British Medical Journal, 301*, 849–856.

Sierles, F. S., Chen, J. J., McFarland, R. E., & Taylor, M. A. (1983). Posttraumatic stress disorder and concurrent psychiatric illness: A preliminary report. *American Journal of Psychiatry, 140*, 1177–1179.

Spreen, O. (1988). *Learning disabled children growing up: A follow-up into adulthood.* New York: Oxford University Press.

Stein, M. B., Kennedy, C. M., & Twamley, E. W. (2002). Neuropsychological function in female victims of intimate partner violence with and without posttraumatic stress disorder. *Biological Psychiatry, 52*, 1079–1088.

Stephen, J., & Masterson, J. (1999). Posttraumatic stress disorder and traumatic brain injury: Are they mutually exclusive? *Journal of Traumatic Stress, 12*(3), 437–453.

Sutker, P. B., Allain, A. N., & Johnson, J. L. (1993). Clinical assessment of long-term cognitive and emotional sequelae to World War II prisoner-of-war confinement: Comparison of pilot twins. *Psychological Assessment, 5*(1), 3–10.

Sutker, P. B., Allain, A. N., & Winstead, D. K. (1987). Cognitive performances in former WWII and Korean-conflict POWs. *VA Practitioner, 4*(6), 77–85.

Sutker, P. B., Galina, Z. H., West, J. A. & Allain, A. N. (1990). Trauma-induced weight loss and cognitive deficits among former prisoners of war. *Journal of Consulting and Clinical Psychology, 58*, 323–335.

Sutker, P. B., Winstead, D. K., Galina, Z. H., & Allain, A. N. (1991). Cognitive deficits and psychopathology among former prisoners of war and combat veterans of the Korean conflict. *American Journal of Psychiatry, 148*, 67–72.

Tarter, R. E., Hegedus, A. M., Winsten, N. E., & Alterman, A. I. (1984). Neuropsychological, personality and familial characteristics of physically abused delinquents. *Journal of the American Academy of Child Psychiatry, 23*, 668–674.

Thygesen, P., Hermann, K., & Willanger, R. (1970). Concentration camp survivors in Denmark persecution, disease, disability, compensation. A 23-year follow-up: A survey of the long-term effects of severe environmental stress. *Danish Medical Bulletin, 17*(3), 65–108.

Trudeau, D. L., Anderson, J., Hansen, L. M., Shagalov, D. N., Schmoller, J., Nugent, S., & Barton, S. (1998). Findings of mild traumatic brain injury in combat veterans with PTSD and a history of blast concussion. *Journal of Neuropsychiatry, 10*, 308–313.

Uddo, M., Vasterling, J. J., Brailey, K., & Sutker, P. (1993). Memory and attention in combat-related PTSD. *Journal of Psychopathology and Behavioral Assessment, 15*, 43–52.

Ursano, R. J., Fullerton, C. S., Epstein, R. S., Crowley, B., Kao, T., Vance, K., Craig, K. J., et al. (1999). Acute and chronic posttraumatic stress disorder in motor vehicle accident victims. *American Journal of Psychiatry, 156*(4), 589–595.

Vasterling, J. J., Brailey, K., Constans, J. I., & Sutker, P. B. (1998). Attention and memory dysfunction in posttraumatic stress disorder. *Neuropsychology, 12*(1), 125–133.

Vasterling, J. J., Duke, L. M., Brailey, K., Constans, J. I., Allain, A. N., & Sutker, P. B. (2002). Attention, learning, and memory performances and intellectual resources in Vietnam veterans: PTSD and no disorder comparisons. *Neuropsychology, 16*, 5–14.

Warden, D. L., Labbate, L. A., Salazar, A. M., Nelson, R., Sheley, E., Staudenmeier, J., & Martin, E. (1997). Posttraumatic stress disorder in patients with traumatic brain injury and amnesia for the event? *Journal of Neuropsychiatry and Clinical Neurosciences, 9*, 18–22.

Watson, P. B. (1990). Posttraumatic stress disorder [Letter to the editor]. *British Journal of Psychiatry*, 156, 910–911.

Watson, P. B., Hoffman, L., & Wilson, G. V. (1988). The neuropsychiatry of posttraumatic stress disorder. *British Journal of Psychiatry, 152*, 164–173.

Weinstein, C. S., Fucetola, R., & Mollica, R. (2001). Neuropsychological issues in the assessment of refugees and victims of mass violence. *Neuropsychological Review, 11*, 131–141.

White, R. F., Feldman, G. G., & Proctor, S. P. (1992). Neurobehavioral effects of toxic exposures. In R. F. White (Ed.), *Clinical syndromes in adult neuropsychology: The practitioner's handbook* (pp. 1–52). Amsterdam: Elsevier Press.

Williams, W. H., Evans, J. J., Wilson, B. A., & Needham, P. (2002). Prevalence of posttraumatic stress disorder after severe traumatic brain injury in a representative community sample. *Brain Injury, 16*(8), 673–679.

Woodward, S. H. (1993). Sleep disturbance in posttraumatic stress disorder. *PTSD Research Quarterly, 4*, 4–7.

Wright, J. C., & Telford, R. (1996). Psychological problems following minor head injury: A prospective study. *British Journal of Clinical Psychology, 35*, 399–412.

Yehuda, R., & Harvey, P. D. (1997). Relevance of neuroendocrine alterations in PTSD to memory-related impairments of trauma survivors. In J. D. Read & D. S. Lindsay (Eds.), *Recollections of trauma: Scientific evidence and clinical practice*

(NATO ASI Series A: Life sciences, Vol. 291, pp. 221–252). New York: Plenum Press.

Yehuda, R., Keefe, R. S., Harvey, P. D., & Levengood, R. A. (1995). Learning and memory in combat veterans with posttraumatic stress disorder. *American Journal of Psychiatry*, *152*, 137–139.

Zalewski, C., Thompson, W., & Gottesman, I. (1994). Comparison of neuropsychological test performance in PTSD, generalized anxiety disorder and control Vietnam veterans. *Assessment*, *2*, 133–142.

Zeitlin, S. B., & McNally, R. J. (1991). Implicit and explicit memory bias for threat in posttraumatic stress disorder. *Behavior Research and Theory*, *29*, 451–457.

Zimering, R. T., Caddell, J. M., Fairbank, J. A., & Keane, T. M. (1993). Posttraumatic stress disorder in Vietnam veterans: An experimental validation of the DSM-III diagnostic criteria. *Journal of Traumatic Stress*, *6*, 327–342.

CHAPTER 13

Neuroimaging Studies in PTSD

JOAN KAUFMAN
DEANE AIKINS
JOHN KRYSTAL

The prevalence of posttraumatic stress disorder (PTSD) is estimated to be between 8% and 9% (Breslau, Davis, Andreski, & Peterson, 1991; Kendler et al., 1995), with rates of PTSD approximately twice as high in females as they are in males (Breslau, Davis, Andreski, Peterson, & Schultz, 1997). PTSD is often a chronic and recurring disorder (Ballenger et al., 2000; Kessler, Sonnega, Bromet, Hughes, & Nelson, 1995) and is associated with high rates of comorbid depression and substance abuse (Giaconia et al., 1995; Marshall et al., 2001; Oquendo et al., 2003). The co-occurrence of these disorders is associated with a worse prognosis (Breslau et al., 1997) and greater risk for suicidality (Giaconia et al., 1995; Oquendo et al., 2003).

Preclinical (e.g. animal) studies of the effects of stress have provided a valuable heuristic for generating hypotheses about the brain structures and neural circuits implicated in the pathophysiology of PTSD and for understanding the high rates of comorbidity observed in patients with this disorder. In this chapter, the first section reviews extant neuroimaging studies: the second section highlights relevant preclinical research; and the last section delineates directions for future investigations.

STRUCTURAL NEUROIMAGING STUDIES OF ADULTS WITH PTSD

Table 13.1 summarizes the methods and results of structural neuroimaging studies in adults with PTSD. There have been 11 studies to date, approximately evenly divided between investigating male and female participants.

TABLE 13.1. Structural MRI Studies in Adults with PTSD

Citation	Sample	Lifetime diagnoses	Trauma	Method	Results
Bremner et al. (1995)	26 PTSD (100% M) 22 NC	68% MDD 76% ALC	Combat	MRI (1.5 T), 3-mm contiguous slices	PTSD < NC R hippocampus (8% reduction)
Gurvits et al. (1996)	7 PTSD (100% M) 7 TC 8 NC	57% MDD 71% ALC	Combat	MRI (1.5 T), 3-mm contiguous slices	PTSD = TC > NC subarachnoidal CSF PTSD < TC = NC L/R hippocampus (26%)
Bremner et al. (1997)	17 PTSD (71% M) 17 NC	86% MDD 71% ALC	Child abuse	MRI (1.5 T), 3-mm contiguous slices	PTSD < NC L hippocampus (12%) PTSD < NC L amygdala (trend only)
Stein et al. (1997)	21 CSA (71% PTSD) 21 NC (100% F)	29% MDD NR ALC[a]	Child abuse	MRI (1.5 T), 4-mm slice, 0.4-mm increments	CSA < NC L hippocampus (5%)
Driessen et al. (2000)	21 BPD (57% PTSD) 21 NC (100% F)	NR MDD[b] NR ALC[c]	Child abuse	MRI (1.5 T), 1.25-mm contiguous slices	BPD+PTSD = BPD-no PTSD < NC L/R hippocampus (16%) BPD+PTSD = BPD-no PTSD < NC L/R amygdala (8%)
Bonne et al. (2001)	10 PTSD (70% F) 27 TC	0% MDD 0% ALC	Mixed[d]	MRI (2.0 T), 1.5-mm contiguous slices, 1 wk and 6 mo posttrauma	PTSD = TC hippocampus, amygdala (1-week assessment) PTSD = TC hippocampus, amygdala (6-month assessment)

Schuff et al. (2001)	18 PTSD (100% M) 19 NC	55% MDD NR ALC[f]	Combat	MRI (1.5 T), 3-mm contiguous slices	PTSD = NC hippocampus PTSD = NC entorhinal cortex
Villarreal et al. (2002)	12 PTSD (83%F) 10 NC	100% MDD 8% ALC	Mixed[e]	MRI (1.5 T), 1.5-mm contiguous slices	PTSD < NC L/R hippocampus (13%, 10%) PTSD < NC white matter/intracranial volume PTSD > NC CSF/intracranial volume
Fennema-Notestine et al. (2002)	11 PTSD (100% F) 11 TC 17 NC	NR MDD[g] NR ALC[h]	Partner violence	MRI (1.5 T), 1.2-mm contiguous slices	PTSD = TC < NC WBV[i], cortical gray, frontal gray, occipital gray, medial temporal lobe gray PTSD = TC = NC hippocampus
Vythilingam et al. (2002)	21 MDD/CA (66% PTSD) 11 MDD—no abuse 14 NC (100% F)	43% ALC (MDD/CA) 27% ALC (MDD/NA)	Child abuse	MRI (1.5 T), 1.5-mm contiguous slices	MDD/CA < MDD – no abuse = NC no abuse L hippocampus (15%)
Gilbertson et al. (2002)	Ex+/Ex- Twins (100% M) 12 Ex+PTSD/Ex- Twins 23 Ex+NoPTSD/Ex- Twins	82%/47% ALC (PTSD) 43%/30% ALC (noPTSD)	Combat	MRI (1.5 T)	Ex+PTSD = Ex- Co-Twin < Ex+NoPTSD = Ex- Co-Twin L/R Hippocampus (4%; 10%)

Notes. PTSD, posttraumatic stress disorder; NC, normal control; TC, trauma control; M, male; F, female; MDD, major depressive disorder; CSA, child sexual abuse; BPD, borderline personality disorder; CA, child abuse; ER, emergency room; WBV, whole brain volume; MTL, mesotemporal lobe; L, left; R, right

[a] CSA > NC on lifetime alcohol use measure. No lifetime alcohol abuse diagnoses reported.

[b] BPD > NC on current depressive symptomatology measure. No lifetime depression diagnoses reported.

[c] BPD > NC on lifetime alcohol use measure. No lifetime alcohol abuse diagnoses reported.

[d] Miscellaneous traumas in adulthood requiring treatment at a hospital emergency room.

[e] Half the participants had a history of child physical and/or sexual abuse; the remaining participants had PTSD secondary to assault, rape, accident, or combat.

[f] Inclusion criteria required individuals with history of alcohol dependence to be abstinent for 5 or more years. Investigator unable to recruit PTSD sample without history of alcohol dependence.

[g] PTSD > TC > NC on rating of current depressive symptomatology. No lifetime depression diagnoses reported.

[h] PTSD = NX > TC on alcohol use in past year. No lifetime alcohol abuse diagnoses reported.

[i] WBV computed using supratentorial cranial vault, a measure of cerebrum and cerebrospinal fluid.

Seven of the 11 studies reported reduced hippocampal volume in patients with PTSD compared with normal controls (Bremner et al., 1995; Bremner, Randall, et al., 1997; Driessen et al., 2000; Gurvits et al., 1996; Stein, Koverola, Hanna, Torchia, & McClarty, 1997; Villarreal et al., 2002; Vythilingam et al., 2002). There are no clear laterality findings across these seven studies, with three studies reporting reduced hippocampal volume only on the left side (Bremner, Randall, et al., 1997; Stein et al., 1997; Vythilingam et al., 2002), one study reporting reduced hippocampal volume only on the right side (Bremner et al., 1995), and three studies reporting reduced hippocampal volume on both sides of the brain (Driessen et al., 2000; Gurvits et al., 1996; Villarreal et al., 2002). All the individuals in the studies who reported reduced hippocampal volume had high rates of lifetime diagnoses of major depressive disorder (MDD) and alcohol dependence, and the majority of individuals in these studies had chronic PTSD.

Bonne and colleagues (Bonne et al., 2001) conducted one of the studies that failed to detect hippocampal volume reduction in association with PTSD. They completed a prospective longitudinal study of adults who experienced acute traumas that required treatment at a hospital emergency room and scanned participants within 1 week of the acute trauma and again 6 months later. Ten of the 37 participants included in the study had developed PTSD at follow-up. The hippocampal volumes of participants who developed PTSD and of those who did not were comparable at baseline and at the 6-month follow-up. These findings suggest that reduced hippocampal volume may be a marker of chronicity and not evident in the early stages of the disease process. Although the inclusion of a normal control comparison group in the study by Bonne and colleagues (Bonne et al., 2001) would have provided greater support for this proposition, as discussed later, findings of studies conducted with pediatric samples are consistent with this view (Carrion et al., 2001; De Bellis, Hall, Boring, Frustaci, & Moritz, 2001; De Bellis et al., 1999; De Bellis et al., 2002). In addition, in neuroimaging studies of adults with MDD, hippocampal volume reductions are significantly more common in adult depressed individuals with recurrent episodes of disorder than in individuals with single episodes of MDD (Bremner, Narayan, et al., 2000; Sheline, Wang, Gado, Csernansky, & Vannier, 1996; Vakili et al., 2000), with degree of hippocampal atrophy found to correlate significantly with lifetime duration of depressive illness (Sheline et al., 1996).

Although the failure to detect hippocampal volume differences in the study by Bonne and colleagues (Bonne et al., 2001) may be due to differences in the chronicity of PTSD symptoms, it may also be due to differences in the comorbid diagnostic profile of the participants. The participants included in the study by Bonne and colleagues had no history of alcohol abuse or dependence (Bonne et al., 2001), in sharp contrast to the studies that reported hippocampal volume reduction in association with PTSD. In one of the other studies that failed to report reduced hippocampal volume, although lifetime diagnoses were not reported, patients with PTSD and controls had consumed a comparable amount of liquor during the previous year (Fennema-Notestine, Stein, Kennedy, Archibald, & Jernigan, 2002). In another study that failed to detect hippocampal volume differences between individuals and controls (Schuff et al., 2001), all individuals with a history of alcohol dependence were required to have been abstinent for 5 or more years for inclusion in the study. Although six of the seven studies that reported reduced hippocampal volume in individuals with PTSD excluded individuals with current alcohol abuse and/or utilized statistical methods to control for lifetime alcohol use (Bremner et al., 1995; Bremner, Randall, et al., 1997; Gurvits et al., 1996; Stein et al., 1997; Villarreal et al., 2002; Vythilingam et al., 2002), the possibility that hippocampal volume reductions in patients with PTSD are related to alcohol use history cannot be entirely ruled out (Agartz, Momenan, Rawlings, Kerich, & Hommer, 1999; Beresford et al., 1999; De Bellis et al., 2000; Laakso et al., 2000).

The other neuroimaging study that failed to detect hippocampal volume differences between individuals and controls was conducted by Gilbertson and colleagues (Gilbertson et al., 2002). These investigators conducted a study with 35 identical twin pairs who were discordant for combat exposure. Twelve of the combat-exposed twins developed PTSD, 23 did not. The twins and their co-twins who had not been exposed to combat were scanned. Combat-exposed twins with PTSD *and* their unexposed co-twins were found to have smaller hippocampal volumes than combat-exposed twins without PTSD and their unexposed co-twins. Given that the identical twins who were not exposed to combat had hippocampal volumes that were comparable to those of their combat-exposed co-twins who developed PTSD and had significantly smaller hippocampi than combat-exposed men who did not develop PTSD, the authors concluded that the reduced hippocampal volume represented a preexisting, inherent vulnerability factor, rather than being a consequence of trauma exposure. This interpretation has to be accepted with caution, however, as the combat-exposed veterans who developed PTSD and their combat-unexposed co-twins were significantly more likely to have a history of alcohol dependence than the combat-exposed veterans who did not develop PTSD and their combat unexposed co-twins (alcohol dependence: Ex+PTSD/Ex-co-twin: 82% and 47% vs. Ex+noPTSD/Ex-co-twin: 43% and 30%). Childhood histories of sexual and physical abuse were also higher in the combat-exposed veterans who developed PTSD and in their combat-unexposed co-twins than in the other twin pairs (child abuse: Ex+PTSD/Ex-co-twin: 29% and 24% vs. Ex+NoPTSD/ex-co-twin: 13% and 9%).

In contrast to the findings reported by Gilbertson and colleagues (2002), in a yet-to-be-published study of dizygotic twin pairs discordant for combat exposure and PTSD diagnosis, combat veterans with PTSD were found to have significantly smaller hippocampal volumes than their dizygotic twins without combat exposure or PTSD (Bremner et al., 2001). Analyses of identical-twin-pair data collected as part of this study are currently underway (Bremner, personal communication, May, 2003), but the preliminary results do not appear to support the conclusions of Gilbertson and colleagues.

Alternatively, in one preclinical study of paternal half-sibling primates raised apart and randomized to various postnatal conditions, estimated heritability for hippocampal size was as high as 54% (Lyons, Yang, Sawyer-Glover, Moseley, & Schatzberg, 2001). This finding is consistent with twin (Kendler et al., 1995; Xian et al., 2000) and family (Davidson, Tupler, Wilson, & Connor, 1998; Reich, Lyons, & Cai, 1996) studies that suggest a genetic liability for exposure to trauma and the development of PTSD, a liability that is shared in part with the genetic risk for the development of MDD and alcohol and substance abuse disorders. It is likely that future neuroimaging studies that incorporate genetic and environmental measures will be most informative in unraveling the pathogenesis of PTSD.

Using the existing databases, it is impossible to definitely determine whether reductions in hippocampal volume in individuals with PTSD are due to predisposing factors, to the stress associated with the precipitating trauma, to altered capacity of the hippocampus to respond to subsequent neuronal assaults, to PTSD symptom persistence, to recurrent depression, or to alcohol consumption (Sapolsky, 2000). Although PTSD, MDD, and alcohol dependence are highly comorbid diagnoses, in most cases the PTSD predates the onset of these other disorders (Breslau et al., 1997; Goldenberg, Mueller, & Fierman, 1995; Kessler et al., 1995). Additional longitudinal studies of individuals with PTSD that start early in the course of the disorder will help to clarify these issues.

MAGNETIC RESONANCE SPECTROSCOPY STUDIES IN ADULTS WITH PTSD

Table 13.2 depicts the methods and results of magnetic resonance spectroscopy (MRS) studies conducted in adults with PTSD. The studies by Villerreal and colleagues (Villarreal et al., 2002) and by Schuff and colleagues (Schuff et al., 2001) included in the table are the same studies cited in the structural neuroimaging section. Although Schuff and colleagues (Schuff et al., 2001) failed to detect structural changes in hippocampal volume in individuals with PTSD, consistent with the other investigators using MRS, neurochemical differences were reported in this region. Specifically, in all three studies using MRS, individuals with PTSD were found to have reduced *N*-acetyl-L-aspartic acid (NAA) and creatine in the hippocampus region when compared with controls (Freeman, Cardwell, Karson, & Komoroski, 1998; Schuff et al., 2001; Villarreal et al., 2002). NAA reduction is typically interpreted as an indication of neuronal loss or damage (De Stefano, Matthews, & Arnold, 1995), with associated loss in neuron number, density, or neuronal metabolism (Birken & Oldendorf, 1989). Creatine reductions are suggestive of decreases in high-

TABLE 13.2. Magnetic Resonance Spectroscopy Studies in Adults with PTSD

Citation	Sample	Trauma	Method	Results
Freeman et al. (1998)	21 PTSD (100% M) 8 NC	Combat	MRS (1.5 T)	PTSD < TC NAA/Cr in medial temporal lobe (right) PTSD < TC Choline/Cr in medial temporal lobe (left)
Schuff et al. (2001)	18 PTSD (100% M) 19 NC	Combat	MRS (1.5 T)	PTSD < NC NAA hippocampus (left, right) PTSD < NC Cr hippocampus (right)
Villarreal et al. (2002)	8 PTSD (25% M) 5 NC	Mixed[a]	MRS (1.5 T)	PTSD < NC NAA hippocampus (left, trend) PTSD < NC Cr hippocampus (left, trend) PTSD < NC Cr occipital (left, right)

NOTES. PTSD, posttraumatic stress disorder; NC, normal control; M, male; MRS, magnetic resonance spectroscopy; NAA, *N*-acetyl-L-aspartic acid; Cr, creatine; T, tesla.
[a] Traumas included child sexual and physical abuse, assault, combat, and witnessing son's death in a fire.

energy phosphate metabolism (Urenjak, Williams, Giadian, & Noble, 1993). These MRS studies are consistent with the results of the structural neuroimaging studies and further suggest a role for the hippocampus in the pathophysiology of PTSD.

Because the individuals included in each of the MRS studies had chronic PTSD and because high rates of lifetime MDD and alcohol dependence were reported in each of the samples, it is impossible to determine whether these neurochemical alterations are predisposing factors for PTSD, are primary disturbances associated with illness onset, or are secondary changes resulting from symptom persistence or the development of co-occurring disorders. Further longitudinal research in this area is warranted as well.

EXPOSURE TO TRAUMATIC STIMULI DURING FUNCTIONAL NEUROIMAGING STUDIES IN ADULTS WITH PTSD

Twelve studies have utilized functional neuroimaging approaches to compare the neural correlates associated with exposure to traumatic stimuli in individuals with PTSD and in trauma controls (Bremner, 1999; Bremner, Narayan, et al., 1999; Bremner, Staib, et al., 1999; Hendler, Rotshtein, & Hadar, 2001; Lanius et al., 2002; Lanius et al., 2001; Lanius et al., 2003; Liberzon et al., 1999; Shin et al., 1997a, 1997b, 1999; Shin et al., 2001; Zubieta et al., 1999). These studies are outlined in Table 13.3. The methodologies utilized in these studies vary considerably. Four studies employed positron emission tomography (PET), three studies used single photon emission computerized tomography (SPECT), and five studies used functional magnetic resonance imagining

TABLE 13.3. Exposure to Traumatic Stimuli during Functional Neuroimaging Studies in Adults with PTSD

Citation	Sample	Trauma	Method	Results[a]
Shin et al. (1997a)	7 PTSD (100% M) 7 TC	Combat	PET—oxygen-15-labeled CO_2 with exposure to neutral, negative, and combat pictures	Different patterns of rCBF changes reported in PTSD and TC participants in each of the conditions No group × condition interactions significant
Shin et al. (1997b)	8 PTSD (100% F) 7 TC	Child sexual abuse	PET—oxygen 15-labeled CO_2 with exposure to traumatic, neutral, and teeth-clenching conditions	Different patterns of rCBF changes reported in PTSD and TC participants in each of the conditions No statistical comparisons between the groups reported
Bremner, Staib, et al. (1999)	10 PTSD (100% M) 10 TC	Combat	PET—oxygen 15-labeled H_2O with combat and neutral slides and combat and neutral sounds	PTSD > TC change rCBF L. inferior parietal (40), R. parahippocampus, R. cerebellum/pons, mid cingulate (23), L. motor cortex (6) during exposure to combat stimuli PTSD < TC change rCBF medial PFC (25), L/R middle temporal gyrus (21, 39), L. thalamus during exposure to combat stimuli
Bremner, Narayan, et al. (1999)	10 PTSD (100% F) 12 TC	Child sexual abuse	PET—oxygen 15-labeled H_2O with traumatic and neutral scripts	PTSD > TC change rCBF L/R superior frontal gyrus (9), L. middle frontal gyrus (6), L/R posterior cingulate (24, 31), L. motor gyrus (4, 6), L. superior temporal gyrus (22) PTSD < TC change rCBF cerebellum, L/R middle occipital gyrus (19), R. supramarginal gyrus (40), R. sensory cortex (1,2), R. inferior frontal gyrus (44), subcallosal gyrus (25), anteromedial frontal gyrus (11), R. fusiform gyrus and inferior temporal gyrus (20), R. hippocampus during traumatic scripts
Liberzon et al. (1999)	14 PTSD (100% M) 11 TC 14 NC	Combat	SPECT—Tc-99m HMPAO with combat sounds and white noise	PTSD > TC = NC amygdala, nucleus accumbens
Shin et al. (1999)	8 PTSD (100% F) 8 TC	Child sexual abuse	PET—oxygen 15-labeled CO_2 with traumatic and neutral scripts	PTSD > TC change rCBF orbitofrontal cortex, anterior temporal poles during traumatic scripts condition

				PTSD < TC change in rCBF anterior and posterior cingulate gyrus, superior and middle frontal gyrus (9, 10, 46), inferior frontal gyrus, superior and middle temporal gyrus, parahippocampal gyrus, inferior parietal lobe during traumatic script
Zubieta et al. (1999)	12 PTSD (100% M) 11 TC 12 NC	Combat	SPECT—Tc-99m HMPAO with combat sounds and white noise	PTSD > TC = NC change rCBF medial PFC (9,10) during combat sounds condition
Lanius et al. (2001)	9 PTSD 9 TC	Child Abuse	fMRI (4.0 T) with traumatic scripts and baseline	PTSD < TC activation L/R thalamus, L/R medial frontal gyrus (10,11), L/R anterior cingulate gyrus (32), R. occipital lobe during traumatic memory
Shin et al. (2001)	8 PTSD (100% M) 8 TC	Combat	fMRI (1.5 T) emotional counting Stroop with combat, generally negative, and neutral words	PTSD > TC R/L anterior insular cortex PTSD < TC R. posterior insular cortex during combat compared with neutral
Hendler et al. (2001)	9 PTSD (100% M) 10 TC	Combat	fMRI (1.5 T) with repeat presentation of combat and neutral pictures	PTSD > TC lateral occipital complex activation to repeat presentations of combat pictures (trend)
Lanius et al. (2002)	7 PTSD (100% F) 10 TC	Child sexual abuse	fMRI (4.0 T) with traumatic scripts and baseline	PTSD > TC superior and middle temporal gyri (38, 39), inferior frontal gyrus (47), occipital lobe (19), parietal lobe precuneus (7), medial frontal gyrus (10), medial cortex (9), and anterior cingulate gyrus (24, 32) PTSD < TC L. parahippocampal gyrus (35), middle frontal gyrus (8), superior temporal gyrus (41,13)
Lanius et al. (2003)	10 PTSD 10 TC	Mixed[b]	fMRI (4.0 T) with baseline and scripts of traumatic, neutral, sad (unrelated to trauma), and anxious (unrelated to trauma) memories	PTSD < TC L/R thalamus, L/R anterior cingulate (24,32) all three mood states PTSD < TC also in the L.superior frotal gyrus (10), L/R inferior frontal gyrus (47,11), parietal lobe—precuneus (7) during traumatic scripts

Notes. PTSD, posttraumatic stress disorder; TC, trauma control; NC, normal control; M, male; F, female; PET, positron emission tomography; SPECT, single photon emission computerized tomography; Tc-99mHMPAO, 99m-technetrium hexamthyl-propyl-amine-oxime; fMRI, functional magnetic resonance imaging; CO_2, carbon dioxide; H_2O, water; rCBF, regional cerebral blood flow; L, left; R, right; PFC, prefrontal cortex; T, tesla.

[a] Numbers in parentheses are Brodmann's areas.

[b] Traumas included child sexual abuse, rape, and motor vehicle accidents.

(fMRI) techniques. Unlike the studies using structural MRI or MRS methodology, most of these studies did not include normal controls but rather trauma controls—individuals with similar traumatic experiences who do not meet criteria for current PTSD. Stimuli included exposure to traumatic and neutral pictures, sounds, single words, or scripts. In some studies, the activation to traumatic stimuli was contrasted with activation to neutral stimuli; in other studies, the activation to traumatic stimuli was compared with a resting baseline.

Table 13.4 summarizes the results of the 12 functional neuroimaging studies that used trauma-exposure paradigms. These studies do not present a coherent picture of the neural correlates associated with exposure to traumatic stimuli. Table 13.4 depicts: (1) the brain regions that were reported to have significantly different activation patters in individuals with PTSD and trauma controls; (2) associated Brodmann's areas, when reported by investigators; (3) the number of studies showing greater activation in patients with PTSD in each area; and (4) the number of studies showing reduced activation in patients with PTSD relative to trauma controls.

Across the 12 studies, 20 different brain regions were identified that distinguished individuals with PTSD from trauma controls, but no brain regions were consistently implicated. The best-replicated finding was increased activation in the motor cortex, with this finding detected in one-third of all studies and likely suggestive of hand clenching in response to traumatic stimuli exposure. Contradictory findings were reported in the majority of other brain regions cited across the different studies. Although altered functioning in regions involved in emotional processing is implicated in the majority of studies, no consistent pattern of findings is evident across the studies. In fact, different patterns of activation have been reported even in studies using the same neuroimaging paradigms (Lanius et al., 2002; Lanius et al., 2001; Lanius et al., 2003; Liberzon et al., 1999; Zubieta et al., 1999). Given variations in neuroimaging methodology and differences in the clinical characteristics of patients with PTSD and trauma controls, it is difficult to draw conclusions from this collection of studies.

ADDITIONAL NEUROIMAGING PARADIGMS IN ADULTS WITH PTSD

Resting Regional Blood Flow

Two studies have been conducted that compare resting regional blood flow in individuals with PTSD and normal controls (Lucey et al., 1997; Sachinvala, Kling, Suffin, Lake, & Cohen, 2000). Both studies utilized SPECT with 99m-technetrium hexamethyl-propyl-amine-oxime (Tc-99HMPAO). One study reported decreased regional blood flow in individuals with PTSD in the superior frontal lobe and caudate (Lucey et al., 1997), and the other study reported increased regional cerebral blood flow in the caudate, right putamen, orbital

TABLE 13.4. Summary of Results of 12 Studies Using Functional Neuroimaging Methods and Exposure to Traumatic Stimuli

Brodmann's area	Brain regions	Number of studies PTSD > TC	Number of studies PTSD < TC
Frontal lobe			
1,2	Sensory cortex		1
6	Motor cortex, middle frontal gyrus,	3	
4,6	motor gyrus, precentral lobule	1	
9	Superior frontal gyrus, medial cortex	2	
10	Superior frontal gyrus		1
8	Middle frontal gyrus		1
9,10,46	Superior and middle frontal gyrus		1
9,10	Medial PFC, medial cortex	2	2
10,11	Medial frontal gyrus		1
11	Anterior medial frontal gyrus		1
	Orbitofrontal	1	
47,11	Inferior frontal gyrus	1	1
44	Inferior frontal		1
Parietal lobe			
40	Inferior parietal, supramarginal gyrus	2	2
	Cuneus	1	
7	Parietal lobe, precuneus	1	1
Temporal lobe			
21,39	Middle temporal gyrus		1
38,39	Superior and middle temporal gyrus		1
41,13	Superior temporal gyrus		1
22	Superior temporal gyrus	2	
20	Fusiform gyrus, inferior temporal gyrus	1	1
	Anterior temporal pole	1	
Occipital lobe, brain stem, cerebellum			
19	Middle occipital gyrus		1
	Occipital lobe	1	1
	Cerebellum	1	1
	Pons	1	1
Subcortical brain regions			
24,32	Anterior cingulate	1	3
	Dorsal anterior cingulate	1	
23	Midcingulate	1	
24,31	Posterior cingulate	2	1
	Thalamus	1	3
	Insular cortex	1	
	Parahippocampus	1	2
	Hippocampus		1
	Amygdala	1	
	Nucleus accumbens	1	

Note. PFC, prefrontal cortex.

cortex, anterior and posterior cingulate, right temporal and parietal regions, and hippocampal regions (Sachinvala et al., 2000). There is no consensus definition of the resting state; it is difficult to control, and it may vary unpredictably (Gusnard & Raichle, 2001). Improved investigation of resting-state blood flow will require human and animal investigation with direct recording of neural activity during resting states to better understand normal resting state physiology and development of theoretical approaches to understand coherence and stability of baseline measures (Gusnard & Raichle, 2001). At present, interpretation of resting-state data is imprecise.

Functional Neuroimaging with an Attention Task

Semple and colleagues conducted three studies using PET in which individuals and controls were scanned during rest and during the performance of an auditory continuous-performance attention task (Semple et al., 1993; Semple et al., 1996; Semple et al., 2000). Participants were presented with a series of 500-Hz tones and instructed to press a button when a target tone was heard. In the first investigation, 6 individuals with PTSD and substance abuse histories and 7 normal controls were studied, and no regional blood flow differences were reported between the two groups during the auditory attention task (Semple et al., 1993). In the second study with a cohort of 8 individuals with PTSD and substance abuse histories and 8 normal controls, individuals with PTSD made more errors than normal controls, and had increased right supramarginal gyrus blood flow (Semple et al., 1996). In the last study, with a cohort of 7 individuals with PTSD and substance abuse histories and 6 normal controls increased blood flow was reported in the PTSD group in the amygdala and left parahippocampal gyrus, and decreased blood flow was reported in the frontal cortex (Semple et al., 2000). Replication of these findings in larger samples, with and without substance abuse histories, is required to better understand the potential mechanisms underlying attention deficits in individuals with PTSD.

Functional Neuroimaging with Working Memory Tasks

Two studies used PET to study working memory in individuals with PTSD (Clark et al., 2003; Shaw et al., 2002). In both studies, participants were instructed to detect neutral target words presented in two colors under fixed and variable target conditions. In the fixed condition participants were to press a button when an a priori defined target word in a given color appeared (e.g., the word "bell" in blue). In the variable-target condition, a target was defined as a consecutive repeat of any word in the attended color. In both studies, patients with PTSD showed reduced activation in the dorsolateral prefrontal cortex when performing the variable-target working-memory portion of the task. Other regional activation differences between individuals and controls were not consistently reported in the two studies. The reduction in dorsolateral prefrontal cortex activation, however, suggests a decreased dependence on executive function in monitoring and manipulating working-memory content in individuals with PTSD.

Functional Neuroimaging with a Masked Faces Paradigm

In an fMRI task, photographic images of fearful, happy, and neutral facial expressions were presented, with fearful and happy expressions shown for 33 milliseconds (target), followed immediately by a 167-millisecond presentation of a neutral expression (mask). The task was administered to 8 Vietnam veterans with current PTSD and 8 veterans in a trauma control group (Rauch et al., 2000). When compared with trauma controls, individuals with PTSD had significantly greater amygdala response during exposure to the masked fearful faces than during exposure to the masked happy faces. No medial frontal activation was evident during this task administration (Rauch et al., 2000). These findings suggest that individuals with PTSD have exaggerated autonomic responses within the amygdala to threat or negative-emotion-related stimuli.

Neuroimaging with a Pharmacological Challenge Paradigm

Bremner and colleagues used PET and [^{18}F]fluorodeoxyglucose to measure brain metabolism in 10 Vietnam veterans with PTSD and 10 healthy age-matched controls following administration of yohimbine or placebo in a randomized, double-blind fashion (Bremner, Innis, et al., 1997). After yohimbine, an alpha-2 adrenergic antagonist, individuals with PTSD had decreased regional cerebral blood flow in the orbitofrontal, parietal, prefrontal, and temporal cortices when compared with normal controls. Yohimbine administration was also associated with anxiety symptoms in individuals, but not in controls. These findings suggest that patients with PTSD have increased norepinephrine (NE) release following yohimbine administration and increased central NE drive, consistent with predictions from preclinical studies of the effects of stress (Francis, Diorio, Liu, & Meaney, 1999; Ladd, Owens, & Nemeroff, 1996; Liu, Caldji, Sharma, Plotsky, & Meaney, 2000).

Receptor Binding Neuroimaging

Bremner and colleagues (Bremner, Innis, et al., 2000) used SPECT imaging with iomazenil to assess benzodiazepine binding in 13 individuals with Vietnam combat-related PTSD and 13 matched normal controls. Individuals with PTSD had reduced benzodiazepine binding in the prefrontal cortex (Brodmann's area 9), with individuals with PTSD showing a 41% reduction in distribution volume (the benzodiazepine receptor binding measure) in this area. No other regions showed receptor binding differences. The authors emphasized that the prefrontal cortex mediates several cognitive and behavioral processes that are relevant to PTSD, including inhibition of cognition, emotions, and behaviors. The reduction in benzodiazepine binding is also consistent with results of preclinical studies that suggest that early stress leads to decreased tone of the inhibitory gamma-aminobutyric acid/benzodiazepine (GABA/BZ) system (Caldji, Francis, Sharma, Plotsky, & Meaney, 2000; Francis, Caldji, Champagne, Plotsky, & Meaney, 1999).

NEUROIMAGING STUDIES IN CHILDREN AND ADOLESCENTS WITH PTSD

Table 13.5 depicts the results of the neuroimaging studies conducted with children and adolescents with PTSD. There have been four structural neuroimaging studies to date (Carrion et al., 2001; De Bellis, Hall, et al., 2001; De Bellis et al., 1999; De Bellis et al., 2002), with one publication reporting repeat longitudinal assessments on a subset of the children who participated in an earlier investigation (De Bellis, Hall, et al., 2001). None of the studies detected evidence of hippocampal atrophy in children and adolescents with PTSD compared with controls (Carrion et al., 2001; De Bellis, Hall, et al., 2001; De Bellis et al., 1999; De Bellis et al., 2002). Group differences in NAA and creatine have not been examined in the hippocampus in pediatric samples (De Bellis, Keshavan, & Harenski, 2001).

Instead of hippocampal atrophy, the children and adolescents with PTSD were found to have smaller intracranial and cerebral volumes than normal controls (Carrion et al., 2001; De Bellis et al., 1999; De Bellis et al., 2002). Intracranial and cerebral volume group differences have not been examined consistently in adult studies, and group differences in whole brain volume are reported in only 1 of the 11 extant adult structural MRI studies (Fennema-Notestine et al., 2002). Two of the pediatric MRI studies also reported increased right, left, and total lateral ventricle volume (De Bellis et al., 1999; De Bellis et al., 2002), and one study reported reduced right frontal lobe volume (Carrion et al., 2001).

In addition, two published pediatric studies reported decreased area of the medial and posterior portions of the corpus callosum (De Bellis et al., 1999; De Bellis et al., 2002). Consistent with these reports, in a recent abstract, psychiatric inpatients with a history of maltreatment were likewise reported to have significant reduction in the medial and caudal portions of the corpus callosum when compared with psychiatric and healthy controls without a history of early child maltreatment (Teicher et al., 2000). Studies with adults have not obtained corpus callosum measurements.

To the best of our knowledge, there is only one published structural MRI study in prepubescent nonhuman primates subjected to early stress (Sanchez, Hearn, Do, Rilling, & Herndon, 1998). Most preclinical studies of early stress have examined the long-term impact of these experiences on brain development in *adult* animals. Interestingly, the study with the young primates also failed to find evidence of hippocampal atrophy. Instead, consistent with the

TABLE 13.5. Neuroimaging Studies in Children and Adolescents with PTSD

Citation	Sample	Lifetime diagnoses	Trauma	Method	Results
DeBellis et al. (1999)	44 PTSD 44 NC	45% MDD 0% ALC	Child abuse	Structural MRI (1.5 T), 1.5-mm contiguous slices	PTSD = NC hippocampus PTSD < NC intracranial volume, cerebral volume, corpus callosum (mid- and posterior areas 4–7) PTSD > NC lateral ventricles
Carrion et al. (2001)	12 PTSD 11 NC	13% MDD 0% ALC	Child abuse	Structural MRI (1.5 T), 1.5-mm contiguous slices	PTSD = NC hippocampus PTSD < NC intracranial volume, cerebral volume, R. frontal lobe Group differences in corpus callosum area not examined
DeBellis et al. (2002)	9 PTSD 9 NC	89% MDD 0% ALC	Child abuse	Structural MRI (1.5 T), 1.5-mm contiguous slices, 2 scans at 2-year interval	PTSD = NC cerebral volume, temporal lobe, amygdala, hippocampus at baseline and 2-year follow-up
DeBellis et al. (2003)	28 PTSD 66 NC	50% MDD 0% ALC	Child abuse	Structural MRI (1.5 T), 1.5-mm contiguous slices	PTSD = NC hippocampus PTSD < NC intracranial volume, cerebral volume, corpus callosum (mid- and posterior areas 4–7) PTSD > NC lateral ventricles
DeBellis et al. (2000)	11 PTSD 11 NC	55% MDD 0% ALC	Child abuse	MRS (1.5 T)	PTSD < NC NAA/Cr ratio anterior cingulate Group differences in hippocampus and other brain regions not reported

Note. PTSD, posttraumatic stress disorder; NC, normal control; MDD, major depressive disorder; MRI, magnetic resonance imaging; NAA, *N*-acetyl-L-aspartic acid; Cr, creatine; ALC, alcohol abuse; T, tesla.

child and adolescent studies described previously, the investigators reported reductions in the medial and caudal portions of the corpus callosum in the juvenile, nonhuman primates subjected to early stress (Sanchez et al., 1998).

The medial and caudal portions of the corpus callosum contain interhemispheric projections from the cingulate, posterior temporal–parietal sensory association cortices, superior temporal sulcus, retrosplenial cortex, insula, and parahippocampal structures (Pandya & Seltzer, 1986). Several of the regions with interhemispheric projections through the medial and caudal portions of the corpus callosum have direct connections with prefrontal cortical areas and are involved in circuits that mediate the processing of emotion and various memory functions—core disturbances observed in individuals with PTSD.

Given the prominence of corpus callosum alterations in children and adolescents with PTSD, our group has conducted a preliminary study using diffusion tensor imaging (DTI) in 8 maltreated children with PTSD and 7 normal controls (Kaufman et al., 2001). DTI can be used to assess the integrity of white matter tracts in the brain. Children with PTSD had significantly greater mean diffusivity in the medial and posterior region of the corpus callosum, a finding that is consistent with the possibility of reduced axonal pruning early in development. There were no group differences in fractional anisotropy, but the two groups were not matched on age, and fractional anisotropy correlated significantly with age ($r = .045$, $p < .05$). When the fractional anisotropy values of the three age- and gender-matched PTSD and control pairs were compared, the children with PTSD had a 23% reduction in fractional anisotropy values (range: 12–39%). This finding is consistent with the possibility of reduced myelination in children with PTSD compared with age-matched controls. We are currently in the process of expanding this pilot initiative to further investigate the role of the corpus callosum in the pathophysiology of PTSD. Corpus callosum assessments should be examined in adults and additional research conducted to examine interhemispheric processing in patients with PTSD.

SUMMARY OF PTSD NEUROIMAGING STUDIES

Reduced hippocampal volume has been reported in 7 of the 11 structural neuroimaging studies of adults with PTSD and in none of the 4 structural neuroimaging studies of children and adolescents with PTSD. In all the studies that reported reduced hippocampal volume, individuals had a chronic course of illness, and high rates of MDD and history of alcohol dependence were reported within the samples. At present, it is impossible to determine whether reductions in hippocampal volume in individuals with PTSD are due to predisposing factors, to the stress associated with the precipitating trauma, to altered capacity of the hippocampus to respond to subsequent neuronal assaults, to PTSD symptom persistence, to recurrent depression, or to alcohol consumption. It is our best guess that all these factors contribute. In addition, as discussed later, an understanding is emerging of developmental factors that appear to contribute to the failure to detect hippocampal volume changes in pediatric cohorts.

MRS studies in adults with PTSD have consistently reported reduced hippocampal NAA and creatine in patients compared with controls. Longitudinal studies are also required to determine whether these changes are primary or secondary to persistence of disorder or onset of additional comorbid psychiatric conditions.

Studies that examine neural correlates of exposure to traumatic stimuli implicate a role for brain regions involved in the processing of emotion in patients with PTSD, but given methodological variations, no coherent patterns of activation in response to traumatic stimuli have been reported across studies. Two studies using functional neuroimaging approaches reported that individuals with PTSD had reduced dorsolateral prefrontal cortex activation compared with controls when completing working memory tasks. Another study reported greater amygdala activation in patients with PTSD after exposure to masked fearful faces, and evidence of altered central norepinephrine and GABA functioning has also been demonstrated via pharmacological challenge and receptor-binding neuroimaging studies. Although some of these findings require replication, the emerging data suggest that core neurochemical systems and neuroanatamical structures involved in the stress response are altered in PTSD.

The corpus callosum findings reported in pediatric samples of patients with PTSD have not been examined in adults with PTSD. The parallel findings in children and adolescents and in prepubescent primates subjected to early stress, however, suggest a potential primary role for interhemispheric processing in the pathophysiology of PTSD and highlight the need for further study of brain connectivity more generally.

PRECLINICAL STUDIES RELEVANT TO UNDERSTANDING NEUROIMAGING FINDINGS

Comorbidity in Patients with PTSD

Preclinical studies suggest that maternal separation, early stress paradigms provide good models for studying the development of anxiety disorders, depression, and alcohol and substance use disorders (Charney, Grillon, & Bremner, 1998; Heim, Owens, Plotsky, & Nemeroff, 1997; Huot, Thrivikraman, Meaney, & Plotsky, 2001; Meaney, Brake, & Gratton, 2002). Maternal separation is associated with increased stress reactivity, decreased exploratory behavior in novel environments, decreased water consumption, and increased ethanol consumption in adult rats (Huot et al., 2001). In addition, early stress alters the development of the mesolimbic dopamine system, which has been proposed as a neurobiological mechanism by which these experiences infer a vulnerability for the development of substance abuse problems. Better understanding of the interrelationships among the systems affected by stress and the behaviors they subserve will provide additional insights into the mechanisms underlying the high rates of comorbidity among PTSD, MDD, and alcohol and substance use disorders.

Gene and Environment Interactions

Several studies have been conducted that suggest that gene and environment interactions are important in understanding the neurobiological effects of stress, with species with more intrinsic reactivity more responsive to the effects of environmental manipulations than species that are less intrinsically reactive (Anisman, Zaharia, Meaney, & Merali, 1998; Steimer, Escorihuela, Fernandez-Teruel, & Driscoll, 1998; Zaharia, Kulczycki, Shanks, Meaney, & Anisman, 1996). For example, in one study, primates with two different genetic variations of the serotonin transporter gene were reared by either peers or parents (Bennett et al., 2002). Animals with the heterozygous alleles who were peer reared had lower cerebrospinal fluid (CSF) 5-hydroxyindoleacetic acid (5-HIAA), the serotonin metabolite, than heterozygous animals who were parent reared and than homozygous animals that were either parent or peer reared. Low CSF 5-HIAA is associated with depression, suicidality, and impulsive aggression—common symptoms observed in individuals with histories of early childhood trauma and/or a diagnosis of PTSD. The inclusion of genetic research approaches in future neuroimaging studies will be invaluable in unraveling the impact of environmental experiences and inherent vulnerability on the development of PTSD and its neural underpinnings. There is a growing appreciation of the role of genetics on the individual's response to trauma and of the influence of environment on the expression of critical genes activated in the stress response. Genes and environment are dynamic in their interactions, and better understanding of the nature of these interactions and their impact on brain development will help to identify novel therapeutic approaches to prevent and/or ameliorate the deleterious effects of extreme stress for vulnerable individuals.

Hippocampus

Preclinical studies of the effects of stress suggest a minimum of three mechanisms by which hippocampal atrophy may develop in individuals with PTSD: neuronal atrophy, neurotoxicity, and neurogenesis. Preclinical studies have found that 3 weeks of exposure to stress and/or stress levels of glucocorticoids can cause neuronal atrophy in the CA3 region of the hippocampus (Watanabe, Gould, & McEwen, 1992; Woolley, Gould, & McEwen, 1990). At this level, glucocorticoids produce a reversible decrease in number of apical dendritic branch points and length of apical dendrites of sufficient magnitude to impair hippocampal-dependent cognitive processes (Watanabe et al., 1992). More sustained stress and/or glucocorticoid exposure can lead to neurotoxicity—actual permanent loss of hippocampal neurons through binding of glutamate to *N*-methyl-D-aspartate (NMDA) receptors. Rats exposed to high concentrations of glucocorticoids for approximately 12 hours per day for 3 months experience a 20% loss of neurons specific to the CA3 region of the hippocampus (Sapolsky, Krey, & McEwen, 1985). Evidence of stress-induced neurotoxicity of cells in this region has been reported in nonhuman primates as well (Sapolsky, 1996; Uno et al., 1994). Reductions in hippocampal volume may also be affected by decreases in neurogenesis that result from decreased expression of brain-derived neurotrophic factor (BDNF) caused by elevated glucocorticoids (Gould & Cameron, 1996). The granule cells in the dentate gyrus of the hippocampus continue to proliferate into adulthood, and neurogenesis in this region is markedly reduced by stress.

Developmental Factors

Emerging findings suggest that multiple developmental factors may be relevant in understanding the absence of hippocampal findings in prepubescent primates subjected to early stress and in children and adolescents with PTSD. For example, there are age-dependent changes in sensitivity to some forms of NMDA receptor blockade: as in preclinical studies of neurotoxicity in corticolimbic regions, cell death has been reported to be minimal or absent prepuberty and reaching peak only in early adulthood (Farber et al., 1995). In addition, in another study, changes in BDNF and NMDA receptors were examined in rats subjected to maternal separation immediately following separation, during a later point in development before weaning, and again during adulthood (Roceri, Hendriks, Racagni, Ellenbroek, & Riva, 2002). As adults, when compared with control animals, rats subjected to early separation showed reduced BDNF baseline levels, smaller changes in BDNF after acute stress, and reduced NMDA receptor subunits in the hippocampus. No changes in BDNF or NMDA receptors were evident immediately following separation or at the other preweaning time point examined. Given these findings, it has been suggested that adverse events during brain maturation may modulate expression of molecular components involved in cellular plasticity within selected brain regions, potentially promoting an increased vulnerability to psychopathology, with some resulting brain changes not evident until later in development or adulthood. Alterations in interhemispheric connectivity may represent an additional mechanism by which early adversity may indicate a vulnerability to later psychopathology and promote additional brain changes observed in later in development.

Amygdala

Studies in animals suggest that the amygdala plays a critical role in the acquisition and elaboration of fear conditioning (Cahill, Weinberger, Roozendaal, & McGaugh, 1999; Davis, 1997). The amygdala is activated during stress by ascending catecholamine neurons originating in the brainstem and by cortical association neurons involved in processing stressful stimuli via direct and indirect medial and orbital prefrontal cortical connections (Lopez, Akil, & Watson, 1999). Neurons of the central nucleus of the amygdala respond positively to glucocorticoids and activate the locus coerelus–norepinephrine (NE) component of the stress system (Lopez et al., 1999). Maternal deprivation is associated with increased amygdala stress responsiveness (Menzaghi, Heinrichs, Pich, Weiss, & Koob, 1993). The preliminary results reported in patients with PTSD are consistent with these preclinical findings.

Prefrontal Cortex

There is growing appreciation of the role of cortical inputs in the stress response (Lopez et al., 1999), with medial prefrontal cortex (PFC), anterior cingulate, and orbital PFC currently understood to play an important role in relaying information from primary sensory and association cortices to subcortical structures involved in the stress response. Medial and orbital PFC are reciprocally interconnected, and each has indirect connections with the hypothalamus and amygdala via inputs to the periaqueductal gray and parabrachial nucleus (An, Bandler, Ongur, & Price, 1998; Krout, Jansen, & Loewy, 1998). The medial and orbital prefrontal cortices also provide direct inputs to the hypothalamus and are reciprocally connected with the amygdala (Ongur, An, & Price, 1998). These prefrontal regions appear to be critical in restraining the acute stress response and facilitating negative feedback inhibition of the stress system (Herman & Cullinan, 1997). Early maternal separation and social isolation have been found to alter the development of efferents to frontal areas believed to be analogous to the medial prefrontal cortex (mPFC) in humans and other primates (Braun, Lange, Metzger, & Poeggel, 2000; Poeggel et al., 1999), reducing negative feedback in the stress response. The preliminary results reported in patients with PTSD are also consistent with these preclinical findings.

Neurochemical Systems

Extensive research has been conducted examining the neurobiological effects of early stress, with these experiences associated with increased central corticotropin releasing hormone and NE drive in adulthood (Francis, Diorio, et al., 1999; Ladd et al., 1996; Liu, Caldji, et al., 2000), and decreased tone of the inhibitory gamma-aminobutyric acid–benzodiazepine (GABA–BZ) system (Caldji et al., 2000; Francis, Caldji, et al., 1999). Emerging findings in patients with PTSD are also consistent with these preclincal findings.

Neuroplasticity

Evidence is emerging that the long-term neurobiological consequences of early stress evident in vulnerable individuals need not be permanent. Cross-fostering experiments in rats subjected to early maternal deprivation suggest that provision of optimal parenting subsequent to the early separation can prevent and/or reverse many of the long-term changes associated with early stress (Anisman et al., 1998; Francis, Diorio, et al., 1999; Liu, Diorio, Day, Francis, & Meaney, 2000). In addition, pharmacological interventions may likewise prevent and/or reverse the neurobiological changes associated with early stress (Magarinos, Deslandes, & McEwen, 1999; McEwen et al., 1997; Plotsky, personal communciation, 1999). Consistent with these preclinical studies, propranolol, a beta-adrenergic blocker, has preliminarily been found to prevent the onset of PTSD in adults when administered after an acute trauma (Pitman et al., 2002), and long-term treatment with a paroxetine, a selective serotonin reuptake inhibitor (SSRI), in addition to promoting symptom reduction, has been found to reverse hippocampal atrophy and memory deficits in patients with PTSD (Vermetten, Vythilingam, Southwick, Charney, & Bremner, 2003).

DIRECTIONS FOR FUTURE RESEARCH

1. The majority of preclinical (e.g. animal) studies investigating the impact of early stress have examined the impact of these experiences on the neurobiology of *adult* animals. More developmental studies of the effects of stress are needed to determine which biological alterations are evident immediately following early stress, which emerge at different developmental stages (e.g. prepuberal, postpubertal, adulthood), and what mechanisms are responsible for the emergence of neurobiological alterations at subsequent points in time.

2. Preclinical studies are needed to identify the mechanisms that promote growth changes in the corpus callosum in juvenile cohorts subjected to early stress and to determine whether corpus callosum atrophy is associated with changes in axon number and/or reductions in myelination.

3. Additional exploration of preclinical studies of stress that model the onset of depression- and anxiety-like behaviors together with the onset of substance use disorders are needed to better understand the mechanisms behind the frequent co-occurrence of PTSD, MDD, and alcohol and/or substance use disorders.

4. Additional longitudinal studies of children, adolescents, and adults immediately following trauma and early in the disease process will help to delineate the primary neuroanatomical and neurochemical disturbances associated with PTSD onset from those that emerge as a consequence of development, PTSD persistence, and/or the onset of co-occurring other psychiatric disorders.

5. Additional studies using standard functional neuroimaging paradigms that can be applied to patients and normal controls are needed. Emphasis should be on the use of paradigms that utilize neural networks hypothesized to be altered in patients with PTSD, such as working memory, affect process-

ing, interhemispheric transfer, attention, startle, and fear-conditioning paradigms.

6. Neuroimaging studies examining central NE and gamma-aminobutyric acid (GABA) should be replicated, and studies examining central corticotropin releasing hormone conducted.

7. Neuoimaging studies should be conducted using candidate gene, twin, sibling-pair, and/or family study designs to better understand the interactions between inherent factors and experiences of extreme stress in the onset of PTSD and the neurobiological alterations associated with the disorder.

8. Given emerging findings that suggest that the quality of the subsequent caregiving environment and some pharmacological interventions can ameliorate and/or reverse neurobiological alterations associated with early stress, additional longitudinal repeat neuroimaging assessments before and after psychosocial (e.g. adoption), and pharmacological interventions are warranted to evaluate neuroplasticity in patients with PTSD.

CONCLUSIONS

PTSD is a common and often unremitting disorder. Preclinical studies suggest that early and/or extreme stress is associated with an increase in central CRH and NE drive, reduced function in the inhibitory GABA/BZ system, and long-term changes in hippocampus, amygdala, and prefrontal regions that are critical in integrating the stress response. The extant neuroimaging data in patients with PTSD support the role of these neurochemical systems and neuroanatomical structures in the pathophysiology of PTSD. The emerging preclinical and clinical literature, however, also highlight the importance of genetic, subsequent environment, comorbid clinical, and developmental factors in understanding the long-term neurobiological sequelae of extreme stress. Careful consideration of these additional factors in future neuroimaging studies will increase our understanding of the neural underpinnings of PTSD, help to identify factors that increase and decrease the likelihood of long-term neurobiological alterations in response to stress, and suggest novel preventive and therapeutic intervention approaches for individuals with PTSD.

REFERENCES

Agartz, I., Momenan, R., Rawlings, R. R., Kerich, M. J., & Hommer, D. W. (1999). Hippocampal volume in patients with alcohol dependence. *Archives of General Psychiatry*, *56*(4), 356–363.

An, X., Bandler, R., Ongur, D., & Price, J. L. (1998). Prefrontal cortical projections to longitudinal columns in the midbrain periaqueductal gray in macaque monkeys [see Comments]. *Journal of Comparative Neurology*, *401*(4), 455–479.

Anisman, H., Zaharia, M. D., Meaney, M. J., & Merali, Z. (1998). Do early-life events permanently alter behavioral and hormonal responses to stressors? *International Journal of Developmental Neuroscience, 16*(3–4), 149–164.

Ballenger, J. C., Davidson, J. R., Lecrubier, Y., Nutt, D. J., Foa, E. B., Kessler, R. C., et al. (2000). Consensus statement on posttraumatic stress disorder from the International Consensus Group on Depression and Anxiety. *Journal of Clinical Psychiatry, 61*(Suppl. 5), 60–66.

Bennett, A. J., Lesch, K. P., Heils, A., Long, J. C., Lorenz, J. G., Shoaf, S. E., et al. (2002). Early experience and serotonin transporter gene variation interact to influence primate CNS function. *Molecular Psychiatry, 7*(1), 118–122.

Beresford, T., Arciniegas, D., Rojas, D., Sheeder, J., Teale, P., Aasal, R., et al. (1999). Hippocampal to pituitary volume ratio: A specific measure of reciprocal neuroendocrine alterations in alcohol dependence. *Journal of Studies on Alcohol, 60*(5), 586–588.

Birken, D. L., & Oldendorf, W. H. (1989). *N-acetyl-L-aspartic acid: A literature review of a compound prominent in 1H-NMR spectroscopic studies of the brain. Neuroscience and Biobehavioral Reviews, 13*, 23–31.

Bonne, O., Brandes, D., Gilboa, A., Gomori, J. M., Shenton, M. E., Pitman, R. K., & Shalev, A. Y. (2001). Longitudinal MRI study of hippocampal volume in trauma survivors with PTSD. *American Journal of Psychiatry, 158*(8), 1248–1251.

Braun, K., Lange, E., Metzger, M., & Poeggel, G. (2000). Maternal separation followed by early social deprivation affects the development of monoaminergic fiber systems in the medial prefrontal cortex of *Octodon degus. Neuroscience, 95*(1), 309–318.

Bremner, J. D. (1999). Alterations in brain structure and function associated with posttraumatic stress disorder. *Seminars in Clinical Neuropsychiatry, 4*(4), 249–255.

Bremner, J. D., Hoffman, M., Reed, L., Afzal, N., Sinead, C., Vaccarino, V., & Goldberg, J. (2001, December). *Hippocampal volume in twins with and without Vietnam combat-related PTSD.* Paper presented at the annual meeting of the American College of Neuorpsychopharmacology, San Juan: Puerto Rico.

Bremner, J. D., Innis, R. B., Ng, C. K., Staib, L. H., Salomon, R. M., Bronen, R. A., et al. (1997). Positron emission tomography measurement of cerebral metabolic correlates of yohimbine administration in combat-related posttraumatic stress disorder. *Archives of General Psychiatry, 54*(3), 246–254.

Bremner, J. D., Innis, R. B., Southwick, S. M., Staib, L., Zoghbi, S., & Charney, D. S. (2000). Decreased benzodiazepine receptor binding in prefrontal cortex in combat-related posttraumatic stress disorder. *American Journal of Psychiatry, 157*(7), 1120–1126.

Bremner, J. D., Narayan, M., Anderson, E. R., Staib, L. H., Miller, H. L., & Charney, D. S. (2000). Hippocampal volume reduction in major depression. *American Journal of Psychiatry, 157*(1), 115–118.

Bremner, J. D., Narayan, M., Staib, L. H., Southwick, S. M., McGlashan, T., & Charney, D. S. (1999). Neural correlates of memories of childhood sexual abuse in women with and without posttraumatic stress disorder. *American Journal of Psychiatry, 156*(11), 1787–1795.

Bremner, J. D., Randall, P., Scott, T. M., Bronen, R. A., Seibyl, J. P., Southwick, S. M., et al. (1995). MRI-based measurement of hippocampal volume in patients with combat-related posttraumatic stress disorder. *American Journal of Psychiatry, 152*(7), 973–981.

Bremner, J. D., Randall, P., Vermetten, E., Staib, L., Bronen, R. A., Mazure, C., et al.

(1997). Magnetic resonance imaging-based measurement of hippocampal volume in posttraumatic stress disorder related to childhood physical and sexual abuse: A preliminary report. *Biological Psychiatry*, *41*(1), 23–32.

Bremner, J. D., Staib, L. H., Kaloupek, D., Southwick, S. M., Soufer, R., & Charney, D. S. (1999). Neural correlates of exposure to traumatic pictures and sound in Vietnam combat veterans with and without posttraumatic stress disorder: A positron emission tomography study. *Biological Psychiatry*, *45*(7), 806–816.

Breslau, N., Davis, G. C., Andreski, P., & Peterson, E. (1991). Traumatic events and posttraumatic stress disorder in an urban population of young adults. *Archives of General Psychiatry*, *48*(3), 216–222.

Breslau, N., Davis, G. C., Andreski, P., Peterson, E. L., & Schultz, L. R. (1997). Sex differences in posttraumatic stress disorder. *Archives of General Psychiatry*, *54*(11), 1044–1048.

Cahill, L., Weinberger, N. M., Roozendaal, B., & McGaugh, J. L. (1999). Is the amygdala a locus of "conditioned fear"? Some questions and caveats. *Neuron*, *23*(2), 227–228.

Caldji, C., Francis, D., Sharma, S., Plotsky, P. M., & Meaney, M. J. (2000). The effects of early rearing environment on the development of GABAA and central benzodiazepine receptor levels and novelty-induced fearfulness in the rat. *Neuropsychopharmacology*, *22*(3), 219–229.

Carrion, V. G., Weems, C. F., Eliez, S., Patwardhan, A., Brown, W., Ray, R. D., & Reiss, A. L. (2001). Attenuation of frontal asymmetry in pediatric posttraumatic stress disorder. *Biological Psychiatry*, *50*(12), 943–951.

Charney, D. S., Grillon, C. G., & Bremner, J. D. (1998). The neurobiological basis of anxiety and fear: Circuits, mechanisms, and neurochemical interations (Part II). *Neuroscientist*, *4*(2), 122–132.

Clark, C. R., McFarlane, A. C., Morris, P., Weber, D. L., Sonkkilla, C., Shaw, M., et al. (2003). Cerebral function in posttraumatic stress disorder during verbal working memory updating: A positron emission tomography study. *Biological Psychiatry*, *53*(6), 474–481.

Davidson, J. R., Tupler, L. A., Wilson, W. H., & Connor, K. M. (1998). A family study of chronic posttraumatic stress disorder following rape trauma. *Journal of Psychiatric Research*, *32*(5), 301–309.

Davis, M. (1997). Neurobiology of fear responses: The role of the amygdala. *Journal of Neuropsychiatry and Clinical Neurosciences*, *9*(3), 382–402.

De Bellis, M. D., Clark, D. B., Beers, S. R., Soloff, P. H., Boring, A. M., Hall, J., et al. (2000). Hippocampal volume in adolescent-onset alcohol use disorders. *American Journal of Psychiatry*, *157*(5), 737–744.

De Bellis, M. D., Hall, J., Boring, A. M., Frustaci, K., & Moritz, G. (2001). A pilot longitudinal study of hippocampal volumes in pediatric maltreatment-related posttraumatic stress disorder. *Biological Psychiatry*, *50*(4), 305–309.

De Bellis, M. D., Keshavan, M. S., Clark, D. B., Casey, B. J., Giedd, J. N., Boring, A. M., et al. (1999). Developmental traumatology: Part II. Brain development. *Biological Psychiatry*, *45*(10), 1271–1284.

De Bellis, M. D., Keshavan, M. S., & Harenski, K. A. (2001). Anterior cingulate N-acetylaspartate/creatine ratios during clonidine treatment in a maltreated child with posttraumatic stress disorder. *Journal of Child and Adolescent Psychopharmacology*, *11*(3), 311–316.

De Bellis, M. D., Keshavan, M. S., Shifflett, H., Iyengar, S., Beers, S. R., Hall, J., &

Moritz, G. (2002). Brain structures in pediatric maltreatment-related posttraumatic stress disorder: A sociodemographically matched study. *Biological Psychiatry*, *52*(11), 1066–1078.

De Stefano, N., Matthews, P. M., & Arnold, D. L. (1995). Reversible decreases in N-acetylaspartate after acute brain injury. *Magnetic Resonance in Medicine*, *34*, 721–727.

Driessen, M., Hermann, J., Stahl, K., Zwann, M., Meier, S., Hill, A., et al. (2000). Magnetic resonance imaging volumes of the hippocampus and the amygdala in women with borderline personality disorder and early traumatization. *Archives of General Psychiatry*, *57*, 1115–1122.

Farber, N. B., Wozniak, D. F., Price, M. T., Labruyere, J., Huss, J., St. Peter, H., & Olney, J. W. (1995). Age-specific neurotoxicity in the rat associated with NMDA receptor blockade: potential relevance to schizophrenia? *Biological Psychiatry*, *38*(12), 788–796.

Fennema-Notestine, C., Stein, B. D., Kennedy, C., Archibald, S., & Jernigan, T. (2002). Brain morphology in female victims of intimate partner violence with and without posttraumatic stress disorder. *Biological Psychiatry*, *51*, 1089–1101.

Francis, D. D., Caldji, C., Champagne, F., Plotsky, P. M., & Meaney, M. J. (1999). The role of corticotropin-releasing factor–norepinephrine systems in mediating the effects of early experience on the development of behavioral and endocrine responses to stress. *Biological Psychiatry*, *46*(9), 1153–1166.

Francis, D., Diorio, J., Liu, D., & Meaney, M. J. (1999). Nongenomic transmission across generations of maternal behavior and stress responses in the rat. *Science*, *286*(5442), 1155–1158.

Freeman, T. W., Cardwell, D., Karson, C. N., & Komoroski, R. A. (1998). In vivo proton magnetic resonance spectroscopy of the medial temporal lobes of subjects with combat-related posttraumatic stress disorder. *Magnetic Resonance in Medicine*, *40*(1), 66–71.

Giaconia, R. M., Reinherz, H. Z., Silverman, A. B., Pakiz, B., Frost, A. K., & Cohen, E. (1995). Traumas and posttraumatic stress disorder in a community population of older adolescents. *Journal of the American Academy of Child and Adolescent Psychiatry*, *34*(10), 1369–1380.

Gilbertson, M., Shenton, M. E., Ciszewski, A., Kasai, K., Lasko, N., Orr, S. P., & Pittman, R. K. (2002). Smaller hippocampal volume predicts pathologic vulnerability to psychological trauma. *Nature Neuroscience*, *5*, 1242–1247.

Goldenberg, I. M., Mueller, T., & Fierman, E. J. (1995). Specificity of substance use in anxiety-disordered subjects. *Comprehensive Psychiatry*, *36*, 319–328.

Gould, E., & Cameron, H. A. (1996). Regulation of neuronal birth, migration and death in the rat dentate gyrus. *Developmental Neuroscience*, *18*(1–2), 22–35.

Gurvits, T. V., Shenton, M. E., Hokama, H., Ohta, H., Lasko, N. B., Gilbertson, M. W., et al. (1996). Magnetic resonance imaging study of hippocampal volume in chronic, combat-related posttraumatic stress disorder. *Biological Psychiatry*, *40*(11), 1091–1099.

Gusnard, D. A., & Raichle, M. E. (2001). Searching for a baseline: Functional imaging and the resting human brain. *Nature Reviews Neuroscience*, *2*(10), 685–694.

Heim, C., Owens, M. J., Plotsky, P. M., & Nemeroff, C. B. (1997). The role of early adverse life events in the etiology of depression and posttraumatic stress disorder: Focus on corticotropin-releasing factor. *Annuals of the New York Academy of Sciences*, *821*, 194–207.

Hendler, T., Rotshtein, P., & Hadar, U. (2001). Emotion–perception interplay in the visual cortex: "The eyes follow the heart." *Cellular and Molecular Neurobiology*, *21*(6), 733–752.

Herman, J. P., & Cullinan, W. E. (1997). Neurocircuitry of stress: central control of the hypothalamo–pituitary–adrenocortical axis. *Trends in Neurosciences*, *20*(2), 78–84.

Huot, R. L., Thrivikraman, K. V., Meaney, M. J., & Plotsky, P. M. (2001). Development of adult ethanol preference and anxiety as a consequence of neonatal maternal separation in Long Evans rats and reversal with antidepressant treatment. *Psychopharmacology (Berl)*, *158*(4), 366–373.

Kaufman, J., Jackowski, M., Staib, L., Schultz, L. R., Douglas-Palumberi, H., Anderson, A., & Krystal, J. (2001, December). *Corpus callosum in maltreated children with PTSD: A diffusion tensor imaging study*. Paper presented at the American College of Neuropsychopharmacology, San Juan, Puerto Rico.

Kendler, K. S., Kessler, R. C., Walters, E. E., MacLean, C., Neale, M. C., Heath, A. C., & Eaves, L. J. (1995). Stressful life events, genetic liability, and onset of an episode of major depression in women. *American Journal of Psychiatry*, *152*(6), 833–842.

Kessler, R. C., Sonnega, A., Bromet, E., Hughes, M., & Nelson, C. B. (1995). Posttraumatic stress disorder in the National Comorbidity Survey. *Archives of General Psychiatry*, *52*(12), 1048–1060.

Krout, K. E., Jansen, A. S., & Loewy, A. D. (1998). Periaqueductal gray matter projection to the parabrachial nucleus in rat [see Somments]. *Journal of Comparative Neurology*, *401*(4), 437–454.

Laakso, M. P., Vaurio, O., Savolainen, L., Repo, E., Soininen, H., Aronen, H. J., & Tiihonen, J. (2000). A volumetric MRI study of the hippocampus in type 1 and 2 alcoholism. *Behavioural Brain Research*, *109*(2), 177–186.

Ladd, C. O., Owens, M. J., & Nemeroff, C. B. (1996). Persistent changes in corticotropin-releasing factor neuronal systems induced by maternal deprivation. *Endocrinology*, *137*(4), 1212–1218.

Lanius, R. A., Williamson, P. C., Boksman, K., Densmore, M., Gupta, M., Neufeld, R. W., et al. (2002). Brain activation during script-driven-imagery-induced dissociative responses in PTSD: A functional magnetic resonance imaging investigation. *Biological Psychiatry*, *52*(4), 305–311.

Lanius, R. A., Williamson, P. C., Densmore, M., Boksman, K., Gupta, M. A., Neufeld, R. W., Gati, J. S., & Menon, R. S. (2001). Neural correlates of traumatic memories in posttraumatic stress disorder: A functional MRI investigation. *American Journal of Psychiatry*, *158*(11), 1920–1922.

Lanius, R. A., Williamson, P. C., Hopper, J., Densmore, M., Boksman, K., Gupta, M., et al. (2003). Recall of emotional states in posttraumatic stress disorder: An fMRI investigation. *Biological Psychiatry*, *53*, 204–210.

Liberzon, I., Taylor, S. F., Amdur, R., Jung, T. D., Chamberlain, K. R., Minoshima, S., et al. (1999). Brain activation in PTSD in response to trauma-related stimuli. *Biological Psychiatry*, *45*(7), 817–826.

Liu, D., Caldji, C., Sharma, S., Plotsky, P. M., & Meaney, M. J. (2000). Influence of neonatal rearing conditions on stress-induced adrenocorticotropin responses and norepinephrine release in the hypothalamic paraventricular nucleus. *Journal of Neuroendocrinology*, *12*(1), 5–12.

Liu, D., Diorio, J., Day, J. C., Francis, D. D., & Meaney, M. J. (2000). Maternal care, hippocampal synaptogenesis and cognitive development in rats. *Nature Neuroscience*, *3*(8), 799–806.

Lopez, J. F., Akil, H., & Watson, S. J. (1999). Neural circuits mediating stress. *Biological Psychiatry*, *46*(11), 1461–1471.

Lucey, J. V., Costa, D. C., Adshead, G., Deahl, M., Busatto, G., Gacinovic, S., et al. (1997). Brain blood flow in anxiety disorders: OCD, panic disorder with agoraphobia, and posttraumatic stress disorder on 99mTcHMPAO single photon emission tomography (SPET). *British Journal of Psychiatry*, *171*, 346–350.

Lyons, D. M., Yang, C., Sawyer-Glover, A. M., Moseley, M. E., & Schatzberg, A. F. (2001). Early life stress and inherited variation in monkey hippocampal volumes. *Archives of General Psychiatry*, *58*(12), 1145–1151.

Magarinos, A. M., Deslandes, A., & McEwen, B. S. (1999). Effects of antidepressants and benzodiazepine treatments on the dendritic structure of CA3 pyramidal neurons after chronic stress. *European Journal of Pharmacology*, *371*(2–3), 113–122.

Marshall, R. D., Olfson, M., Hellman, F., Blanco, C., Guardino, M., & Struening, E. L. (2001). Comorbidity, impairment, and suicidality in subthreshold PTSD. *American Journal of Psychiatry*, *158*(9), 1467–1473.

McEwen, B. S., Conrad, C. D., Kuroda, Y., Frankfurt, M., Magarinos, A. M., & McKittrick, C. (1997). Prevention of stress-induced morphological and cognitive consequences. *European Neuropsychopharmacology*, *7*(Suppl. 3), S323–S328.

Meaney, M. J., Brake, W., & Gratton, A. (2002). Environmental regulation of the development of mesolimbic dopamine systems: A neurobiological mechanism for vulnerability to drug abuse? *Psychoneuroendocrinology*, *27*(1–2), 127–138.

Menzaghi, F., Heinrichs, S. C., Pich, E. M., Weiss, F., & Koob, G. F. (1993). The role of limbic and hypothalamic corticotropin-releasing factor in behavioral responses to stress. *Annals of the New York Academy of Sciences*, *97*, 142–154.

Ongur, D., An, X., & Price, J. L. (1998). Prefrontal cortical projections to the hypothalamus in macaque monkeys [see Comments]. *Journal of Comparative Neurology*, *401*(4), 480–505.

Oquendo, M. A., Friend, J. M., Halberstam, B., Brodsky, B. S., Burke, A. K., Grunebaum, M. F., et al. (2003). Association of comorbid posttraumatic stress disorder and major depression with greater risk for suicidal behavior. *American Journal of Psychiatry*, *160*(3), 580–582.

Pandya, D. N., & Seltzer, B. (1986). The topography of commisural fibers. In F. Lepore, M. Ptito, & H. H. Jasper (Eds.), *Two hemispheres—one brain: Functions of the corpus callosum* (Vol. 17, pp. 47–74.). New York: Liss.

Pitman, R. K., Sanders, K. M., Zusman, R. M., Healy, A. R., Cheema, F., Lasko, N. B., et al. (2002). Pilot study of secondary prevention of posttraumatic stress disorder with propranolol. *Biological Psychiatry*, *51*(2), 189–192.

Poeggel, G., Lange, E., Hase, C., Metzger, M., Gulyaeva, N., & Braun, K. (1999). Maternal separation and early social deprivation in *Octodon degus*: Quantitative changes of nicotinamide adenine dinucleotide phosphate–diaphorase–reactive neurons in the prefrontal cortex and nucleus accumbens. *Neuroscience*, *94*(2), 497–504.

Rauch, S. L., Whalen, P. J., Shin, L. M., McInerney, S. C., Macklin, M. L., Lasko, N.

B., et al. (2000). Exaggerated amygdala response to masked facial stimuli in posttraumatic stress disorder: A functional MRI study. *Biological Psychiatry*, *47*(9), 769–776.

Reich, J., Lyons, M., & Cai, B. (1996). Familial vulnerability factors to posttraumatic stress disorder in male military veterans. *Acta Psychiatrica Scandinavica*, *93*(2), 105–112.

Roceri, M., Hendriks, W., Racagni, G., Ellenbroek, B. A., & Riva, M. A. (2002). Early maternal deprivation reduces the expression of BDNF and NMDA receptor subunits in rat hippocampus. *Molecular Psychiatry*, *7*(6), 609–616.

Sachinvala, N., Kling, A., Suffin, S., Lake, R., & Cohen, M. (2000). Increased regional cerebral perfusion by 99mTc hexamethyl propylene amine oxime single photon emission computed tomography in posttraumatic stress disorder. *Military Medicine*, *165*(6), 473–479.

Sanchez, M. M., Hearn, E. F., Do, D., Rilling, J. K., & Herndon, J. G. (1998). Differential rearing affects corpus callosum size and cognitive function of rhesus monkeys. *Brain Research*, *812*(1–2), 38–49.

Sapolsky, R. M. (1996). Stress, glucocorticoids, and damage to the nervous system: The current state of confusion. *Stress*, *1*(1), 1–19.

Sapolsky, R. M. (2000). Glucocorticoids and hippocampal atrophy in neuropsychiatric disorders. *Archives of General Psychiatry*, *57*(10), 925–935.

Sapolsky, R. M., Krey, L. C., & McEwen, B. S. (1985). Prolonged glucocorticoid exposure reduces hippocampal neuron number: Implications for aging. *Journal of Neuroscience*, *5*(5), 1222–1227.

Schuff, N., Neylan, T. C., Lenoci, M. A., Du, A. T., Weiss, D. S., Marmar, C. R., & Weiner, M. W. (2001). Decreased hippocampal N-acetylaspartate in the absence of atrophy in posttraumatic stress disorder. *Biological Psychiatry*, *50*(12), 952–959.

Semple, W. E., Goyer, P. F., McCormick, R., Compton-Toth, B., Morris, E., Donovan, B., et al. (1996). Attention and regional cerebral blood flow in posttraumatic stress disorder patients with substance abuse histories. *Psychiatry Research*, *67*(1), 17–28.

Semple, W. E., Goyer, P. F., McCormick, R., Donovan, B., Muzic, R. F., Jr., Rugle, L., et al. (2000). Higher brain blood flow at amygdala and lower frontal cortex blood flow in PTSD patients with comorbid cocaine and alcohol abuse compared with normals. *Psychiatry*, *63*(1), 65–74.

Semple, W. E., Goyer, P., McCormick, R., Morris, E., Compton, B., Muswick, G., et al. (1993). Preliminary report: Brain blood flow using PET in patients with posttraumatic stress disorder and substance-abuse histories. *Biological Psychiatry*, *34*(1–2), 115–118.

Shaw, M. E., Strother, S. C., McFarlane, A. C., Morris, P., Anderson, J., Clark, C. R., & Egan, G. F. (2002). Abnormal functional connectivity in posttraumatic stress disorder. *NeuroImage*, *15*(3), 661–674.

Sheline, Y. I., Wang, P. W., Gado, M. H., Csernansky, J. G., & Vannier, M. W. (1996). Hippocampal atrophy in recurrent major depression. *Proceedings of the National Academy of Sciences of the United States of America*, *93*(9), 3908–3913.

Shin, L. M., Kosslyn, S. M., McNally, R. J., Alpert, N. M., Thompson, W. L., Rauch, S. L., & Macklin, M. L. (1997a). Visual imagery and perception in posttraumatic stress disorder: A positron emission tomographic investigation. *Archives of General Psychiatry*, *54*(3), 233–241.

Shin, L. M., McNally, R. J., Kosslyn, S. M., Thompson, W. L., Rauch, S. L., Alpert, N. M., et al. (1997b). A positron emission tomographic study of symptom provocation in PTSD. *Annals of the New York Academy of Sciences*, *821*, 521–523.

Shin, L. M., McNally, R. J., Kosslyn, S. M., Thompson, W. L., Rauch, S. L., Alpert, N. M., et al. (1999). Regional cerebral blood flow during script-driven imagery in childhood sexual abuse-related PTSD: A PET investigation. *American Journal of Psychiatry*, *156*(4), 575–584.

Shin, L. M., Whalen, P. J., Pittman, R. K., Bush, G., Macklin, M. L., Lasko, N., et al. (2001). An fMRI study of anterior cingulate function in posttraumatic stress disorder. *Biological Psychiatry*, *50*, 932–942.

Steimer, T., Escorihuela, R. M., Fernandez-Teruel, A., & Driscoll, P. (1998). Long-term behavioural and neuroendocrine changes in Roman high-(RHA/Verh) and low-(RLA-Verh) avoidance rats following neonatal handling. *International Journal of Developmental Neuroscience*, *16*(3–4), 165–174.

Stein, M. B., Koverola, C., Hanna, C., Torchia, M. G., & McClarty, B. (1997). Hippocampal volume in women victimized by childhood sexual abuse. *Psychological Medicine*, *27*(4), 951–959.

Teicher, M. H., Anderson, S. L., Dumont, Y., Ito, C. A., Glod, C., Vaituzis, C., & Giedd, J. N. (2000, October). *Childhood neglect attenuates development of the corpus callosum*. Society of Neuroscience Conference, New Orleans, LA.

Uno, H., Eisele, S., Sakai, A., Shelton, S., Baker, E., DeJesus, O., & Holden, J. (1994). Neurotoxicity of glucocorticoids in the primate brain. *Hormones and Behavior*, *28*(4), 336–348.

Urenjak, J., Williams, S. R., Giadian, D. G., & Noble, M. (1993). Proton nuclear magnetic resonance spectroscopy unambiguously identifies different neuronal cell types. *Journal of Neuroscience*, *13*, 981–989.

Vakili, K., Pillay, S. S., Lafer, B., Fava, M., Renshaw, P. F., Bonello-Cintron, C. M., & Yurgelun-Todd, D. A. (2000). Hippocampal volume in primary unipolar major depression: A magnetic resonance imaging study. *Biological Psychiatry*, *47*(12), 1087–1090.

Vermetten, E., Vythilingam, M., Southwick, S. M., Charney, D. S., & Bremner, J. D. (2003). Long-term treatment with paroxetine increases verbal declarative memory and hippocampal volume in posttraumatic stress disorder. *Biological Psychiatry*, *54*(7), 693–702.

Villarreal, G., Hamilton, D. A., Petropoulos, H., Driscoll, I., Rowland, L. M., Griego, J. A., et al. (2002). Reduced hippocampal volume and total white matter volume in posttraumatic stress disorder. *Biological Psychiatry*, *52*(2), 119–125.

Vythilingam, M., Heim, C., Newport, J., Miller, A. H., Anderson, E., Bronen, R., et al. (2002). Childhood trauma associated with smaller hippocampal volume in women with major depression. *American Journal of Psychiatry*, *159*(12), 2072–2080.

Watanabe, Y., Gould, E., & McEwen, B. S. (1992). Stress induces atrophy of apical dendrites of hippocampal CA3 pyramidal neurons. *Brain Research*, *588*(2), 341–345.

Woolley, C. S., Gould, E., & McEwen, B. S. (1990). Exposure to excess glucocorticoids alters dendritic morphology of adult hippocampal pyramidal neurons. *Brain Research*, *531*(1–2), 225–231.

Xian, H., Chantarujikapong, S. I., Scherrer, J. F., Eisen, S. A., Lyons, M. J., Goldberg, J., et al. (2000). Genetic and environmental influences on posttraumatic stress disorder, alcohol and drug dependence in twin pairs. *Drug and Alcohol Dependence*, *61*(1), 95–102.

Zaharia, M. D., Kulczycki, J., Shanks, N., Meaney, M. J., & Anisman, H. (1996). The effects of early postnatal stimulation on Morris water-maze acquisition in adult mice: Genetic and maternal factors. *Psychopharmacology (Berl)*, *128*(3), 227–239.

Zubieta, J. K., Chinitz, J. A., Lombardi, U., Fig, L. M., Cameron, O. G., & Liberzon, I. (1999). Medial frontal cortex involvement in PTSD symptoms: A SPECT study. *Journal of Psychiatric Research*, *33*(3), 259–264.

CHAPTER 14

Psychobiological Laboratory Assessment of PTSD

MATTHEW J. FRIEDMAN

During the past 20 years a number of experimental laboratory procedures have been utilized to distinguish individuals with posttraumatic stress disorder (PTSD) from those without the disorder. Such procedures can be divided into baseline assessments and provocative tests. In all cases, research with these various techniques has significantly advanced our understanding of the unique pathophysiology of this disorder. In no case, however, has a research protocol achieved the status of a routine clinical assessment technique. The major reason for this is that PTSD-related abnormalities are generally found within the normal clinical range and, therefore, can be detected only in comparison with non-PTSD control groups. A second reason is that inconsistent findings from one research laboratory to the next, with respect to some measures, have cast doubt on the general utility of such tests at this time. A third reason is that most psychobiological research to date has focused primarily on military veterans and to a lesser extent on women exposed to sexual trauma as adults or children. There have been too few psychobiological observations on survivors of nonmilitary or nonsexual trauma. Furthermore, there have been too few observations on females, children, non-Caucasians, and non-European Americans.

Despite these considerations, I believe that there are many reasons to hope that accurate, inexpensive, and clinically useful laboratory techniques for assessing PTSD will be developed within the foreseeable future. Because other chapters have focused on psychophysiological, neuropsychological, and neuroimaging assessment, I focus in this chapter on laboratory measurement of neurotransmitters, neuropeptides, and neurohormones.

THE HUMAN STRESS RESPONSE AND THE PATHOPHYSIOLOGY OF PTSD

First, it is important to establish a conceptual framework by considering the human stress response. The human stress system has evolved for coping, adaptation, and preservation of the species. It encompasses central and peripheral nervous systems, the endocrine system, and the immunological system. The amygdala plays a key role in coordinating the response to stress or threat through activation of the hypothalamic–pituitary–adrenocortical (HPA) and the locus coeruleus–norepinephrine-sympathetic (LC–NE) systems. Corticotropin releasing factor (CRF) plays a strategic role because it activates not only HPA, LC–NE, and immunological mechanisms but also a complex cascade of reactions involving many other neurotransmitter, neurohormonal, immunological, and metabolic mechanisms, including adrenergic, serotonergic, opioid, glutamatergic, GABA-ergic, cholinergic, and cytokine systems (Chrousos, 1998; McEwen, 1998). (It is important to keep in mind that CRF may also initiate more fine-grained actions involving only the HPA, only the LC–NE, or only other specific immunological or neurobiological systems. In the face of an overwhelming stressor, however, it is not unreasonable to consider CRF from the present standpoint, as the principal neurohormonal mover in the complex spectrum of actions that characterize the human stress response.)

PTSD results when a traumatic experience overwhelms the capacity of an individual's stress system. Failure to cope with the demands of traumatic stress might take a number of forms, such as inability to mobilize an adequate response, inability to achieve normal recovery, and inability to calibrate the magnitude of the stress response to the actual psychobiological demands of the traumatic situation.

From this perspective, PTSD exemplifies the human stress response gone wrong. As a result of the organism's failure to cope and recover, key psychobiological functions are altered. Dysregulation of the HPA, LC–NE and immune systems produces many secondary abnormalities that are mediated through a cascade of downstream mechanisms. In chronic PTSD, a new balance is achieved in the face of such stable psychobiological alterations. Countermeasures are brought into play to compensate for (1) the failure to mount an adequate response; (2) the failure to shut off activated mechanisms in order to achieve normal recovery; (3) the failure to habituate to repeated challenges of the same kind; and (4) the failure to calibrate subsequent stress system responses to realistic demands of the situation (Friedman, 2002; Friedman & McEwen, 2004). McEwen (1998) has called the process of achieving stability in the face of such altered neurobiological mechanisms *allostasis*, whereas the price of achieving such stability in the face of these deleterious functional alterations is called *allostatic load*. As I discuss later, allostatic load in chronic PTSD has already been detected in a number of key systems shown in Table 14.1, such as HPA, LC–NE, serotonergic, opioid, and endocrinological sys-

TABLE 14.1. Biological Abnormalities Associated with PTSD

Neurobiological system	Specific indicator	Abnormality
HPA	CRF	Increased
	ACTH	Variable findings
	Cortisol	Variable findings
	DHEA	Reduced
	DHEA/cortisol	Reduced?
	GR receptors	Supersensitivity?
Adrenergic	Tonic norepinephrine/epinephrine	Increased
	Phasic norepinephrine/epinephrine	Increased
	NPY (tonic and phasic)	Reduced
	Dopamine	Increased
	Galanin	Unknown (possibly reduced)
Serotonin	$5HT_{1A}$ receptor function	Unknown (possibly reduced)
	$5HT_{2A}$ receptor function	Unknown (possibly elevated)
Opioid	Beta-endorphin/enkephalin	Mixed findings generally indicative of systemic dysregulation
Glutamatergic	NMDA, non-NMDA, metabotropic receptors	Unknown
GABA-ergic	$GABA_A$ receptors, benzodiazepine receptors	Unknown (possibly blunted)
Substance P	Substance P	Unknown (possibly blunted)
Thyroid	T_3, T_4, TSH	$\uparrow T_3$, $\uparrow T_4$, $\uparrow T_3/T_4$, $\downarrow$TSH
Gonadal	Testosterone	Mixed results
	Estrogen	Unknown
Growth	GH	Tonic GH unchanged; decreased GH activation by clonidine and levodopa
Immunological	Cell-mediated immunity	Immunosuppression
	Cytokine levels	Increased inflammatory cytokines (IL-1, IL-2, IL-6, TNF)

Note. HPA, hypothalamic–pituitary–adrenocortical; CRF, corticotropin releasing factor; ACTH, adrenocorticotropic hormone; DHEA, dehydropiandosterone; GR, glutocorticoid receptor; 5HT, 5-hydroxytryptamine (serotonin); NMDA, *N*-methyl-D-aspartate; GABA, gamma amino butyric acid; T_3, triiodothyronine; T_4, thyroxine; GH, growth hormone; IL, interleukin; TNF, tissue necrosis factor.

tems. Based on laboratory findings, it is reasonable to expect that allostatic load will also be detected in glutamatergic, GABA-ergic, immunological, and other mechanisms, as well. More information on such abnormalities can be found elsewhere (Friedman, 1999; Friedman, Charney & Deutch, 1995; Charney, 2004; Morgan et al., 2003).

HYPOTHALAMIC–PITUITARY–ADRENOCORTICAL SYSTEM

A large body of evidence indicates that HPA abnormalities figure prominently in the pathophysiology of PTSD. Investigations have focused mostly on CRF release, cortisol levels, and glucocorticoid receptor sensitivity.

Corticotropin Releasing Factor

CRF initiates both the HPA and LC–NE systems, as well as other neurotransmitter, neurohormonal, metabolic, and immunological responses. Studies with male combat veterans and premenopausal survivors of childhood sexual abuse have detected elevated cerebrospinal fluid CRF levels and enhanced hypothalamic release of CRF among people with PTSD compared with those without (Baker et al., 1999; Bremner et al., 1997; Yehuda et al., 1996). Mixed results have been found with respect to the ACTH response to CRF (Heim, Newport, Bonsall, Miller, & Nemeroff, 2001; Smith et al., 1989).

Cortisol Levels

Findings on urinary free cortisol levels are mixed. Earlier studies with male combat veterans and elderly male and female Holocaust survivors generally found reduced 24-hour urinary cortisol levels in those with PTSD compared with trauma survivors without PTSD. Other studies with male veterans have shown no difference. More recent investigations, mostly with premenopausal women and traumatized children, have found the opposite (i.e., elevated urinary cortisol levels) among those with PTSD (see reviews by Heim et al., 2001; Rasmusson & Friedman, 2002; Rasmusson et al., 2001; Yehuda, 1999).

To complicate the picture even more, the same patient may exhibit remarkable fluctuations in urinary cortisol during a single hospitalization. Mason, Giller, Kosten, and Wahby (1990) measured urinary cortisol levels in hospitalized combat veterans with PTSD at admission, midpoint, and discharge. Many veterans with low urinary cortisol at admission exhibited high levels several weeks later during that phase of the hospitalization that included therapeutic reexposure of patients to stressful traumatic memories of the Vietnam War. After more weeks had passed, these same veterans reexhibited low urinary cortisol prior to discharge. The investigators proposed that baseline

HPA function can fluctuate dramatically in response to external (stressful) circumstances.

Dehydroepiandosterone

In addition to releasing cortisol, ACTH also stimulates the release of dehydroepiandosterone (DHEA) from the adrenal cortex. Both hormones are secreted episodically and synchronously in response to ACTH (Rosenfeld et al., 1971). DHEA antagonizes the actions of cortisol and other glucocorticoids (Browne, Wright, Porter, & Svec, 1992). Rasmusson and associates (Rasmusson et al., in press) suggested that through cortisol antagonism, DHEA release protects against the effects of excessive adrenocortical activation. Morgan (2001), working with military special forces personnel exposed to a severely stressful training exercise, suggested that DHEA/cortisol ratios may represent a useful measure of psychobiological resilience.

Glucocorticoid Receptor Sensitivity

HPA balance is maintained by a negative feedback system. CRF produces ACTH secretion, which promotes cortisol release from the adrenal cortex. The hypothalamus monitors the amount of circulating cortisol through its glucocorticoid receptors. When a sufficient number of these receptors are occupied by cortisol, CRF secretion is inhibited. This negative feedback mechanism prevents blood cortisol levels from getting too high. When cortisol levels are too low, however, and an insufficient number of hypothalamic glucocorticoid receptors are occupied, CRF is released until the proper blood cortisol level is achieved.

An important theory concerning HPA function in PTSD, derived mostly from Yehuda's work (see Yehuda, 1997, 1999), suggests that there is a stable neurohormonal equilibrium marked by low cortisol, an increase in the number (e.g., upregulation) of glucocorticoid receptors, and enhanced negative feedback of the HPA system due to supersensitivity of these same glucocorticoid receptors detected by the dexamethasone suppression test (DST). The paradox of this elegant model is that, despite lower cortisol levels, the system may act as if there were excessive HPA activity because of the supersensitivity of the glucocorticoid receptors. Indeed, many of the research findings presented here are consistent with the hypothesis that HPA activity is elevated, not reduced, in PTSD.

To summarize, HPA function appears to be dysregulated in PTSD, although variable experimental findings make it impossible to specify a unitary pattern of abnormalities at this time. Many findings suggest enhanced HPA activity due to some combination of elevated CRF activity, glucocorticoid receptor sensitivity, and, in some cases, elevated cortisol levels. Reports vary regarding whether hypocortisolism in PTSD is or is not associated with glucocorticoid receptor supersensitivity. Such variability may reflect tonic (e.g., baseline), as well as phasic (e.g., stress-induced episodic), HPA abnormalities, the magnitude of an individual's stress response at the time of measurement, methodological issues regarding the collection and assay of blood or urine samples, and/or gender-related differences in neurohormonal factors affecting CRF, cortisol levels, or glucocorticoid receptor sensitivity.

ADRENERGIC ABNORMALITIES IN PTSD

Because the LC–NE system is activated during the human stress response (Cannon, 1932), it is not surprising that PTSD has been associated with both tonic and phasic alterations of catecholaminergic function.

Tonic Adrenergic Activity

Twenty-four-hour urinary norepinephrine and epinephrine have been measured in male combat veterans, male and female Holocaust survivors, and female sexual abuse victims. Results in many, but not all, studies have shown elevated catecholamine levels among individuals with PTSD compared with both trauma exposed/no-PTSD and nonexposed controls (see Southwick et al., 1999, for references). Elevated CSF norepinephrine levels have also been detected (Geracioti et al., 2001).

It would be expected that increased catecholamine levels would produce a compensatory reduction (or down-regulation) of adrenergic receptors. This effect has been shown in research on both alpha-2 and beta adrenergic receptors. Two studies (with combat veterans and traumatized children, respectively) have shown reduced platelet alpha-2 binding sites among individuals with PTSD compared with controls (Perry, 1994; Perry, Giller, & Southwick, 1987). In addition, there is evidence that beta adrenergic receptors are also down-regulated (Lerer, Gur, Bleich, & Newman, 1994).

Phasic Adrenergic Activity

A variety of challenge studies have consistently demonstrated excessive phasic adrenergic responses among individuals with PTSD. In addition to physiological hyperreactivity, exposure to psychological stressors has been associated with abrupt elevations in plasma epinephrine and norepinephrine, respectively, in two studies with combat veterans with PTSD (Blanchard, Kolb, Prins, Gates, & McCoy, 1991; McFall, Murburg, Ko, & Veith, 1990).

Yohimbine, an alpha-2 adrenergic receptor antagonist, has been an important pharmacological probe in studies on phasic adrenergic activity. Yohimbine enhances adrenergic activity by blocking the inhibitory presynaptic alpha-2 receptor, thereby enhancing presynaptic release of norepinephrine. An investigation with Vietnam combat veterans found that among the participants with PTSD, yohimbine elicited panic attacks, combat-related flashbacks, and elevated brain adrenergic metabolism in contrast to veterans without PTSD, who did not exhibit such abnormalities (Bremner, Innis, et al., 1997; Southwick et al., 1997).

Thus studies on catecholamine function indicate that the major adrenergic abnormality in PTSD is a hyperreactive phasic response, although alterations in tonic activity have also been detected.

Neuropeptide Y

Neuropeptide Y (NPY) is a neuropeptide found in adrenergic neurons that is released along with norepinephrine during intense activation of the adrenergic system by yohimbine or excessive exercise (Pernow, 1988; Rasmusson et al., 2000). It apparently enhances the efficiency of adrenergic transmission in the sympathetic nervous system (Colmers & Bleakman, 1994) and appears to have a profound anxiety-reducing effect (Kask, Rago, & Harro, 1996). Of particular relevance to our previous discussion of HPA function, anxiolytic doses of NPY also antagonize the anxiogenic and other actions of CRF, making NPY a potential major moderator of the intensity of the human stress response (Britton et al., 1997). NPY is, therefore, an important neuropeptide to consider in PTSD because it is released during intense phasic activation of the adrenergic system and because it is a potent antagonist of CRF.

Veterans with PTSD exhibited significantly lower baseline NPY levels, as well as a blunted NPY response to yohimbine, in comparison with non-PTSD controls (Rasmusson et al., 2000). This result is consistent with animal studies showing reduced NPY inhibition of adrenergic function following chronic stress (Corder, Castagne, Rivet, Mormede, & Gaillard, 1992). Indeed, it is possible that hypoactive NPY function contributes both to adrenergic hyperreactivity and increased CRF activity in PTSD (Rasmusson & Friedman, 2002).

Dopamine

Amygdala activation by uncontrollable stress in laboratory animals produces activation of medial prefrontal cortex dopamine release but inhibition of release by the nucleus accumbens. This suggests that dopaminergic mechanisms play a role in the stress response that is both complicated and not well understood at this time (Charney, 2004). In the few published clinical studies with participants with PTSD, both urinary and plasma dopamine concentrations have been elevated (Hamner & Diamond, 1993; Lemieux & Coe, 1995; Yehuda et al., 1994).

Galanin

Galanin is a neuropeptide, found in 80% LC–NE noradrenergic neurons, that is released during activation. It reduces both LC and amygdala activation (Gentleman et al., 1989; Holmes & Crawley, 1995; Perez, Wynic, Steiner, &

Mufson, 2001). Like NPY, galanin appears to have anxiolytic effects and to antagonize the anxiogenic effects of stress when administered to rats (Bing, Moller, Engel, Soderpal, & Heilig, 1993; Charney, 2004; Moller, Sommer, Thorsell, & Heilig, 1999). Thus it appears that the net amount of stress-inducted anxiety will depend on how much NPY and galanin are available to offset the anxiogenic impact of norepinephrine. There are currently no studies on galanin with humans under stress or with PTSD, so this hypothesis has yet to be tested (Charney, 2004).

SEROTONERGIC SYSTEM

The serotonergic system has important reciprocal relationships with both the HPA and LC–NE systems. Excessive HPA activity associated with chronic life stress or PTSD produces down-regulation of 5-HT_{1A} receptors (which have anxiolytic effects) and upregulation of 5-HT_{2A} receptors (which are anxiogenic), resulting in abnormal neurotransmission in key limbic nuclei (Charney, 2004; McEwen, 1998; Southwick et al., 1999). There also may be synergistic interactions between $5HT_{1A}$ receptors and the GABA/benzodiazepine (GABA/BZ) system (Charney, 2004).

Clinical studies have shown that patients with PTSD exhibit a number of abnormalities associated with low 5-HT, such as impulsivity, rage, aggression, depression, panic, obsessional thoughts, and chemical dependency (Friedman, 1990).

The first two drugs to receive U.S. Federal Drug Administration approval as indicated treatments for PTSD are the selective serotonin reuptake inhibitor (SSRI) antidepressants sertraline and paroxetine. Among their other actions, SSRIs produce amelioration in all three symptom clusters of PTSD. Other antidepressants that affect serotonergic function, such as nefazadone and amitriptyline, have also shown efficacy in PTSD. Given the complexity of the serotonergic system with its large number of distinctive receptor types, it can be expected that in the future research will provide a better understanding of different roles played by the various serotonergic receptor systems in modulating the human stress response.

ENDOGENOUS OPIOIDS

CRF also activates the opioid peptide beta-endorphin, which reciprocally inhibits both the adrenergic and HPA components of the human stress response. The few studies on opioid activity in PTSD suggest that there may be both tonic and phasic abnormalities. Abnormal baseline opioid function has been detected among individuals with PTSD, although the specifics of such findings have varied from study to study. Elevated cerebrospinal fluid beta-endorphin levels were observed in male combat veterans with PTSD (Baker et al., 1997).

Studies on plasma beta-endorphin show mixed results: higher levels among Croatian women with PTSD due to the trauma of war (Sabioncello et al., 2000); normal levels in male combat veterans (Baker et al., 1997); and lower levels in a different cohort of combat veterans with PTSD (Hoffman, Watson, Wilson, & Montgomery, 1989). There is also evidence that exposure of people with PTSD to relevant trauma-related stimuli (e.g., Vietnam veterans with PTSD viewing combat scenes) produces an abrupt phasic elevation in circulating opioid levels (Pitman, van der Kolk, Orr, & Greenberg, 1990).

GLUTAMATERGIC SYSTEMS

Glutamate is an amino acid that is the brain's primary excitatory amino acid. It is rapidly mobilized during stressful or threatening situations and mediates almost all rapid excitatory transmission in the brain. Glutamatergic mechanisms are key to cognitive functions such as perception, appraisal, conditioning, extinction, and memory. Fear conditioning, sensitization, and resistance to extinction, all of which are mediated at *N*-methyl-D-aspartate (NMDA) synapses, are altered in PTSD (Charney, Deutch, Krystal, Southwick, & Davis, 1993) Information processing is disrupted with respect to learning and cognition. Memory function may be altered in the direction of excessive recall (e.g., intrusive recollections) or problems with retrieval (e.g., amnesia). Finally, dissociation, an abnormality that is beginning to be understood as a very important posttraumatic symptom, appears to represent a disruption of glutamatergic function (Chambers et al., 1999; Krystal, Bennett, Bremner, Southwick, & Charney, 1995). It appears likely that medication that normalizes neurotransmission at NMDA, non-NMDA, and metabotropic glutamate receptors may produce benefits for individuals with chronic PTSD.

GABA–BENZODIAZEPINE SYSTEM

In direct contrast to glutamate, gamma-aminobutyric acid (GABA) is the brain's major inhibitory neurotransmitter. The anxiolytic action of benzodiazepines is exerted primarily at $GABA_A$ receptors. A great deal of animal research shows that inescapable stress and anxiety are associated with reduced benzodiazepine receptor binding in the cortex and, possibly, the hippocampus (Weizman et al., 1989; Nutt & Malizia, 2001).

Human neuroimaging studies have shown reduced cortical and subcortical benzodiazepine receptor binding associated with PTSD and panic disorder (Bremner, Innis, White, et al., 2000; Bremner, Innis, Southwick, et al., 2000; Malizia et al., 1998). An important, unanswered question is whether such findings indicate a stress-induced down-regulation of benzodiazepine receptor binding or stress-induced alteration in GABA-ergic transmission that affects benzodiazepine receptor binding (Charney, 2004).

SUBSTANCE P

Based on their neuroanatomic distribution, it appears likely that substance P neurons are activated during the human stress response and have reciprocal interactions with the LC–NE system. Safe substance P antagonists have been synthesized and, in one randomized trial, the substance P antagonist MK-869 was as effective an antidepressant as the SSRI paroxetine (Kramer et al., 1998). Research with this class of medications certainly seems to offer possibilities for important clinical and conceptual advances in PTSD.

HYPOTHALAMIC–PITUITARY–THYROID AXIS

Thyroid-stimulating hormone (TSH) promotes thyroid gland secretion of thyroxine (T4), as well as conversion of T4 to the more metabolically active triiodothyronine (T3). Studies with combat veterans have demonstrated elevations in both T3 and T4. Such increases were positively associated with PTSD severity (Mason et al., 1995; Wang & Mason, 1999). Furthermore, unpublished observations on women with PTSD related to childhood sexual abuse (CSA), show higher T3 and lower TSH in comparison with female CSA survivors without PTSD (Friedman et al., 2001).

HYPOTHALAMIC–PITUITARY–GONADAL AXIS

Increased HPA activity suppresses all aspects of gonadal function, including secretion of gonadotropin-releasing hormone from the hypothalamus, follicle stimulating and luteinizing hormones from the pituitary, and estradiol and testosterone from the reproductive organs. There appears to be a direct hypothalamic–testicular pathway through which CRF suppresses testosterone secretion (Charney, 2004). Clinical studies in which testosterone was measured in people with PTSD have produced mixed findings. Elevated serum (Mason et al., 1990), unchanged serum (Bauer, Priebe, Graef, & Keurten, 1994), and reduced cerebrospinal fluid (Mulchahey et al., 2001) testosterone levels have been detected among male combat veterans with PTSD.

Estrogen may have an important role in the human stress response and may in part be responsible for the fact that PTSD prevalence is twice as great in women as in men (Kessler, Sonnega, Bromet, Hughes, & Nelson, 1995). Animal studies indicate that acute administration of estradiol reduces ACTH secretion and stress responsiveness. More prolonged estrogen treatment, however, enhances HPA activity (Charney, 2004; Stroud, Salovey, & Epel, 2002; Young, Altemus, Parkison, & Shastry, 2001). The mechanism of action of estrogen appears to be on CRF or ACTH secretion rather than directly on the adrenal cortex (Charney, 2004). Estrogen also has complex actions on serotonin activity (McEwen, 2002). Despite these intriguing findings, the role of estrogen in the development of PTSD awaits systematic scientific investigation.

GROWTH AXIS

Increased HPA activity interferes with growth axis function through inhibition of growth hormone release, as well as through suppression of growth at target tissues. Vietnam combat veterans with and without PTSD showed no difference in growth hormone levels (Laudenslager et al., 1998). Another study, in which PTSD was not measured, may be relevant. Sexually and physically abused boys (not assessed for PTSD) exhibited a blunted growth hormone response to both clonidine and levodopa, in contrast to nonabused control participants.

THE IMMUNE SYSTEM

Because blood levels of lymphocyte or natural killer (NK) cells vary according to the dynamics of catecholamine and glucocorticoid secretion, I limit this brief review to functional measures of immunological activity such as NK cytotoxicity per cell, assays of cell proliferation, and the cytokine response to specific antigens (Dhabhar & McEwen, 1997). More comprehensive reviews can be found elsewhere (see Dougall & Baum, 2004; Schnurr & Jankowski, 1999). The results in people with chronic PTSD are mixed. Extrapolating from findings associated with chronic stress syndrome (Chrousos, 1998; McEwen, 1998), one would expect to observe immunosuppression in individuals with chronic PTSD. Surprisingly, enhanced immunological function has actually been found more often than immunosuppression. Three studies on veterans with chronic PTSD observed higher cutaneous cell-mediated immunity and higher cytokine levels among those with PTSD, compared with a non-PTSD group (Burges-Watson, Muller, Jones, & Bradley, 1993; Laudenslager et al., 1998; Spivak et al., 1997). In a fourth report, however, immunological activation by antigens was no different among veterans with PTSD than among controls (Boscarino & Chang, 1999). Finally, Boscarino (1997) found that male Vietnam combat veterans with PTSD appeared to have reduced immunological function because they reported higher prevalence of non-sexually-transmitted infectious disease than non-PTSD veterans.

Given the complexity of the immune system and given that both tonic and phasic abnormalities have been found in people with PTSD in most biological systems investigated, one way to reconcile these diverse findings is to postulate that there is both a tonic state of immunosuppression and an episodic or phasic state characterized by enhanced immunological function.

PSYCHOBIOLOGICAL ASSESSMENT OF PTSD: A GAME PLAN FOR THE FUTURE

Table 14.1 summarizes all of the information presented thus far about psychobiological abnormalities associated with PTSD. There is no doubt that in the future many gaps in current knowledge will be filled, and many current controversies will be resolved. I wish to present here an overall strategy for assessing the functional capacity of the stress system in individuals. Application of such an approach need not wait until after someone has been exposed to a devastating traumatic event. As I have stated elsewhere, such an approach could be part of an overall health maintenance or preventive public health strategy through which a person's vulnerability to or resilience against traumatic stress might be evaluated in advance (Friedman, 2002).

Baseline Assessment

Such an approach would begin with a psychobiological assessment protocol that would focus on the primary components of the stress response rather than on downstream mechanisms. It might be a two-stage process measuring both baseline and elicited stress system measures. The first stage, analogous to a serum lipid profile for detecting individuals at greatest risk for heart disease, might consist of baseline serum or urinary indicators of HPA, LC–NE, serotonergic, opioid, and immunological function (see Table 14.2). Abnormal levels of any of these stress system components might identify those individuals most vulnerable (or resilient) to develop PTSD following traumatization.

As noted earlier, baseline measurement of almost any single biological marker, listed in Table 14.1, is unlikely to be very informative because it is liable to fall within the normal clinical range. A better strategy might be to consider some pattern of abnormalities that, taken together, give a better indication of the magnitude of allostatic load produced by PTSD. Returning to our serum lipid profile example, the cholesterol/high-density-lipoprotein (HDL) ratio is much more informative than either value alone. The possible utility of such an approach was recognized during the early days of PTSD biological research in which Mason, Giller, and colleagues (Mason, Giller, Kosten, & Harkness, 1988) suggested that the urinary norepinephrine/cortisol ratio might be a more useful indicator than either value by itself. Given the variability in urinary cortisol findings in more recent research, this no longer seems like a promising index. On the other hand, the DHEA/cortisol ratio or the norepinephrine/NPY + galanin ratio might prove to have clinical utility in the future.

Provocative Tests

Because the hallmark of PTSD is hyperreactivity, the second stage of stress system assessment might be a series of provocative tests to probe the functional capacity of the stress system itself. This would be analogous to a treadmill test to detect heart disease or a glucose tolerance test to detect diabetes mellitus in medical practice. Such provocative tests (shown in Table 14.2) might include (1) *in vivo* stress paradigms to assess mobilization of HPA, LC–NE, serotonergic, opioid, and immunological components of the stress response; (2) the dexamethasone suppression test to assess glucocorticoid receptor sensitivity; (3) yohimbine provocation to assess LC–NE function; (4) antigen provocation to assess humoral or cell-mediated immunity; or (5) other provocative tests. Should abnormalities be detected either at baseline or following provocation, the next question would be whether they can be corrected with pharmacological and/or behavioral treatment. Posttreatment assessment would subsequently determine whether the therapeutic intervention produced improvement in the psychobiological abnormalities previously detected (Friedman, 2002).

Thus I have outlined a systematic assessment strategy that utilizes psychobiological tools to determine the resilience or vulnerability of individuals to traumatic stress. It also detects the magnitude and characteristics of allostatic load borne by individuals who currently suffer from PTSD.

TABLE 14.2. A Psychobiological Assessment Strategy

Baseline assessment	HPA function:	CRF, ACTH, cortisol, DHEA, DHEA/cortisol ratio
	LC–NE function:	Norepinephrine, epinephrine, dopamine, NPY, galanin, norepinephrine/NPY + galanin ratio
	Other:	Serotonin, opioid, glutamatergic, GABA-ergic, substance P, thyroid, gonadal, and growth axis function
Provocative tests	*In vivo* stress paradigms to assess mobilization of:	HPA, LC–NE, other functions (per step 1)
	Dexamethasone suppression:	Glucocorticoid receptor sensitivity
	Yohimbine provocation:	LC–NE and NPY response
	Immunological provocation:	Humoral and cell-mediated immunity
Periodically repeat steps 1 and 2 for:		People exposed to traumatic stress
		People in high-risk professions
Treatment:	Correct abnormalities detected in steps 1, 2, or 3.	

Note. Adapted from Friedman (2002).
HPA, hypothalamic–pituitary–adrenocortical; CRF, corticotropin releasing factor; ACTH, adrenocorticotropic hormone; DHEA, dehydroepiandosterone; NPY, neuropeptide Y; GABA, gamma aminobutyric acid; LC–NE, locus ceruleus/norepinephrine.

Recent research with U.S. Special Forces military personnel provides a concrete example of this approach. Morgan and associates (Morgan et al., 2001; Morgan et al., 2000) monitored the stress response among military personnel exposed to an extremely stressful training experience at Fort Bragg, North Carolina. They showed that individuals who were best able to mobilize NPY tolerated the experience and performed better than those unable to achieve comparable NPY levels. These results suggest that stress-induced NPY mobilization may be an important index of resilience against PTSD. The clinical question raised by such findings is whether people with lower capacity to mobilize NPY under stressful circumstances might benefit from treatment with a (yet to be developed) medication that mobilizes NPY activity.

Indications for Repeated Psychobiological Assessment

There are a number of professions in which individuals are routinely exposed to potentially traumatic events in the course of their normal duties; these include soldiers, police, firefighters, emergency medical personnel, and disaster/refugee mental health clinicians. For such individuals, it would be appropriate to periodically repeat the baseline assessments and provocative tests (e.g., step 3 in Table 14.2). For the same reason that people at risk for heart disease have their serum lipid profiles repeated annually as part of routine health maintenance, people in these high-risk professions should have steps 1 and 2 repeated periodically, because they are at greater risk to develop PTSD. Furthermore, it might be advisable, as a matter of military policy, to repeat steps 1 and 2 following any major deployment to a war zone or for peacekeeping operations.

Assessment of Chronic PTSD

Whereas the emphasis in prevention and assessment of acutely traumatized individuals focuses exclusively on primary components of the human stress response (e.g., CRF, HPA, LC–NE, and probably immunological mechanisms), the focus in chronic PTSD may include downstream mechanisms. Such an assessment might also emphasize procedures to detect secondary neurotransmitter (e.g., 5-HT, dopamine, GABA-ergic, glutamatergic, substance P) or hormonal (e.g., thyroid, gonadotropic, growth hormone) abnormalities.

Assessment goals in chronic PTSD would be similar to laboratory assessment for any disorder. Step 1 and step 2 measurements would provide a clinical baseline against which any progress in treatment might be evaluated. Furthermore, such an approach would provide clinicians with a rational basis for choosing specific therapeutic targets and would enable them to choose a treatment strategy that focuses primarily on the HPA, LC–NE, serotonergic, or some other biological system that has been altered by the allostatic burden of PTSD.

SUMMARY

I began this brief chapter with a description of the human stress system as the context within which to understand neurotransmitter, neuropeptide, and neurohormonal alterations associated with PTSD. Then I reviewed the current empirical evidence concerning psychobiological abnormalities associated with PTSD. Finally, I proposed a conceptual approach to psychobiological assessment consisting of both baseline measurements and provocative tests. Because it appears that no single psychobiological alteration distinguishes PTSD from other psychiatric disorders, the current challenge is to search for a distinctive pattern of psychobiological abnormalities that sets PTSD apart from other disorders and to translate such laboratory findings into useful and feasible clinical diagnostic procedures.

REFERENCES

Baker, D. G., West, S. A., Nicholson, W. E., Ekhator, N. N., Kasckow, J. W., Hill, K. K., et al. (1999). Serial CSF corticotropin-releasing hormone levels and adrenocortical activity in combat veterans with posttraumatic stress disorder. *American Journal of Psychiatry, 156*, 585–588.

Baker, D. G., West, S. A., Orth, D. N., Hill, K. K., Nicholson, W. E., Ekhator, N. N., et al. (1997). Cerebrospinal fluid and plasma [beta]-endorphin in combat veterans with posttraumatic stress disorder. *Psychoneuroendocrinology*, 22, 517–529.

Bauer, M., Priebe, S., Graef, K. J., & Keurten, I. (1994). Psychosocial and endocrine abnormalities in refugees from East Germany: II. Serum levels of cortisol, prolactin, luteinizing hormone, follicle stimulating hormone and testosterone. *Psychiatry Research, 51*, 75–85.

Bing, O., Moller, C., Engel, J. A., Soderpal, B., & Heilig, M. (1993). Anxiolytic-like action of centrally administered galanin. *Neuroscience Letters, 164*, 17–20.

Blanchard, E. B., Kolb, L. C., Prins, A., Gates, S., & McCoy, G. C. (1991). Changes in plasma norepinephrine to combat-related stimuli among Vietnam veterans with posttraumatic stress disorder. *Journal of Nervous and Mental Disease, 179*, 371–373.

Boscarino, J. A. (1997). Diseases among men 20 years after exposure to severe stress: Implications for clinical research and medical care. *Psychosomatic Medicine, 59*, 605–614.

Boscarino, J. A., & Chang, J. (1999). Electrocardiogram abnormalities among men with stress-related psychiatric disorders: Implications for coronary heart disease and clinical research. *Annals of Behavioral Medicine, 21*, 227–234.

Bremner, J. D., Innis, R. B., Ng, C. K., Chin, K., Staib, L. H., et al. (1997). PET measurement of central metabolic correlates of yohimbine administration in posttraumatic stress disorder. *Archives of General Psychiatry, 54*, 146–156.

Bremner, J. D., Innis, R. B., Southwick, S. M., Staib, L., Zoghbi, S., & Charney, D.S. (2000). Decreased benzodiazepine receptor binding in prefrontal cortex in combat-related posttraumatic stress disorder. *American Journal of Psychiatry, 157*, 1120–1126.

Bremner, J. D., Innis, R. B., White, T., Fujita, M., Silbersweig, D., Goddard, A. W., et al. (2000). SPECT [I-123] iomazenil measurement of the benzodiazepine receptor in panic disorder. *Biological Psychiatry*, *47*, 96–106.

Bremner, J. D., Licinio, J., Darnell, A., Krystal, J. H., Owens, M. J., Southwick, S. M., et al. (1997). Elevated CSF cortocotropin-releasing factor concentrations in posttraumatic stress disorder. *American Journal of Psychiatry*, *154*, 624–629.

Britton, K. T., Southerland, S., Van Uden, E., Kirby, D., Rivier, J., & Koob, G. (1997). Anxiolytic activity of NPY receptor agonists in the conflict test. *Psychopharmacology*, *132*, 6–13.

Browne, E. S., Wright, B. E., Porter, J. R., & Svec F. (1992). Dehydroepiandrosterone: Antiglucocorticoid action in mice. *American Journal of Medical Science*, *303*, 366–371.

Burges-Watson, I. P., Muller, H. K., Jones, I. H., & Bradley, A. J. (1993). Cell-mediated immunity in combat veterans with posttraumatic stress disorder. *Medical Journal of Australia*, *159*, 513–516.

Cannon, W. B. (1932). *The wisdom of the body*. New York: Norton.

Chambers, R. A., Bremner, J. D., Moghaddam, B., Southwick, S., Charney, D. S., & Krystal, J. H. (1999). Glutamate and TSD: Toward a psychobiology of dissociation. *Seminars in Clinical Neuropsychiatry*, *4*, 274–281.

Charney, D. S. (2004). Psychobiological mechanisms of resilience and vulnerability: Implications for the successful adaptation to extreme stress. *American Journal of Psychiatry, 161,* 195–216.

Charney, D. S., Deutch, A., Krystal, J. H., Southwick, S. M., & Davis, M. (1993). Psychobiological mechanisms of posttraumatic stress disorder. *Archives of General Psychiatry*, *50*, 294–305.

Chrousos, G. P. (1998). Stressors, stress and neuroendocrine integration of the adaptive response: The 1997 Hans Selye Memorial Lecture. *Annals of the New York Academy of Sciences*, *851*, 311–334.

Colmers, W., & Bleakman, D. (1994). Effects of neuropeptide Y on the electrical properties of neurons. *Trends in Neuroscience*, *17*, 373–379.

Corder, R., Castagne, V., Rivet, J. M., Mormede, P., & Gaillard, R.C. (1992). Central and peripheral effects of repeated stress and high NaCl diet on neuropeptide Y. *Physiology and Behavior*, *52*, 205–210.

Dhabhar, F., & McEwen, B. S. (1997). Acute stress enhances while chronic stress suppresses cell-mediated immunity: A potential role for leukocyte trafficking. *Brain Behavior and Immunology*, *11*, 286–306.

Dougall, A. L., & Baum, A. (2004). Psychoneuroimmunology and trauma. In P. P. Schnurr & B. L. Green (Eds.), *Trauma and health: Physical health consequences of exposure to extreme stress* (pp. 129–156). Washington, DC: American Psychological Association.

Friedman, M. J. (1990). Interrelationships between biological mechanisms and pharmacotherapy of posttraumatic stress disorder. In M. E. Wolf & A. D. Mosnaim (Eds.), *Posttraumatic stress disorder: Biological mechanisms and clinical aspects* (pp. 204–225). Washington, DC: American Psychiatric Press.

Friedman, M. J. (Ed.). (1999). Progress in psychobiological research on PTSD. *Seminars in Clinical Neuropsychiatry*, *4*, 229–316.

Friedman, M. J. (2002). Future pharmacotherapy for PTSD: Prevention and treatment. *Psychiatric Clinics of North America*, *25*, 427–442.

Friedman, M. J., Charney, D. S., & Deutch, A. Y. (Eds.). (1995). *Neurobiological and clinical consequences of stress: From normal adaptation to posttraumatic stress disorder*. Philadelphia, PA: Lippincott-Raven.

Friedman, M. J., McDonagh-Coyle, A., Jalowiec, J. E., Wang, S., Fournier, D. A., McHugo, G. (2001, December). Neurohormonal findings during treatment of women with PTSD due to CSA. In M. J. Friedman (Chair), *PTSD-CSA treatment: Psychological, physiological, and hormonal responses*. Symposium conducted at the meeting of the International Society for Traumatic Stress Studies, New Orleans, LA.

Friedman, M. J., & McEwen, B. S. (2004). Posttraumatic stress disorder, allostatic load, and medical illness. In P. P. Schnurr & B. L. Green (Eds.), *Trauma and health: Physical health consequences of exposure to extreme stress* (pp. 157–188). Washington, DC: American Psychological Association.

Gentleman, S. M., Alkai, F., Bogerts, B., Herrero, M. T., Polak, J. M., & Roberts, G. W. (1989). Distribution of galanin-like immunoreactivity in the human brain. *Brain Research, 505*, 311–315.

Geracioti, T. D., Jr., Baker, D. G., Ekhator, N. N., West, S. A., Hill, K. K., Bruce, A. B., et al. (2001). CSF norepinephrine concentrations in posttraumatic stress disorder. *American Journal of Psychiatry, 158*, 1227–1230.

Hamner, M. B., & Diamond, B. I. (1993). Elevated plasma dopamine in posttraumatic stress disorder: A preliminary report. *Biological Psychiatry, 33*, 304–306.

Heim, C., Newport, D. J., Bonsall, R., Miller, A. H., & Nemeroff C. B. (2001). Altered pituitary-adrenal axis responses to provocative challenge tests in adult survivors of childhood abuse. *American Journal of Psychiatry, 158*, 575–581.

Hoffman, L., Watson, P. D., Wilson, G., & Montgomery, J. (1989). Low plasma β-endorphin in posttraumatic stress disorder. *Australian and New Zealand Journal of Psychiatry, 23*, 268–273.

Holmes, P. V., & Crawley, J. N. (1995). Coexisting neurotransmitters in central noradrenergic neurons. In F. E. Bloom & D. J. Kupfer (Eds.), *Psychopharmacology: The fourth generation of progress* (pp. 347–353). New York: Raven Press.

Kask, A., Rago, L., & Harro, J. (1996). Anxiogenic-like effect of the neuropeptide Y Y1 receptor antagonist BIBP3226: Antagonism with diazepam. *European Journal of Pharmacology, 317*, R3–R4.

Kessler, R. C., Sonnega, A., Bromet, E., Hughes, M., & Nelson, C. B. (1995). Posttraumatic stress disorder in the National Comorbidity Survey. *Archives of General Psychiatry, 52*, 1048–1060.

Kramer, M. S., Cutler, N., Feighner, J., Shrivastava, R., Carman, J., & Sramek, J. J., et al. (1998). Distinct mechanism for antidepressant activity by blockade of central Substance P receptors. *Science, 281*, 1640–1645.

Krystal, J., Bennett, A. L., Bremner, J. D., Southwick, S. M., & Charney, D. S. (1995). Toward a cognitive neuroscience of dissociation and altered memory functions in posttraumatic stress disorder. In M. J. Friedman, D. S. Charney, & A. Y. Deutch (Eds.), *Neurobiological and clinical consequences of stress: From normal adaptation to posttraumatic stress disorder* (pp. 239–269). Philadelphia: Lippincott-Raven.

Laudenslager, M. L., Aasal, R., Adler, L., Berger, C. L., Montgomery, P. T., Sandberg, E., et al. (1998). Elevated cytotoxicity in combat veterans with long-term posttraumatic stress disorder: Preliminary observations. *Brain, Behavior, and Immunity, 12*, 74–79.

Lemieux, A. M., & Coe, C. L. (1995). Abuse-related PTSD: Evidence for chronic neuroendocrine activation in women. *Psychosomatic Medicine*, *57*, 105–115.

Lerer, B., Gur, E., Bleich, A., & Newman, M. (1994). Peripheral adrenergic receptors in PTSD. In M. M. Murburg (Ed.), Catecholamine function in posttraumatic stress disorder: Emerging concepts. *Progress in psychiatry* (No. 42, pp. 257–276). Washington, DC: American Psychiatric Press.

Malizia, A. L., Cunningham, V. J., Bell, C. J., Liddle, P. F., Jones, T., & Nutt, D. J. (1998). Decreased brain GABA(A)-benzodiazepine receptor binding in panic disorder: Preliminary results from a quantitative PET study. *Archives of General Psychiatry*, *55*, 715–720.

Mason, J. W., Giller, E. L., Kosten, T. R., & Harkness, L. L. (1998). Elevation of urinary norepinephrine/cortisol ratio in posttraumatic stress disorder. *Journal of Nervous and Mental Disease*, *176*, 498–502.

Mason, J. W., Giller, E. L., Kosten, T. R., & Wahby, V. S. (1990). Serum testosterone levels in posttraumatic stress disorder patients. *Journal of Traumatic Stress*, *3*, 449–457.

Mason, J. W., Wang, S., Yehuda, R., Bremner, J. D., Riney, S. J., & Lubin, H. (1995). Some approaches to the study of the clinical implications of thyroid alterations in posttraumatic stress disorder. In M. J. Friedman, D. S. Charney, & A. Y. Deutch (Eds.), *Neurobiological and clinical consequences of stress: From normal adaptation to posttraumatic stress disorder* (pp. 367–380). Philadelphia: Lippincott-Raven.

McEwen, B. S. (1998). Protective and damaging effects of stress mediators. *New England Journal of Medicine*, *338*, 171–179.

McEwen, B. (2002). Estrogen actions throughout the brain. *Recent Progress in Hormone Research*, *57*, 357–384.

McFall, M. E., Murburg, M. M., Ko, G. N., & Veith, R. C. (1990). Autonomic responses to stress in Vietnam combat veterans with posttraumatic stress disorder. *Biological Psychiatry*, *27*, 1165–1175.

Moller, C., Sommer, W., Thorsell, A., & Heilig, M. (1999). Anxiogenic-like action of galanin after intra-amygdala administration in the rat. *Neuropsychopharmacology*, *21*, 507–512.

Morgan, C. A. III. (2001, May). *Predicting performance: What we can learn from psychobiological studies of humans participating in highly stressful military training*. Paper presented at the meeting of the Society for Biological Psychiatry, New Orleans, LA.

Morgan, C. A., Krystal, J. H., & Southwick, S. M. (2003). Toward early pharmacologic posttraumatic stress intervention. *Biological Psychiatry*, *53*, 834–843.

Morgan, C. A., III, Wang, S., Rasmusson, A., Hazlett, G., Anderson, G., & Charney, D. S. (2001). Relationship among plasma cortisol, catecholamines, neuropeptide Y, and human performance during exposure to uncontrollable stress. *Psychosomatic Medicine*, *63*, 412–422.

Morgan, C. A., III, Wang, S., Southwick, S. M., Rasmusson, A., Hazlett, G., Hauger, R. L., & Charney, D. S. (2000). Plasma neuropeptide-Y concentrations in humans exposed to military survival training. *Biological Psychiatry*, *47*, 902–909.

Mulchahey, J. J., Ekhator, N. N., Zhang, H., Kasckow, J. W., Baker, D. G., & Geracioti, T. D. (2001). Cerebrospinal fluid and plasma testosterone levels in posttraumatic stress disorder and tobacco dependence. *Psychoneuroendocrinology*, *26*, 273–285.

Nutt, D. J., & Malizia, A. L. (2001). New insights into the role of the GABA(A)-benzodiazepine receptor in psychiatric disorder. *British Journal of Psychiatry, 179*, 390–396.

Perez, S. E., Wynic D., Steiner, R. A., & Mufson, E. J. (2001). Distribution of galaninergic immunoreactivity in the brain of the mouse. *Journal of Comparative Neurology, 434*, 158–185.

Pernow, J. (1988). Co-release and functional interactions of neuropeptide Y and noradreneraline in peripheral sympathetic vascular control. *Acta Physiologica Scandinavia* (Suppl. 568), 1–56.

Perry, B. D. (1994). Neurobiological sequelae of childhood trauma: PTSD in children. In M. M. Murburg (Ed.), *Catecholamine function in posttraumatic stress disorder: Emerging concepts* (pp. 233–255). Washington, DC: APA Press.

Perry, B. D., Giller, E. L., & Southwick, S. M. (1987). Altered platelet alpha2 adrenergic binding sites in posttraumatic stress disorder. *American Journal of Psychiatry, 144*, 1511–1512.

Pitman, R. K., van der Kolk, B. A., Orr, S. P., & Greenberg, M. S. (1990). Naloxone-reversible analgesic response to combat-related stimuli in posttraumatic stress disorder. *Archives of General Psychiatry, 47*, 541–544.

Rasmusson, A. M., & Friedman, M. J. (2002). The neurobiology of PTSD in women. In R. Kimerling, P. C. Ouimette, & J. Wolfe (Eds.), *Gender and PTSD* (pp. 43–75). New York: Guilford Press.

Rasmusson, A. M., Hauger, R. L., Morgan, C. A., Bremner, J. D., Charney, D. S., & Southwick, S. M. (2000). Low baseline and yohimbine-stimulated plasma neuropeptide (NPY) levels in combat-related PTSD. *Biological Psychiatry, 47*, 526–639.

Rasmusson, A. M., Lipschitz, D. S., Wang, S., Hu, S., Vojvoda, D., Bremner, J. D., Southwick, S. M., et al. (2001). Increased pituitary and adrenal reactivity in premenopausal women with PTSD. *Biological Psychiatry, 50*, 965–977.

Rasmusson, A. M., Vasek, J., Lipschitz, D. S., Vojvoda, D., Mustone, M. E., Shi, Q., et al. (in press). Increased release of the adrenal antiglucorticoid dehydroepiandrosterone (DHEA) in premenopausal women with PTSD. *Neuropsychopharmacology.*

Rosenfeld, R. S., Hellman, L., Roffwarg, H., Weitzman, E. D., Fukushima, D. K., & Gallagher, T. F. (1971). Dehydroisoandrosterone is secreted episodically and synchronously with cortisol by normal man. *Journal of Clinical Endocrinology, 33*, 87–92.

Sabioncello, A., Kocijan-Hergigonja, D., Rabatic, S., Tomasic, J., Jeren, T., Matijevic, L., et al. (2000). Immune, endocrine, and psychological responses in civilians displaced by war. *Psychosomatic Medicine, 62*, 502–508.

Schnurr, P. P., & Jankowski, M. K. (1999). Physical health and posttraumatic stress disorder: Review and synthesis. *Seminars in Clinical Neuropsychiatry, 4*, 295–304.

Smith, M. A., Davidson, J. R. T., Ritchie, J. C., Kudler, H. S., Lipper, S., Chappell, P., et al. (1989). The corticotropin-releasing hormone test in patients with posttraumatic stress disorder. *Biological Psychiatry, 26*, 349–355.

Southwick, S. M., Krystal, J. H., Bremner, J. D., Morgan, C. A., Nicolaou, A. L., Nagy, L. M., et al. (1997). Noradrenergic and serotonergic function in posttraumatic stress disorder. *Archives of General Psychiatry, 54*, 749–758.

Southwick, S. M., Paige, S. R., Morgan, C. A., Bremner, J. D., Krystal, J. H., &

Charney, D. S. (1999). Adrenergic and serotonergic abnormalities in PTSD: Catecholamines and serotonin. *Seminars in Clinical Neuropsychiatry*, *4*, 242–248.

Spivak, B., Shohat, B., Mester, R., Avraham, S., Gil-As, I., Bleich, A., et al. (1997). Elevated levels of serum interleukin-1β in combat-related posttraumatic stress disorder. *Biological Psychiatry*, *42*, 345–348.

Stroud, L. R., Salovey, P., & Epel, E. S. (2002). Sex differences in stress responses: Social rejection versus achievement stress. *Biological Psychiatry*, *52*, 318–327.

Wang, S., & Mason, J. (1999). Elevations of serum T3 levels and their association with symptoms in World War II veterans with combat-related posttraumatic stress disorder: Replication of findings in Vietnam combat veterans. *Psychosomatic Medicine*, *61*, 131–138.

Weizman, R., Weizman, A., Kook, K. A., Vocci, F., Deutsch, S., & Paul, S. M. (1989). Repeated swim stress alters brain benzodiazepine receptors measured in vivo. *Journal of Pharmacology and Experimental Therapeutics*, *249*, 701–707.

Yehuda, R. (1997). Sensitization of the hypothalamic-pituitary-adrenal axis in posttraumatic stress disorder. *Annals of the New York Academy of Sciences*, *821*, 57–75.

Yehuda, R. (1999). The neuroendocrinology of posttraumatic stress disorder with recent neuroanatomic findings. *Seminars in Clinical Neuropsychiatry*, *4*, 256–265.

Yehuda, R., Giller, E. L., Southwick, S. M., Kahana, B., Boisneau, D., Ma, X., & Mason, J. W. (1994). Relationship between catecholamine excretion and PTSD symptoms in Vietnam combat veterans and holocaust survivors. In M. M. Murburg (Ed.), *Catecholamine function in posttraumatic stress disorder: Emerging concepts* (pp. 203–220). Washington, DC: American Psychiatric Press.

Yehuda, R., Levengood, R. A., Schmeidler, J., Wilson, S., Guo, L. S., & Gerber, D. (1996). Increased pituitary activation following metyrapone administration in posttraumatic stress disorder. *Psychoneuroendrocrinology*, *21*, 1–16.

Young, E. A., Altemus, M., Parkison, V., & Shastry, S. (2001). Effects of estrogen antagonists and agonists on the ACTH response to restraint stress in female rats. *Neuropsychopharmacology*, *25*, 881–891.

PART IV

Physical Health, Substance Use Disorder, and Bereavement

CHAPTER 15

Trauma, PTSD, and Physical Health

Clinical Issues

TODD C. BUCKLEY
BONNIE L. GREEN
PAULA P. SCHNURR

Although the relationship between stress and physical health has a fairly rich empirical history (Selye, 1955), the literature on explicit examination of the impact of trauma and posttraumatic stress disorder (PTSD) on physical health is much younger. However, since the previous edition of this volume, research examining the interaction between trauma, PTSD, and physical health has expanded considerably; so much so that an exhaustive review of this work might make for a book in its own right. Thus we aim here to distill this expanding literature down to the most essential concepts that have a bearing on clinical research, clinical assessment, and treatment planning in service delivery settings.

Indeed, when examining how trauma, PTSD, and physical health relate to one another, one need not think about the matter long before a number of interesting questions are raised: Does the experience of psychological trauma have an adverse effect on physical health? Is the relationship between trauma and physical health mediated by one's response to that trauma (i.e., PTSD)? Can receiving a terminal medical diagnosis serve as a criterion A stressor in the same manner as time-limited events such as rape or combat? As one might gather from these questions, this chapter aims to cover two conceptual areas. First, we examine how trauma and PTSD may play a causal role in instigating poor health outcomes. Second, we discuss how psychiatric disturbance, PTSD in particular, manifests in the aftermath of medical events.

TRAUMA AND PTSD AS CAUSAL AGENTS IN POOR PHYSICAL HEALTH

Early papers on this topic were largely descriptive in nature; however, several recent review papers have outlined conceptual models that are driving empirical work in this area in a more theoretical way (Schnurr & Jankowski, 1999; Schnurr & Green, 2004). We briefly outline a theory proposed by Schnurr and colleagues that lays out a causal model for explaining trauma, PTSD, and physical health relationships. Then we review the empirical evidence that bears on the model.

In short, the model is based on the premise that the experience of psychological trauma in and of itself rarely leads directly to poor health outcomes. The exception to this is cases in which physical injury or other biological insult occurs in conjunction with the psychological trauma; for example, in motor vehicle accident victims or prisoners of war. The model specifically asserts that psychological trauma that is profound enough to result in psychiatric disturbance—operationally defined as a PTSD diagnosis—results in concomitant behavioral, physiological, and attentional changes that tax the physical capacity of the individual to adaptively cope with his or her environment in a manner that promotes good physical health. In this respect, PTSD is seen as the major mediator between trauma exposure and health outcomes (as assessed by a variety of methods). Indeed, as can be seen in the literature reviewed herein, both trauma exposure and PTSD bear negative correlations with a variety of measures of health. The model explicitly predicts this, as trauma exposure is a prerequisite condition for the development of PTSD. As such, studies that find either trauma exposure or PTSD to be correlated with physical health are concordant with the model. However, the strongest test of the model is undertaken when both trauma and PTSD are measured simultaneously in quantitative analysis and PTSD accounts for a large portion of the statistical variance in the relationship between trauma and health (Taft, Stern, King, & King, 1999).

This model regards the behavioral and physiological disturbances known to accompany PTSD as processes that contribute to allostatic load, a concept noted by McEwen (2000). Allostatic load is a construct related to the amount of deviation from homeostasis in repeated adaptations to stress, which thereby taxes biological systems in an organism. In this respect, the physiological disturbances (e.g., potentiated cardiovascular responding to stress) and the behavioral disturbances (e.g., excess alcohol consumption) that often accompany PTSD present challenges to the maintenance of homeostasis in the organism and facilitate poor health status. A fuller explication of the model is beyond the scope of this chapter. More explicit details of this model can be found in Schnurr and Green (2004). In addition, more explicit details of PTSD and allostatic processes can be found in Friedman and McEwen (2004). We now turn to the empirical evidence in support of the model.

Self-Reported Health

In recent years, several empirical papers have emerged that suggest that having chronic PTSD places one at risk for poor physical health in a number of organ systems (Boscarino, 1997; Boscarino & Chang, 1999). Although studies also offer compelling evidence that trauma exposure correlates with health outcomes (Felitti et al., 1998; Golding, Cooper, & George, 1997), it appears that much of this relationship is mediated by psychiatric disturbance, most notably PTSD, in the aftermath of such trauma (Friedman & Schnurr, 1995; Schnurr & Jankowski, 1999). Specifically, among studies that examine indices of trauma exposure only (i.e., no assessment of PTSD) and indices of physical health, the general finding is one of poorer health among those who are trauma exposed than among comparable groups of individuals with no trauma history (e.g., Felitti et al., 1998). However, when studies examine the effect of both trauma exposure and PTSD on physical health, they generally find that PTSD mediates much of the relationship between trauma exposure and indices of physical health (Boscarino & Chang, 1999). Thus we focus primarily on the relationship between PTSD and physical health.

Data demonstrating a link between PTSD and physical health come from a variety of research methodologies. For example, in descriptive studies in which self-report measures of physical health are obtained, individuals with PTSD report a greater number of specific symptoms (e.g., back pain), diagnostic conditions (e.g., hypertension), and impairment relative to comparable groups without PTSD (Beckham et al., 1998; Kulka et al., 1990; Wagner, Wolfe, Rotnitsky, Proctor, & Erikson, 2000). In addition, evidence suggests that individuals with PTSD rate the level of role-functioning impairment associated with physical morbidity as greater than do either the general population or other psychiatric groups (Zatzick et al., 1997; Zayfert, Dums, Ferguson, & Hegel, 2002).

Although comparisons in such studies are generally made between individuals with PTSD and well-adjusted comparison groups, recent data such as those presented by Zayfert et al. (2002) suggest that PTSD imparts a negative impact on perceived physical health at a greater magnitude than other psychiatric disorders known to correlate with physical health outcomes. Moreover, these data are consistent with studies that have examined the impact of PTSD on harder health end points (e.g., myocardial infarction). That is to say, studies also suggest that PTSD has a more negative impact on health than other anxiety or affective disorders when assessed via objective indicators (Boscarino & Chang, 1999), a point we return to shortly.

In a particularly large study, the Centers for Disease Control and Prevention's Vietnam Experiences Study, it was found that a lifetime diagnosis of PTSD was associated with increased risk of self-reported cardiovascular disorders, infectious diseases, respiratory disorders, digestive conditions, and endocrine/metabolic disorders (Boscarino, 1997). Although most studies of this sort have been done with male veterans, a study with Australian firefighters revealed a very similar pattern of findings to those from the CDC study (McFarlane, Atchinson, Rafalowicz, & Papay, 1994), as did a study with female veterans with PTSD (Wolfe, Schnurr, Brown, & Furey, 1994). In addition to Wolfe et al. (1994), other studies that have utilized exclusively female samples to examine the relationship between PTSD and self-reported health have also consistently found that PTSD is associated with poorer ratings of health (Kimerling, Clum, & Wolfe, 2000; Zoellner, Goodwin, & Foa, 2000).

Physician-Diagnosed Medical Problems

In a complementary line of investigation, physician-diagnosed medical problems are found to be more frequent among those who carry a diagnosis of chronic PTSD relative to comparison groups without PTSD (Beckham et al., 1998; Boscarino & Chang, 1999; Schnurr, Spiro, & Paris, 2000). The study by Schnurr et al. (2000) is noteworthy because of its longitudinal design. In a long-term follow-up of World War II and Korean War veterans (*N* 900), the authors found that the presence of significant PTSD symptoms was associated with elevated rates of arterial, lower gastroinestinal, dermatological, and musculoskeletal conditions. Boscarino and Chang (1999) found that PTSD was associated with myocardial infarction and atrioventricular conduction problems as assessed by electrocardiogram (ECG) findings.

Studies of clinical samples with chronic PTSD also suggest elevated rates of physical morbidity relative to what one would expect in the general population. For example, both Beckham et al. (1998) and Buckley, Mozley, Bedard, Dewulf, and Greif (in press) have found elevated rates of physician-diagnosed medical problems in individuals presenting for mental health treatment in PTSD clinics within Veterans Affairs Medical Center hospitals. It is important to note that studies in this domain routinely control for potential variables such as years of cigarette smoking, age, body mass, and other well-established predictors of health when examining the effect of PTSD. Even after accounting for such variables, the effect of PTSD on physician-diagnosed medical problems remains statistically robust (Beckham et al., 1998; Schnurr & Spiro, 1999; Schnurr et al., 2000).

Health Care Utilization

As one might expect from the literature reviewed, a population that is at higher risk for physical morbidity is certainly bound to use more health-care services than the general population. Recent data certainly support this point. In fact, when one considers that PTSD is among the most prevalent psychiatric disorders (Kessler, Sonnega, Bromet, Hughes, & Nelson, 1995) and that the rate of health-care utilization for physical morbidity among individuals with PTSD is greater than for most other psychiatric conditions (Greenberg et al. 1999; Schnurr, Friedman, Sengupta, Jankowski, & Holmes, 2000), the cost to the health-care system is quite large.

Studies in this domain suggest that relative to both nonpsychiatric controls and other psychiatric comparison groups, PTSD is associated with elevated rates of health-care utilization for physical morbidity (Deykin et al., 2001; Greenberg et al., 1999). For example, using case-control methods, Deykin et al. (2001) found that among a group of veterans classified as high utilizers, the rates of PTSD were markedly elevated relative to a group of individuals classified as low utilizers. Importantly, the authors of this study excluded health-care visits to mental health clinics in their analysis. They also excluded medical interventions that required multiple visits (e.g., dialysis) in their categorization of utilization. After such controls, PTSD still bore a correlation to overall utilization rates. In a related vein, Walker et al. (2003) reported on 1,225 women in a large metropolitan health maintenance organization and found that among women with high levels of PTSD symptoms the health-care costs were nearly double those of women with low PTSD symptom levels. Although this study included mental health costs in the analyses, an itemized analysis according to health-care specialty revealed that the effect for utilization held up in non-mental-health sectors. These studies are concordant with a larger literature documenting that individuals who are victims of sexual crimes or battery use health-care resources at greater rates (for physical morbidity) relative to comparable groups of nontraumatized individuals (e.g., Koss, Woodruff, & Koss, 1991; Norris, Kaniasty, & Scheer 1990).

PTSD in Specialty Health Clinics

To this point, we have reviewed studies that seek to address the relationship between PTSD and physical health by examining groups that differ in their psychiatric status. That is to say, these studies examine health indices as a function of PTSD-positive or PTSD-negative status (e.g., Buckley & Kaloupek, 2001). Another manner in which to examine the link between trauma, PTSD, and health is to examine the rates of trauma and PTSD among individuals with known medical diagnoses (e.g., HIV) vis-à-vis comparison samples who are physically well. Generally speaking, there is much less of this type of research, and definitive statements cannot be drawn at this time. However, there is some evidence to suggest that the rates of trauma and PTSD are elevated among patients seeking care in medical specialty clinics. This is true for sexually transmitted diseases (Kimerling et al., 1999), functional gastrointestinal problems (e.g., IBS; Delvaux, Denis, & Allemand, 1997), pain conditions (Goldberg, 1994), and HIV (Allers & Benjack, 1991).

Summary of PTSD and Physical Health Studies

These multiple areas of investigation point in unison to the fact that having a diagnosis of PTSD is a risk factor for physical morbidity and that the effect does not seem constrained to one organ system (Friedman & Schnurr, 1995; Schnurr & Jankowski, 1999). In light of these findings, investigators have begun searching for causal mechanisms that may account for the PTSD and physical health correlation. In the sections to follow, we review potential mechanisms of action that may account for this relationship. A comment worthy of note before proceeding, however, is that in such research one needs to account for physical health problems associated with index trauma, in addition to those that develop over time in conjunction with mental health disturbance. Specifically, it is tempting to attribute much of the physical morbidity seen in PTSD populations to the trauma itself rather than to PTSD. Given the often-violent nature of trauma, it is not uncommon for individuals to experience injury and biological insults during the course of their trauma, which may result in longer term health problems. Indeed, some of the PTSD–physical health morbidity correlation is accounted for by this phenomenon. However, longitudinal studies and studies wherein trauma exposure is controlled suggest that the majority of the variance in the PTSD–physical health relationship is not accounted for by physical injury incurred at time of the index trauma (see Friedman & Schnurr, 1995; Schnurr & Jankowski, 1999).

MECHANISMS OF ACTION LINKING PTSD TO PHYSICAL HEALTH

Broadly speaking, two processes hold the most promise in terms of explaining the PTSD–physical health correlations. That is to say, two processes seem to play the most profound role in allostatic load among individuals with PTSD. First, some have hypothesized that, due to the "stress reactive" nature of PTSD, continual engagement of the physiological stress response system places individuals with chronic PTSD at risk for the progression of health problems. More specifically, some of have asserted that repeated responding to stressors with augmented sympathetic nervous system output and disturbed HPA-axis functioning places individuals with PTSD at undue risk for physical morbidity (Buckley & Kaloupek, 2001; Friedman & McEwen, 2004). Indeed, several laboratory studies suggest that individuals with PTSD show augmented sympathetic responses to stress challenges relative to control groups (Blanchard & Buckley, 1999). The second of the two allostatic processes involves the greater frequency of adverse health behaviors (e.g., smoking, lack of exercise, etc.) that seem to be more prevalent among individuals with PTSD than in those without PTSD.

Physiological Disturbances in PTSD

A compelling line of research suggests that the two major arms of the stress response system are disrupted among individuals with PTSD; namely, the sympathetic nervous system and the hypothalamic–pituitary–adrenocortical (HPA) axis. These disturbances can play a role in the progression of disease processes and, indeed, correlate with other physiological mechanisms considered surrogate measures of health. For example, elevated basal catecholamine levels (McFall, Veith, & Marburg, 1992) and abnormal hypothalamic–pituitary–adrenal (HPA) functioning (Yehuda, Giller, Southwick, Lowy, & Mason, 1991) have been noted, such that individuals with PTSD will show augmented sympathetic reactivity to stress provocation. A large literature supplements these studies and documents that, when exposed to trauma cues, individuals with PTSD showed greater sympathetic arousal (as indexed by greater heart rate and skin conductance reactivity) than both traumatized and nontraumatized comparison groups without PTSD (Blanchard et al., 1996; Keane et al., 1998). Such physiological disturbances have been considered mechanisms of disease progression for cardiovascular problems. Indeed, chronic PTSD has been associated with elevated resting heart rate (Buckley & Kaloupek, 2001), ECG-determined presence of nonfatal myocardial infarction (Boscarino & Chang, 1999), and low heart rate variability (Cohen et al., 1997). In total, such findings suggest that allostatic processes might hold explanatory power in addressing the PTSD–health correlation (Friedman & McEwen, 2004).

Many of these findings are particularly noteworthy with respect to their relationship to cardiovascular health. The findings of low-heart-rate variability (Cohen et al., 1997) and elevated basal heart rate (Buckley & Kaloupek, 2001), respectively, suggest that among individuals with chronic PTSD there may be an increased rate of premature mortality due to cardiovascular disease. Although some data support this proposition (Boscarino & Chang, 1999), longer term prospective studies with chronic samples are needed to further evaluate this prediction. In short, most studies that examine surrogate measures of health or statistical predictors of mortality have found that PTSD has a negative effect on health status.

Health Behaviors

The second proposed mechanism that might link PTSD to physical health outcomes is the comorbidity of PTSD with adverse lifestyle behaviors (Schnurr & Spiro, 1999). Indeed, a number of different health behaviors, both adverse and preventive, might provide a mediational link between PTSD and markers of health (cardiovascular health in particular). For example, PTSD is associated with high rates of alcohol abuse and dependence comorbidity (e.g., Kessler et al., 1995; Kulka et al., 1990). It is well documented that alcohol consumption of greater than three drinks per day is associated with increased blood pressure and heart rate, as well as with increased mortality from coronary artery disease and stroke (Hillbom & Juvela, 1996). PTSD is also associated with markedly elevated rates of nicotine use (Lasser et al., 2000). These influences point to ways in which PTSD can have an indirect relationship on cardiovascular health (Schnurr & Spiro, 1999).

A question invariably raised by many studies that examine PTSD and adverse health behaviors such as smoking is the question of whether PTSD predisposes one to substance abuse or whether substance abuse and dependence increase risk for trauma exposure and PTSD. Research generally supports the former notion (Stewart & Conrod, 2003). That is to say, when PTSD and substance use are comorbid, it is most often the case that the PTSD diagnosis predates the substance-use-disorder diagnosis. Such findings support the notion that individuals with PTSD often use substances for affect regulation purposes. In a particularly well-done prospective study on this matter, Breslau, Davis, and Schultz (2003) followed more than 1 thousand 21- to 30-year-olds over a 10-year period of time to assess the longitudinal course of trauma exposure and PTSD. Among individuals with PTSD at study entry, the 10-year incidence of nicotine use and illicit substance use was much greater than among trauma-exposed individuals without PTSD and individuals not exposed to trauma. Studies such as those cited here suggest that the onset of PTSD often precedes the adoption of unhealthy lifestyle habits that put one at risk for physical morbidity.

Although most examinations of PTSD and health behaviors have focused on adverse health behaviors (e.g., smoking), few have looked at preventive health behaviors (e.g., exercise). In a recent study, however, Buckley et al. (in press) found that individuals with PTSD had poor sleep hygiene habits, exercise habits, and other general self-care habits relative to what would be considered appropriate by contemporary health-care recommendations.

Trauma, PTSD, and Sexually Transmitted Disease Risk

Several studies suggest that exposure to trauma and PTSD elevates the risk for engaging in behavior that facilitates the spread of sexually transmitted diseases. For example, Stiffman, Dore, Earls, and Cunningham (1992) found an association between PTSD and higher incidence of risk behaviors. In a related vein, Rotheram-Borus, Koopman, and Bradley (1989) found odds ratios of 5.9 that youths with symptoms of PTSD would use intravenous drugs. Similar conclusions have been reached in studies that examine trauma exposure and HIV-risk behavior (Cunningham, Stiffman, Dore, & Earls 1994). These studies suggest that having PTSD places one at risk for the acquisition of communicable disease via risky health behaviors that are entirely preventable.

PTSD and Adherence to Medical Regimens

Another way in which PTSD might affect physical health outcomes is via its effect on adherence to medical regimens. Specifically, the presence of PTSD may very well impede adherence to prescribed medical regimens for the primary physical problem that is associated with PTSD, thereby increasing risk for serious adverse events or even mortality due to lack of medical compliance. Although not much work has been done in this regard, it is worthy of comment here, as it is an area in need of further investigation. (Although a literature exists on the association of many psychological factors and their role in nonadherence, we focus exclusively on PTSD.)

A study by Shemesh et al. (2001) points to the importance of assessing for PTSD in the context of ongoing medical care for life-threatening problems. In following a group of patients after myocardial infarction (MI) who were being treated with captopril (an angiotensin-converting enzyme [ACE] inhibitor often prescribed for severe post-MI), the authors found that PTSD symptoms related to the index MI were negatively associated with adherence as assessed by pill counts at follow-up. Although correlational, this finding is compelling because lack of compliance with captropril was associated with mortality during follow-up.

Similar findings regarding the relationship of PTSD to compliance with medical regimens has been noted for individuals who are positive for HIV and who receive psychiatric care in outpatient AIDS clinics (Cohen, Alfonso, Hoffman, Milau, & Carrera, 2001) and for those who receive treatment for heroin dependence (Hien, Nunes, Levin, & Fraser, 2000). Studies such as these suggest that even if individuals are being treated for a primary medical problem, screening for trauma exposure and PTSD should be considered (and extensively followed if necessary), as the presence of such problems may compromise adherence to medical regimens.

Discussion of PTSD and Physical Health Findings

As one can see, allostatic processes have intuitive and empirical appeal in explaining the PTSD–physical health correlation. In fact, based on the extant empirical literature, one can make a case that it is probably a combination of both stress-induced physiological disturbances and a profile of adverse lifestyle behaviors common to PTSD that accounts for the PTSD and physical morbidity correlations. The work that has examined the impact of PTSD on physical health suggests that the average level of overall self-care and physical morbidity among individuals with PTSD is quite poor. This conclusion is based on the high rate of endorsement of health risk behaviors (e.g., smoking and alcohol abuse), the relatively low frequency of preventive health behaviors such as exercise and medical screening, findings of basal and stress-induced physiological disturbances, and a higher incidence of specific medical conditions relative to the general population. Moreover, the amount of role-functioning impairment and health-care utilization for physical morbidity is markedly elevated in this psychiatric population (Walker et al., 2003; Zayfert et al., 2002).

With respect to the clinical relevance of the findings reviewed thus far, the data suggest that, although individuals with PTSD present to mental health settings seeking psychiatric treatment for PTSD symptoms, assessment of physical morbidity and lifestyle behaviors is an issue that warrants attention from a treatment planning perspective. It is not uncommon for individuals with chronic PTSD to need services from several medical subspecialties concurrently. Data such as these also suggest that educational and behavioral interventions aimed at health promotion (wellness groups) may have a role in the secondary prevention of physical morbidity in this high-risk population.

It is important to consider that, above and beyond structured interview and self-report inventories of psychiatric symptoms, inclusion of assessment materials that bear on self-care, health behaviors, and role-functioning impairment are important to consider when doing evaluations with trauma survivors. Certainly much of this can be accomplished with open clinical interviewing, but instruments are available that can also serve this purpose well. The Short Form-36 (SF-36; Ware, Snow, Kosinski, & Gandek, 1997) for example, serves as a useful adjunctive measure to gauge role functioning impairment due to physical morbidity and pain problems. The Alcohol Use Disorders Identification Test (AUDIT; Saunders, Aasland, Babor, de la Fuente, & Grant, 1993) can be used as a quantitative measure of recent alcohol use. It has been used to screen for alcohol problems and performs well across genders and racial groups. Likewise, the Drug Abuse Screening Test (DAST; Skinner, 1982) is a 10-item screening instrument developed by the Addiction Research Foundation that indicates the degree of drug abuse-related problems over the previous 12 months (Skinner, 1982). These measures, and others similar to them, should be considered in the context of doing PTSD evaluations that also involve the administration of instruments geared at more traditional psychiatric symptoms.

MEDICAL ILLNESS AS A CRITERION A EVENT

In examining the historical roots of PTSD, the diagnosis has focused on individuals' responses to discrete events of a horrific nature that are no longer threatening in the present time. For example, long before the diagnosis of PTSD was formally recognized in DSM-III (American Psychiatric Association, 1980) terms such as "shellshock" described psychiatric disturbances that were linked to exposure to a life-threatening event that occurred in the past (combat). Such clinical descriptions map closely to the current DSM-IV (American Psychiatric Association, 1994) construct of PTSD. In the early stages of research on PTSD, such conceptualizations of the stressor criterion and the concomitant psychiatric disturbance continued with an exclusive tendency toward examining psychiatric disturbance in response to discrete events, most notably rape and combat exposure.

In recent years, however, interest has been increasing in the possibility that receiving medical diagnosis of a life-threatening illness (e.g., lung cancer) may serve as a criterion A stressor. Stressors such as this have been labeled "information stressors" by Green and colleagues (Green et al., 1998), as they differ from more "classically" defined criterion A stressors that involve acute and imminent threat to life and physical integrity. Indeed, DSM-IV explicitly allows for such a stressor (receiving a medical diagnosis) to serve as the foundation for a PTSD assessment and subsequent diagnosis (American Psychiatric Association, 1994). With this explicit recognition in DSM-IV, one might conclude that any argument over whether such events are capable of producing comparable patterns of psychiatric disturbance relative to more "classic" criterion A traumas is a moot point. However, we submit that the debate is far from resolved.

The applicability of PTSD as a psychiatric construct to individuals diagnosed with chronic or terminal medical illnesses is complicated because of the ambiguity of the stressor (Kangas, Henry, & Bryant, 2002). More specifically, it is difficult to disentangle the effects of receiving the diagnosis from ongoing, and often aversive, medical treatment, as well as future-oriented concerns about recurrence and mortality. By way of contrast, assessing PTSD symptoms in response to a single-index event (e.g., motor vehicle accident) allows one to anchor symptom onset and changes to a single point in time. Such single-index traumas also allow for relatively straightforward determinations of pathological processes in patients from whom imminent threat regarding their trauma is long over. However, how does one easily resolve such assessment questions with cancer survivors? Is it appropriate to consider "sense of foreshortened future" as a "psychiatric" symptom in an individual recently diagnosed with breast cancer? Certainly such a phenomenon would seem to be different from a sense of foreshortened future for a physically healthy individual who witnessed a physical attack on someone else several years prior. Sticking with the breast cancer example, how might one go about determining whether or a person is having difficulty with PTSD-related reexperiencing symptoms or is appropriately worrying about future-oriented outcomes of having the cancer diagnosis?

Life-Threatening Illness as a Criterion A Stressor

There are two fundamental ways in which life-threatening illness is different from more traditional stressors. First, the threat from such events is not from the external environment, as in events such as disasters, rape, combat, and automobile accidents. Rather, it arises internally, so that the threat and the individual cannot be separated. This fact may make the experience qualitatively different from one in which the threat arises from the outside. Second, once a person has been treated for his or her illness and survived, the ongoing stressor may not be the memory of the past event but rather the threat that in the future the illness may recur or be exacerbated, with death resulting. Conceptualized this way, the threat is not primarily in the past but in the future. With the exception of such illnesses as MI or seizure disorder, in which the acute onset may also be life threatening, the immediate "death encounter" in the majority of life-threatening illnesses is not experienced in the initial episode but, rather, looms ahead. This type of threat is more vague than the moment of immediately imminent death that one might experience with a mugging or a rape. However, certain aspects of treatment for these illnesses, for example, surgery, may be stressful in their own right and perceived as a "death encounter."

Prior to beginning our studies of breast cancer survivors, one of us (B. L. G.) noted that the threat associated with cancer is primarily the *information* that one has the disease. In this sense, the diagnosis of cancer is similar to learning that one has been exposed to radioactive or toxic chemical contamination (Green, Lindy, & Grace, 1994). The "stressor" in these cases is the information that one has been exposed or has cancer or heart damage, which is learned after the fact. In such cases, the nature of the threat is quite vague. These differences in the nature and source of threat have important diagnostic implications. Specifically, the intrusive images and thoughts about the threat may not be actual recollections of the event(s), such as the precise moment of receiving the news that one has cancer, but more future-oriented ruminations about possible recurrence, manifestation of physical problems, or death.

Cancer

Interest in the psychiatric impact of cancer has been an active area of research interest and funding. One of the primary reasons for this is the growing numbers of cancer survivors. With some cancers (e.g., Hodgkin's disease and testicular cancer), the vast majority of individuals treated will be cured of the illness. Most patients live for extended periods of time with the disease. To achieve these advances however, treatments have become more aggressive, lengthy, and toxic. As a result, cancer has become a chronic illness for many survivors.

A number of studies show that receiving a diagnosis of cancer causes significant psychological distress. For example, Derogatis et al. (1983) found that 47% of a cross-section of cancer patients met criteria for a psychiatric disorder, in comparison with 12–13% estimated for the general population. Although many studies examine a number of psychosocial aspects related to the cancer experience, we focus exclusively on those with a bearing on PTSD. Research in this area has generally taken the approach of measuring PTSD symptoms by way of self-report questionnaires or of more formally assessing PTSD diagnostic status with structured clinical interviews. The overwhelming majority of the studies in this area have focused on female samples of breast cancer survivors, with a few studies examining pediatric or mixed-gender adult populations (Kangas et al., 2002).

With respect to studies that examine self-reported PTSD symptoms, the majority of the studies find low to moderate numbers of individuals experiencing some level of symptoms as assessed by symptom checklists. For example, among a sample of 244 breast cancer survivors, Bleicker, Pouwer, van der Ploeg, Leer, and Ader (2000) found that 16% of the sample had high intrusive symptoms and 15% had high avoidance symptoms at 2 months postsurgery, as assessed by the Impact of Event Scale. A number of similar studies find a range of symptom reports generally in the moderate range (e.g., Brewin, Watson, McCarthy, Hyman, & Dayson, 1998; Butler, Koopman, Classen, & Spiegel, 1999; Hampton & Frombach, 2000). Virtually dozens of studies have employed this type of methodology, and all have arrived at similar conclusions (see Kangas et al. 2002). Such studies suggest that some level of psychological distress following cancer diagnoses is quite common. However, the specificity with which these symptoms map onto the construct of the PTSD diagnosis is less clear. Specifically, among cancer survivors, appropriate future-oriented rumination is often mistaken for a "reexperiencing" symptom (Green et al., 1998). Likewise, the aversive physical side effects of both the specific disease state and the often aggressive treatment regimens can be mistakenly counted as PTSD hyperarousal symptoms. Clearly, such instances of counting symptoms toward a PTSD diagnosis are not warranted in cancer survivors. Studies that employ stricter diagnostic criteria by way of structured clinical interviews can shed light on this topic, an issue we cover in the paragraphs to follow.

Among studies that have utilized structured clinical interviews, the rates of PTSD among cancer survivors have ranged somewhat. However, it is fair to say that in the majority of studies the prevalence of diagnosable PTSD is fairly low (Kangas et al., 2002). Some studies have employed strict diagnostic criteria in an effort to disentangle symptoms that are due to physical problems and interventions related to the index diagnosis of cancer as opposed to those that are secondary to a psychiatric disturbance (Green et al., 1998). Specifically, Green et al. (1998) used decision rules that avoided counting future-oriented concerns as reexperiencing symptoms (which might result in false-positive PTSD diagnoses). In this way, they found that only 1.9% of a sample of 160 women with early-stage breast cancer would meet current PTSD diagnosis (average of 6 months posttreatment). Moreover, they found a 3% lifetime (postcancer) rate of PTSD among the same sample of women.

The findings of Green et al. (1998) are concordant with other studies that have employed structured diagnostic interviews. For example, Alter et al. (1996) found a 4% current rate of PTSD among a sample of women with mixed cancers who were on average more than 4 years posttreatment. In some studies, the rates of current PTSD have ranged as low as 0% (Mundy et al., 2000). Such findings are concordant with results from studies that use self-report instruments in sophisticated ways in order to arrive at diagnostic judgments (Cordova, Stadts, Hann, Jacobsen, & Andrykowski, 2000; Andryowski, Cordova, McGrath, Sloan, Kenady, 2000). In total, the research with cancer survivors suggest that PTSD is possible but, fortunately, not very prevalent.

Investigators have speculated that cancer in the young may fit better (conceptually) with the PTSD stressor criterion because the threat of death is happening "off time." Studies investigating this phenomenon have looked at rates of PTSD in both children with cancer and their parents. Thus we treat these studies of pediatric cancer survivors separately.

Alter and colleagues (1992) examined the incidence of PTSD in three patient groups who were an average of about 5 years posttreatment: adolescent survivors of cancer, their mothers, and adult breast cancer survivors. As part of the multicenter DSM-IV field trial for PTSD, this was the only site that examined medical illness as a stressor event. The authors reported current and lifetime prevalence rates of cancer-related PTSD of 4% and 16%, respectively, for adult survivors (Alter et al., 1996), 30% and 46% for mothers, and 33% and 54% for adolescent survivors. No differences were found related to time since treatment or stage of illness.

An exploratory study by Stuber, Meeske, Gonzales, Houskamp, and Pynoos (1994) evaluated 30 childhood cancer survivors, 8–19 years old, who were disease-free and at least 22 months posttreatment. Participants were assessed for the presence of PTSD symptoms using the Reaction Index (RI), and they answered six questions about their subjective appraisal of the intensity and difficulty of treatment. The authors found that 5 (17%) of the survivors reported posttraumatic stress symptoms in the moderate range and that 9 (30%) had mild symptoms. Appraisal of treatment intensity was significantly correlated with severity of symptoms, although there was some suggestion that age at time of treatment moderated this effect. Symptoms in children over age 7 at the time of diagnosis appeared to be related to objective aspects of treatment (such as duration), whereas for younger children, subjective appraisal of treatment intensity was more highly related to distress. As with other studies, time since treatment, type of tumor, and perceived life threat were not significantly correlated with severity of symptoms.

Taken as a whole, current studies in this area suggest that, although PTSD can occur as a function of diagnosis and treatment of cancer in adults, it may affect only a small number of patients. The higher rates of PTSD symptomatology in pediatric cancer survivors indicate that age may be an important risk factor and may also put individuals at risk for chronic problems. The most important challenge facing the clinician in doing a psychiatric evaluation with cancer survivors is accurately differentiating between symptoms that are truly psychiatric in nature and those that are appropriate to coping with a medical illness and aversive treatment regimens. We return to this point in more detail shortly.

In summary, cancer may be qualitatively different from more traditional PTSD stressor events in a number of ways. These include the fact that the threat is internal rather than external and that it is ongoing, chronic, and future oriented. Thus the focus of the survivor is on the future rather than the past. On the other hand, many aspects overlap as well, for example, the news about having a potentially deadly illness can be sudden and unexpected, the treatment may be traumatic, and many of the mental and emotional processes for avoiding and integrating the experiences are likely similar. The anxiety and arousal associated with the information and certainly with some of the associated procedures may be quite similar, as well, along with the disruption in relationships brought on by the knowledge that one has had an experience that others may not be able to understand or find equally frightening. Thus PTSD is possible but not very common in this population.

PTSD Subsequent to Myocardial Infarction

Unlike receiving a medical diagnosis of which one had been unaware or free of symptoms, as is the case with receiving a cancer diagnosis, the experience of having a life-threatening medical problem with an abrupt onset (e.g., myocardial infarction) can be particularly frightening, with obvious imminent life threat and other defining features more typically associated with the DSM-IV criterion A definition of a traumatic stressor. As such, one might imagine that PTSD would be more likely in the aftermath of unexpected myocardial infarctions (MIs) than in response to other medical diagnoses.

Consistent with such conjecture are data presented by Ginzburg, Solomon, and Bleich (2002), who found that at approximately 7 months post-MI, roughly 15% of their sample met criteria for PTSD. Notable among their results was the fact that repressive coping style (measured less than 1 month post-MI) was negatively associated with rates of PTSD at 7-month follow-up. That is to say, those who tended to minimize the physical impact of their MI had better psychiatric adjustment. Such findings are consistent with more general emotional adjustment findings that suggest that the denial of the impact of MI seems to correlate with good emotional adjustment post-MI.

Van Driel & Op den Velde (1995) also examined the rates of PTSD in 23 consecutive admissions for first-incident MI. At the 2-year follow-up, no patients had received a diagnosis of PTSD, and only one had partial PTSD, during the first year post-MI (5 patients died during follow-up, and hence their psychiatric status was unknown). Kutz and colleagues examined PTSD symptoms in 100 patients 6 to 18 months (average 14 months) post-MI (Kutz, Shabtai, Solomon, Neumann & David, 1994), using a self-report questionnaire for PTSD symptoms. They found "probable" chronic PTSD in 16% of their sample and "probable" acute PTSD (lasting less than 6 months and not present at time of evaluation) in 9% of the sample, yielding a 25% lifetime risk. In 19 (76%) of the participants with chronic PTSD, the disorder appeared within 3 months of their MI. Prior MI, cardiac-related hospitalization, and prior PTSD of noncardiac origin increased risk of MI-related PTSD, as did greater anticipation of subsequent MI-caused disability. The strong association between concern over disability and PTSD prompted the researchers to suggest that denial or only mild apprehension at the time of MI may be adaptive in the long term. They also found that PTSD may play a central role in the tendency of this population to seek emergency medical help. Almost half (47%) of patients who reported repeated visits to emergency settings for "feeling another heart attack" met symptom criteria for PTSD, as opposed to 20% of those who did not utilize emergency medical services.

Doerfler, Pbert, and DeCosimo (1994) assessed 50 men 6 to 12 months following hospitalization for first MI or coronary artery bypass graph

(CABG) surgery using self-report methods. Using DSM-III-R criteria applied to an algorithm on self-report data, 4 patients (8%) met full criteria for PTSD. Although the researchers cautioned that corroboration using interview data was warranted, they concluded that PTSD may represent an unrecognized problem for some men who sustain an MI or undergo CABG surgery. These rates of PTSD are similar to those in other studies that examine individuals who survived acute cardiac events (Kutz, Garb, & David, 1988).

In summary, studies examining MI-related PTSD suggest that a small number of adults may be at potential risk for this disorder (although at slightly higher rates than with cancer). Although rates of PTSD associated with most life-threatening illnesses in general are too low to warrant routine screening for the disorder, MI may represent a special case. Clinical data suggest that denial in the early period post-MI may be important for recovery. Thus patients who experience acute emotional distress in this period are not only more likely to develop later PTSD but may also be at greater risk for poor recovery or death from their disease, and they should receive further evaluation. Nonetheless, the low rates of PTSD in such studies are encouraging as affective disturbance post-MI is generally predictive of increased mortality.

ASSESSING PTSD FOLLOWING LIFE-THREATENING ILLNESS

One general concern in assessing psychological symptoms or disorders in a medical population is the differentiation between symptoms characteristic of the stress response and those typically produced by the illness or treatment. For example, pain related to surgery can cause sleeplessness and irritability. Radiotherapy and chemotherapy cause fatigue and lethargy, as well as depressed mood. Difficulty concentrating can result from a variety of treatments and medications. As with the diagnosis of other psychiatric disorders in persons with medical illnesses, it may be difficult to identify the source of the symptom. Thus, in the case of PTSD following medical illness events, the differential diagnosis is not only between PTSD and other psychiatric disorders but also between PTSD and the medical conditions that have served as the source of stress.

A second concern regarding assessment of PTSD in this context relates to potential differences in intrusive thinking. For example, Green et al. (1998) assessed PTSD via the Structured Clinical Interview for DSM-III-R (SCID). The first question on this schedule is whether the event (which was defined for participants as "your cancer diagnosis and treatment," specifically focusing on aspects that they had defined as most stressful during this period) came back to them "suddenly and vividly when you didn't want it to." About one-third of the participants in this study answered yes to this question, but, for some, the content of the images and thoughts was ruminative and future oriented, rather than a recollection of past events. Most of these women reported thinking constantly and involuntarily about the fact that they had this potentially deadly disease. Other women had actual recollections, such as picturing the doctor telling her that her biopsy showed a malignancy or being wheeled into surgery. This distinction applied to dreaming as well. Their distress at reminders and their avoidance symptoms were similar to those found with other types of stressors.

With regard to the denial and numbing symptoms, life-threatening illness poses particular problems for the symptom of "foreshortened future." To begin with, this symptom has not been well defined in adults. In cancer populations, for example, the SCID question "has (the trauma) changed the way you think about the future?" nearly always elicited a positive response. Yet, for the most part, the changes reported seemed to indicate appropriate and healthy adaptation (e.g., enjoying the present more because the future is not guaranteed, putting one's affairs in order, talking to children about one's will). These types of responses should not count as indications of a pathological sense of foreshortened future.

With regard to the arousal symptom of hypervigilance, this often takes a different form in cancer survivors than in survivors of other types of traumas. Rather than being hyperalert to their surroundings, these individuals became hyperalert to their physical health and any bodily changes that might signal that the cancer was recurring. Thus this symptom may resemble hypochondriasis in a medically ill population. For example, participants with this symptom reported examining themselves for additional lumps, sometimes many times a day, or far more often than appropriate for routine monitoring. Hypervigilance in medical populations should be counted as a psychiatric symptom only when it appears related to fear of external environmental threats or to medical issues and is above and beyond appropriate levels of concern given the available medical data (e.g., performing several self-examinations per day for breast lumps when physician's recommendations are for examinations with considerably lower frequency).

ASSESSMENT OF TRAUMA AND PTSD IN PRIMARY CARE

The findings just described have important implications for assessment. Clearly, individuals who have been traumatized and those with PTSD make disproportionate use of the medical system. They are more likely to be seen in health-care settings than their nonexposed counterparts and more likely to be seen in primary care or medical emergency settings than in the mental health sector. Thus, as Kamerow, Pincus and MacDonald (1986) suggest, the primary care setting is a potentially useful one in which to identify and assess potential trauma victims so that they will receive appropriate care.

Given the high prevalence of trauma survivors in medical settings, primary care providers should be trained to be sensitive to the presence of trauma exposure in their patients. A trauma history should be an integral part of medical history taking and is especially important in persons with high distress and/or in those who are frequent users of health-care resources. Because of the high-risk health behaviors frequently engaged in by those with trauma and PTSD, screening for these behaviors may be useful as well. Identifying those at risk for poor health and threatening health practices is an essential ingredient in any intervention strategy.

In spite of these findings, however, a number of studies have now documented low rates of inquiry even about ongoing or current domestic violence in primary care settings (e.g., Rodriguez, Bauer, McLoughlin, & Grumbach, 1999). And qualitative studies suggest that female patients may be hesitant to disclose violence when physicians do not ask (Bauer, Rodriguez, Quiroga, & Flores-Ortiz, 2000). This combination suggests that current violence is likely to go undetected without explicit efforts on the part of the provider to inquire. Past trauma is even less likely to be addressed, yet most patients favor routine inquiry about prior sexual and physical abuse (Friedman, Samet, Roberts, Hudlin, & Hans, 1992).

Although it is tempting to suggest that one or two general questions could be used by busy physicians to do a quick screening in these settings, this approach has a number of drawbacks. It is clear at this point, first, that use of words such as "rape," "abuse," and so forth, reduce endorsement, as individuals may be reluctant to label as abusive those acts committed by known others such as parents or boyfriends (Resnick, Falsetti, Kilpatrick & Freedy, 1996). These terms are not used in any of the recent instruments for obtaining general trauma history information (Norris & Hamblen, Chapter 3, this volume). Rather, detailed questions about specific behaviors are required to learn whether certain of these experiences have occurred (Resnick et al., 1996). Furthermore, individuals or patients will not necessarily volunteer information about specific events to open-ended questions ("has anything terrible, frightening, etc., ever happened to you?") nor respond to list of possible examples of events with events *not* on the list. Again, this suggests the importance of asking about each important event. The most efficient strategy would be to employ one of the self-report measures reviewed by Norris and Hamblen (Chapter 3, this volume), or others (e.g., Kriegler et al., 1992; MacIan & Pearlman, 1992) to query for a *range* of events. Self-report inquiry requires no physician time (a receptionist can include the form in an intake packet, although it may be appropriate to have the patient put it into an sealed envelope on completion). The use made of such a measure would be up to the individual physician. He or she would have the option of only reviewing the report, of asking the patient whether he or she wanted to discuss anything reported, or of asking additional questions about the events reported to get a clinical sense of their potential connection, psychologically or temporally, with the physical complaints or condition for which the patient has sought help. Self-report measures may be more comfortable for the physician, who may not be completely at ease inquiring about specific details of past abuse, especially in the sexual arena. It is important to note, however, that it may be better not to ask at all if the questions are designed in such a way as to discourage reporting of emotionally salient experiences. Further, physicians need to be clear about how they will respond to such reports—by gathering more details, suggesting referral to mental health colleagues, and so forth. Often the most devastating aspect of early trauma is that others did not protect the person from trauma or abuse or denied or minimized the importance of what was reported. To repeat this in a medical setting would be very unhelpful as well.

Little is known at this time about screening for PTSD in primary care. Only a few studies have addressed this issue, although more are certainly under way. Studies in primary care have suggested that about 8–9% of individuals in primary care screen positive for PTSD (Stein et al., 2000; Krupnick, 2002). However, both of these studies found that universal screening for trauma and PTSD was a relatively low-yield endeavor in terms of those who followed through with full diagnostic assessments and treatment.

The field is beginning to develop short screening measures for PTSD with good sensitivity and specificity. In the Krupnick (2002) study, the 8-item screen developed by Breslau and colleagues (Breslau et al., 1999) was used to assess probable PTSD. Participants were rescreened 1 or 2 weeks later. Of those who rescreened positive, all but 1 met criteria for PTSD at clinical interview, indicating good validity for the screener and suggesting that sequential screening was an excellent way to identify PTSD.

Overall, it seems important to develop better approaches to screening and referral for patients with trauma exposure and PTSD seen in non-mental-health settings, especially relatively short screening questions for interviews or questionnaires for primary care settings. If physicians want to include a few trauma history questions in their screening, we urge them to ask inclusive questions that do not "label" the behavior with such terms as "rape" and "abuse" (Resnick et al., 1996). We recommend separate questions for sexual trauma, physical trauma (including examples of parents and spouse), serious accident, serious illness, and combat.

Going forward, it seems important to be clear about the purposes of screening for trauma and for PTSD. These would include, but not be limited to, intervention for current violence (e.g., reporting to authorities), helping providers and patients understand better the patient's current health picture, and determining whether the patient needs mental health treatment and whether he or she is psychologically ready to accept the diagnosis and the need for treatment.

SUMMARY

In recent years, dozens of studies have examined the connections between trauma, PTSD, and physical health from a variety of angles. In short, the most prominent research areas investigated include: (1) How trauma and PTSD play a role in instigating poor physical health, and (2) how medical diagnoses and interventions can serve as criterion A stressors that precipitate a PTSD diagnosis. The extant data suggest that trauma, and PTSD more specifically, do indeed raise the risk of individuals engaging in a profile of unhealthy lifestyle habits that increases the risk for physical morbidity. In addition, the physiological disturbances common to the disorder also seem to put individuals at increased health risk. These two factors drive an increased morbidity rate and a concomitant increase in health-care utilization, making PTSD a burden to the health-care system. Medical diagnoses and events such as cancer diagnosis and onset of myocardial infarctions can serve as criterion A stressors that lead to PTSD. Fortunately, the prevalence rates of PTSD subsequent to these events is low. However, careful attention is warranted in cases in which such distress may be present as psychiatric disturbance related to the index medical diagnosis can adversely affect the medical outcome and create impairment in the psychosocial aspects of a patient's life. These two ways in which PTSD relates to medical morbidity require that clinicians and researchers broaden their scope of focus beyond that of traditional psychiatric symptoms and examine PTSD in the context of an individual's entire mental and physical health profile.

REFERENCES

Allers, C., & Benjack, K. J. (1991). Connections between childhood abuse and HIV infection. *Journal of Counseling and Development*, *70*(2), 309–313.

Alter, C. L., Pelcovitz, D., Axelrod, A., Goldenberg, B., Harris, H., Meyers, B., et al. (1996). Identification of PTSD in cancer survivors. *Psychosomatics*, *37*, 137–143.

Alter, C. L., Pelcovitz, D., Axelrod, A., Goldenberg, B., Septimus, A., Harris, H., et al. (1992, October). *The identification of PTSD in cancer survivors*. Paper presented at the meeting of the Academy of Psychosomatic Medicine, San Diego, CA.

American Psychiatric Association. (1980). *Diagnostic and statistical manual of mental disorders* (3rd ed.). Washington, DC: Author.

American Psychiatric Association. (1994). *Diagnostic and statistical manual of mental disorders* (4th ed.). Washington, DC: Author.

Andryowski, M. A., Cordova, M. J., McGrath, P. C., Sloan, D. A., & Kenady, D. E. (2000). Stability and change in posttraumatic stress disorder symptoms following breast cancer treatment: A 1-year follow-up. *Psycho-Oncology*, *9*, 69–78.

Bauer, H. M., Rodriguez, M. A., Quiroga, S. S., & Flores-Ortiz, Y. G. (2000). Barriers to health care for abused Latina and Asian immigrant women. *Journal of Health Care for the Poor and Underserved*, *11*, 33–44.

Beckham, J. C., Moore, S. D., Feldman, M. E., Hertzberg, M. A., Kirby, A. C., & Fairbank, J. A. (1998). Health status, somatization, and severity of postraumatic stress disorder in Vietnam combat veterans with posttraumatic stress disorder. *American Journal of Psychiatry*, *155*, 1565–1569.

Blanchard, E. B., & Buckley, T. C. (1999). Psychophysiological assessment and PTSD. In P. Saigh & D. Bremner (Eds.), *Posttraumatic stress disorder: A comprehensive text* (pp. 248–266). Needham, MA: Allyn & Bacon.

Blanchard, E. B., Hickling, E. J., Buckley, T. C., Taylor, A. E., Vollmer, A. J., & Loos, W. R. (1996). The psychophysiology of motor vehicle accident related posttraumatic stress disorder: Replication and extension. *Journal of Consulting and Clinical Psychology*, *64*, 742–751.

Bleicker, E. M. A, Pouwer, F., van der Ploeg, H. M., Leer, J. H., & Ader, H. J. (2000). Psychological distress two years after diagnosis of breast cancer: Frequency and prediction. *Patient Education and Counseling*, *40*, 209–217.

Boscarino, J. A. (1997). Diseases among men 20 years after exposure to severe stress: Implications for clinical research and medical care. *Psychosomatic Medicine*, *59*, 605–614.

Boscarino, J. A., & Chang, J. (1999). Electrocardiogram abnormalities among men with stress-related psychiatric disorders: Implications for coronary heart disease and clinical research. *Annals of Behavioral Medicine*, *21*, 227–234.

Breslau, N., Davis, G. C., & Schultz, L. R. (2003). Posttraumatic stress disorder and the incidence of nicotine, alcohol, and other drug disorders in persons who have experienced trauma. *Archives of General Psychiatry*, *60*, 289–294.

Breslau, N., Peterson, E. L., Kessler, R. C., & Schultz, L. R. (1999). Short screening scale for DSM-IV posttraumatic stress disorder. *American Journal of Psychiatry*, *156*, 908–911.

Brewin, C. R., Watson, M., McCarthy, S., Hyman, P., & Dayson, D. (1998). Intrusive memories and depression in cancer patients. *Behaviour Research and Therapy*, *36*, 1131–1142.

Buckley, T. C., & Kaloupek, D. G. (2001). A meta-analytic examination of basal cardiovascular activity in PTSD. *Psychosomatic Medicine*, *63*, 585–594.

Buckley, T. C., Mozley, S., Bedard, M., Dewulf, A. C., & Greif, J. (in press). Preventive health behaviors, health risk behaviors, physical morbidity, and health-related role functioning impairment in a consecutive series of treatment-seeking PTSD patients. *Military Medicine*.

Butler, L. D., Koopman, C., Classen, C., & Spiegel, D. (1999). Traumatic stress, life events, and emotional support in women with metastatic breast cancer: Cancer-related traumatic stress symptoms associated with past and current stressors. *Health Psychology*, *18*, 555–560.

Cohen, H., Kotler, M., Matar, M. A., Kaplan, Z., Miodownik, H., & Cassuto, Y. (1997). Power spectral analysis of heart rate variability in posttraumatic stress disorder patients. *Biological Psychiatry*, *41*, 627–629.

Cohen, M. A., Alfonso, C. A., Hoffman, R. G., Milau, V., & Carrera, G. (2001). The impact of PTSD on treatment adherence in persons with HIV infection. *General Hospital Psychiatry*, *23*, 294–296.

Cordova, M. J., Studts, J. L., Hann, D. M., Jacobsen, P. B., & Andrykowski, M. A. (2000). Symptom structure of PTSD following breast cancer. *Journal of Traumatic Stress*, *13*, 301–319.

Cunningham, R. M., Stiffman, A. R., Dore, P., & Earls, F. (1994). The association of physical and sexual abuse with HIV risk behaviors in adolescence and young adulthood: Implications for public health. *Child Abuse and Neglect*, *18*, 233–245.

Delvaux, M., Denis, P., & Allemand, H. (1997). Sexual abuse is more frequently reported by IBS patients than by patients with organic digestive diseases or controls: Results of a multicentre inquiry. *European Journal of Gastroenterology and Hepatology*, *9*(4), 345–352.

Derogatis, L. R., Morrow, G. R., Fetting, J., Penman, D., Piasetsky, S., Schmale, A. M., Henrichs, M., & Carnicke, C. L. M. (1983). The prevalence of psychiatric disorders among cancer patients. *Journal of the American Medical Association, 249*, 751–757.

Deykin, E. Y., Keane, T. M., Kaloupek, D. G., Fincke, G., Rothendler, J., Siegfried, M., & Creamer, K. (2001). Posttraumatic stress disorder and the use of health services. *Psychosomatic Medicine, 63*, 835–841.

Doerfler, L. A., Pbert, L., & DeCosimo, D. (1994). Symptoms of posttraumatic stress disorder following myocardial infarction and coronary artery bypass surgery. *General Hospital Psychiatry, 16*, 193–199.

Felitti, V. J., Anda, R. F., Nordenberg, D., Williamson, D. F., Spitz, A. M., Edwards, V., et al. (1998). Relationship of childhood abuse and household dysfunction to many of the leading causes of death in adults: The adverse childhood experiences (ACE) study. *American Journal of Preventative Medicine, 14*(4), 245–258.

Friedman, L. S., Samet, J. H., Roberts, M. S., Hudlin, M., & Hans, P. (1992). Inquiry about victimization experiences: A survey of patient preferences and physician practices. *Archives of Internal Medicine, 152*, 1186–1190.

Friedman, M. J., & McEwen, B. S. (2004). Posttraumatic stress disorder, allostatic load, and medical illness. In P. P. Schnurr & B. L. Green (Eds.), *Trauma and health: Physical health consequences of exposure to extreme stress* (pp. 157–188). Washington, DC: American Psychological Association.

Friedman, M. J., & Schnurr, P. P. (1995). The relationship between trauma, posttraumatic stress disorder, and physical health. In M. J. Friedman, D. S. Charney, & A. Y. Deutch (Eds.), *Neurobiological and clinical consequences of stress: From normal adaptation to PTSD* (pp. 507–524). Philadelphia: Lippincott-Raven.

Ginzburg, K., Solomon, Z., & Bleich, A. (2002). Repressive coping style, acute stress disorder, and posttraumatic stress disorder after myocardial infarction. *Psychosomatic Medicine, 64*, 748–757.

Goldberg, R. T. (1994) Childhood abuse, depression, and chronic pain. *Clinical Journal of Pain, 10*(4), 277–281.

Golding, J. M., Cooper, M. L., & George, L. K. (1997). Sexual assault history and health perceptions: Seven general population studies. *Health Psychology, 16*, 417–425.

Green, B. L., Lindy, J. D., & Grace, M. C. (1994). Psychological effects of toxic contamination. In R. J. Ursano, B. G. McCaughey, & C. S. Fullerton (Eds.), *Individual and community responses to trauma and disaster* (pp. 154–176). Cambridge, UK: Cambridge University Press.

Green, B. L., Rowland, J. H., Krupnick, J. L., Epstein, S. A., Stockton, P., Stern, N. M, et al. (1998). Prevalence of posttraumatic stress disorder in women with breast cancer. *Psychosomatics, 39*, 102–111.

Greenberg, P. E., Sisitsky, T., Kessler, R. C., Finkelstein, S. N., Berndt, E. R., Davidson, J. R., et al. (1999). The economic burden of anxiety disorders in the 1990s. *Journal of Clinical Psychiatry, 60*, 427–435.

Hampton, M. R., & Frombach, I. (2000). Women's experience of traumatic stress in cancer treatment. *Health Care for Women International, 21*, 67–76.

Hien, D. A., Nunes, E., Levin, F. R., & Fraser, D. (2000). Posttraumatic stress disorder and short-term outcome in early methadone maintenance treatment. *Journal of Substance Abuse Treatment, 19*(10), 31–37.

Hillbom, M., & Juvela, S. (1996). Alcohol and risk for stroke. In S. Zakhari & M.

Wassef (Eds.), *Alcohol and the cardiovascular system* (pp. 63–84). Bethesda, MD: National Institutes of Health.

Kamerow, D. B., Pincus, H. A., & MacDonald, D. I. (1968). Alcohol abuse, other drug abuse and mental disorders in medical practice: Prevalence, costs, recognition, and treatment. *Journal of the American Medical Association, 255*, 2054–2057.

Kangas, M., Henry, J. L., & Bryant, R. A. (2002). Posttraumatic stress disorder following cancer: A conceptual review. *Clinical Psychology Review, 22*, 499–524.

Keane, T. M., Kolb, L. C., Kaloupek, D. G., Orr, S. P., Blanchard, E. B., Thomas, R. G., et al. (1998). Utility of psychophysiological measurement in the diagnosis of posttraumatic stress disorder: Results from a Department of Veterans Affairs cooperative study. *Journal of Consulting and Clinical Psychology, 66*, 914–923.

Kessler, R. C., Sonnega, A., Bromet, E., Hughes, M., & Nelson, C. B. (1995). Posttraumatic stress disorder in the National Comorbidity Survey. *Archives of General Psychiatry, 52*, 1048–1060.

Kimerling, R., Calhoun, K. S., Forehand, R., Armistead, L. Morse, E., Morse, P., et al. (1999) Traumatic stress in HIV-infected women. *AIDS Education and Prevention, 11*(4), 321–330.

Kimerling, R., Clum, G. A., & Wolfe, J. (2000). Relationships among trauma exposure, chronic posttraumatic stress disorder symptoms and self-reported health in women: Replication and extension. *Journal of Traumatic Stress, 13*, 115–128.

Koss, M. P., Woodruff, W. J., & Koss, P. G. (1991). Criminal victimization among primary care medical patients: Prevalence, incidence, and physician usage. *Behavioral Sciences and the Law, 9*, 85–96.

Kriegler, J. A., Blake, D. D., Schnurr, P., Bremner, J. D., Zaidi, L. Y., & Krinsley, K. (1992). *The early trauma interview*. Boston: National Center for Posttraumatic Stress Disorder.

Krupnick, J. L. (2002, November). Interpersonal psychotherapy groups with low-income women with PTSD. In N. Talbot (Chair), *Emerging findings on psychotherapies for PTSD in community settings*. Symposium conducted at the meeting of the International Society for Traumatic Stress Studies, Baltimore, MD.

Kulka, R. A., Schlenger, W. E., Fairbank, J. A., Hough, R. L., Jordan, B. K., Marmar, C. R., & Weiss, D. S. (1990). *Trauma and the Vietnam War generation: Report of findings from the National Veterans Readjustment Study*. New York: Brunner/Mazel.

Kutz, I., Garb, R., & David, D. (1988). Posttraumatic stress disorder following myocardial infarction. *General Hospital Psychiatry, 10*, 169–176.

Kutz, I., Shabtai, H., Solomon, Z., Neumann, M., & David, D. (1994). Posttraumatic stress disorder in myocardial infarction patients: Prevalence study. *Israeli Journal of Psychiatry and Related Science, 31*(1), 48–56.

Lasser, K., Boyd, J. W., Woolhandler, S., Himmelstein, D. U., McCormick, D., & Bor, D. H. (2000). Smoking and mental illness: A population-based prevalence study. *Journal of the American Medical Association, 284*, 2606–2610.

MacIan, P. S., & Pearlman, L. A. (1992). Development and use of the TSI Life Event Questionnaire. *Treating Abuse Today: The International Newsjournal of Abuse, Survivorship and Therapy*, 2(1), 9–11.

McEwen, B. S. (2000). Allostasis and allostatic load. In G. Fink (Ed.), *Encyclopedia of stress* (Vol., pp. 143–150). San Diego, CA: Academic Press.

McFall, M. E., Veith, R. C., & Murburg, M. M. (1992). Basal sympathodadrenal function in posttraumatic stress disorder. *Biological Psychiatry, 31*, 1050–1056.

McFarlane, A. C., Atchinson, M., Rafalowicz, E., & Papay, P. (1994). Physical symptoms in posttraumatic stress disorder. *Journal of Psychosomatic Research*, *38*(7), 715–726.

Mundy, E. A., Blanchard, E. B., Cirenza, E., Gargiulo, J., Maloy, B., & Blanchard, C. G. (2000). Posttraumatic stress disorder in breast cancer patients following autologous bone marrow transplantation or conventional cancer treatments. *Behaviour Research and Therapy*, *38*, 1015–1027.

Norris, F. H., Kaniasty, K. Z., & Scheer, D. A. (1990). Use of mental health services among victims of crime: Frequency, correlates, and subsequent recovery. *Journal of Consulting and Clinical Psychology*, *58*, 538–547.

Resnick, H. S., Falsetti, S. A., Kilpatrick, D. G., & Freedy, J. R. (1996). Assessment of rape and other civilian trauma-related PTSD: Emphasis on assessment of potentially traumatic events. In T. W. Miller (Ed.), *Theory and assessment of stressful life events. International Universities Press stress and health series* (pp. 235–271). Madison, CT: International Universities Press.

Rodriguez, M. A., Bauer, H. M., McLoughlin, E., & Grumbach, K. (1999). Screening and intervention for intimate partner abuse: Practices and attitudes of primary care physicians. *Journal of the American Medical Association*, *282*, 468–474.

Rotheram-Borus, M. J., Koopman, C., & Bradley, J. S. (1989). Barriers to successful AIDS prevention programs with runaway youth. In J. D. Woodruff, D. Doherty, & J. G. Athey (Eds.), *Troubled adolescents and HIV infection* (pp. 37–55). Washington, DC: Georgetown University, Child Development Center, Child and Adolescent Service System Program Technical Assistance Center.

Saunders, J. B., Aasland, O. G., Babor, T. F., de la Fuente, J. R., & Grant, M. (1993). Development of the Alcohol Use Disorders Identification Test (AUDIT): WHO collaborative project on early detection of persons with harmful alcohol consumption: II. *Addiction*, *88*, 791–804.

Schnurr, P. P., Friedman, M. J., Sengupta, A., Jankowski, M. K., & Holmes, T. (2000). PTSD and utilization of medical treatment services among male Vietnam veterans. *Journal of Nervous and Mental Disease*, *188*, 496–504.

Schnurr, P. P., & Green, B. L. (2004). Understanding relationships among trauma, PTSD, and health outcomes. In P. P. Schnurr & B. L. Green (Eds.), *Trauma and health: Physical health consequences of exposure to extreme stress* (pp. 247–274). Washington, DC: American Psychological Association.

Schnurr, P. P., & Jankowski, M. K. (1999). Physical health and posttraumatic stress disorder: Review and synthesis. *Seminars in Clinical Neuropsychiatry*, *4*(4), 295–304.

Schnurr, P. P., & Spiro, A. (1999). Combat exposure, posttraumatic stress disorder symptoms, and health behaviors as predictors of self-reported physical health in older veterans. *Journal of Nervous and Mental Disease*, *187*, 353–359.

Schnurr, P. P., Spiro, A., & Paris, A. H. (2000). Physician-diagnosed medical disorders in relations to PTSD symptoms in older male military veterans. *Health Psychology*, *19*, 91–97.

Selye, H. (1955). Stress and disease. *Science*, *122*, 625–631.

Shemesh, E., Rudnick, A., Kaluski, E., Milovanov, O., Salah, A., Alon, D., et al. (2001). A prospective study of posttraumatic stress symptoms and nonadherence in survivors of a myocardial infarction (MI). *General Hospital Psychiatry*, *23*, 215–222.

Skinner, H. A. (1982). The drug abuse screening test. *Addictive Behaviors*, *7*, 363–371.

Stein, M. B., McQuaid, J. R., Pedrelli, P., Lenox, R., & McCahill, M. E. (2000). Posttraumatic stress disorder in the primary care medical setting. *General Hospital Psychiatry*, *22*, 261–269.

Stewart, S. H., & Conrod, P. J. (2003). Psychosocial models of functional associations between posttraumatic stress disorder and substance use disorder. In P. Ouimette & P. J. Brown (Eds.), *Trauma and substance abuse: Causes, consequences, and treatment of comorbid disorders* (pp. 29–55). Washington DC: American Psychological Association.

Stiffman, A. R., Dore, P., Earls, F., & Cunningham, R. (1992). The influence of mental health problems on AIDS-related risk behaviors in young adults. *Journal of Nervous and Mental Disease*, *180*, 314–320.

Stuber, M. L., Meeske, K., Gonzalez, S., Houskamp, B., & Pynoos, R. (1994). Posttraumatic stress after childhood cancer: I. The role of appraisal. *Psycho-Oncology*, *3*, 305–312.

Taft, C. T., Stern, A. S., King, L. A., & King, D. W. (1999). Modeling physical health and functional health status: The role of combat exposure, posttraumatic stress disorder, and personal resource attributes. *Journal of Traumatic Stress*, *12*(1), 3–23.

van Driel, R. C., & Op den Velde, W. (1995). Myocardial infarction and posttraumatic stress disorder. *Journal of Traumatic Stress*, *8*(1), 151–159.

Wagner, A. M., Wolfe, J., Rotnitsky, A., Proctor, S. P., & Erikson, D. J. (2000). An investigation of the impact of posttraumatic stress disorder on physical health. *Journal of Traumatic Stress*, *13*(1), 41–55.

Walker, E. A., Katon, W., Russo, J., Ciechanowski, P., Newman, E., & Wagner, A. W. (2003). Health care costs associated with posttraumatic stress disorder symptoms in women. *Archives of General Psychiatry*, *60*, 369–374.

Ware, J. E., Snow, K. K., Kosinski, M., & Gandek, B. (1997). *SF-36 Health Survey: Manual and interpretation guide*. Boston: New England Medical Center.

Wolfe, J., Schnurr, P. P., Brown, P. J., & Furey, J. (1994). Posttraumatic stress disorder and war zone exposure as correlates of perceived health in female Vietnam war veterans. *Journal of Consulting and Clinical Psychology*, *62*(6), 1235–1240.

Yehuda, R., Giller, E. R., Southwick, S. M., Lowy, M. T., & Mason, J. W. (1991). Hypothalamic–pituitary–adrenal dysfunction in posttraumatic stress disorder. *Biological Psychiatry*, *30*, 1031–1048.

Zatzick, D. F., Marmar, C. R., Weiss, D. S., Browner, W. S., Metzler, T. J., Golding, J. M., et al. (1997). Posttraumatic stress disorder and functioning and quality of life outcomes in a nationally representative sample of male Vietnam veterans. *American Journal of Psychiatry*, *154*(12), 1690–1695.

Zayfert, C., Dums, A. R., Ferguson, R. J., & Hegel, M. T. (2002). Health functioning impairments associated with posttraumatic stress disorder, anxiety disorders, and depression. *Journal of Nervous and Mental Disease*, *190*(4), 233–240.

Zoellner, L. A., Goodwin, M. L., & Foa, E. B. (2000). PTSD severity and health perceptions in female victims of sexual assault. *Journal of Traumatic Stress*, *13*(4), 635–649.

CHAPTER 16

Assessment of Trauma, PTSD, and Substance Use Disorder

A Practical Guide

LISA M. NAJAVITS

The wish to escape pain through alcohol and drugs occurs across cultures and across history (Lowinson, Ruiz, Millman, & Langrod, 1997). Trauma and substance use disorder (SUD) thus represent a natural pairing. One victim of childhood physical and sexual abuse said, "When I was twelve I had my first drink, and I knew immediately this was my answer. I felt relaxed for the first time in my life. I became an instant alcoholic." Substances are also used by trauma perpetrators, whether they are under the influence while committing harm (many violent assaults are committed while intoxicated) or whether they use a substance to sedate the victim (Bureau of Justice Statistics, 1992). Community-wide traumatic disasters are also known to lead to increased substance use, including the September 11, 2001, attacks, Hurricane Hugo, and the Oklahoma City bombing (Clark, 2002; North et al., 1999). Various populations tend to have particularly high rates of trauma and SUD, including women, teens, prisoners, the homeless, gays and lesbians, veterans, rescue workers such as firefighters and police, victims of domestic violence, and prostitutes (e.g., Davis & Wood, 1999; Jacobsen, Southwick, & Kosten, 2001; Najavits, Weiss, & Shaw, 1997; North et al., 2002; Substance Abuse and Mental Health Services Administration (SAMHSA), 2001; Smith, North, & Spitznagel, 1993; Tarter & Kirisci, 1999; Teplin, Abram, & McClelland, 1996).

Posttraumatic stress disorder (PTSD), the psychiatric disorder most directly related to trauma, is highly associated with SUD. In the United States, among men with PTSD, 51.9% are estimated to have alcohol use disorder and 34.5% have drug use disorder (lifetime rates); for women the rates are 27.9%

and 26.9%, respectively (Kessler, Sonnega, Bromet, Hughes, & Nelson, 1995). Their clinical needs are urgent and serious. Those with the dual diagnosis have worse outcomes than those with either disorder alone, higher rates of subsequent trauma, and a more severe clinical profile, including other Axis I and II disorders, medical problems, HIV risk, legal problems, lower work functioning, suicidality, and self-harm (Brady, Killeen, Saladin, Dansky, & Becker, 1994; Hien, Nunes, Levin, & Fraser, 2000; Najavits, Gastfriend, et al., 1998; Najavits et al., 1997; Ouimette, Finney, & Moos, 1999). Misuse of substances may represent reenactment of trauma, whether conscious or not: an act of harming the body that echoes familiar traumatic experiences; giving up on oneself after having been violated by others; or playing the role of the marginalized "bad one" or rebel (Najavits, 2002b; Teusch, 2001). It is notable that one of the major predictors of both trauma and SUD is a family history of these—the repeating cycle over generations of this seemingly inexorable combination (Kendler, Davis, & Kessler, 1997; Yehuda, Schmeidler, Wainberg, Binder-Brynes, & Duvdevani, 1998).

THE PROBLEM OF UNDERDIAGNOSIS

Accurate assessment is thus essential. It is the precursor to effective treatment, without which the patient may not receive adequate attention to one or both disorders. Of particular challenge is the fact that, quite unique among Axis I disorders, both PTSD and SUD are highly prone to minimization, whether through lying, denial, or the shame and guilt inherent in both. Patients may say, "Growing up, I was blamed for the sexual abuse, so I learned never to talk about it"; or "I hid my cocaine use from others, but also from myself; I couldn't admit I had a problem." Moreover, both PTSD and SUD were quite late in joining the mainstream of the mental health field. PTSD was established as a diagnosis only in 1980, with Freud's disavowal of trauma as "fantasy" contributing to a lack of attention to PTSD for much of the 20th century (Herman, 1992). SUD, though a diagnostic category, was often ignored by mental health clinicians, viewed as a surface issue rather than a genuine clinical concern, and addressed primarily through grassroots 12-step movements (Najavits & Weiss, 1994).

The systemic neglect of both PTSD and SUD have historically resulted in a lack of adequate assessment and a marked separation of the two fields that only lately has begun to improve. A culture of exclusion continues to exist, with many mental health clinicians believing they cannot adequately assess or treat SUD and many SUD clinicians believing they cannot assess or treat PTSD (Najavits, 2002b; Read, Bollinger, & Sharansky, 2002). More and more, there is recognition that a no-wrong-door approach is the most helpful (Clark, 2002). Regardless of how they enter the system, patients should be assessed for both disorders and provided with treatment. Split systems, in which a patient who uses substances is rejected from mental health programs until abstinent or in which the patient with mental health issues is rejected from substance abuse treatment until stabilized, are believed to be less effective than integrated or concurrent treatment, according to most current experts (Brady, 2001; Ouimette & Brown, 2002). Yet it remains the case that *most* SUD patients are not adequately assessed for PTSD nor given treatment for it (Brown, Stout, & Gannon-Rowley, 1998; Dansky, Roitzsch, Brady, & Saladin, 1997; Hyer, Leach, Boudewyns, & Davis, 1991; Najavits, Sullivan, Schmitz, Weiss, & Lee, 2004). Many mental health clinicians, similarly, may fail to assess and treat SUD or, alternatively, may take an overly harsh stance, such as withholding treatment unless the patient agrees to attend Alcoholics Anonymous or terminating treatment if a patient relapses. Newer approaches to SUD, such as harm reduction, offering the patient choices, and an emphasis on support rather than confrontation, may be unfamiliar to some mental health clinicians (Fletcher, 2001; Marlatt, Tucker, Donovan, & Vuchinich, 1997). Yet these modifications of standard SUD treatment may be especially helpful for dual diagnosis patients in general and for those with PTSD specifically (Marlatt et al., 1997; Najavits, 2002b).

The lack of assessment of both disorders occurs for other reasons as well. Gender, for example, plays a role. Some women who do not fit the classic image of addicts—such as professional women, college women, housewives, and middle- and upper-class women—are underassessed for SUD (Najavits, 2002c). Men may be underassessed for PTSD, particularly civilian men who experienced physical or sexual abuse (which violate the image of the masculine role), crime witnessing, or victimization, which may not be recognized as traumatic in subcultures in which these events are common (Lisak, 1994). Establishing norms for measures based solely on dominant gender or ethnic group also has historically resulted in a lack of accurate assessment. For example, SUD measures were normed primarily on men and may be less accurate for women, who are known to become addicted more quickly and with lower levels of use than men (Mendelson & Mello, 1998; Najavits, 2002c). The reality is that both PTSD and SUD tend to be underdiagnosed according to empirical studies, and it remains a public health concern to increase valid assessment of them (Brown et al., 1998; Dansky et al., 1997; Davidson, 2001; Hyer et al., 1991; Najavits, 2002c).

The goal of this chapter is to provide a practical assessment guide for clinicians in both the mental health and substance abuse fields. Three topics are addressed: (1) myths, (2) suggestions for the assessment of PTSD and SUD, and (3) resources.

MYTHS

Perhaps because of the historic schism between the fields of PTSD and SUD, several misperceptions persist about diagnosis of the disorders. Before discussing assessment strategies, it may be helpful to describe some of these.

"Labels aren't good for patients; it's better not to give a PTSD or SUD diagnosis." This view tends to be held by staff without formal training in psychopathology, such as domestic violence advocates, paraprofessional addiction counselors, and nonclinicians. Some may distrust the mental health field as a system of social control, coercion, or hierarchy. Others may simply view diagnosis as outside their realm of training. They are well intentioned in their attempt not to impose views on patients or disempower them, particularly as those with the dual diagnosis of PTSD/SUD are often marginalized by society. This perspective also arises from a legacy of some very real diagnostic distortions, such as misuse of the label "borderline personality disorder," which became notoriously pejorative and inaccurately applied to patients with PTSD (Herman, 1992). However, it is borne out by clinical experience that accurate labeling of PTSD and SUD is, in fact, usually highly therapeutic. Most experts view the diagnoses as beneficial guides to treatment planning that are important to identify early (Brady, 2001; Brown et al., 1998; Davidson, 2001; Jacobsen et al., 2001; Ouimette & Brown, 2002; Triffleman, 1998). The diagnoses provide a framework that helps organize patients' experience to promote recovery. One SUD patient, on learning about her PTSD diagnosis, said:

> At first I thought, "Oh no, not another condition," but then I was relieved to find I had something with a name. I thought it was just me—I'm crazy. But I can deal with this now. It's different when you don't know, but when you find out, it's like a person with cancer—you can work on it. Now I can put down the cocaine and work on what's behind it. (quoted in Najavits, 2002c)

For many patients with SUD, learning about the PTSD diagnosis allows them to view their addiction in a new light, as a way to cope with overwhelming emotional pain (particularly as the PTSD usually occurs first; Jacobsen et al., 2001; Najavits et al., 1997). They may feel less alone, less "crazy," and more understanding of themselves. Indeed, the majority of patients with SUD who are educated about PTSD report that they want treatment for it (Brown et al., 1998; Najavits et al., 2004). Similarly, the SUD diagnosis can reduce denial and minimization. Exploring the definition of SUD can help move the patient out of debates with clinicians or family members, and into the more objective realm of how SUD is defined in DSM-IV. Reading it on paper can make it more acceptable. Of course, for all patients, sensitivity to how they react to the diagnoses and careful education are key. A collaborative stance is also important, rather than just asserting the clinicians' views.

"SUD itself is trauma or PTSD." This view arises from the observation that addiction can be extremely destructive. It causes physical and psychological harm, and it leaves the patient feeling out of control, all of which parallel the trauma experience. However, though SUD is highly destructive, it does not meet criteria for trauma or PTSD. Trauma is generally understood to be unpredictable and occurring from some force external to the patient—another person, a natural disaster, an accident, or combat, for example. Substance

abuse relies on the person picking up the drink or drug. Also, the PTSD and SUD criteria have little or no overlap (American Psychiatric Assocation, 1994). Ultimately, clear use of the terms "SUD," "trauma," and "PTSD" conveys respect for patients' experience. To merge terms until they become undifferentiated does not do justice to the importance and character of each. One can help a patient understand the destructiveness of SUD without resorting to the conceptual imprecision of merging terms that each have their own meaning.

"Assessing for trauma is enough." In many clinical settings, at least some assessment of trauma occurs on intake. For example, asking patients if they have a history of physical, sexual, or emotional abuse is part of the Addiction Severity Index, one of the most widely used assessment tools in the addiction field (Najavits, Weiss, Reif, et al., 1998). Assessing for PTSD, however, is much more rare (Danksy, Roitzsch, Brady, & Saladin, 1997), and, indeed, some clinicians simply equate trauma with PTSD. Yet trauma itself is not a diagnosis; it is an event that may or may not still cause problems for the patient. Most people who experience a trauma do not develop PTSD (Kessler et al., 1995). According to a literature review by Ruzek, Polusny, and Abueg (1998), the diagnosis of PTSD is associated with SUD much more than with trauma per se. Effective treatment thus requires assessment of whether the patient is actually experiencing problems from the trauma, such as nightmares, flashbacks, hypervigilance, and intense distress when reminded of the event. One cannot assume that the trauma no longer creates problems for the patient, nor the opposite, that trauma is always problematic. Accurate assessment of both trauma and PTSD is key. Also, it is important to have a clear understanding of their definitions. Some believe that trauma means "any upsetting event" or that emotional abuse counts as a trauma in DSM-IV (American Psychiatric Association, 1994). In fact, in DSM-IV, trauma must involve some sort of physical harm, whether experienced, confronted, or witnessed. It also involves an emotional response at the time: It is not just an event (e.g., a car accident) but also the experience of fear, helplessness, or horror.

"SUD means . . . use of drugs/amount of use/how the substance is used." Clinicians sometimes use idiosyncratic definitions of SUD. For example, alcohol may be viewed as acceptable because it is legal and socially sanctioned, whereas illegal drugs may be regarded as more pathological. Or the clinician may try to ascertain the amount or form of alcohol or drug use and make a judgment from that. For example, three drinks per week is fine, but drinking every day is not; or, drinking with others is acceptable but drinking alone is not. However, the essential feature of SUD is not the presence or amount of substance use per se, nor whether it is taken alone or with others, nor based on the patient's motivation (e.g., to get "wasted," to relax). Rather, it is based on criteria such as physiological impact (tolerance, withdrawal), inability to stop using, and its consequences (whether the substance use causes demonstrable problems—legal, medical, social, psychiatric, or vocational—yet the person continues to use anyway). One may have opinions on what is healthy or socially acceptable, but a diagnosis of

SUD requires evaluation of specific criteria. The definitions are complex, filling 97 pages of DSM-IV, and clinicians may not have formal training in addiction. Yet it is important to provide patients with an accurate diagnosis of SUD rather than an ill-informed or moral judgment, which for so long was part of society's historical response to it.

"*I need to wait until the patient is through substance use and withdrawal before assessing PTSD.*" This is a fascinating and complex issue. The idea is that substance use or withdrawal may either dampen PTSD symptoms (thus obscuring the diagnosis, i.e., false negatives) or increase PTSD symptoms (thus inflating rates of the diagnosis, i.e., false positives; Read et al., 2002; Ruzek et al., 1998). Thus it is sometimes said that until 4 to 6 weeks of abstinence are achieved, PTSD or other mental disorders should not be diagnosed. However, there appear to be no studies at this point on whether, in fact, the diagnosis of PTSD during substance use or withdrawal is less accurate after a period of abstinence. Although some psychiatric disorders can indeed be confusing to assess clearly in the context of substance use or withdrawal (e.g., depression, generalized anxiety), the PTSD diagnosis appears quite robust through these states, even if some symptoms intensify or diminish (Pamela Brown, Paige Ouimette, personal communications, March 31, 2003). Thus the PTSD diagnosis may be more stable and accurate in the context of SUD than are other Axis I diagnoses, highlighting the point that all dual diagnoses are not the same (Weiss, Najavits, & Mirin, 1998). Moreover, from a clinical perspective, it is problematic to wait before diagnosing PTSD. Many patients with the dual diagnosis are unable to achieve such a stable period of abstinence, and their difficulty may arise in part from inadequate attention to PTSD. Clinically, the most sensible approach appears to be to assess for trauma and PTSD immediately and to reconfirm the diagnosis, if needed, once the patient achieves sustained abstinence.

SUGGESTIONS FOR THE ASSESSMENT OF PTSD AND SUD

Several suggestions may help guide the assessment of this dual diagnosis.

Choose Measures Based on the Question of Interest and Practical Considerations

Numerous measures are available for PTSD and SUD. Selection depends on the goal of the assessment (e.g., screening, diagnosis, clinical work, research, outcome assessment), as well as on the practical limitations of the assessment context. For example, it is easy to recommend that all patients be given the best available assessment of both disorders, such as the Structured Clinical Interview for DSM-IV (Spitzer, Williams, & Gibbon, 1997); yet in many settings, this is impossible due to heavy workloads, lack of training in psychopathology or assessment, and some patients' unwillingness or inability to answer lengthy questioning. Moreover, only a few trauma/PTSD measures have been validated in SUD samples (e.g., Bernstein, 2000; Coffey, Dansky, Falsetti, Saladin, & Brady, 1998; El-Bassel et al., 1998), but most have not. In general, it is better to pursue some assessment, even in a limited fashion, than to take an all-or-none stance (i.e., state-of-the-art rigorous assessment or no assessment).

Tables 16.1 and 16.2 provide key areas of assessment for both PTSD and SUD, with examples of measures. To obtain actual measures, see "Resources for Assessment," the final section of this chapter. Many are in the public domain, free, and can be directly downloaded from online sources. Note that SUD measures span a wide range of questions, including screening for SUD, diagnosis of SUD, level of substance use, verification of substance use, negative consequences of SUD, motivation for SUD treatment, acute medical detoxification issues, and cognitions. Similarly, for PTSD, questions might include screening, diagnosis, other trauma-related diagnoses, other trauma-related symptoms, and cognitions. No one measure or set of measures can be recommended for all purposes, but the following guidelines may be helpful.

SUD treatment programs are typically interested in adding trauma and PTSD assessment, as they are already well versed in SUD. They usually seek short self-report measures that do not require interviewer time or formal training. Many programs are underfunded and understaffed, and the chief aim is to add assessment without additional burden. Many SUD clinicians do not have access to computers or training in assessment, and thus searching for measures may be impractical. "Do more and do it better" is a continual demand on SUD treatment staff (Gustafson, 1991). Suggested measures follow, with emphasis on those that are brief (i.e., approximately one page) and that can be obtained and distributed for free.

- For a *trauma screen*, consider the Stressful Life Experiences Screening (Stamm et al., 1996), which can be downloaded from *www.isu.edu/~bhstamm/tests.htm*, along with scoring and psychometric information.
- For assessment of *PTSD*, consider the PTSD Checklist—Civilian version (Weathers, Litz, Herman, Huska, & Keane, 1993), which translates the DSM-IV PTSD definition into a pencil-and-paper format and requires no training to administer; it too can be downloaded from *www.isu.edu/~bhstamm/tests.htm*.
- For *trauma-related symptoms*, a widely used free measure is the Trauma Symptom Checklist-40, which can be downloaded from *www.johnbriere.com* (click "TSC-40"), including scoring information and psychometric information. Other measures, some of which can be ordered from Psychological Assessment Resources (800-331-TEST) for a fee, are also described on that site, including versions for children and adolescents.

TABLE 16.1. Areas of Substance Use Disorder Assessment

<u>Screening for substance use disorder</u>

Key question: Might the patient have a substance use disorder?

Examples of measures: For alcohol—Michigan Alcohol Screening Test (Seltzer, 1971); for drugs—Drug Abuse Screening Test (Skinner, 1982)

Notes: Brief, requires little or no training, some available online or in community programs (e.g., National Alcohol Screening Day).

<u>Diagnosis of substance use disorder</u>

Key question: Does the patient truly have a substance use disorder?

Examples of measures: Structured Clinical Interview for DSM-IV (Spitzer et al., 1997); Mini-International Neuropsychiatric Interview (Sheehan et al., 1998)

Notes: Alcohol and drug use disorders have separate diagnostic criteria. Training in both the measure and diagnostic criteria are required (usually DSM-IV, but may be ICD-9 or other system). Interrater reliability usually needs to be established. Most measures are interview based, but some self-report computerized versions also exist.

<u>Level of substance use</u>

Key question: What, how much, and how often is the patient using?

Examples of measures: Addiction Severity Index (McLellan et al., 1992); Timeline Follow-Back (Sobell & Sobell, 1992)

Notes: For clinical practice, the clinician often simply asks the three questions at each session: What type of substances have you used in the past week? How much of each (e.g., number of drinks)? How often for each? More formal measures are typically used for research. Related are measures of *cravings* for substances (see Abrams, 2000, for a review).

<u>Verification of substance use</u>

Key question: Is the patient telling the truth about use?

Examples of measures: Biological measures include urinalysis testing (home kit or laboratory), breath alcohol testing, and blood or hair analysis. Collateral informant measures involve corroboration by family members or others (Maisto, Sobell, & Sobell, 1982).

Notes: Accuracy of biological measures depend in part on how long ago the patient used (e.g., alcohol may be detected only within a few hours, whereas marijuana may be detected days later). Random testing and chain-of-custody procedures enhance accuracy. Collateral informant measures require the patient's written consent.

<u>Negative consequences of substance use</u>

Key question: How is the substance use affecting the patient's life?

Examples of measures: Inventory of Drug Use Consequences (Tonigan & Miller, 2002); Addiction Severity Index (McLellan et al., 1992)

Notes: Typical areas of assessment include impact of substance on legal, psychiatric, social, vocational, medical, and family functioning.

<u>Motivation for substance abuse treatment</u>

Key question: How motivated is the patient to engage in substance abuse treatment?

Examples of measures: Stages of Change Readiness and Treatment Eagerness Scale (Miller & Tonigan, 1994); University of Rhode Island Change Assessment Scale

Notes: The widely used *stages of change* model evaluates the patient's readiness in terms of stages (e.g., precontemplation, action, maintenance).

(continued)

TABLE 16.1. (*continued*)

Acute detoxification issues

Key question: Does the patient have any immediate medical issues related to addiction that need attention?

Examples of measures: Clinical Institute Withdrawal Assessment (Sullivan, Sykora, Schneiderman, Naranjo, & Sellers, 1989).

Notes: A patient who has had heavy abuse of alcohol or prescription medication usually needs medical evaluation and treatment prior to stopping. Referral can be made to a detoxification program or to an outpatient physician or psychiatrist who can evaluate the patient's needs.

Cognitive measures

Key question: How does the patient view the addiction?

Examples of measures: Beliefs about Substance Use (Wright, 1992); Cocaine Expectancy Questionnaire (Jaffe & Kilbey, 1994)

Notes: These are used to evaluate patients' reasons for using substances and their expectations about their ability to stop using.

Mental health treatment programs typically seek to add SUD measures. Because there are so many different types of SUD assessment, per Table 16.1, it is beyond the scope of this chapter to review them. However, mental health clinicians may not be aware that there is an extraordinary amount of material on SUD assessment and treatment that can be obtained free from the government, either downloaded from the Internet or ordered by phone. Because SUD is a major public health problem (indeed the most common lifetime Axis I disorder; Kessler et al., 1994), there is probably more available on SUD than any other psychiatric disorder. (See the "Resources for Assessment" section of this chapter.)

Research programs usually seek state-of-the-art measures and have readily available staff and training. Depending on the research questions, there may be need for rigorous interview-based diagnostic measures (such as the SCID), outcome assessment, and description of the sample. (See the "Resources for Assessment" section for ways to obtain psychometric information on SUD and PTSD measures). Also, a helpful method is to read research reports related to one's work and to obtain measures that others have used. For example, outcome research articles on the dual diagnosis of PTSD/SUD typically use the Structured Clinical Interview for DSM-IV (Spitzer et al., 1997), the Addiction Severity Index (McLellan et al., 1992), and the Timeline Follow-Back (Sobell & Sobell, 1992). By adopting these, one can more readily compare results with the existing literature. Other research considerations for SUD assessment include the need to establish whether psychoactive medications are taken as prescribed and to corroborate self-report of substance use with biological or collateral confirmation (see the section in Table 16.1, "Verification of Substance Use"). These considerations may also apply to clinical settings.

TABLE 16.2. Areas of Trauma/PTSD Assessment

Trauma

Key question: Did the patient experience a trauma?

Examples of measures: Trauma History Questionnaire (Green, 1996); Stressful Life Experiences Screening (Stamm et al., 1996)

Notes: In addition to identifying the events a patient experienced (e.g., rape, assault, accident), a good trauma measure also evaluates the other trauma criteria of DSM-IV (e.g., presence of fear, helplessness, or horror).

PTSD

Key question: Does the patient meet criteria for PTSD (the disorder most directly associated with trauma)?

Examples of measures: Clinician-Administered PTSD Scale (Blake et al., 1995); PTSD Checklist (Weathers et al., 1993); Modified PTSD Symptom Scale (Falsetti, Resnick, Resick, & Kilpatrick, 1993)

Notes: The PTSD diagnosis requires that the person meet criteria for having experienced a trauma. Some measures include this; others do not. Thus a trauma measure would be needed (see previous section of this table). Some PTSD measures are interview; others are self-report measures that take less time.

Other trauma-related diagnoses

Key question: Does the patient have other disorders related to trauma? These include acute stress disorder, dissociative disorders, and disorders of extreme stress—not otherwise specified (NOS).

Examples of measures: Structured Interview for Disorders of Extreme Stress—NOS (Pelcovitz, van der Kolk, Roth, Mandel, & Kaplan, 1997); Structured Clinical Interview for DSM-IV (Spitzer et al., 1997)

Notes: For complex diagnoses such as dissociative disorders, interviews are typically recommended.

Other trauma-related symptoms

Key question: Does the patient have other symptoms related to trauma? These include self-harm, dissociation, sexuality problems, and relationship problems, such as distrust.

Examples of measures: Trauma Symptom Checklist-40 (Elliott & Briere, 1990); Trauma Symptom Checklist for Children (Briere, 1996)

Notes: These measures may be especially helpful for clinical purposes and for outcome assessment because they provide levels of symptoms (rather than the yes/no format of many diagnostic measures). Also, trauma-related symptoms are broader than diagnostic criteria, and thus useful to measure, even if the patient meets criteria for PTSD or other diagnoses.

Cognitive measures

Key question: How has trauma affected the patient's beliefs?

Example of measure: World Assumptions Scale (Janoff-Bulman, 1989); Traumatic Stress Institute Belief Scale (1996)

Notes: Such scales address trauma-related beliefs, such as safety, trust, and loss.

Recognize the Complexity of the SUD Diagnosis

The SUD diagnosis is quite complex, requiring evaluation based on the substance (e.g., alcohol vs. cocaine), an understanding of remission categories (early full, early partial, sustained full, and sustained partial, depending on when and how many criteria the patient meets); and knowledge of symptoms of withdrawal and tolerance (which vary based on the substance). The complexity of the SUD diagnosis helps explain why it is so difficult to locate simple self-report diagnostic measures for SUD, as well as ones that evaluate both alcohol and drug use. Thus measures often come in two separate forms for alcohol and drugs (e.g., the Michigan Alcohol Screening Test for alcohol vs. the Drug Abuse Screening Test for drugs, Seltzer, 1971; Skinner, 1982; and the SCID alcohol module vs. the SCID drug use disorder module, Spitzer et al., 1997). SUD also does not usually lend itself to a direct translation into self-report format, in contrast to the PTSD diagnosis, which can easily be made into a short self-report (e.g., the PTSD Checklist; Weathers et al., 1993). Adding another layer of complexity is the assessment of nonsubstance addictions such as gambling, Internet use, sex, shopping, and other addictions, each of which has its own assessment measures (Lowinson et al., 1997).

When Assessing Trauma in Patients with SUD, "Less Is More"

In general, most assessment procedures assume that more information is better and that interviews (compared with self-report) obtain the best results. With SUD patients, the opposite may hold. When assessing trauma in this highly impulsive population, destabilization may occur if patients are asked to provide extensive details, which may evoke high levels of emotion that can lead to increased substance use or other unsafe behavior. Coffey et al. (2002), for example, found that substance cravings increase when patients are exposed to trauma memories. Indeed, studies of exposure therapy in this population, which ask patients to describe trauma in detail, have had mixed results (Brady, Dansky, Back, Foa, & Caroll, 2001; Ruzek et al., 1998; Keane, 1995; Ruzek et al., 1998; Solomon, Gerrity, & Muff, 1992), unless there is careful selection of patients (Coffey, Dansky, & Brady, 2002) or adaptation of exposure therapy for SUD (Najavits, Schmitz, Gotthardt, & Weiss, in press). Although an assessment of trauma is not exposure therapy per se, it is similar in potentially evoking intense emotions in patients who may not be prepared to cope with them and who may not be in a treatment context to process them sufficiently. The principle "first do no harm" applies to assessment as much as to treatment. Even if patients want to describe details of their trauma history, they often underestimate the level of emotion that results, and thus the assessor must serve as gatekeeper and limit the information to safe bounds. Thus it is suggested that only very basic trauma information be obtained at intake. A brief trauma screen, for example, does not require the patient to identify a great deal of detail. Later, if a patient is in an ongoing therapy and the timing is appropriate, it may become an important part of the therapy to explore details of the trauma. At intake, however, it may be best to ask only the information needed for the specific *purpose* of the assessment. Routinely asking patients for intrusive detail is not justified. For example, if the goal is to screen patients for possible PTSD, the assessor simply needs to know the trauma that the patient currently perceives as the "worst" or the "most upsetting." That trauma can be described in a word or phrase (e.g., "rape" or "stabbing"), from which the assessor may choose to conduct an assessment of PTSD. A related issue is whether to use an interview or written self-report format for trauma assessment. Results at this point are unclear. For example, one study found better results for interview (Bastiaens & Kendrick, 2002; another found better results for a checklist (Najavits, Weiss, Reif, et al., 1998). For some patients, it may be more difficult to say aloud to the assessor that one has been raped, for example, than to mark it on a checklist. The shame and embarrassment are more acute in an interview. Asking patients to use a written checklist increases their privacy and may be less destabilizing. It is suggested, however, that such a checklist be completed on site in the clinical setting, rather than filled out at home. It seems to work well to have the patient fill out the form in the waiting room with instructions to stop and ask for help if it becomes too upsetting.

Obtain Age-Appropriate Measures for Children and Adolescents

Measures of PTSD and SUD are now available for children and adolescents. A recent review of trauma measures for these age groups is provided by Ohan and Myers (2002), for example. For substance abuse, see recent reviews by Miller, Westerberg, and Waldron (1995) and Tarter and Kirisci (1999). See the "Resources for Assessment" section to obtain Treatment Improvement Protocol #31, Screening and Assessing Adolescents for Substance Use Disorders.

Consider the Context of the Assessment

For this dual diagnosis population, there may be contextual issues that affect honesty about SUD, PTSD, or both.

- A patient with SUD who reports high levels of psychiatric disturbance (e.g., depression, suicidality) may be refused entry into SUD treatment until stabilized; thus the patient may minimize such symptoms.
- A patient with PTSD who receives disability benefits for the disorder may not want to report a decrease in symptoms for fear of losing the benefits.
- A patient with SUD who reports recent substance use may be evicted from housing, lose custody of her children, or be fired from a job. SUD

is often inadequately addressed in rescue professions, for example, such as fire and police forces, because a diagnosis of SUD can result in removal from duty.

- Adolescents may fear restriction from friends or normal activities if they report substance use honestly.
- In some settings, such as prison or the military, reporting trauma perpetrated by those in power may result in punishment to the victim (Janofsky & Schemo, 2003).
- A patient going into surgery may not reveal a history of SUD for fear of obtaining inadequate pain medication, which is often restricted even if the patient has been abstinent for many years.

In short, various circumstances may lead to either increased or decreased reporting of PTSD or SUD symptoms. In the assessment, such contextual factors should be identified.

Know and Warn Patients of the Legal Implications of Assessment

Both PTSD and SUD may involve legal issues to a greater degree than other Axis I disorders. For example, SUD legal issues include drug dealing charges, driving under the influence, loss of custody of children, use of illegal drugs, and using while on the job. In a prison setting, if patients in treatment admit using a substance, they may have time added to their sentences. A helpful document from the federal government includes sample consent forms for SUD information, as separate consent may be needed for SUD assessment given the sensitivity of the information (Technical Assistance Protocol #13; see "Resources for Assessment"). Trauma assessment may, in some states, evoke mandatory reporting such that the clinician is required to report to authorities the name of and other information about a trauma perpetrator, even if the event was decades ago and the patient does not want the information reported. Another issue relevant to PTSD is the need for legal deposition prior to therapy for a patient who may want to initiate legal proceedings against a perpetrator; otherwise the therapist may be accused of creating false memories. For both PTSD and SUD, patients may not be aware that their records may be obtained by court order, even if the assessor assured them of confidentiality. Clinicians, particularly those in private practice or with little cross-training in both disorders, may inadvertently misinform or fail to inform patients of these various legal dilemmas. In research settings, some investigators are not aware that they can apply for a certificate of confidentiality for federally funded studies, which provides the highest level of protection of records, including from court orders (above and beyond standard institutional protections). Researchers can obtain information about the certificate from the institute that provided their funding.

Be Aware of Common Misdiagnoses

Misdiagnosis may involve errors of commission, omission, or both. An error of commission is giving a diagnosis that is not accurate (e.g., borderline personality disorder rather than PTSD, even though only the latter actually fits the patient). An error of omission is giving a diagnosis that is accurate but neglecting additional diagnoses that also may be present (e.g., a patient has both borderline personality disorder and PTSD, but receives only one of these diagnoses). As noted earlier, both PTSD and SUD are biased in the direction of being underdiagnosed. In addition to carefully assessing for both disorders, it is also important to ensure that additional psychiatric diagnoses, both Axis I and II, are accurate. Some common misdiagnoses for this population include the following.

- *Affective and anxiety disorders (e.g., depression, bipolar disorder, generalized anxiety disorder).* Affective disorders often co-occur with PTSD or SUD, and because they typically have less stigma and clearer medication regimens, they are more likely to be diagnosed. Yet such disorders may be secondary to PTSD or SUD or may be substance induced. For children and adolescents, attention-deficit/hyperactivity disorder may also be misdiagnosed.
- *Borderline personality disorder* (BPD). This diagnosis is known for being misused in place of a PTSD diagnosis (Herman, 1992). However, with growing recognition of this problem, some clinicians go to the opposite extreme, believing that BPD does not exist and that any patient who presents with such symptoms actually has PTSD. Both BPD and PTSD are legitimate diagnoses, and patients who have one do not automatically either have nor not have the other (Gunderson & Sabo, 1993). For example, in a sample of patients with SUD and PTSD, only about one-third also had BPD (Najavits, Weiss, Shaw, & Muenz, 1998); and vice versa, among patients with BPD and SUD, about one-third also had PTSD (Linehan et al., 1999).
- *Antisocial personality disorder* (ASP). Comparable to BPD, ASP may be diagnosed when, in fact, PTSD and SUD are more accurate. There is a clear gender pattern, with more males diagnosed with ASP and more females with BPD.

The best way to guard against misdiagnosis is to screen for major Axis I and II disorders. Asking the patient whether psychiatric symptoms occur only when using, only during withdrawal, or only when abstinent may also be helpful (Weiss et al., 1998). However, some patients will be unable to answer such questions because they have been using substances for so long that they cannot identify a period of nonuse. Finally, even the notion of "dual" diagnosis is a misnomer, as many patients with PTSD and SUD have additional co-occurring disorders, including affective disorders, other anxiety disorders, and Axis II disorders (Brady et al., 1994).

Be Prepared for Memory Problems

Patients with either disorder, or their combination, may have substantial memory problems. Indeed, patients with PTSD may use substances either as a way to forget trauma ("drinking to forget"; Stewart, 1997) or to remember (Ruzek et al., 1998). In PTSD, the issue of memory accuracy has received a great deal of research. A task force of the American Psychological Association came to the conclusion that although most trauma survivors remember all or part of what happened to them, there may be gaps in their memories, and pseudomemories are possible as well (i.e., memories the patient believes are accurate but that are not). They provide several helpful guidelines, including the precepts that hypnosis should not be used to uncover trauma memories and that clinicians need to maintain separate roles (e.g., forensic assessor from clinician) (Alpert et al., 1998). At least one study (Whitfield, 1998) found that patients with this dual diagnosis had difficulty remembering trauma and suggests that "soft signs" may be important to note, such as reenactments. In SUD, chronic use, acute use, withdrawal, and the tendency to deny or minimize use (conscious or not) all can impair memory. The assessor may need to be especially diligent in establishing rapport. It is also important not to assume that patients are willfully withholding information, although under some conditions this may occur.

Give Patients Feedback about Assessment Results

As described, the diagnoses of PTSD and SUD can be helpful for patients to understand that they are not alone and not "crazy." Diagnoses provide a way for patients to better understand their experiences, which can aid the recovery process. Some symptoms, too, even if not a full-blown disorder, may warrant discussion. For example, dissociation, depersonalization, and transient psychotic symptoms that may occur in severe PTSD or SUD may be very frightening to the patient. Learning that these occur in people with the dual diagnosis can help. It is thus suggested that patients be provided with an explanation of what was found in the assessment, if they want to know.

The Assessor's Style Is Important, Balancing Kindness with Directness

The assessor's style may determine the accuracy of information obtained. Given the stigma of both PTSD and SUD, patients often fear being judged, treated harshly, or misunderstood (Read et al., 2002). In some settings, they may have had very negative experiences with incompetent or uncaring professionals (Jennings, 1994). One study found that more than half of patients with this dual diagnosis report shame and blame as barriers to treatment (Brown et al., 1998). Paranoia is also commonly associated with both disorders and may increase distrust of professionals and systems. Several traits are thus central. First, the assessor needs to be kind. This means being nonjudgmental, even when hearing about difficult scenarios such as sex-for-drugs exchanges or drug dealing. Second, the assessor needs to be comfortable asking direct and "taboo" questions that patients may not want to address (e.g., How much are you using? Are you using around your children?). Some clinicians are much stronger at support than at directness and may unwittingly collude with the patient's illness by not asking such questions. Finally, the assessor needs to avoid power struggles and give the patient as much control as possible. Powerlessness is inherent in both trauma and SUD (Najavits, 2002b). Thus, it is suggested that the patient be given as much control as possible in the assessment process. This may include asking the patients' permission throughout the interview ("I'd like to ask you now about your level of substance use—is that okay with you?"), informing the patient that they can stop at any point, and checking how the patient is doing ("Is this okay so far?").

"Own" One's Countertransference

Both PTSD and SUD may evoke countertransference in the assessor. PTSD, for example, may stir painful identification with the patient's suffering, anger at patients' victimization, or distancing based on not wanting to feel vulnerable (Najavits, 2002a; Pearlman & Saakvitne, 1995; Wilson & Lindy, 1994). SUD, too, can evoke a range of responses, including hopelessness that the patient will ever improve and judgment of a lifestyle that may be far removed from the clinician's world (Imhof, 1991; Najavits et al., 1995). Although these issues are more often discussed with regard to treatment, they may also occur during assessment. Providing assessors with support and open discussion may help improve the assessment process.

If a Patient Is Intoxicated, Delay the Assessment

It is a serious mistake to attempt assessment if the patient shows up high or drunk. The patient is less likely to be accurate, the assessment may be more prone to upset the patient, and it can reinforce substance use. It is thus standard in SUD clinical settings that neither assessment nor treatment occurs unless the patient is sober. This does not mean that the patient must have a period of abstinence before assessment, but rather that the assessment will not proceed if the patient is visibly intoxicated. The assessor is responsible for calling a family member or taxi service to pick up the patient and for not allowing the patient to drive home under the influence. Even if the patient denies being intoxicated, it is the assessor's evaluation that determines how the situation is handled. Being kind but firm is key (e.g., "I will be happy to talk with you tomorrow, once you're no longer high").

Note That Prominence of PTSD Symptoms May Vary Based on Substance of Abuse

Some studies have evaluated PTSD symptom clusters in relation to SUD, with results varying based on the SUD population. For example, Stewart, Conrod, Pihl, and Dongier (1999) found that alcohol dependence correlated with PTSD arousal scores, anxiolytic dependence with arousal and numbing scores, and analgesic dependence with arousal, intrusions, and numbing scores (see also McFall, Mackay, & Donovan, 1992, for similar results). Najavits, Runkel, et al. (2003) found arousal the most common PTSD symptom cluster among cocaine-dependent patients. Also, those with the dual diagnosis differ from patients with PTSD alone in their symptoms. Saladin, Brady, Dansky, and Kilpatrick (1995) found that those with the dual diagnosis had more avoidance and arousal symptoms and more sleep disturbance than a PTSD-alone group. Brown (2000) found PTSD re-experiencing symptoms a key predictor of SUD relapse.

RESOURCES FOR ASSESSMENT

Online

A Web search with any key terms or combination ("assessment," "screen," "PTSD," "trauma," "substance abuse") will yield hundreds of hits. The resources listed here were selected because they offer (1) reputable sources, such as government or academic institutions; (2) extensive information, such as listings of measures and how to obtain them; and (3) searchable online databases, clearinghouses, free materials, and other resources.

Substance Use Disorders

NATIONAL INSTITUTE ON ALCOHOL ABUSE AND ALCOHOLISM (NIAAA)

The website *www.niaaa.nih.gov/publications/* provides a table listing more than 85 measures related to alcoholism, many of which can be directly downloaded. It describes target populations, administration characteristics (e.g., self-report, number of questions, training required), psychometric and scoring information, how to obtain or download the measures, and references. Measures that can be downloaded include, for example, the Addiction Severity Index, the Alcohol Dependence Scale, the Alcohol Effects Questionnaire, and the Denial Rating Scale. Also, *www.niaaa.nih.gov/publications/assess1.htm* provides an overview of alcohol assessment (e.g., general considerations, such as giving clients feedback).

UNIVERSITY OF NEW MEXICO CENTER ON ALCOHOLISM, SUBSTANCE ABUSE, AND ADDICTIONS

The website *http://casaa.unm.edu/inst/inst.html* (click "downloads") provides a wide variety of scales related to substance abuse that can be directly downloaded.

SUBSTANCE ABUSE AND MENTAL HEALTH SERVICES ADMINISTRATION (SAMHSA)

The website *http://store.health.org* (or 800-729-6686) provides a catalogue from which one can order free publications and products on addiction topics. Of particular relevance are the "knowledge application product" (KAP) keys and "quick guides," which provide brief, user-friendly assessment tools for clinicians.

The website *www.health.org* (National Clearinghouse for Alcohol and Drug Information) is one of the most widely known addiction resources, offering free publications, referral resources, and searchable online databases (*www.health.org/dbases*). It provides journal article information (e.g., enter "assessment" to search on that topic).

The website *http://samhsa.gov/centers/clearinghouse/clearinghouses.html* provides links to federal information clearinghouses, including those of the Center for Substance Abuse Treatment, the Center for Substance Abuse Prevention, the Center for Mental Health Services, Department of Health and Human Services, Centers for Disease Control and Prevention, Department of Justice, and many others. Each clearinghouse provides numerous online resources such as free publications, databases, and referrals.

The website *http://www.samhsa.gov* (click "publications," then "substance abuse treatment resources," then "TIE-treatment improvement exchange forum") provides free substance abuse assessment, prevention, and treatment resources that can be either downloaded or ordered free as hard copies. It includes the following:

- Click on "CSAT TIPS" for the *Treatment Improvement Protocol (TIP)* series of more than 35 guides written specifically for clinicians. Each provides a state-of-the-art consensus statement on best practices for a particular topic and includes a wide variety of materials that can be photocopied, such as assessment tools. Several focus on assessment, such as TIP 16 (Alcohol and Other Drug Screening of Hospitalized Trauma Patients), TIP 9 (Assessment and Treatment of Patients with Coexisting Mental Illness and Alcohol and Other Drug Abuse), and TIP 31 (Screening and Assessing Adolescents for Substance Use Disorders).
- Click on "CSAT TAPS" for the *Technical Assistance Publications (TAP)* series of more than 20 guides that provide information on practical is-

sues in the substance abuse field. For example, relevant to assessment are TAP 18 (Checklist for Monitoring Alcohol and Other Drug Confidentiality Compliance) and TAP 21 (Addiction Counseling Competencies: The Knowledge, Skills and Attitudes of Professional Practice).

- Click on "Private online resources" for links to more than 60 professional and nonprofit organizations devoted to addictions.
- Click on "Federal online resources" for links to more than 20 federal agencies relevant to addictions.

NATIONAL INSTITUTE ON DRUG ABUSE

Clicking "Publications" on *www.nida.nih.gov* provides publications that can be downloaded or ordered, including assessment tools, information on specific drugs of abuse, treatment manuals (which may include assessments), posters, and videos.

FREE ALCOHOL SCREENING

By answering questions online at *www.alcoholscreening.org*, based on the Alcohol Use Disorders Identification Test (Babor & Grant, 1989), respondents can obtain immediate feedback on their likelihood of having an alcohol problem. Referral information is also provided. Sponsored by Boston University and Join Together (a community-based drug prevention program).

HOME-TEST KITS FOR SUBSTANCE USE

Various companies provide low-cost home testing kits for urinalysis that can evaluate use of numerous substances. For testing alcohol use, a breathalyzer is typically used. Local pharmacies may stock both types of tests. Also, online, a search under the terms "drug test" or "breathalyzer" will locate numerous companies that offer these products. One example is *www.drugtestsuccess.com* (or 888-280-4194). A central source is *www.thomasregister.com*, which provides a table of different companies (enter the term "alcohol drug test").

Trauma/PTSD

NATIONAL CENTERS FOR PTSD

Clicking "assessment" on *www.ncptsd.org* provides tables on measures, including target group, administration (e.g., number of items, format), psychometrics, scoring, and information on obtaining them. Topics include assessment of trauma exposure, adult PTSD self-report, adult PTSD interviews, and child measures.

FREE TRAUMA/PTSD MEASURES

The website *www.isu.edu/~bhstamm/tests.htm* provides several free measures for trauma screening and PTSD assessment, including the Stressful Life Experiences Screening (Stamm et al., 1996) and the PTSD Checklist (Weathers et al., 1993).

The website *www.johnbriere.com* provides the Trauma Symptom Checklist–40 (click "TSC-40"), a free measure of trauma-related symptoms. Other trauma/PTSD measures by Briere are also described on the site, which can be ordered from Psychological Assessment Resources (800-331-TEST).

Books

Examples of books include the following:

Substance Use Disorders

Juhnke, G. A. (2002). *Substance abuse assessment and diagnosis: A comprehensive guide for counselors and helping professionals*. New York: Brunner-Routledge.

Murphy, L. L., & Impara, J. C. (1996). *Buros desk reference: Assessment of substance abuse*. Lincoln, NE: Buros Institute of Mental Measurements.

Perrin, E. B., & Koshel, J. (1997). *Assessment of performance measures for public health, substance abuse, and mental health*. Washington, DC: National Academy Press.

Trauma/PTSD

Briere, J. (1997). *Psychological assessment of adult posttraumatic states*. Washington, DC: American Psychological Association.

Carlson, E. B. (1997). *Trauma assessments: A clinician's guide*. New York: Guilford Press.

Pynsent, P. B., Fairbank, J. C. T., & Carr, A. J. (1994). *Outcome measures in trauma*. Burlington, MA: Butterworth-Heinemann.

Community Screenings

National outreach effort. Community-based annual screenings for alcohol and anxiety disorders (including PTSD) at local libraries, schools, workplaces, and clinics. See *www.mentalhealthscreening.org* for information, dates, and locations.

REFERENCES

Abrams, D. B. (2000). Transdisciplinary concepts and measures of craving: Commentary and future directions. *Addiction, 95*, S237–S246.

Alpert, J. L., Brown, L. S., Ceci, S. J., Courtois, C. A., Loftus, E. F., & Ornstein P. A. (1998). Final report of the American Psychological Association working group on investigation of memories of child abuse. *Psychology, Public Policy, and Law, 4*(4), 931–1068.

American Psychiatric Association. (1994). *Diagnostic and statistical manual of mental disorders* (4th ed.). Washington, DC: Author.

Babor, T. F., & Grant, M. (1989). From clinical research to secondary prevention: International collaboration in the development of the Alcohol Use Disorders Identification Test (AUDIT). *Alcohol Health and Research World, 13*(4), 371–374.

Bastiaens, L., & Kendrick, J. (2002). Trauma and PTSD among substance-abusing patients. *Psychiatric Services, 53*, 634.

Bernstein, D. P. (2000). Childhood trauma and drug addiction: Assessment, diagnosis, and treatment. *Alcoholism Treatment Quarterly, 18*, 19–30.

Blake, D., Weathers, F., Nagy, L., Kaloupek, D., Gusman, F., Charney, D., & Keane, T. (1995). The development of a Clinician-Administered PTSD Scale. *Journal of Traumatic Stress, 8*, 75–90.

Brady, K., Dansky, B., Back, S., Foa, E., & Caroll, K. (2001). Exposure therapy in the treatment of PTSD among cocaine-dependent individuals: Preliminary findings. *Journal of Substance Abuse Treatment, 21*, 47–54.

Brady, K. T. (2001). Comorbid posttraumatic stress disorder and substance use disorders. *Psychiatric Annals, 31*, 313–319.

Brady, K. T., Killeen, T., Saladin, M. E., Dansky, B. S., & Becker, S. (1994). Comorbid substance abuse and posttraumatic stress disorder: Characteristics of women in treatment. *American Journal on Addictions, 3*, 160–164.

Briere, J. (1996). Psychometric review of the Trauma Symptom Checklist-40. In B. H. Stamm (Ed.), *Measurement of stress, trauma, and adaptation*. Lutherville, MD: Sidran Press.

Brown, P. J. (2000). Outcome in female patients with both substance use and posttraumatic stress disorders. *Alcoholism Treatment Quarterly, 18*, 127–135.

Brown, P. J., Stout, R. L., & Gannon-Rowley, J. (1998). Substance use disorders–PTSD comorbidity: Patients' perceptions of symptom interplay and treatment issues. *Journal of Substance Abuse Treatment, 14*, 1–4.

Bureau of Justice Statistics. (1992). *Criminal victimization in the US, 1992*. Washington, DC: Author.

Clark, H. W. (2002, January). *Meeting overview*. Paper presented at the Trauma and Substance Abuse Treatment Meeting, Center for Substance Abuse Treatment, Bethesda, MD.

Coffey, S. F., Dansky, B. S., & Brady, K. T. (2002). Exposure-based, trauma-focused therapy for comorbid posttraumatic stress disorder–substance use disorder. In P. Ouimette & P. J. Brown (Eds.), *Trauma and substance abuse: Causes, consequences, and treatment of comorbid disorders* (pp. 209–226). Washington, DC: American Psychological Association Press.

Coffey, S. F., Dansky, B. S., Falsetti, S. A., Saladin, M. E., & Brady, K. T. (1998). Screening for PTSD in a substance abuse sample: Psychometric properties of a modified version of the PTSD Symptom Scale Self-Report. *Journal of Traumatic Stress*, *11*, 393–399.

Coffey, S. F., Saladin, M. E., Drobes, D. J., Brady, K. T., Dansky, B. S., & Kilpatrick, D. G. (2002). Trauma and substance cue reactivity in individuals with comorbid posttraumatic stress disorder and cocaine or alcohol dependence. *Drug and Alcohol Dependence*, *65*, 115–127.

Danksy, B. S., Roitzsch, J. C., Brady, K. T., & Saladin, M. E. (1997). Posttraumatic stress disorder and substance abuse: Use of research in a clinical setting. *Journal of Traumatic Stress*, *10*, 141–148.

Davidson, J. R. T. (2001). Recognition and treatment of posttraumatic stress disorder. *Journal of the American Medical Association*, *286*, 584–588.

Davis, T. M., & Wood, P. S. (1999). Substance abuse and sexual trauma in a female veteran population. *Journal of Substance Abuse Treatment*, *16*, 123–127.

El-Bassel, N., Schilling, R. F., Ivanoff, A., Chen, D. R., Hanson, M., & Bidassie, B. (1998). Stages of change profiles among incarcerated drug-using women. *Addictive Behaviors*, *23*, 389–394.

Elliott, D. M., & Briere, J. (1990). *Predicting molestation history in professional women with the Trauma Symptom Checklist (TSC-40)*. Paper presented at the Western Psychological Association, Los Angeles, CA.

Falsetti, S. A., Resnick, H. S., Resick, P. A., & Kilpatrick, D. G. (1993, June). The Modified PTSD Symptom Scale: A brief self-report measure of posttraumatic stress disorder. *Behavior Therapist*, 161–162.

Fletcher, A. (2001). *Sober for good: New solutions for drinking problems—Advice from those who have succeeded*. Boston: Houghton Mifflin.

Green, B. (1996). Trauma History Questionnaire. In B. H. Stamm (Ed.), *Measurement of stress, trauma, and adaptation* (pp. 366–369). Lutherville, MD: Sidran Press.

Gunderson, J. G., & Sabo, A. N. (1993). The phenomenological and conceptual interface between borderline personality disorder and PTSD. *American Journal of Psychiatry*, *150*(1), 19–27.

Gustafson, J. (1991). Do more . . . and do it better: Staff-related issues in the drug treatment field that affect the quality and effectiveness of services. *NIDA Research Monograph*, *106*, 53–62.

Herman, J. L. (1992). *Trauma and recovery*. New York: Basic Books.

Hien, D. A., Nunes, E., Levin, F. R., & Fraser, D. (2000). Posttraumatic stress disorder and short-term outcome in early methadone maintenance treatment. *Journal of Substance Abuse Treatment*, *19*, 31–37.

Hyer, L., Leach, P., Boudewyns, P. A., & Davis, H. (1991). Hidden PTSD in substance abuse inpatients among Vietnam veterans. *Journal of Substance Abuse Treatment*, *8*, 213–219.

Imhof, J. (1991). Countertransference issues in alcoholism and drug addiction. *Psychiatric Annals*, *21*, 292–306.

Jacobsen, L. K., Southwick, S. M., & Kosten, T. R. (2001). Substance use disorders in patients with posttraumatic stress disorder: A review of the literature. *American Journal of Psychiatry*, *158*, 1184–1190.

Jaffe, A. J., & Kilbey, M. M. (1994). The Cocaine Expectancy Questionnaire (CEQ): Construction and predictive validity. *Psychological Assessment*, *6*, 18–26.

Janoff-Bulman, R. (1989). *World Assumptions Scale*. Unpublished manuscript, University of Massachusetts, Amherst.

Janofsky, M., & Schemo, D. J. (2003, March). Women recount life as cadets: Forced sex, fear and silent rage. *The New York Times*, pp. 1, 19.

Jennings, A. (1994). On being invisible in the mental health system. *Journal of Mental Health Administration, 21,* 374–387.

Keane, T. M. (1995). The role of exposure therapy in the psychological treatment of PTSD. *Clinical Quarterly (National Center for Posttraumatic Stress Disorder), 5*(1), 3–6.

Kendler, K. S., Davis, C. G., & Kessler, R. C. (1997). The familial aggregation of common psychiatric and substance use disorders in the National Comorbidity Survey: A family history study. *British Journal of Psychiatry*, *170*, 541–548.

Kessler, R. C., McGonagle, K. A., Zhao, S., Nelson, C. B., Hughes, M., & Eshleman, S. (1994). Lifetime and 12-month prevalence of DSM-III-R psychiatric disorders in the United States: Results from the national comorbidity survey. *Archives of General Psychiatry*, *51*, 8–19.

Kessler, R. C., Sonnega, A., Bromet, E., Hughes, M., & Nelson, C. B. (1995). Posttraumatic stress disorder in the national comorbidity survey. *Archives of General Psychiatry*, *52*, 1048–1060.

Linehan, M. M., Schmidt, H., Dimeff, L. A., Craft, J. C., Kanter, J., & Comtois, K. A. (1999). Dialectical behavior therapy for patients with borderline personality disorder and drug dependence. *American Journal on Addictions*, *8*, 279–292.

Lisak, D. (1994). The psychological impact of sexual abuse: Content analysis of interviews with male survivors. *Journal of Traumatic Stress*, *7*(4), 525–548.

Lowinson, J., Ruiz, P., Millman, R., & Langrod, J. (Eds.). (1997). *Substance abuse: A comprehensive textbook* (3rd ed.). Baltimore: Williams & Wilkins.

Maisto, S. A., Sobell, L. C., & Sobell, M. B. (1982). Corroboration of drug abuser's self-reports through the use of multiple data sources. *American Journal of Drug and Alcohol Abuse*, *83*(9), 301–308.

Marlatt, G., Tucker, J., Donovan, D., & Vuchinich, R. (1997). Help-seeking by substance abusers: The role of harm reduction and behavioral–economic approaches to facilitate treatment entry and retention. In L. Onken, J. Blaine, & J. Boren (Eds.), *Beyond the therapeutic alliance: Keeping the drug-dependent individual in treatment* (pp. 44–84). Rockville, MD: U.S. Department of Health and Human Services.

McFall, M. E., Mackay, P. W., & Donovan, D. M. (1992). Combat-related posttraumatic stress disorder and severity of substance abuse in Vietnam veterans. *Journal of Studies on Alcohol*, *53*, 357–362.

McLellan, A. T., Kushner, H., Metzger, D., Peters, R., Smith, I., Grissom, G., et al. (1992). The fifth edition of the Addiction Severity Index. *Journal of Substance Abuse Treatment*, *9*, 199–213.

Mendelson, J. H., & Mello, N. K. (1998). Diagnostic evaluation of alcohol and drug abuse problems in women. *Psychopharmacology Bulletin*, *34*(3), 279–281.

Miller, W. R., & Tonigan, J. S. (1994). *Assessing drinkers' motivation for change: The Stages of Change Readiness and Treatment Eagerness Scale (SOCRATES)*. Unpublished manuscript, Center on Alcoholism, Substance Abuse, and Addictions, University of New Mexico, Albuquerque, NM.

Miller, W. R., Westerberg, V. S., & Waldron, H. B. (1995). Evaluating alcohol problems in adults and adolescents. In R. K. Hester & W. R. Miller (Eds.), *Handbook of alcoholism treatment approaches: Effective alternatives* (2nd ed., pp. 61–88). Needham Heights, MA: Allyn & Bacon.

Najavits, L. M. (2002a). Clinicians' views on treating posttraumatic stress disorder and substance use disorder. *Journal on Substance Abuse Treatment*, *22*, 79–85.

Najavits, L. M. (2002b). *Seeking Safety: A treatment manual for PTSD and substance abuse*. New York: Guilford Press.

Najavits, L. M. (2002c). *A woman's addiction workbook*. Oakland, CA: New Harbinger.

Najavits, L. M., Gastfriend, D. R., Barber, J. P., Reif, S., Muenz, L. R., Blaine, J., et al. (1998). Cocaine dependence with and without posttraumatic stress disorder among subjects in the NIDA Collaborative Cocaine Treatment Study. *American Journal of Psychiatry*, *155*, 214–219.

Najavits, L. M., Griffin, M. L., Luborsky, L., Frank, A., Weiss, R. D., Liese, B. S., et al. (1995). Therapists' emotional reactions to substance abusers: A new questionnaire and initial findings. *Psychotherapy*, *32*, 669–677.

Najavits, L. M., Runkel, R., Neuner, C., Frank, A., Thase, M., Crits-Christoph, P., & Blane, J. (2003). Rates and symptoms of PTSD among cocaine-dependent patients. *Journal of Studies on Alcohol*, *64*, 601–606.

Najavits, L. M., Schmitz, M., Gotthardt, S., & Wiess, R. D. (in press). Seeking Safety plus Exposure Therapy—revised: An outcome study in men with PTSD and substance dependence. *Journal of Psychoactive Drugs*.

Najavits, L. M., Sullivan, T. P., Schmitz, M., Weiss, R. D., & Lee, C. S. N. (2004). Treatment utilization of women with PTSD and substance dependence. *American Journal on Addictions*, *13*, 1–10.

Najavits, L. M., & Weiss, R. D. (1994). The role of psychotherapy in the treatment of substance use disorders. *Harvard Review of Psychiatry*, *2*, 84–96.

Najavits, L. M., Weiss, R. D., Reif, S., Gastfriend, D. R., Siqueland, L., Barber, J. P., et al. (1998). The Addiction Severity Index as a screen for trauma and posttraumatic stress disorder. *Journal of Studies on Alcohol*, *59*, 56–62.

Najavits, L. M., Weiss, R. D., & Shaw, S. R. (1997). The link between substance abuse and posttraumatic stress disorder in women: A research review. *American Journal on Addictions*, *6*, 273–283.

Najavits, L. M., Weiss, R. D., Shaw, S. R., & Muenz, L. R. (1998). "Seeking Safety": Outcome of a new cognitive-behavioral psychotherapy for women with posttraumatic stress disorder and substance dependence. *Journal of Traumatic Stress*, *11*, 437–456.

North, C. S., Nixon, S. J., Shariat, S., Mallonee, S., McMillen, J. C., Spitznagel, E. L., & Smith, E. M. (1999). Psychiatric disorders among survivors of the Oklahoma City bombing. *Journal of the American Medical Association*, *282*, 755–762.

North, C. S., Tivis, L., McMillen, J. C., Pfefferbaum, B., Spitznagel, E. L., Cox, J., et al. (2002). Psychiatric disorders in rescue workers after the Oklahoma City bombing. *American Journal of Psychiatry*, *159*, 857–859.

Ohan, J. L., & Myers, K. (2002). Ten-year review of rating scales: IV. Scales assessing trauma and its effects. *Journal of the American Academy of Child and Adolescent Psychiatry*, *41*, 1401–1422.

Ouimette, P., & Brown, P. J. (2002). *Trauma and substance abuse: Causes, consequences, and treatment of comorbid disorders*. Washington, DC: American Psychological Association Press.

Ouimette, P. C., Finney, J. W., & Moos, R. H. (1999). Two-year posttreatment functioning and coping of substance abuse patients with posttraumatic stress disorder. *Psychology of Addictive Behaviors*, *13*, 105–114.

Pearlman, L. A., & Saakvitne, K. W. (1995). *Trauma and the therapist: Countertransference and vicarious traumatization in psychotherapy with incest survivors.* New York: Norton.

Pelcovitz, D., van der Kolk, B. A., Roth, S. H., Mandel, F. S., & Kaplan S. (1997). Development of a criteria set and a structured interview for disorders of extreme stress (SIDES). *Journal of Traumatic Stress, 10,* 3–16.

Read, J. P., Bollinger, A. R., & Sharansky, E. (2002). Assessment of comorbid substance use disorder and posttraumatic stress disorder. In P. Ouimette & P. J. Brown (Eds.), *Trauma and substance abuse: Causes, consequences, and treatment of comorbid disorders* (pp. 111–125). Washington, DC: American Psychological Association Press.

Ruzek, J. I., Polusny, M. A., & Abueg, F. R. (1998). Assessment and treatment of concurrent posttraumatic stress disorder and substance abuse. In V. M. Follette, J. I. Ruzek, & F. R. Abueg (Eds.), *Cognitive-behavioral therapies for trauma* (pp. 226–255). New York: Guilford Press.

Saladin, M. E., Brady, K. T., Dansky, B. S., & Kilpatrick, D. G. (1995). Understanding comorbidity between PTSD and substance use disorders: Two preliminary investigations. *Addictive Behaviors, 20,* 643–655.

Seltzer, M. L. (1971). The Michigan Alcohol Screening Test: The quest for new diagnostic instrument. *American Journal of Psychiatry, 127,* 1653–1658.

Sheehan, D., Lecrubier, Y., Harnett Sheehan, K., Amorim, P., Janavs, J., Weiller, E., et al. (1998). The Mini-International Neuropsychiatric Interview (M.I.N.I.): The development and validation of a structured diagnostic psychiatric interview for DSM-IV and ICD-10. *Journal of Clinical Psychiatry, 59,* 22–33.

Skinner, H. A. (1982). Drug Abuse Screening Test. *Addictive Behavior, 7,* 363–371.

Smith, E. M., North, C. S., & Spitznagel, E. L. (1993). Alcohol, drugs, and psychiatric comorbidity among homeless women: An epidemiologic study. *Journal of Clinical Psychiatry, 54*(3), 82–87.

Sobell, L. C., & Sobell, M. B. (1992). Timeline Follow-Back: A technique for assessing self-reported alcohol consumption. In R. Litten & J. Allen (Eds.), *Measuring alcohol consumption* (pp. 41–72). New York: Humana Press.

Solomon, S. D., Gerrity, E. T., & Muff, A. M. (1992). Efficacy of treatments for posttraumatic stress disorder. *Journal of the American Medical Association, 268,* 633–638.

Spitzer, R. L., Williams, J. B. W., & Gibbon, M. (1997). *Structured Clinical Interview for DSM-IV—Patient Version.* New York: Biometrics Research Institute.

Stamm, B. H., Rudolph, J. M., Dewane, S., Gaines, N., Gorton, K., McNeil, F., et al. (1996, November). *Stressful Life Experiences Screening Instrument Short and Long Forms.* Poster presented at the 12th annual conference of the International Society for Traumatic Stress Studies, San Francisco.

Stewart, S. H. (1997). Trauma memory and alcohol abuse: Drinking to forget? In J. D. Read & D. S. Lindsay (Eds.), *Recollections of trauma: Scientific evidence and clinical practice* (pp. 461–467). New York: Plenum Press.

Stewart, S. H., Conrod, P. J., Pihl, R. O., & Dongier, M. (1999). Relations between posttraumatic stress symptom dimensions and substance dependence in a community-recruited sample of substance-abusing women. *Psychology of Addictive Behaviors, 13,* 78–88.

Substance Abuse and Mental Health Services Administration. (2001). *A provider's introduction to substance abuse treatment for lesbian, gay, bisexual, and transgender individuals*. Rockville, MD: U.S. Department of Health and Human Services.

Sullivan, J. T., Sykora, K., Schneiderman, J., Naranjo, C. A., & Sellers, E. M. (1989). Assessment of alcohol withdrawal: The revised Clinical Institute Withdrawal Assessment for Alcohol scale (CIWA-AR). *British Journal of Addiction, 84*, 1353–1357.

Tarter, R. E., & Kirisci, L. (1999). Psychological evaluation of alcohol and drug abuse in youth and adults. In P. J. Ott & R. E. Tarter (Eds.), *Sourcebook on substance abuse: Etiology, epidemiology, assessment, and treatment* (pp. 212–226). Needham Heights, MA: Allyn & Bacon.

Teplin, L. A., Abram, K. M., & McClelland, G. M. (1996). Prevalence of psychiatric disorders among incarcerated women: I. Pretrial detainees. *Archives of General Psychiatry, 53*, 505–512.

Teusch, R. (2001). Substance abuse as a symptom of childhood sexual abuse. *Psychiatric Services, 52*, 1530–1532.

Tonigan, J. S., & Miller, W. R. (2002). The Inventory of Drug Use Consequences (InDUC): Test–retest stability and sensitivity to detect change. *Psychology of Addictive Behaviors, 16*, 165–168.

Traumatic Stress Institute Belief Scale. (1996). Unpublished measure. South Windsor, CT: Traumatic Stress Institute.

Triffleman, E. (1998). An overview of trauma exposure, posttraumatic stress disorder, and addictions. In H. R. Kranzler & B. J. Rounsaville (Eds.), *Dual diagnosis and treatment: Substance abuse and comorbid medical and psychiatric disorders* (pp. 263–316). New York: Marcel Dekker.

Weathers, F. W., Litz, B. T., Herman, D. S., Huska, J. A., & Keane, T. M. (1993). *The PTSD Checklist (PCL): Reliability, validity, and diagnostic utility*. Paper presented at the International Society for Traumatic Stress Studies, San Antonio, TX.

Weiss, R. D., Najavits, L. M., & Mirin, S. M. (1998). Substance abuse and psychiatric disorders. In R. J. Frances & S. I. Miller (Eds.), *Clinical textbook of addictive disorders* (2nd ed., pp. 291–318). New York: Guilford Press.

Whitfield, C. L. (1998). Internal evidence and corroboration of traumatic memories of child sexual abuse and addictive disorders. *Sexual Addiction and Compulsivity, 5*, 269–292.

Wilson, J. P., & Lindy, J. D. (Eds.). (1994). *Countertransference in the treatment of PTSD*. New York: Guilford Press.

Wolfe, J., & Kimmerling, R. (1997). In J. P. Wilson & T. M. Keane (Eds.), *Assessing psychological trauma and PTSD* (pp. pp. 192–238). New York: Guilford Press.

Wright, F. D. (1992). *Beliefs about substance use*. Philadelphia, PA: Unpublished manuscript, University of Pennsylvania, Center for Cognitive Therapy.

Yehuda, R., Schmeidler, J., Wainberg, M., Binder-Brynes, K., & Duvdevani, T. (1998). Vulnerability to posttraumatic stress disorder in adult offspring of Holocaust survivors. *American Journal of Psychiatry, 155*, 1163–1171.

CHAPTER 17

Assessing Traumatic Bereavement

BEVERLEY RAPHAEL
NADA MARTINEK
SALLY WOODING

The idea of traumatic loss, of bereavements that are associated with traumatic stress as well as grief, has come to increasing prominence in recent times. These concepts have been linked to the understanding of the impact of horrific and profound traumatic deaths, such as those caused by terrorism, murder and other violent incidents on a mass scale, as well as individual circumstances of the death of a loved one (Raphael & Martinek, 1997; Raphael & Wooding, 2004). A core issue is that in some cases the *circumstances* of death in and of themselves represent a horrific and shocking encounter with death and thus lead to a traumatic stress reaction. For those bereaved in this way, the reactive processes of grief and those of traumatic stress make the response to the death and loss more "stressful," complex, and difficult to resolve. The impact of the traumatic stressor may lock the person to the death itself, its circumstance, horror, and images, and to the issue of personal survival in the face of terror, violence, and mass destruction. Grief and grieving may not be possible until later or not at all.

The study of response to mass deaths of this kind has generally been understood or researched only in terms of the traumatic stress/posttraumatic stress disorder (PTSD) phenomenology, with little attention to the bereavement impact and outcomes. For instance, in the recent wave of studies on the impact of September 11, 2001, only two studies at the time of this writing mentioned the losses and their impact (Galea et al., 2002; Schlenger et al., 2002).

Nevertheless, media portrayals of rituals of recognition, remembrance, and memorialization have powerfully identified the needs of those bereaved.

And specialized counseling has also been provided for them (Harvey, personal communication, 2002; Rynearson, personal communication, 2002). There is clearly a need to better understand the response to such traumatic loss, both for early intervention and management of the impact of mass violence (National Institute of Mental Health, 2001, Ritchie et al., 2001) as well as for the optimum management of such circumstances of violent and untimely deaths when they affect smaller numbers of people or individuals.

This chapter builds on earlier knowledge and conceptualization (Raphael, 1983; Raphael, 1986; Raphael & Martinek, 1997). It reviews work that has been reported since that time, including evolving understanding of abnormal, complicated, and chronic patterns of grief and new and emerging research on acute stress reactions, acute stress disorder (ASD), and PTSD as they may be relevant in this context. It also discusses quite specific research such as that of Prigerson et al. (1999), who developed diagnostic criteria for what was called "traumatic grief" and has now been renamed again as complicated grief disorder, as this term better reflects the broader clinical syndrome. This nomenclature has led to some confusion in this field. Concepts of chronic or abnormal grief (Raphael & Minkov, 1999) and those of coexistent grief and trauma or traumatic grief are further elaborated. This chapter examines the range of abnormalities of grief and the special issues of individual bereavement after individual traumatic deaths, such as homicide (Rynearson, 2002). Instruments, measures, and other assessment tools that can facilitate the assessment of reactions to trauma, loss, and traumatic loss are also reviewed. Implications for clinical assessment, clinical intervention, and management are briefly considered. As well, the needs for research development of this field are delineated.

CONCEPTUALIZATION OF TRAUMATIC STRESS, GRIEF, AND TRAUMATIC BEREAVEMENT

Trauma in the psychological sense was conceptualized by Freud (1920/1959) as following such external events as could lead to the mental apparatus being "flooded with large amounts of stimulus" that had "broken through the protective shield of the ego." These experiences could lead to "traumatic neuroses," with phenomena of fixation to the trauma and repetitions. Grief was described by Freud in *Mourning and Melancholia* (1917/1957). It involved preoccupation with thoughts of the dead person when he or she was alive, review of memories, and withdrawal bit by bit of bonds to the deceased. It involved "turning away from every effort not connected with thoughts of the dead" (p. 153). Thus, Freud saw these two psychological and phenomenological responses as different.

Lindemann's classic presentation of acute grief described symptoms and abnormal patterns of grief in those bereaved by what were likely to have been traumatic circumstances of death following the Coconut Grove nightclub fire

(Lindemann, 1944). He did not separate the two sets of phenomena, but his classical description of grief was influential, and the normal bereavement phenomena were not clarified until studies such as those of Parkes (1971) and Bowlby (1980). Thus it is possible that grief and trauma were seen as grief in this description if Lindemann's report is taken as that of "acute grief."

On the other hand, Horowitz's influential work with traumatic stress syndromes (Horowitz, 1976) included normal bereavement as a stressor and thus bereavement as a traumatic stress syndrome, whether or not the loss had come through traumatic death circumstances. The Impact of Event Scale (Horowitz, Wilner, & Alvarez, 1979) measured intrusive, reexperiencing, and avoidant phenomena but did not encompass the pathognomonic phenomena of grief and bereavement, namely, the yearning, longing, and pining of separation distress. Trauma and grief were thus not conceptualized or clarified separately in these studies or formulations.

Nevertheless, clinical and research studies were beginning to identify the elements of traumatic stress and grief as different reactions to specific stressors, particularly in more prospectively oriented studies.

Raphael and Maddison (1976), in studies of recently bereaved widows, reported on the "traumatic circumstances" of deaths that were risk factors for more adverse health outcomes, possibly because of a "traumatic neurosis" related to these circumstances that interfered with the grief process.

Rynearson (1984), in his clinical descriptions of bereavement following homicide, also highlighted the presence of posttraumatic stress phenomena, as well as bereavement phenomena. This work has been further extended in his intervention programs, which we discuss later. Similarly, studies of sudden infant death syndrome bereavements reported posttraumatic stress, as well as bereavement phenomena (Dyregov & Mattheisen, 1987), and that this was associated with more adverse outcomes than in those bereaved by stillbirth and neonatal deaths.

The study by Green, Grace, and Gleser (1985) of the survivors of the Beverly Hills Supper Club fire assessed the impact of bereavement, life threat, and other stressors that were part of the disaster experience. They also reported that in their outreach to survivors they found traumatic stress and bereavement to operate separately and that they required specific interventions, the trauma often having to be dealt with first before the grief could be worked with (Lindy, Green, Grace, & Tichener, 1983). McFarlane (1988a, 1988b) also assessed these stressor effects in researching the impact of Australian bush fires, but none of the researchers reported on the phenomenology of the bereavement over time.

The most important research to identify clearly these distinctions was that of Pynoos and colleagues (Pynoos, Frederick, et al., 1987; Pynoos, Nader, Frederick, Gonda, & Stuber, 1987). These workers studied a group of schoolchildren following a sniper attack at a school. They developed measures and assessed these children using a Grief Reaction Inventory of 9 items and a

Traumatic Stress Reaction Index of 16 items. They found that the severity of exposure to life threat correlated with high symptom levels on the Traumatic Stress Reaction Index. Closeness to a child who died correlated with scores on the Grief Index. They observed that sometimes these two sets of phenomenology were manifested independently, whereas at other times there was an interplay between the two. Life threat and traumatic stress reactive processes were likely to be associated with development of PTSD; loss was likely to be associated with a depressive episode or adjustment reaction and worry about a separation from someone close, such as a sibling, was associated with persisting anxiety about such separation (Pynoos, Frederick, et al., 1987; Pynoos, Nader, et al., 1987).

With an adult population, Schut, Keijser, Van Den Bout, and Dijhuis (1991) studied posttraumatic stress symptomatology in a group of bereaved people. Symptomatology was usually related to more shocking circumstances of the death. The researchers did not follow or differentiate patterns of traumatic stress and bereavement phenomena, however.

PHENOMENA IN CLINICAL AND RESEARCH STUDIES

Comparing traumatic stress and grief through clinical observations and findings from research studies can provide a useful template against which to examine new findings in this field.

Tables 17.1–17.4 present these phenomena in terms of cognitive processes, affective reactions, avoidance phenomena, and arousal phenomena. The comparison tables highlight differences, but it is recognized that experience of these phenomena and observations of them may not be so clear-cut in the reality of such acute and traumatic losses. They are, however, useful concepts for clinical assessment in such settings.

Cognitive Processes and Repetitive Phenomena

The preoccupations of those *traumatically stressed* are with the death and its circumstances; the death encounter; gruesome, horrific scenes of death; personal life threat; and so forth. These images and preoccupations are associated with intense anxiety, fear related to the trauma, repetition of the shock and horror, and the reexperiencing of the traumatic aspects of the event.

The *preoccupations of the bereaved* are with the lost person. The images that intrude are of the dead person when he or she was alive, and there is a yearning and longing for him or her to return. In the case of a traumatic bereavement, the images are likely to be of the dead person as dead, of the horrific nature of this death, and it may be difficult for the images of the person alive and longed for to be experienced in the process of grieving. These phenomena are presented in Table 17.1.

TABLE 17.1. Cognitive Phenomena of Posttraumatic Reactions and Bereavement

Posttraumatic phenomena	Bereavement phenomena
• Intrusions of *scene of trauma* (e.g., death) not associated with yearning or longing • Associated with distress, anxiety at image • Preoccupation with the *traumatic event* and circumstances of it • *Memories* usually of the *traumatic* scene • Reexperiencing of threatening aspects of the event	• Image of *lost person* constantly comes to mind (unbidden or bidden) • Associated with yearning or longing • Distress that person is not there • Preoccupation with the *lost person* and intense images of him or her • *Memories of person* associated with affect relevant to memory (often positive) • Reexperiencing of *person's presence,* as though he or she were still there (e.g., hallucinations of sound, touch, sight)

Affective Reactions

In the case of *traumatic stress reactive processes*, anxiety is predominately about the threat, about the death encounter. There is fear related to what happened, to threat and danger, and to the possibility of its return. It is precipitated by and specific to what happened and to reminders of the event.

In *normal bereavement* the anxiety is separation anxiety and is specific to separation from the lost person. It is about the absence of that person and is precipitated by his or her failure to return and the possibility of the future without him or her. Yearning, pining, and longing—if they occur in the case of traumatic stress—are for the world to be as it was, for the trauma not to have occurred. Yearning and longing are pathognomonic of bereavement and are for the lost person. They are triggered by reminders of her or him and are painful and intense. Sadness and nostalgia are part of grief but are rarely found with traumatic stress, unless they are related to concurrent losses. These phenomena are summarized in Table 17.2.

Avoidance Phenomena

Avoidance phenomena are seen as one of the key elements of *traumatic stress reactive processes*. The person wishes to avoid reminders, and this avoidance may be active or take the form of numbing of feeling, difficulty talking of what happened, or withdrawnal from others. In normal *bereavement* that is not related to traumatic deaths, the bereaved persons seek reminders of the loved ones, such as treasured memories, places, photos, objects, and so forth. They may try to avoid reminders of the person's absence, not of the person himself or herself. Although they try to mitigate the painful pangs of grief, they also recognize that this expression is part of the reaction to the loss and a "necessary" experience. They may seek the support of others and talk of the lost person. Those traumatized may wish to talk of the circumstances or may avoid such talk. Numbing and denial may, of course, be an integral part of both sets of reactive processes. See Table 17.3 for a summary of avoidance phenomena.

Arousal Phenomena

Both those psychologically traumatized and those bereaved are likely to experience high levels of arousal unless dissociation and denial supervene. This arousal diminishes over time unless negative trajectories appear, foreshadowing pathologies in these spheres. Arousal in those traumatized by an encounter with life threat and death is oriented to such threat and danger, and individuals scan the environment for danger. They are alert to it, demonstrate an exaggerated startled response, and overreact to cues related to the trauma.

Those bereaved (but not traumatized) are also hyperaroused, but they scan their environment not for threat but for the lost person or cues to them. They search for the lost person in familiar places, and they overrespond to cues, misperceiving the person's presence, image, touch, or voice. These comparisons are summarized in Table 17.4.

TABLE 17.2. Affective Phenomena

Posttraumatic phenomena	Bereavement phenomena
	Anxiety
• Anxiety is the principal affect	• Anxiety, when present, is *separation* anxiety
• And is *general* and generated by threat	• Is specific and generated by separation from lost person
• Fearful of *threat/danger*	• Is generated by imagined future without lost person
• Precipitated by *reminders, intrusions*	• Precipitated by his or her *failure to return*
Yearning/longing	
• These are not prominent features	• Yearning for lost person
• Not person oriented; if occurs, is for things to have been as they were before—for the return of "innocence of death" and the sense of personal invulnerability	• Is intense, painful, profound • Is triggered by reminders of him or her • Yearning for him or her to return, to be there
	Sadness
• Sadness not commonly described	• Sadness frequent and profound
• Nostalgia for event not described	• Feelings of nostalgia common and persistent

TABLE 17.3. Avoidance Phenomena

Posttraumatic phenomena	Bereavement phenomena
• *Avoids* reminders of event, including places • Attempts to lessen affect; numbing, lessened feelings generally • May have great difficulty talking of event during avoidance times, although at others may be powerfully driven to talk of the experience (but not person) • Withdrawal from others (protective of self)	• May search for and *seek out* places of familiarity, *treasured objects* (e.g., linking objects, photos and images) • May try to *avoid reminders of the absence* of the lost person • May try to *mitigate* pangs of grief but only temporarily, including distracting, but also seeks to express grief as normal • May be very driven to talk of lost relationship and lost person • May seek others for support or to talk of deceased

Other Phenomena

Observations suggest that there are basic psychobiological and sociocultural differences in terms of traumatic stress reactions and grief reactions. However, the systematic study of these reactive processes from the earliest stages is only now developing. Changes over time are seen as reflecting normal phenomena that may be resolving, continuing, and worsening. Some of these psychophysiological phenomena are discussed below.

Nevertheless, one set of early observations is worthy of comment. Charles Darwin (1872), in his work *The Expression of Emotion in Man and Animals* differentiated the reactions to traumatic threat and danger and those of grief in terms of the facial expression.

He described the reactions that occur on witnessing or experiencing something horrific, something associated with fear and threat, and reactions associated with grief. The differing facial expressions and facial muscles used are described and fit well with many portrayals of trauma and grief. These are summarized in Table 17.5.

TABLE 17.4. Arousal Phenomena

Posttraumatic phenomena	Bereavement phenomena
• *Oriented to threat* and danger	• Oriented to lost person
• General *scanning and alertness to danger,* fearfulness	• General *scanning* of *environment for lost one or cues* of him or her
• Exaggerated *startle* response (i.e., response to minimal threat)	• Generates *searching* behavior
• Overresponse to cues of trauma	• Overresponse to cues of lost person

TABLE 17.5. Other Phenomena: Signs of Reactive Process

Posttraumatic phenomena	Bereavement phenomena
• Occur on witnessing something horrific, torture, etc., fear and threat • "probably that horror would generally be accompanied by *strong contraction of the brow*, but as far as fear is one of the elements, the *eyes and mouth* would be *opened*, and the *eyebrows raised*—as far as antagonistic action of the corrugations permitted this movement" (pp. 322–323) • "*Contraction of platysma* does add greatly to the expression of fear" (p. 317) • Eyes somewhat staring • Pupils may be dilated	• "Contraction of the grief muscles . . . appears to be common to all the races of mankind" (p. 185) • *Obliquity of the eyebrows* contraction of central fascia of frontal muscle • Inner ends of eyebrows (p. 188) puckered into bunch • Transverse furrows across the middle part of the forehead • *Depression of corners of mouth* Mouth closed Corners drawn downward and outward (pp. 201–202) Curved mouth concavely downward

Note. Page numbers are from Darwin (1872/1998).

DEVELOPMENTS RELEVANT TO TRAUMATIC BEREAVEMENT

The concept of "traumatic grief" was developed by Prigerson et al. (1997) in a reexamining and revaluation of their concept of complicated grief disorder. Prigerson et al.'s work clearly described abnormal and chronic patterns of grief in patients studied 6 months and more following the deaths of their loved ones. This concept showed reactive processes that continued with phenomena such as ongoing preoccupation with images of the loved one who had died and feelings of being unable to manage without the dead person. This complicated grief was seen as traumatic because of the presence of separation distress related to the loss and a type of traumatic distress related to the loss of a long-standing and apparently dependent relationship. This pattern of relationship has been identified elsewhere as increasing the risk of complicated and adverse bereavement outcomes (Raphael, 1977; Parkes & Weiss, 1983). Prigerson et al. (1997) suggest, in line with this, that a traumatic loss is one that "disrupts a person's sense of safety and control" and that it causes a "loss of sense of identity and purpose." Clearly, this definition differs from the life threat/death encounter that leads to traumatic stress reactions as described previously and from the key criterion A necessary for the diagnosis of ASD and PTSD, the pathological sequelae of such exposure.

Elsewhere, Jacobs and Prigerson (2000) make it clear that "central to their concept of 'Traumatic Grief' is separation anxiety," and, more recently still, they have returned to use the term "complicated grief disorder" (Prigerson, personal communication, 2002; Gray, Prigerson, & Litz, 2004).

Nevertheless, in a series of studies of complicated grief or traumatic grief, Prigerson and her colleagues (1997, 1999) have shown that this syndrome can be distinguished from anxiety and depression syndromes even though strongly linked to adverse outcomes in terms of physical or mental health. They also found it to be associated with heightened suicidal ideation.

At around the same time, Horowitz et al. (1997) described complicated grief disorder as a syndrome. This had many features in common with Prigerson's complicated grief disorder, or traumatic grief (Prigerson et al., 1999). Table 17.6 describes some common symptoms of complicated grief disorder and traumatic grief.

Both these syndromes are distinct from postbereavement-related morbidity of anxiety and depressive disorders. Careful examination of these patterns and time lines shows that those syndromes reflect many symptoms of normal acute grief, continuing in chronic, intense, and disabling ways. Although avoided grief is part of Horowitz's syndrome, in many other ways the two are similar (see Table 17.6).

Middleton, Burnett, Raphael, and Martinek (1996) and Middleton, Moylan, Raphael, and Martinek (1998) studied and analyzed bereavement phenomena over time, using a measure developed by factor analysis of bereavement phenomena from other significant studies. The measure of 17 Core Bereavement Items (the CBI) showed changes over time in the studies of bereaved adults, assessed at 1 month and at 10 weeks and followed over 6 or 7 months and 13 months. This measure showed changes over time on the core bereavement phenomena and differences between those bereaved through

TABLE 17.6. Assessing Grief: Common Symptoms of Complicated Grief Disorder and Traumatic Grief

	Complicated grief disorder (Horowitz et al., 1997)	Traumatic grief[a] (Prigerson et al., 1999, Table 2, p. 71)
Cognitive		
Intrusive thoughts/fantasies	+	+
Yearning	+	+
Affective		
Emptiness/loneliness	+	+
Anger/irritability	–	+
Overwhelming emotion	+	–
Behavioral		
Avoidance	+	–
Sleep disturbance	+	+
Poor adaptation at work, socially, etc.	+	+

[a]Now complicated grief.

death of a parent, a spouse, or a child, the latter being the most intense. A similar study in the elderly showed the value of a related measure of the phenomenology of bereavement with the elderly (Byrne & Raphael 1994). Sound psychometric properties were established for this measure (Burnett, Middleton, Raphael, & Martinek, 1997). In these and other studies of these phenomena, it was found that about 9% showed continuing high levels of bereavement-related distress/symptoms that continued beyond 3–4 months and 13 months or more.

The major dimensions of phenomena in the CBI are in three factors:

1. *Images and Thoughts*, with seven items of cognitions about the person who is lost (e.g., "Do you find yourself preoccupied with images or memories of *X*?"; "Do you find yourself thinking of reunion with *X*?").
2. *Acute Separation*, with five items including yearning and focusing on the lost person (or arousal oriented to the person and searching; e.g., "Do you find yourself pining for/yearning for *X*?"; "Do you find yourself looking for *X* in familiar places?"; "Do you feel distress/pain if for any reason you are confronted with the reality that *X* is not present/not coming back?").
3 *Grief*, with five items of affective response to reminders of the lost person, including sadness (e.g., "Do reminders of *X*, such as photos, situations, music, places, etc., cause you to feel longing for *X*?"; "Do reminders of "*X*" such as photos, situations, music, places, etc., cause you to feel loneliness?"; "Do reminders of *X*, such as photos, situations, music, places, etc., cause you to feel sadness?").

This pattern could be seen as a form of chronic grief or abnormal grief, but not as specifically related to any traumatic stress component (Raphael & Minkov, 1999). As can be seen, there are common symptoms with those described by Prigerson et al. (1999) and Horowitz et al. (1997), as described previously.

Prigerson et al. (1999) after establishing diagnostic criteria for traumatic grief and reiterating their findings (Prigerson & Jacobs, 2001), have more recently renamed their syndrome "complicated grief" (Prigerson, 2002, personal communication; Gray et al., 2004). This is helpful as it removes some of the confusion that arose with this term and clarified its difference from traumatic stress and bereavement co-occurring in response to traumatic, violent, and horrific deaths. Gray et al. (2003) clearly distinguish the difference between these patterns and those of PTSD syndrome and draw from the conceptualizations of Raphael and Martinek (1997). Furthermore, the authors argue against an overarching loss as trauma framework, such as that suggested by Green (2000), which they see as failing to adequately take into account the unique biological, psychological, and social–behavioral aspects of the bereavement reaction. Nevertheless, as these authors and Prigerson's (1997) earlier studies demonstrate, morbid outcomes and correlates are frequent, including increased risk of suicide and impact on quality of life and adverse physical health events. Furthermore, when recent bereavements were assessed for PTSD and complicated grief, the authors reported a level of comorbidity between these syndromes (Gray et al., 2004).

Studies of homicide victims' bereavements and development of intervention programs for these has been the focus of important programs such as those of Rynearson (2001) on restorative storytelling as a bereavement intervention following bereavement through violent deaths. Rynearson showed that the trauma associated with homicide deaths was such that, even if the bereaved was not present at the death, traumatic images and intrusions and other phenomena related to its circumstances were still likely to disrupt and complicate the grieving process. Bereaved affected in this way were likely to be so affected by this trauma that it was often only later that they could engage in supportive bereavement-focused interventions to progress with their grieving (Rynearson, 2001).

TRAUMATIC BEREAVEMENTS: PATTERNS OF TRAUMATIC STRESS AND GRIEF OVER TIME

The actual high levels of distress and other reactive phenomena that may appear with either traumatic stress or grief reactions or a combination of these need to be considered in context, and any assessment process needs to take such a context into account, as should any proposal for intervention.

Acute and Emergency Contexts and Assessment

In the acute circumstance of such loss, horror, disbelief, fear, a sense of unreality, and dissociative response may all be considered as a normal reaction to what has happened. And this is of course the more so when there is ongoing violence, threat, danger, and uncertainty. In the instance of a terrorist attack or other mass violence, key principles of *response* would include containing the threat and ensuring survival, as far as is possible, of those who have not been killed. Triage of the acutely and severely injured who have a chance of survival is part of this. Even in more individual circumstances of homicide, chaos, fear, and uncertainty may prevail, especially in those homicides that occur in family or personal settings. The aims of ensuring survival, safety, security, and shelter of those surviving are the first requirements. Compassionate outreach and practical and human responses are the core elements of these earliest responses.

Identifying those who are affected and assessing their basic needs flows on from this and may be part of triage, rescue, and the provision of places of security. Registration of those separated from loved ones, who may or may not be deceased, is the first step in identifying those who may need more detailed subsequent assessment and follow-up.

The principles of a "psychological first aid" were described by Raphael (1977) and have been linked to such triage in terms of the mental state of the affected person or persons, identifying those who are so highly *aroused* that this is threatening to their functioning, who are showing the *behaviors* that place themselves or others at high risk, or whose *cognition* is impaired (either from organic or psychologically induced effects). Thus, in the emergency, a brief, clinically based assessment of these aspects of functioning may indicate a person acutely in need of more in-depth assessment and care. Protection from harm, containment and support to decrease arousal, and giving comfort may all help. Those who are separated from loved ones (e.g., children, partner, parents) whom they fear may be deceased may demonstrate intense searching behaviors, which may be fruitless and place themselves and others at further risk.

Provision of Accurate Up-to-Date Information

As soon as feasible, it is important to give those separated from loved ones knowledge of where they are or what has happened to them. Information provision is an intervention of significance at this time, as others and those traumatically bereaved may need assessment of their physical, social, cultural, and mental health needs continuing through this process.

Assessment in the Period of the Following Days and Weeks

Continuing assessment in the early stages of traumatic bereavement is part of accumulating data and documentation of key parameters relevant for acute management, identification of risk, and follow-up for care. Here the key themes of "therapeutic assessment" start the linkage to a chain of staged assessments and actions:

- Has a loved one died, or is he or she missing?
- What is known of the circumstances of the death? Is it likely that these, in and of themselves, constitute a traumatic stressor?
- What will be the official processes (including legal) required in terms of confirming the death and the dead person's identity? How may these affect those bereaved? (for instance, disaster victim identification processes, criminal investigations, the actuality or otherwise of the death and state of the remains)?
- What are the cultural and social requirements for those bereaved with regard to the deceased and their remains, and will these be able to be fulfilled?
- What processes exist for those bereaved that will assist their capacity to deal with the traumatic grief (for instance, social networks, personal

strengths and resources, community support, acknowledgment, and recognition of the traumatic event and subsequent need to grieve)?

Thus assessment commences, first informally, and then more formally linked to information systems and required processes. It is only later that it can link with continuity to a more *formal assessment* process, usually after the first week or weeks following the emergency, depending on whether or not the emergency is still ongoing. For if it is, or if the bereaved faces, as is more usual than not, many other stresses, the psychological mode at this early stage may be that of survival. Psychological, as well as physical, survival needs must be recognized. These may explain some of the bereaved's focus on action rather than expression of feeling, or appearing "in control" or "unaffected." For the bereaved, this may not be a time when he or she can either deal with the trauma or allow the grief free rein.

Assessment of Reactive Processes

The next stage, clinically based assessment, needs to take further into account the possible changes over time that may indicate vulnerability and need for preventive or treatment interventions, either at this time or subsequently. These should be provided in effective, compassionate, and acceptable ways.

Assessment entails the concept of therapeutic assessment.

Assessment of the Circumstances of the Death

This first step allows for assessment of reactions to the circumstances of the death as a potential traumatic stressor, including whether or not they would meet criterion A of an ASD/PTSD diagnosis in DSM-IV and whether dissociation, intrusive repetition of these traumatic circumstances, avoidance and numbing responses, or heightened arousal and its associated phenomena are present. It will also be possible to monitor from such a baseline (be it ASD or not) the progress and change of these phenomena over time. The ongoing presence of high levels of these phenomena, particularly to the level of ASD, persistent dissociative phenomena, or persistent rumination on the circumstances (4 weeks on), may be predictive of chronic PTSD in this domain (Murray, Ehlers, & Mayou, 2002).

Assessment of the Relationship between the Bereaved and the Deceased

A history of this relationship allows the bereaved to talk of their loved one and assessment of the phenomena of preoccupation—yearning, longing and separation distress, and sadness and review of memories—the psychological processes of grief.

The presence of these phenomena and the changes over time will enable an assessment of the reactive processes of grieving for the lost person. It will allow assessment of whether or not there are persisting high levels of bereavement-related distress, 4 weeks or more on, which may be related to heightened risk of chronic grief.

It will also provide the basis for assessment of the nature of the relationship with the deceased and whether intense dependence in the relationship or high levels of ambivalence will further complicate the grieving process, perhaps leading to complicated grief or other pathologies. Previous studies have established the relevance of these risk factors for adverse bereavement outcomes (Vachon, Lyall, & Rogers, 1980; Parkes & Weiss, 1983; Raphael, 1977).

Assessment of Events Since the Death

Assessment of events since the death allows further clarification of changes over time, additional stressors, social support, and progress or lack of progress and the degree to which the bereaved may be ready to deal with their psychological needs in relation to the death and its circumstances, as well as the loss.

It is of interest that intense and prolonged initial distress, as for instance with ASD (Bryant & Harvey, 1997) or as indicated by Weisaeth's (1989) work in Norway, has been predictive of later PTSD. Similarly, Vachon et al. (1980) reported that high levels of acute distress in grieving widows is predictive of chronic grief, as Middleton (1996) also demonstrated with bereaved adults following the death of parents, partners, and most particularly children.

Structured Assessment by Measures and Tests

Although it is clear from the preceding that it may be extremely difficult, and at times ethically constrained, for systematic assessment using reliable and valid measures to take place in the earliest days or weeks, the need to expand knowledge in this field and to ensure replication of findings and evaluation of interventions is also crucial.

Extensive reviews of PTSD measures form a core aspect of this volume and are covered elsewhere. Structured assessment of the traumatic stress components might range from psychophysiological measures such as reactivity to scripted imagery to the neuroendocrine studies of cortisol and cortisol challenge (Davidson, 2002). It will also be useful, when acceptable and possible, to explore changes from the acute phase over time, in terms of functional brain scans, examining areas such as the hippocampus (Hull, 2002), which has been implicated in studies of chronic rather than evolving posttraumatic stress disorder.

Similarly, with bereavement, a recent review (Hall & Irwin, 2001) has examined neuroendocrine and psychoimmune studies of bereavement, showing the impact on immune function of acute bereavement and the variable patterns of cortisol response (more related to depression), and of functional brain scanning that shows reactions to experimentally induced sadness and, again, depressive aspects.

None of these findings, except perhaps those of psychophysiological reactions to scripted imagery in PTSD or the specific impact of the trigger of the lost person, will as yet contribute in reliable and valid ways to assessment.

Standardized psychological questionnaires and measures for PTSD are well reviewed in this volume.

For acute emergencies and their sequelae, brief measures that are reliable and valid in terms of the phenomena described will be of most value. Thus measures such as that reported by Brewin et al. (2002), the Acute Stress Disorder Scale/Measure of Bryant and Harvey (1997), or measures such as those proposed by Murray et al. (2002) and Pynoos, Nader, et al. (1987) have provided useful measures for children such as the Child Posttraumatic Stress Reaction Index. Pynoos, Frederick, et al.'s (1987) and Pynoos, Nader, et al.'s (1987) Grief Reaction Index has established validity with children and has been used in such acute and longer term circumstances (Pynoos, Frederick, et al., 1987; Laor et al., 2002).

For bereavement, measures used in acute settings, such as the Core Bereavement Items (CBI; Middleton et al., 1996; Burnett et al., 1997), are particularly useful, as are the Texas Revised Inventory of Grief (TRIG; Faschingbauer, 1987), the Inventory of Complicated Grief (ICG; Prigerson et al., 1995), or indeed the phenomenological measures used by Jacobs et al. (1987). These have been well reviewed by Niemeyer and Hogan (2001). The problem with each and all of these traumatic stress and grief measures is that they do not adequately define the phenomena listed in the tables in this chapter and thus may fail to clarify either acute or evolving phenomena of traumatic stress and grief or, indeed, their differentiation and interaction, their changes over time, and their linkages with emerging pathologies, either general or specific. Research proposed with a Web-based model of survey such as Litz, Gray, Bryant, and Adler (2002), although of value, may also fail to make these needed clarifications.

CONCLUSION

There is clearly a need to recognize and respond to traumatic stress and loss, to traumatic bereavements and evolving vulnerabilities, and to pathologies associated with these. It is vital to understand the patterns and correlates of the strengths and personal growth that follow mourning. The field needs systematic research to inform the understanding of the morbidity that arises as a consequence of mass violence or the resilience and personal strengths that may help people to adapt.

The assessments delineated herein have been derived from responses to such emergencies, from research and the issues that arise in the aftermath of traumatic loss. Like all assessments, they should be empathetic to the needs of those so profoundly affected by such tragedies. They should "do no harm." And they should provide the basis for programs of prevention and care. To achieve these goals and lead to better outcomes, research and assessment methods need to be responsive to such acutely distressing circumstances, compassionate in their implementation, culturally sensitive, and scientifically appropriate, with the utilization of qualitative and quantitative, as well as clinical, social, and biological, data.

REFERENCES

Bowby, J. (1980). *Attachment and loss: Vol. 3. Loss, sadness, and depression*. London: Hogarth Press.

Brewin, C. R., Rose, S., Andrews, B., Green, J., Tata, P., McEvedy, C., et al. (2002). Brief screening instrument for posttraumatic stress disorder. *British Journal of Psychiatry*, *181*, 158–162

Bryant, R. A., & Harvey, A. G. (1997). Acute stress disorder: A critical review of diagnostic issues. *Clinical Psychology Review*, *17*, 757–773.

Burnett, P., Middleton, W., Raphael, B., & Martinek, N. (1997). Measuring core bereavement phenomena. *Psychological Medicine*, *27*, 49–57.

Byrne, G. J., & Raphael, B. (1994). A longitudinal study of bereavement phenomena in recently widowed elderly men. *Psychological Medicine*, *24*, 411–421.

Darwin, C. (1998). *The expression of emotion in men and animals* (3rd ed.). London: HarperCollins. (Original work published 1872)

Davidson, J. R. T. (2002). Surviving disaster: What comes after the trauma? *British Journal of Psychiatry*, *181*, 366–368.

Dyregov, A., & Mattheisen, S. B. (1987). Anxiety and vulnerability in parents following the death of an infant. *Scandinavian Journal of Psychology*, *28*, 16–25.

Faschingbauer, T. R., Zisook, S., & DeVaul, R. (1987). The Texas Revised Inventory of Grief. In S. Zisook (Ed.), *Biopsychosocial aspects of grief and bereavement* (pp. 111–124). Washington, DC: American Psychiatric Press.

Freud, S. (1957). Mourning and melancholia. In *Collected papers* (Vol. 4). New York: Basic Books. (Original work published 1917)

Freud, S. (1959). *Beyond the pleasure principle*. New York: Bantam. (Original work published 1920)

Galea, S., Ahern, J., Resnick, H., Kilpatrick, D., Bucuvalas, M., Gold, J., et al. (2002). Psychological sequelae of the September 11 terrorist attacks in New York City. *New England Journal of Medicine*, *346*, 982–987.

Gray, M. J., Prigerson, H. G., & Litz, B. T. (2004). Conceptual and definitional issues in complicated grief. In B. T. Litz (Ed.), *Early intervention for trauma and traumatic loss* (pp. 65–84). New York: Guilford Press.

Green, B. L. (2000). Traumatic loss: Conceptual and empirical links between trauma and bereavement. *Journal of Personal and Interpersonal Loss*, *5*, 1–17.

Green, B. L., Grace, M. C., & Gleser, G. L. (1985). Identifying survivors at risk: Long-term impairment following the Beverly Hills Supper Club fire. *Journal of Consulting and Clinical Psychology*, *53*, 672–678.

Hall, M., & Irwin, M. (2001). Physiological indices of functioning in bereavement. In M. S. Stroebe, R. O. Hannson, W. Stroebe, & H. Schut (Eds.), *Handbook of bereavement research: Consequences, coping, and care* (pp. 473–492). Washington, DC: American Psychological Association.

Horowitz, M. J. (1976). *Stress response syndromes*. New York: Aronson.

Horowitz, M. J., Siegel, B., Holen, A., Bonanno, G. A., Milbrath, C., & Stinson, C. H. (1997). Diagnostic criteria for complicated grief disorder. *American Journal of Psychiatry*, *154*, 904–910.

Horowitz, M., Wilner, N., & Alvarez, W. (1979). Impact of Event Scale: A measure of subjective stress. *Psychosomatic Medicine*, *41*, 209–218.

Hull, A. M. (2002). Neuroimaging findings in post-traumatic stress disorder: Systematic review. *British Journal of Psychiatry*, *181*, 102–110.

Jacobs, S., Kasl, O., Ostfeld, A., Berkman, L., Kosten, T., & Charpentier, P. (1987). The measurement of grief: Bereaved verus nonbereaved. *Hospice Journal*, *2*, 21–36.

Jacobs, S., & Prigerson, H. (2000). Psychotherapy of traumatic grief: A review of evidence for psychotherapeutic treatments. *Death Studies*, *24*, 479–496.

Laor, N., Wolmer, L., Kora, M., Yucel, D., Spirman, S., & Yazgan, Y. (2002). Posttraumatic, dissociative and grief symptoms in Turkish children exposed to the 1999 earthquakes. *Journal of Nervous and Mental Disease*, *190*(12), 824–832.

Lindemann, E. (1944). Symptomatology and management of acute grief. *American Journal of Psychiatry*, *101*, 141–148.

Lindy, J. D., Green, B. L., Grace, M., & Tichener, J. (1983). Psychotherapy with survivors of the Beverly Hills Supper Club fire. *American Journal of Psychotherapy*, *37*, 593–610.

Litz, B. T., Gray, M. J., Bryant, R. A., & Adler, A. B. (2002). Early intervention for trauma: Current status and future directions. *Clinical Psychology: Science and Practice*, *9*(2), 112–134.

McFarlane, A. C. (1988a). The longitudinal course of posttraumatic morbidity: The range of outcomes and their predictors. *Journal of Nervous and Mental Disease*, *176*, 30–39.

McFarlane, A. C. (1988b). The phenomenology of posttraumatic stress disorders following a natural disaster. *Journal of Nervous and Mental Disease*, *176*, 22–29.

Middleton, W. (1996). *The phenomenology of bereavement and the process of resolution*. Unpublished doctoral dissertation, University of Queensland.

Middleton, W., Burnett, P., Raphael, B., & Martinek, N. (1996). The bereavement response: A cluster analysis. *British Journal of Psychiatry*, *169*, 167–171.

Middleton, W., Moylan, A., Raphael, B., & Martinek, N. (1998). A longitudinal study comparing bereavement phenomena in recently bereaved spouses, adults, children and parents. *Australian and New Zealand Journal of Psychiatry*, *32*, 235–241.

Murray, J., Ehlers, A., & Mayou, R. A. (2002). Dissociation and posttraumatic stress disorder: Two prospective studies of road traffic accident survivors. *British Journal of Psychiatry*, *180*, 363–368.

National Institute of Mental Health. (2001). *Mental health and mass violence: Evidence-based early psychological intervention for victims/survivors of mass violence. A workshop to reach consensus on best practices* (NIH Publication No. 02-5138). Washington, DC: U.S. Government Printing Office.

Niemeyer, R. A., & Hogan, N. S. (2001). Quantitative or qualitative?: Measurement issues in the study of grief. In M. S. Stroebe, R. O. Hansson, W. Stroebe, & H. Schut (Eds.), *Handbook of bereavement research: Consequences, coping, and care* (pp. 89–118). Washington, DC: American Psychological Association.

Parkes, C. M. (1971). The first year of bereavement: A longitudinal study of the reaction of London widows to the death of their husbands. *Psychiatry, 33*, 444–467.

Parkes, C. M., & Weiss, R. S. (1983). *Recovery from bereavement*. New York: Basic Books.

Prigerson, H. G., Bierhals, A. J., Kasl, S. V., Reynolds, C. F., Shear, M. K., Day, N., et al. (1997). Traumatic grief as a risk factor for mental and physical morbidity. *American Journal of Psychiatry, 154*, 616–623.

Prigerson, H. G., & Jacobs, S. C. (2001). Traumatic grief as a distinct disorder: A rationale, consensus criteria, and a preliminary empirical test. In M. S. Stroebe, R. O. Hansson, W. Stroebe, & H. Schut (Eds.), *Handbook of bereavement research: Consequences, coping, and care* (pp. 613–646). Washington, DC: American Psychological Association.

Prigerson, H. G., Maciejewski, P., Newson, J., Reynolds, C. F., Bierhals, A. J., Miller, M., et al. (1995). Inventory of complicated grief: A scale to measure maladaptive symptoms of loss. *Psychiatry Research, 59*, 65–79.

Prigerson, H. G., Shear, M. K., Jacobs, S. C., Reynolds, C. F., Maciejewski, P. K., Davidson, J. R. T., et al. (1999). Consensus criteria for traumatic grief: A preliminary empirical test. *British Journal of Psychiatry, 174*(1), 67–73.

Pynoos, R. S., Frederick, C., Nader, K., Arroyo, W., Steinberg, A., Eth, S., et al. (1987). Life threat and posttraumatic stress in school-age children. *Archives of General Psychiatry, 44*, 1057–1063.

Pynoos, R. S., Nader, K., Frederick, C., Gonda, L., & Stuber, M. (1987). Grief reactions in school-age children following a sniper attack at school. *Israeli Journal of Psychiatry and Related Sciences, 24*, 53–63.

Raphael, B. (1977). The Granville train disaster: Psychological needs and their management. *Medical Journal Australia, 1*, 303–305.

Raphael, B. (1983). *Anatomy of bereavement*. New York: Basic Books.

Raphael, B. (1986). *When disaster strikes*. New York: Basic Books.

Raphael, B., & Maddison, D. C. (1976). The care of bereaved adults. In O. W. Hill (Ed.), *Modern trends in psychosomatic medicine* (pp. 491–506). London: Butterworth.

Raphael, B., & Martinek, N. (1997). Assessing traumatic bereavement and posttraumatic stress disorder. In J. P. Wilson & T. M. Keane (Eds.), *Assessing psychological trauma and PTSD* (pp. 373–395). New York: Guilford Press.

Raphael, B., & Minkov, C. (1999). Abnormal grief. *Current Opinion in Psychiatry, 12*, 99–102.

Raphael, B., & Wooding, S. (2004). Early mental health interventions for traumatic loss in adults. In B. T. Litz (Ed.), *Early intervention for trauma and traumatic loss* (pp. 147–178). New York: Guilford Press.

Ritchie, E. (2001). *Summary of consensus statement*. First annual Consensus Workshop on Mass Violence and Early Intervention Conference, Virginia. *http://www.nimh.nih.gov/Publicat/massviolence.pdf*

Rynearson, E. K. (1984). Bereavement after homicide: A descriptive study. *American Journal of Psychiatry, 141*, 1452–1454.

Rynearson, E. K. (2001). *Retelling violent death*. Philadelphia: Brunner-Routledge.

Schlenger, W. E., Caddell, J. M., Ebert, L., Jordan, B. K., Rourke, K. M., Wilson, D., et al. (2002). Psychological reactions to terrorist attacks: Findings from the National Study of Americans' reactions to September 11. *Journal of the American Medical Association, 288*(5), 581–588.

Schut, H. A. W., Keijser, J. D., Van Den Bout, J., & Dijhuis, J. H. (1991). Posttraumatic stress symptoms in the first years of conjugal bereavement. *Anxiety Research, 4*, 225–234.

Vachon, M. L., Lyall, W. A., & Rogers, J. (1980). A controlled study of self-help interventions for widows. *American Journal of Psychiatry, 137*, 1380–1384.

Weisaeth, L. (1989). The stressors and the posttraumatic stress syndrome after an industrial disaster. *Acta Psychiatrica Scandinavica* (Suppl. 355), 25–37.

PART V

Psychosocial Development and Gender Issues

CHAPTER 18

Assessing Traumatic Experiences in Children and Adolescents

Self-Reports of DSM PTSD Criteria B–D Symptoms

KATHLEEN O. NADER

In the past two decades, a number of instruments and subscales have been developed and revised to reflect a growing knowledge of children's posttraumatic reactions. It has become clear that multiple methods, measures, and sources of information are important in accurately assessing children (Nader, 2003). Researchers have begun to identify the important variables and mediating factors associated with children's traumatic reactions and symptoms, to measure the success of treatment methods, to examine the differences between varied traumatic experiences, and to assess long-term results of trauma and treatment (Greenwald, 2002; La Greca, Silverman, Vernberg, & Roberts, 2002; Nader, 2001). Nevertheless, understanding childhood traumatic reactions has been limited or confused by (1) the lack of detailed information about children prior to their traumatic experiences, (2) mixed methods, sample size, and study results, (3) unidentified mediating variables, (4) the need to identify the changing nature of symptoms over time, and (5) the lack of detailed studies of children before and after traumas and at intervals across the life span (Nader, 2003).

A number of issues affect the accuracy of assessment of children's posttraumatic reactions, including selection (e.g., random, matched, self); preparation for and the method of measurement (e.g., training, interviewers, interview style); event issues (e.g., briefing, phase of response, type of trauma); and child issues (e.g., culture, age, temperament, attachment style, history, family circumstances; Fletcher, 2003; Nader, 2001, 2003; Webb, 2004). Examining the exact effects of any single element is complicated by the interaction of elements.

THREE DECADES OF ASSESSING TRAUMA IN YOUTH

Prior to 1980, the assessment of childhood traumatic response was accomplished primarily through clinical case examination (Carey-Trefzer, 1949; Bloch, Silber, & Perry, 1956; Bergen, 1958; Lacey, 1972; Newman, 1976; Green, 1983) and/or review of case records (Levy, 1945). Clinicians most often reported case observations and parent or teacher reports of children's reactions. Terr's examination of children following a school bus kidnapping (Terr, 1979, 1981, 1983) and other studies of children exposed to violence and disaster (Eth & Pynoos, 1985) demonstrated the effectiveness of interviewing children directly regarding their experiences and responses. However, the need for a more systematic statistical analysis of children's traumatic reactions resulted in the application of a number of research instruments. These instruments included measures of depression (e.g., Birleson Depression Inventory; Birleson, 1981), anxiety (e.g., Children's Manifest Anxiety Scale; Reynolds & Richmond, 1978), fear (e.g., Fear Survey Schedule for Children; Ollendick, 1983), and "caseness" (Rutter's Scale; Rutter & Graham, 1967; Elander & Rutter, 1996) and measures of trauma that apply adult scales to children (e.g., the Impact of Event Scale; Horowitz, Wilner, & Alvarez, 1979; see also Weiss, Chapter 7, this volume). After a sniper opened fire on a crowded elementary school playground in south central Los Angeles in 1984, the necessity for an emergency revision of Calvin Frederick's 16-item Adult Post Traumatic Stress Reaction Index marked the emergence of posttraumatic stress disorder (PTSD) scales for children (Frederick, 1985; Pynoos et al., 1987).

In the past several years, in addition to the measures for school-age children's and adolescents' self-reports of symptoms, a number of measures, interviews, and methods have been developed to assess other aspects of trauma in youth. Among these are measures for assessing exposure rates and levels and complicated trauma and traumatic grief reactions; adult reports; observational methods; and measurements of dissociation, functioning, neurobiology, comorbid disorders, associated symptoms, and child attributes (e.g., development, culture, temperament, type, self-esteem, coping, life satisfaction, trait anxiety). Because of space constraints, these measures, their psychometric properties, and other issues (multiple measure assessment, multiple sources of information, varied contexts, the nature of the interview, the nature of the event) are discussed in a separate publication (Nader, 2003). This chapter briefly delineates some of the main aspects of child and adolescent trauma assessment and briefly describes youth self-report measures of DSM PTSD criteria B–D symptoms (American Psychiatric Association, 1994) and sometimes additional symptoms.

MULTIMETHOD ASSESSMENT

Comprehensive assessment of children includes collecting information from multiple sources and in multiple contexts (e.g., from parents, children, and other sources; at school or day care, with caregivers, and in clinical settings; Reynolds & Kamphaus, 1998; Scheeringa, Peebles, Cook, & Zeanah, 2001). Self-reports, caregiver reports, naturalistic observations, and structured laboratory observations all have their advantages and disadvantages (Rothbart & Bates, 1998). Because no single source can provide complete and accurate data and because children behave and respond differently in different contexts, comprehensive assessment requires multiple sources of data (Achenbach & Rescorla, 2001; Briere, 1996; Friedrich, Jaworski, Huxsahl, & Bengtson, 1997; Reich & Earls, 1987; Reynolds & Kamphaus, 1998; Sternberg et al., 1993; Weissman et al., 1987). Not only are certain behaviors situation specific, but different observers may perceive and interpret behaviors differently (Reynolds & Kamphaus, 1998). Moreover, some researchers have found that reliability increases when using multiple assessment sessions with the same protocol (Rothbart & Bates, 1998).

The Source of Information

Establishing the presence or absence of a symptom or trait for clinical or research purposes may be based on information from a single source or counted as present if reported by either adult or child (Costello, Angold, March, & Fairbank, 1998). As discussed previously, no single source can provide complete and accurate information regarding youth and their traumatic reactions (Achenbach & Rescorla, 2001; Briere, 1996; Friedrich et al., 1997; Reich & Earls, 1987; Reynolds & Kamphaus, 1998; Sternberg et al., 1993; Weissman et al., 1987). In the event that one group must be chosen, Weissman et al. (1987) recommended interviewing the children. In order to fully understand the nature of childhood traumatic response, however, information from multiple sources must be examined and collected over time. Children generally report more symptoms for themselves than others report for them. Adult raters and scale agreement have generally been lowest for internalizing symptoms and highest for the more observable externalizing symptoms (Achenbach & Rescorla, 2001; Nader, 2003; Reynolds & Kamphaus, 1998).

Event Factors

In addition to child characteristics (e.g., age at onset of the trauma, current age, pubertal stage, personality, temperament, attachment style, cognitive and coping skills, and support systems) and family history and style (e.g., early and subsequent experience, culture, socioeconomic status, and family lifestyle), the nature of the traumatic experience—the type of event; the manner in which it unfolds; its intensity, duration, and phase; the degree of threat or loss; the personal meaning of the event and its individual episodic moments; and its link to other issues in the child's life—also help to shape traumatic reactions, reporting, responses to treatment, and recovery (Fletcher, 2003; Nader, 2003). For ongoing traumas, the phase of the event itself is important to recognize. When events are ongoing, numbing and avoidance may be prevalent. Symptoms may be warded off or ignored because there might be more to endure. When the event is perceived to be over rather than ongoing or when the numbing wears off, there may be a reassessment of the experience, its results, and one's role in it; of beliefs and expectations; and of the meaning of events and interactions. In order to cope, the youth may unwittingly intersperse periods of numbing and avoidance between phases of reexperiencing and arousal or between attempts to face aspects of his or her experience and response (Nader, 1997, 2003; Realmuto et al., 1992).

Identifying Variables

> [C]omplexly determined outcomes cannot be predicted with high precision from only one or a few antecedents.
>
> —NESSELROADE (1995, p. 345)

In order to fully and accurately understand symptom endorsement and scale scores, it is essential to examine the appropriate variables (before, during, and after the event) that may contribute to specific posttraumatic reactions. Assessing too many variables risks having to combine trivial variables with overly elaborate relationships in order to make them theoretically interesting. Too few risks that variables will be defined so inclusively that they conceal relationships (Nesselroade, 1995).

The field of childhood trauma would benefit greatly from appropriately obtained, detailed information about children prior to their exposures to traumatic events (Nader, 2003). In addition to the need to examine trauma in relationship to preexisting child attributes, experiences, and circumstances is the need to understand that, especially for children, some characteristics are in an ongoing state of change (Roberts & DelVecchio, 2000). Moreover, more than one kind of change or continuity needs to be examined over time (e.g., amount, group placement, a set of variables, and an individual in comparison to self; Caspi & Roberts, 2001). From childhood to adolescence, youths vary widely in the amount of continuity or change they exhibit. Change is affected by environmental, biosocial, genetic, and historical factors, as well as experiential factors (Caspi & Roberts, 2001).

Differences or levels of traumatic reactions may not be statistically or clinically significant until the effects of variables such as cultural attitudes, weight, subgroup, or pubertal stage are identified (De Bellis et al., 1999). Some symptoms may appear only after prolonged or intense exposure. For example, dissociation has been found to be related to age, gender, and duration and severity of sexual abuse (Friedrich et al., 1997).

Symptoms (e.g., intrusive reexperiencing) may appear, increase, or decrease in response to specific experiences (e.g, indirect witnessing, media exposure, worry about another) or other variables (e.g., location, denial, culture; Briere, 1996; Elliot & Briere, 1994; Nader, Pynoos, Fairbanks, Al-Ajeel, & Al-Asfour, 1993; Nader, 2003; Pfefferbaum et al., 1999; Richters & Martinez, 1991; Singer, Anglen, Song, & Lunghofer, 1995). It may be necessary to distinguish between symptoms associated with different variables (e.g., trauma vs. grief dreams or play) or to determine the nature of the response (e.g., initial fear or ongoing response, coping strategy or trauma symptom; Fletcher, 2003; Nader, 1997; Stallard, Velleman, Langsford, & Baldwin, 2001). Some symptoms (e.g., fear, cognitive impairment) may be reduced by reducing other symptoms (e.g., sleep disturbance or bad dreams; Krakow et al., 2001). Over time, some symptoms may transform into behavioral patterns, vulnerabilities, inhibitions, or styles of assessment and decision making (Danieli, 1998). Consequently, the ongoing effects of trauma may go unnoticed if only traditional scales and measures are used.

Identifying the subtypes and characteristics of children (e.g., size, temperament, age, gender), the traumatic experience (e.g., type and timing), and the child's history (e.g., heredity, experience, family structure, SES) that affect outcomes may prevent the canceling out of effects. For example, Lipschitz, Morgan, and Southwick (2002) described two biological subtypes of traumatized youths: those with high and those with reduced autonomic responsiveness (see also Biederman et al., 1990, on behavioral inhibition).

When appropriate personal variables (e.g., personality, personal experience, cultural heritage, family secrets, and family support systems) are excluded from the analysis, effects may be attributed to trauma that are in fact a result of other variables or variable combinations (Nader, 2003; Pinderhughes, 1998). For example, when determining the differences among traumatized children related to some characteristics (e.g., gender) or experiences (e.g., exposure to violence), it is essential to control for the effects of personality characteristics (e.g., inhibition, lack of control, and reactivity) that have been associated with gender and the later presence or absence of specific symptoms over time (e.g., aggression, externalizing symptoms; Biederman et al., 1990; Caspi, Henry, McGee, Moffitt, & Silva, 1995; Rothbart & Bates, 1998). In assessing the effects of treatment and the course of recovery, recognizing the effects of these variables may explain variations in response over time (Nader, 2003).

METHOD AND PREPARATION FOR MEASUREMENT

The Nature of the Interview

As one aspect of a full evaluation, children's posttrauma screening instruments have been administered (1) in direct interviews with children (structured, semistructured, or combined methods; Angold et al., 1995; Harrington et al., 1988); (2) by mail or other distribution for completion and return; and (3) by issuing it to groups of children to complete. Children's responses may be subject to conscious and unconscious distortions primarily in the direction of greater social desirability (Nader, 1997; Piers & Herzberg, 2002). Conducting in-person interviews, rather than having the child complete the instrument, seems to increase the sensitivity of the measurement (Jones & Ribbe, 1991). Reich and Earls (1990) found interviewing children by phone economical, saving both time and money and permitting continued contact with respondents at a distance. However, when comparing matched groups of children interviewed by phone or in person using the Diagnostic Interview for Children and Adolescents (DICA), the telephone group as a whole reported fewer symptoms than the in-person group. In a recent study (Todd, Joyner, Heath, Neuman, & Reich, 2003) using the Missouri Assessment of Genetics Interview for Children (MAGIC; Reich & Todd, 2002a; a revision of the DICA), differences in phone and in-person interviews for parents and adolescents were not significant (none were conducted for younger children). Establishing good rapport with the respondent is essential to truthful and timely completion of a scale regardless of the format used to obtain information (Reynolds & Kamphaus, 1998; Reich & Todd, 2002b).

Training

Although varying amounts of training have been recommended for the different instruments, in general, greater accuracy, better concordance with clinical diagnoses and with other raters, and better therapeutic results have been reported for trained interviewers (Jones & Ribbe, 1991). Scheeringa et al. (2001) found that trained raters were better able than parents to identify some symptoms in children (e.g., reactivity to reminders and restricted range of affect). Some interview methods (e.g., unstructured or semistructured) require more training than others (e.g., structured; Angold et al., 1995).

Specialized methods are often essential to use in interviewing victims of trauma. For example, understanding the respondent's state of mind and issues of closure are crucial to effective and harmless interviews. A variety of harmful effects (e.g., worsened symptoms, suicides and suicide attempts, murder, severe depressions, and acute psychotic episodes) have resulted from interviews conducted by untrained, poorly trained, unskilled, or culturally ignorant interviewers (Mayou, Ehlers, & Hobbs, 2000; Nader, 1997; Ruzek & Watson, 2001; Raphael & Wilson, 2001; Swiss & Giller, 1993).

Preliminary Briefing

Preliminary briefing is an essential part of preparation for assessment and/or intervention with children following traumatic events. Knowing the details of the traumatic event—including those identified by police, news, and eyewitness reports of the event—enables the researcher to recognize aspects of symptomatic response and variables affecting response and to have a sense of the child's accuracy of recall (Nader, 1997, 2003).

Translations

Translations of instruments may be necessary for cultural adaptation (Nader, 2003). Canino and Bravo (1999) list five dimensions for cultural equivalence: semantic (the meaning of questions), content (relevance of the content to the target population), technical (e.g, applicability of the assessment format), conceptual (construct validity; e.g., whether scores relate to measurable dysfunction), and criterion (similar interpretation of results in relation to established cultural norms). Karno, Burnam, Escobar, Hough, and Eaton (1983) recommend a system of translation and "back translation" (to the original language) for accuracy. Several back translations and retranslations may be necessary. Having a bilingual translator who matches the target population's understanding of terminology is more informative in the back translation process (Nader, 1997, 2003).

Symptom Ratings and Question Order

Rating systems (e.g., to rate presence, frequency, intensity, duration, or a combination) vary across measures (Nader, 1997, 2003). Independent of frequency, the intensity of some symptoms has predicted a PTSD diagnosis or a child's functional impairment (Carrion, Weems, Ray, & Reiss, 2002). For other symptoms, frequency has predicted impairment. Thus using both frequency and intensity ratings may promote rating accuracy and distinguish symptoms occurring in response to stress from those resulting from traumatization. In order to clearly establish the course and nature of childhood traumatic response, it may be necessary to assess changes in symptoms and development of behavioral patterns over time as well as onset, duration, frequency, and intensity of symptoms.

In assessing symptoms endorsed by children, it is important to be cognizant of developmental issues. Some behaviors are common at specific phases of development but signal disturbances at other age levels (Hornstein & Putnam, 1992; Putnam, 1993; Friedrich et al., 1997). Children (especially young children) may respond to cues from the interviewer when answering questions. It is essential that the child sense a willingness to hear any answer and that there are no wrong answers. When there are open-ended questions or questions asking for a general list of results (e.g., "Has anything really bad ever happened to you?"), asking the open-ended question and waiting for an answer before giving specific examples or making specific probes can be helpful.

With children and adolescents, in addition to the need for clearly specified terms, definitions, and formulas for endorsing assessment items, it is essential to define age-appropriate developmental expectations and thresholds of symptom-level impairment (Scheeringa et al., 2001). For some children, icons may set a more playful, less serious tone and may subtly suggest that a lighter atmosphere is sought. Young or regressed youths tend to take things literally and concretely, may be easily focused on one train of thought or emotion, and may be particularly vulnerable to the interviewer's tone or subtle/unconscious suggestions. Youths have exhibited concern regarding the judgments of their peers, their symptoms, and their symptom levels. Therefore, opening questions or statements and interview format may be of particular importance when assessing youths (Nader, 2003).

APPLICABILITY OF DSM CRITERIA B–D

Researchers continue to debate the nature of childhood traumatic response and the applicability of DSM criteria A–D (Fletcher, 2003; Nader, 2003). A number of studies have identified children with subsyndromal but clinically significant PTSD (Carrion et al., 2002; Daviss et al., 2000; Vila, Porsche, & Mouren-Simeoni, 1999; Scheeringa et al., 2001). Research is needed to examine the changing nature of symptoms over time and the complexity of reactions to ongoing or multiple traumas.

Among the concerns and recommendations with regard to criteria B–D are (1) adjustment of criteria C and D for children (Carrion et al., 2002); (2) the study of childhood PTSD as a continuous variable (Fletcher, 2003; Putnam, 1998); (3) a greater focus on the effects of trauma that lead to referral for clinical services (e.g., functioning; Angold, Costello, Farmer, Burns, & Erkanli, 1999; La Greca et al., 2002); (4) recognition of delayed impairment that may occur months or years later; (5) confirmation of the predictive value of individual symptoms (Carrion et al., 2002); and (6) resolution of the overlap in some symptoms (e.g., sleep impairment and reexperiencing; Wolfe & Birt, 2002b; Nader, 2003).

CHILD INTERVIEWS

Interviewing children directly may be most effective (1) after physical needs are met and a sense of safety is restored (Nader, 1999a; Scheeringa & Zeanah, 1995); and (2) when the interviewer is appropriately knowledgeable and deemed caring and trustworthy by the children. Children may be traumatized by their experiences, yet they may not report the full range of PTSD symptoms (Carrion et al., 2002; Nader & Fairbanks, 1994). Additionally, over time, children may minimize their symptoms, thinking that other children are no longer symptomatic, or that they should not be symptomatic after months have passed. Symptoms or their link to a trauma may become less overt. For example, earlier symptoms or traumatic impressions may later translate into vulnerabilities or behavior patterns (Nader, 2001, 2003).

Age and Development

Age and developmental influences affect children's appraisals of threat, abilities to report symptoms and experiences, assignment of meaning to aspects of the event, emotional and cognitive coping, capacities to tolerate their reactions, and abilities to address secondary life changes (James, 1994; Nader, 2001; Pynoos & Nader, 1993). Very young children's preverbal or barely verbal capacities render them unable to report their subjective experiences (Scheeringa & Zeanah, 1995). Studies of young children have underscored the need for collecting information from multiple sources (Scheeringa et al., 2001). Between 18 months and 2 years of age, children begin to use symbolic play and language to represent experience (Piaget, 1952) and to demonstrate their perceptual memories (Terr, 1985). Children under age 5 have been best assessed by a combination of observation, questions during or directions regarding play, and supplemental information from adult caretakers (Nader, 2003; Scheeringa et al., 2001).

When relying on self-reports or peer ratings to gather data, researchers must speak the language of their informants (McCrae & John, 1992). Instruments have been adapted for specific age groups through rewording of questions, breaking down of questions into simpler units for younger children, and use of age-related answering systems. Children under the age of 8 may have difficulty with the concept of time, even when the time is narrowed to the preceding month. They may also have difficulty with the complexities of a 5-point scale. Symptom and exposure criteria altered from the current DSM-IV criteria may be helpful for accurately diagnosing infants and children (Carrion et al., 2002; Scheeringa & Zeanah, 1995; Scheeringa et al., 2001).

In addition to age, the ability to report or respond to rating scales may be affected by emotional sophistication or how "streetwise" the child is. Pubertal development rather than age may distinguish groups of children (Carrion et al., 2002). As mentioned earlier, the order of questions, as well as wording and the contributions of the interviewer (e.g., focus, acceptance, tone of questions), may be particularly important for children.

Cultural Issues

Children's ethnic, religious, and cultural backgrounds have been relatively understudied in relation to traumatic reactions (La Greca et al., 2002). Moreover, comparisons have sometimes been confounded by the presence of other variables (e.g., numbers and levels of traumatic exposures, SES, or other risk factors; Costello, Keeler, & Angold, 2001; Fletcher, 2003; Mash & Dozois, 2003; Silverman & La Greca, 2002). Cultural and religious beliefs influence the manner in which individuals respond to traumas and to treatment (McGoldrick, 1998). Cultural beliefs and attitudes affect a number of issues important to the measurement of childhood trauma, such as the way questions are interpreted, values, expectations (e.g., of behaviors after a death or disaster), gender roles and valued behaviors, issues of trust, establishing a time frame, and the admission and expression of emotions (Marsella, Friedman, Gerrity, & Scurfield, 1996; Mills, 2001; Nader, Dubrow, & Stamm, 1999; Shiang, 2000). Cultural backgrounds may contribute to the risk and protective factors following traumatic events (Rabalais, Ruggiero, & Scotti, 2002). Cultural and religious differences shape the meaning attributed to the event; reactions to helping professionals; acknowledgement or silence about injuries and reactions; the response to loss; the need for action, inaction, or reclusion; the methods of restoring safety; the management of anxiety; the support for or suspicion of one another; and more. Religious or spiritual beliefs may influence or dictate responses to crises. As sources of comfort and as anchors, they may mitigate traumatic reactions, or they may promote a sense of hopelessness and helplessness (Hines, 1998; Tully, 1999).

In addition to their effects on a youth's willingness to share information, cultural values may provide an awareness of desired or expected responses. The number of weeks, months, or years it takes for a person to reveal the extent of personal traumatic reactions varies by culture (Kinzie, 1993). In some cultures (e.g., Cambodian, Chinese, Arabic), voicing mental health problems may shame or stigmatize (Kinzie, 1993; Shiang, 2000). In some cultures, complaining of physical symptoms instead of emotional ones allows the elicitation of social support without the stigmatization and shame of a mental problem (Shiang, 2000). Emotional expressions, conceptualizations, and word meanings differ from society to society (Mills, 2001).

TRAUMA QUESTIONNAIRES

Differences in trauma questionnaires are affected by format, age range, authors' theoretical beliefs, research findings, and the desire to be either brief or thorough (Nader, 2003). The length of each interview or time for scale completion is affected by the length of the questionnaire, the degree of a child's symptomatic presentation, and the rater's or interviewee's interactional or contemplative style (Egger & Angold, 2004). Interviews with children and research findings continue to reveal the need to reword, arrange, add to, and effectively present questions in order to best assess children and to make the process easier for them. Trauma measures for school-age children and adolescents presented in this section include those that assess DSM-IV trauma (and sometimes additional symptoms), trauma measures that include child abuse, and comprehensive measures of PTSD and other disorders. Several of the instruments were undergoing revision or psychometric testing before publication of this chapter. All of the measures presented here have demonstrated acceptable to excellent psychometric properties (Nader, 2003).[1]

[1] Due to space contraints, the psychometric properties of the current versions of scales and interviews presented here can be found in Nader (2003).

Trauma Symptoms: School-Age Children and Adolescents

Child's Reaction to Traumatic Events Scale—Revised

Age range: 6–18 years; *translation*: Spanish; *format*: child completion or semistructured interview.

The Child's Reaction to Traumatic Events Scale (CRTES; Jones, 1994, 1995, 2002a) was a revision of the Impact of Events Scale for Children (IES-C). The most recent version (CRTES-R; Jones, Fletcher, & Ribbe, 2002) is a 23-item self-report measure. It now includes arousal symptoms based on HIES arousal symptoms, as well as the original avoidance and intrusion symptoms. The revised CRTES uses a 4-point frequency rating scale: *not at all* (0); *rarely* (1); *sometimes* (3); and *often* (5). A score of 28 or higher on the two main subscales is recommended for making a diagnosis of PTSD (Jones, 2002b). Distress scores for the new arousal items on the CRTES-R are being tested. The scale is being updated for DSM-IV. (The CRTES-R is available from Russell T. Jones, Department of Psychology, Stress and Coping Lab, 4102 Derring Hall, Virginia Tech University, Blacksburg, VA 24060.)

Child Report of Posttraumatic Symptoms

Age range: 5–17 years; *translations*: Bosnian, Dutch, German, Italian, Persian, Spanish; *associated scales*: PROPS, LITE; *format*: child completion, structured phone interview.

The Child Report of Posttraumatic Symptoms (CROPS; Greenwald, 1996, 1997) is a 26-item scale that includes DSM-IV PTSD criteria and additional symptoms (Fletcher, 1996; American Psychiatric Association, 1994). It can be used with or without an identified trauma. The child is asked to rate the validity of symptom-endorsing statements, over the preceding week, on a scale of 0–2 (*none*, *some*, *lots*; Greenwald & Rubin, 1999; Wiedemann & Greenwald, 2000). Scores are continuous rather than subdivided into diagnostic algorithms. (The CROPS is available from Sidran Institute; sidran@sidran.org; *www.sidran.org*; 200 E. Joppa Road, Suite 207, Towson, MD 21286; phone: 410-825-8888; fax: 410-337-0747, 1-888-825-8249.)

Clinician-Administered PTSD Scale for Children and Adolescents (CAPS-CA)

Age range: 8–17 years; *translation*: German; *format*: semistructured child interview.

The Clinician-Administered PTSD Scale for Children (CAPS-CA; Nader, Kriegler, Blake, & Pynoos, 1994; Nader et al., 1996; Nader et al., 2004) is an instrument developed to measure DSM-IV PTSD and associated symptoms in children and adolescents. It provides a method to evaluate the frequency, intensity, and reporting validity of individual symptoms toward a current or lifetime diagnosis of PTSD, as well as social, developmental, and scholastic functioning. Two 5-point rating scales (frequency and intensity) accompany each item. The scale provides a practice section and optional picture (icon) response scales (Nader, Blake, & Kriegler, 1994; Newman et al., 1997). (The CAPS-CA is available from *ncptsd@ncptsd.org* or from Western Psychological Services [WPS], 12031 Wilshire Blvd., Los Angeles, CA 90025-1251; phone: 310-478-2061 or 800-648-8857; fax: 310-478-7838.)

Child Posttraumatic Stress Reaction Index and Additional Questions

Age range: 7–17 years; *translations*: Canadian French, Croatian, Kuwaiti Arabic, Norwegian, Vietnamese; *associated scales*: CPTS-RI-Parent, EQ, CPTSR-PI; *format*: semistructured child interview.

The Child Posttraumatic Stress Reaction Index (CPTS-RI; Frederick, Pynoos & Nader, 1992) is a 20-item scale, and the Additional Questions (AQ; Nader, 1999b) has 11 main questions and 48 probe or clarification questions. CPTS-RI items include some of the DSM-IV PTSD symptoms from each of three main subscales and two associated features (guilt and regression). The AQ includes other DSM-IV items. A 5-point Likert frequency rating scale ranges from *none* (0) to *most of the time* (4). For the 20-item index, the scoring system establishes a level of PTS (Nader, 1993, 1999b). (Available from *measures@twosuns.org*)

My Worst Experience Survey

Age range: 8–17 years; *associated scales*: Life Events; *format*: child completion–individually, in a group, or in semistructured interview.

My Worst Experience Survey (MWES; National Center for Study of Corporal Punishment and Alternatives in Schools, 1992; Hyman, Zelikoff, & Clarke, 1988) consists of a preliminary inquiry (Part I) about the worst experience and the child's rating of how upsetting it was; a page of possible worst experiences (e.g., abuse, death of significant other, disaster, personal or family problems, illness, divorce, robbery, or kidnapping); and indications of with whom they occurred and their duration, frequency, and impact. Part II is a 105-item checklist based on DSM-III-R and DSM-IV criteria for PTSD and research studies regarding traumatic stress in children (Berna, 1993; Kohr, 1995). The rating system for these instruments is a 5-point Likert scale ranging from *one time* (1) to *all of the time* (5). Scores range from 0 to 525. (The MWES is available from Western Psychological Services [WPS], 12031 Wilshire Blvd., Los Angeles, CA 90025-1251; phone: 310-478-2061 or 800-648-8857; fax: 310-478-7838.)

UCLA PTSD Index for DSM-IV

Age range: 7–18 years; *associated scales*: PTSD, Reminders of Loss, Exposure, parent scales; *format*: completed by child/parent or semistructured interview.

UCLA PTSD Index for DSM-IV (UPID; Pynoos, Rodriguez, Steinberg, Stuber, & Frederick, 1998) includes 26 exposure questions, 1 dissociative item, 19 items for the 17 DSM-IV PTSD symptoms, and 2 associated features (guilt and fear of recurrence). The 20-item child scale and 22-item adolescent scale (including two alternatively worded questions for criteria D2, aggression, and C7, view of the future) have now been combined into a single scale. Items are rated on a 4-point frequency scale ranging from *none* to *most* of the time. The CPTS-RI is a precursor to this scale. A two-page instruction sheet is available (Rodriguez, 2001). (The UPID is available from Alan Steinberg, *ASteinberg@mednet.ucla.edu*)

When Bad Things Happen

Age range: 8–19 years; *translations*: Armenian, Hebrew, Spanish; *format*: child completion; *associated scales*: Parent Report of Child's Stress Reaction, DOSE, TTTc, YAUTC, WVS, Child and Parent PTSD Interviews.

The When Bad Things Happen scale (WBTH, R4; Fletcher, 1991, 1992) includes four questions to assess DSM criterion A, 56 questions (2–6 questions per criterion item) to assess DSM reexperiencing, numbing/avoidance, and arousal, and 2–5 questions to assess each of 11 categories of associated symptoms. Items are scored on a 3-point scale (*lots*, *some*, *never*; or the reverse). A rating scale with a coding key accompanies the scale, assisting computation of the DSM-III or -IV diagnosis or a continuous score. A computer-scoring diskette and a tape to assist younger children in completing the instrument are available. (WBTH is available from Kenneth Fletcher, Psychiatry Department, University of Massachusetts Medical Center, 55 Lake Avenue North, Worcester, MA 01655; *Kenneth.Fletcher@umassmed.edu*.)

Trauma and Child Abuse

The three measures presented here have been used to assess trauma symptoms in abused children. The Angie/Andy Cartoon Trauma Scales include symptoms of complex trauma. The CITES-2 defines a traumatic event. The TSCC does not link responses to a specific, defined event (Wolfe & Birt, 2002a).

Angie/Andy Cartoon Trauma Scales

Age range: 6–11 years; *format*: semistructured child interview.

The Child Rating Scales of Exposure to Interpersonal Abuse (CRS-EIA), now called the Angie/Andy Cartoon Trauma Scales (ACTS; Praver, Pelcovitz, & DiGiuseppe, 1994, 1998), is a 44-item clinician-administered scale. It was generated from research on abuse and community violence, complicated trauma (van der Kolk, Roth, Pelcovitz, & Mandel, 1992; Herman, 1992a, 1992b), and the Levonn (Richters & Martinez, 1990), a cartoon-based measure. In the ACTS, either a girl (Angie) or a boy (Andy) has been exposed to four forms of violence: sexual abuse, physical abuse, witnessing family violence, and community violence. The ACTS employs a 4-point thermometer rating scale measuring *never* (1), *just a few times* (2), *some of the time* (3) and *a lot of the time* (4). Five sample cartoons depicting one of the four frequency ratings are repeated until the child responds correctly. An introductory note provides methods of checking to see if the child understands and of encouraging the child's responses. (The ACTS is available from F. Praver, *drpraver@cs.com*; fax: 516 671-3269.)

Children's Impact of Traumatic Events Scale—2

Age range: 8–16 years; *format*: semistructured child interview—child completion is possible; *associated scales*: HVF, CPEQ.

The Children's Impact of Traumatic Events Scale—Revised (CITES-2; Wolfe & Gentile, 2003) is a 78-item measure for sexually abused children's PTSD symptoms, attributions, perceptions of social reactions, and some symptoms of complicated trauma. It also permits the examination of trauma factors, social reactions, and other subjective responses common to traumatized children in general (Wolfe & Birt, 2002b). The CITES-2 is intended to be scored as a continuous measure; however, it can also be used to examine DSM-IV PTSD symptom criteria and diagnostic status. Items are rated on a 3-point scale from 0–2 (*not true*, *somewhat true* or *very true*). A scoring diskette is available. (The CITES-2 is available from Vicky Veitch Wolfe, Child and Adolescent Centre, 346 South Street, London Health Sciences Centre, London, Ontario, Canada, N6A 4G5, or *wolfev@lhsc.on.ca*.)

Trauma Symptom Checklist for Children

Age range: 8–16 years; *translations*: Cambodian; *format*: child completion; *associated scales*: Detailed Assessment of Posttraumatic Stress (DAPS; for 17- or 18-year-olds and older; Briere, 2001)

The Trauma Symptom Checklist for Children (TSCC; Briere, 1989, 1996) is a 54-item scale intended for use in the evaluation of children who have experienced traumatic events such as childhood physical and sexual abuse, victimization by peers (e.g., physical or sexual assault), major losses, the witnessing of violence to others, and natural disasters. Subscales are not intended to provide a diagnosis of specific disorders (e.g., PTSD or dissociative disorder). The scale is rated on a 4-point Likert frequency format ranging from *never* (0) to *almost all of the time* (3). Scores are cumulative for each subscale. Normative data are available (Briere, 1996; Evans & Briere, 1994; Friedrich, 1995; Singer et al., 1995). (The TSCC is available from Psychological Assessment Resources Inc., phone: 1-800-331-TEST).

PTSD and Other Disorders

Among the disorders found in association with PTSD are attention deficit disorder (ADD), attention-deficit/hyperactivity disorder (ADHD), conduct disorder (CD), oppositional defiant disorder (ODD), depressive disorders (e.g., major or not otherwise specified), phobias (e.g., social or specific), and anxiety disorders (e.g., separation; Carrion et al., 2002; Ford, 2002; Greenwald, 2002; Weinstein, Staffelbach, & Biaggio, 2000). Two of the scales that measure psychiatric disorders in children are described here.

Child and Adolescent Psychiatric Assessment

Age range: 9–17 years; *parent interview*: included (for ages 6–17); *format*: semistructured with structured questions and ratings; *relevant subscales*: Family Structure; Life Events; PTSD; other disorders; *training*: required and essential.

The Child and Adolescent Psychiatric Assessment (CAPA; v. 4.2; Angold, Cox, Prendergast, Rutter, & Simonoff, 2000) combines both respondent- and interviewer-based methods of assessment. It is based on DSM-III, DSM-IV, ICD-9, and draft ICD-10 glossaries, as well as a variety of additional symptoms of psychopathological interest (e.g., among PTSD symptoms: emotional responses, somatic responses, intervention fantasies). Items that are involved in more than one diagnosis are represented in only one place. Symptoms are rated for intensity, frequency, and duration on scales from 2 to 5 points (e.g., 0 = absent; 2 = present to a specified degree; 3 = more pervasively or intensely present as defined; Angold et al., 2000; Angold et al., 1995). The reference period is 3 months unless DSM criteria require otherwise. A symptom is counted whether reported by parent or child (Costello et al., 1998). After a symptom has been thoroughly investigated (e.g., reports of the context, aggravating and ameliorating factors, and consequences of the symptom; observation of the child in the interview), all the information obtained is used to match the subject's symptom description (i.e., behavior, emotion, or thought) to detailed glossary definitions and levels of severity. Questions are asked verbatim. The interviewer is expected to continue appropriate questioning until all the necessary information for making a rating has been obtained (Angold et al., 1995). (CAPA is available from Adrian Angold, Center for Developmental Epidemiology, Department of Psychiatry and Behavioral Sciences, Duke University Medical Center, Box 3454, Durham, NC, 27710-3454)

Missouri Assessment of Genetics Interview for Children

Age range: 7–12 and 13–18 years; *translations*: English, Spanish, Lebanese Arabic; *relevant subscales*: Home Environment; Sibling Relations; Peer Relations; Psychosocial Stressors; Perinatal and Early Life; PTSD; other disorders; *format*: semistructured interview; *training*: required.

The Missouri Assessment of Genetics Interview for Children (MAGIC) is a new version of the Diagnostic Interview for Children and Adolescents (DICA; Earls, Reich, & Jung, 1988; Reich & Kaplan, 1994). The DICA-R (Reich, Taibleson, & Shayka, 1992) was revised to create the MAGIC in 1997 (Reich & Todd, 1997, 2002a, 2002b). MAGIC disorders include the criteria of both DSM-III-R and DSM-IV so that studies using either can be compared with current studies. Six versions of the MAGIC include age-specific language and examples: Child Version (ages 7–12); Adolescent Version (13–17); Young Adult version (18–25); Adult Version (26+); Parent Version (to ask parents about their children ages 7–17). A number of rating scales are used. Web-based computer programs for the versions are now available (Reich & Todd, 2002b). MAGIC items are included in the manual. Like the DICA-R, the MAGIC includes an initial question and specified probe questions (sometimes required and sometimes optional; Reich & Todd, 2002b). (The MAGIC is available from Wendy Reich, Department of Child Psychiatry, Campus Box 8134, Washington University School of Medicine, St. Louis, MO 63110; *wendyr@twins.wustl.edu*.)

CONCLUSIONS

Because of developmental variables, assessing children's traumatic reactions is significantly different from assessing those of adults. The manner in which symptoms may manifest or be reported varies by age group. Aspects of the child, his or her circumstances, the traumatic event, the rater, the assessment measures, and the methods of interview all affect the accuracy of assessment. Multiple methods, measures, and sources of information are important in accurately assessing children. School-age children and adolescents generally report more symptoms for themselves than others report for them. Adult raters and scale agreement have generally been highest for the more observable externalizing symptoms.

The time it takes for scale or interview completion is affected by the degree of a child's symptomatic response and presentation, the rater's or interviewee's interactional or contemplative style, and the length of the questionnaire. Shorter scales may be quicker and easier to administer, whereas scales and interviews with probe or additional questions for each item permit endorsement of symptoms missed due to wording issues or state of mind. The longer measures allow exploration of the accuracy of initial responses.

Findings regarding children's reactions have sometimes been contradictory. Identifying all appropriate mediating variables in examining youths' responses to traumatic events may help to explain some of the differences in findings. Moreover, accurate long-term assessment will necessitate delineating the changing nature of children's symptoms over time, as well as the symptoms not currently listed for a diagnosis of PTSD. For example, methods are needed for assessing whether and how initial childhood reactions translate into behavioral patterns, life choices, vulnerabilities, and inhibitions. Routine and intermittent school assessments of a number of child characteristics, large samples, long-term studies, and better identification of all of the outcomes of childhood traumatic experience would improve knowledge and benefit the affected children.

ACKNOWLEDGMENTS

Sincere appreciation is extended to Dr. John Wilson for his continued patience and encouragement and for his help in obtaining copies of many of the articles sought for this chapter. My thanks to his students, Michael Doherty, Deb Tyson, and others, for gathering articles. I am grateful to the publishers and authors who provided copies of their scales, interviews, measures, manuals, and sometimes papers for my review. I also extend my gratitude to M. Conant and A. Spencer for their valuable feedback.

REFERENCES

Achenbach, T. M., & Rescorla, L. A. (2001). *Manual for the ASEBA School-Age Forms and Profiles*. Burlington, VT: University of Vermont, Research Center for Children, Youth, and Families.

American Psychiatric Association. (1994). *Diagnostic and statistical manual of mental disorders* (4th ed.). Washington, DC: American Psychiatric Association.

Angold, A., Costello, E., Farmer, E., Burns, B., & Erkanli, A. (1999). Impaired but undiagnosed. *Journal of the American Academy of Child and Adolescent Psychiatry, 38*(2), 129–137.

Angold, A., Cox, A., Prendergast, M., Rutter, M., & Simonoff, E. (2000). *Child and Adolescent Psychiatric Assessment (CAPA)*. (Available from Adrian Angold, Center for Developmental Epidemiology, Department of Psychiatry and Behavioral Sciences, Duke University Medical Center, Box 3454, Durham, NC, 27710-3454)

Angold, A., Prendergast, M., Cox, A., Harrington, R., Simonoff, E., & Rutter, M. (1995). The Child and Adolescent Psychiatric Assessment. *Psychological Medicine, 25*, 739–753.

Bergen, M. (1958). The effect of severe trauma on a four-year-old child. *Psychoanalytic Study of the Child, 23*, 407–429.

Berna, J. M. (1993). *The worst experiences of adolescents from divorced and separated parents and the stress responses to those experiences*. A dissertation submitted to Temple University Graduate Board, Philadelphia, PA.

Biederman, J., Rosenbaum, J., Hirshfield, D., Faraone, S., Bolduc, E., Gersten, N., et al. (1990). Psychiatric correlates of behavioral inhibition in young children with and without psychiatric disorders. *Archives of General Psychiatry*, *47*, 21–26.

Birleson, P. (1981). The validity of depressive disorder in childhood and the development of a self-rating scale: A research report. *Journal of Child Psychology and Psychiatry*, *22*, 73–88.

Bloch, D., Silber, E., & Perry, S. (1956). Some factors in the emotional reaction of children to disaster. *American Journal of Psychiatry*, *113*, 416–422.

Briere, J. (1989). *Trauma Symptom Checklist for Children (TSCC)*. (See Briere, 1996).

Briere, J. (1996). *Trauma Symptom Checklist for Children (TSCC) professional manual*. Odessa, FL: Psychological Assessment Resources.

Briere, J. (2001). *Detailed Assessment of Posttraumatic Stress (DAPS) professional manual*. Odessa, FL: Psychological Assessment Resources.

Canino, G., & Bravo, M. (1999). The translation and adaptation of diagnostic instruments for cross-cultural use. In D. Shaffer, C. Lucas, & J. Richters (Eds.), *Diagnostic assessment in child and adolescent psychopathology* (pp. 285–298). New York: Guilford Press.

Carey-Trefzer, C. (1949). The results of a clinical study of war-damaged children who attended the Child Guidance Clinic, the Hospital for Sick Children, Great Ormond Street, London. *Journal of Mental Science*, *95*, 535–559.

Carrion, V. G., Weems, C. F., Ray, R. D., & Reiss, A. L. (2002). Toward an empirical definition of pediatric PTSD: The phenomenology of PTSD symptoms in youth. *Journal of the American Academy of Child and Adolescent Psychiatry*, *41*(2), 166–173.

Caspi, A., Henry, B., McGee, R. O., Moffitt, T. E., & Silva, P. A. (1995). Temperamental origins of child and adolescent behavior problems: From age three to age fifteen. *Child Development*, *66*, 55–68.

Caspi, A., & Roberts, B. W. (2001). Personality development across the life course: The argument for change and continuity. *Psychological Inquiry*, *12*(2), 49–66.

Costello, E. J., Angold, A., March, J., & Fairbank, J. (1998). Life events and posttraumatic stress: The development of a new measure for children and adolescents. *Psychological Medicine*, *28*, 1275–1288.

Costello, E. J., Keeler, G. P., & Angold, A. (2001). Poverty, race/ethnicity, and psychiatric disorder: A study of rural children. *American Journal of Public Health*, *91*(9), 1494–1498.

Danieli, Y. (1998). *International handbook of multigenerational legacies of trauma*. New York: Plenum Press.

Daviss, W. B., Mooney, D., Racusin, R., Ford, J. D., Fletscher, A., & McHugo, G. J. (2000). Predicting posttraumatic stress after hospitalization for pediatric injury. *Journal of American Academy of Child and Adolescent Psychiatry*, *59*(5), 576–583.

De Bellis, M., Keshavan, M., Clark, D., Casey, B., Giedd, H., Boring, A., et al. (1999). Developmental traumatology: Part II. Brain development. *Biological Psychiatry*, *45*, 1271–1284.

Earls, F., Reich, W., & Jung, K. G. (1988). Psychopathology in children of alcoholic and antisocial parents. *Alcohol Clinical Experimental Research*, *12*, 481–487.

Egger, H. L., & Angold, A. (2004). The Preschool Age Psychiatric Assessment. In R. Del Carmen-Wiggins & A. Carter (Eds.), *A handbook of infant and toddler mental assessment* (pp. 223–243). New York: Oxford University Press.

Elander, J., & Rutter, M. (1996). Use and development of the Rutter Parents' and

Teachers' Scales. *International Journal of Methods in Psychiatric Research, 6,* 63–78.

Elliott, D., & Briere, J. (1994). Forensic sexual abuse evaluations of older children: Disclosures and symptomatology. *Behavioral Sciences and the Law, 12,* 261–277.

Eth, S., & Pynoos, R. (1985). Developmental perspectives on psychic trauma in children. In D. Schetky & E. Benedek (Eds.), *Child psychiatry and the law.* New York: Brunner/Mazel.

Evans, J. J., & Briere, J. (1994, January). *Reliability and validity of the Trauma Symptom Checklist for children in a normal sample.* Paper presented at the Conference on Child Maltreatment, San Diego, CA.

Fletcher, K. (1991). *Parent report of the Child's Reaction to Stress.* (Available from Kenneth Fletcher, PhD, Psychiatry Department, University of Massachusetts Medical Center, 55 Lake Avenue North, Worcester, MA 01655; *Kenneth.Fletcher@umassmed.edu*)

Fletcher, K. (1992). *When Bad Things Happen Scale.* (See Fletcher, 1992).

Fletcher, K. E. (1996). Childhood posttraumatic stress disorder. In E. J. Mash & R. A. Barkley (Eds.), *Child psychopathology* (1st ed., pp. 242–275). New York: Guilford Press.

Fletcher, K. E. (2003). Childhood posttraumatic stress disorder. In E. J. Mash & R. A. Barkley (Eds.), *Child psychopathology* (2nd ed., pp. 330–371). New York: Guilford Press.

Ford, J. D. (2002). Traumatic victimization in childhood and persistent problems with oppositional defiance. *Journal of Aggression, Maltreatment and Trauma, 6*(1), 25–58.

Frederick, C. (1985). Selected foci in the spectrum of posttraumatic stress disorders. In J. Laube & S. A. Murphy (Eds.), *Perspectives on disaster recovery* (pp. 110–130). East Norwalk, CT: Appleton-Century-Crofts.

Frederick, C., Pynoos, R. S., & Nader, K. O. (1992). Childhood Post-Traumatic Stress Reaction Index (CPTS-RI). (Available from *measures@twosuns.org*)

Friedrich, W. (1995). Evaluation and treatment: The clinical use of the Child Sexual Behavior Inventory: Commonly asked questions. *American Professional Society on the Abuse of Children (APSAC) Advisor, 8*(1), 1, 17–20.

Friedrich, W., Jaworski, T. M., Huxsahl, J. E., & Bengtson, B. S. (1997). Dissociative and sexual behaviors in children and adolescents with sexual abuse and psychiatric histories. *Journal of Interpersonal Violence, 12*(2), 155–171.

Green, A. (l983). Dimensions of psychological trauma in abused children. *Journal of the American Academy of Child Psychiatry, 22,* 231–237.

Greenwald, R. (1996). The information gap in the EMDR controversy. *Professional Psychology: Research and Practice, 27*(1), 67–72.

Greenwald, R. (1997). *Child and Parent Reports of Post-traumatic Symptoms (CROPS and PROPS).* (Available from Sidran Institute; *sidran@sidran.org*; *www.sidran.org*; 200 E. Joppa Road, Suite 207, Towson, MD 21286 USA, Phone: 410-825-8888, Fax: 410-337-0747, 1-888-825-8249)

Greenwald, R. (Ed.). (2002). *Trauma and juvenile delinquency: Theory, research, and interventions.* New York: Haworth Press.

Greenwald, R., & Rubin, A. (1999). Brief assessment of children's posttraumatic symptoms: Development and preliminary validation of parent and child scales. *Research on Social Work Practice, 9,* 61–75.

Harrington, R., Hill, J., Rutter, M., John, K., Fudge, H., Zoccolillo, M., & Weissman, M. M. (1988). The assessment of lifetime psychopathology: A comparison of two interviewing styles. *Psychological Medicine*, *18*, 487–493.

Herman, J. (1992a). Complex PTSD: A syndrome in survivors of prolonged and repeated trauma. *Journal of Traumatic Stress*, *5*(3), 377–391.

Herman, J. (1992b). A new diagnosis. In J. L. Herman (Ed.), *Trauma and recovery* (pp. 115–127). New York: Basic Books.

Hines, P. M. (1998). Climbing up the rough side of the mountain: Hope, culture, and therapy. In M. McGoldrick (Ed.), *Re-visioning family therapy* (pp. 78–89). New York: Guilford Press.

Hornstein, N. L., & Putnam, F. W. (1992). Clinical phenomenology of child and adolescent dissociative disorders. *Journal of the American Academy of Child and Adolescent Psychiatry*, *31*, 1077–1085.

Horowitz, M., Wilner, N., & Alvarez, W. (1979). Impact of Event Scale: A measure of subjective stress. *Psychosomatic Medicine*, *41*, 209–218.

Hyman, I., Zelikoff, W., & Clarke, J. (1988). *School Trauma Survey—Student Form*. National Center for the Study of Corporal Punishment and Alternatives in the Schools (NCSCPAS), Philadelphia, PA: Temple University.

James, B. (1994). *Handbook for treatment of attachment-trauma problems in children*. Lexington, MA: Lexington Books.

Jones, R. T. (1994). *Child's Reaction to Traumatic Events Scale* (CRTES). A self-report traumatic stress measure. (see Jones, Fletcher, & Ribbe, 2002)

Jones, R. T. (1995). *Child's Reaction to Traumatic Events Scale* (CRTES). A self-report traumatic stress measure. (see Jones, Fletcher, & Ribbe, 2002)

Jones, R. T. (2002a). *Child's Reaction to Traumatic Events Scale* (CRTES). A self-report traumatic stress measure. (see Jones, Fletcher, & Ribbe, 2002)

Jones, R. T. (2002b). *Revision of distress levels for the Child's Reaction to Traumatic Events Scale*. Unpublished manuscript.

Jones, R. T., Fletcher, K., & Ribbe D. R. (2002). Child's Reaction to Traumatic Events Scale—Revised (CRTES-R): A self-report traumatic stress measure. (Available from Russell T. Jones, PhD, Professor, Department of Psychology, Stress and Coping Lab, 4102 Derring Hall, Virginia Tech University, Blacksburg, VA 24060)

Jones, R. T., & Ribbe, D. P. (1991). Child, adolescent and adult victims of residential fire. *Behavior Modification*, *15*(4), 560–580.

Karno, M., Burnam, A., Escobar, J. I., Hough, R. L., & Eaton, W. W. (1983). Development of the Spanish-language version of the National Institute of Mental Health Diagnostic Interview Schedule. *Archives of General Psychiatry*, *40*, 1183–1188.

Kinzie, J. D. (1993). Posttraumatic effects and their treatment among southeast Asian refugees. In J. Wilson & B. Raphael (Eds.), *The international handbook of traumatic stress syndromes* (pp. 311–319). New York: Plenum Press.

Kohr, M. (1995). *Validation of the My Worst Experience Survey*. An unpublished doctoral dissertation, Temple University, Philadelphia, PA.

Krakow, B., Hollifield, M., Johnston, L., Koss, M., Schrader, R., Warner, T.D., et al. (2001). Imagery rehearsal therapy for chronic nightmares in sexual assault survivors with posttraumatic stress disorder. *Journal of the American Medical Association*, *286*(5). Retrieved September 2, 2002, from *jama.ama-assn.org/issues/v286n5/abs/joc10245.html*.

Lacey, G. N. (1972). Observations on Aberfan. *Journal of Psychosomatic Research, 16*, 257–260.

La Greca, A. M., Silverman, W. K., Vernberg, E. M., & Roberts, M. C. (Eds.). (2002). *Helping children cope with disasters and terrorism.* Washington, DC: American Psychological Association.

Levy, D. M. (1945). Psychic trauma of operations in children. *American Journal of Diseases of Children, 69*, 7–25.

Lipschitz, D. S., Morgan, C. A., & Southwick, S. M. (2002). Neurobiological disturbances in youth with childhood trauma and in youth with conduct disorder. *Journal of Aggression, Maltreatment and Trauma, 6*(1), 149–174.

Marsella, A. J., Friedman, M. J., Gerrity, E. T., & Scurfield, R. M. (Ed.). (1996). *Ethnocultural aspects of posttraumatic stress disorder: Issues, research, and clinical applications.* Washington, DC: American Psychological Association.

Mash, E. J., & Dozois, D. (2003). Child psychopathology: A developmental systems perspective. In E. J. Mash & R. A. Barkley (Eds.), *Child psychopathology* (2nd ed., pp. 3–71). New York: Guilford Press.

Mayou, R. A., Ehlers, A., & Hobbs, M. (2000). Psychological debriefing for road traffic accident victims: Three-year follow-up of a randomized controlled trial. *British Journal of Psychiatry, 176*, 589–593.

McCrae, R. R., & John, O. P. (1992). An introduction to the five-factor model and its applications. *Journal of Personality, 60*, 175–215.

McGoldrick, M. (1998). A framework for re-visioning family therapy. In M. McGoldrick (Ed.), *Re-visioning family therapy* (pp. 3–19). New York: Guilford Press.

Mills, S. (2001). The idea of different folk psychologies. *International Journal of Philosophical Studies, 9*(4), 501–519.

Nader, K. (1993). Instruction manual, Childhood PTSD Reaction Index (rev., English version). (Available from *measures@twosuns.org*)

Nader, K. (1997). Assessing traumatic experiences in children. In J. Wilson & T. Keane (Eds.), *Assessing psychological trauma and PTSD* (pp. 291–348). New York: Guilford Press.

Nader, K. (1999a). *Psychological first aid for trauma, grief and traumatic grief* (3rd ed.). Austin, TX: Two Suns.

Nader, K. (1999b). *Additional Questions.* (Available from measures@twosuns.org)

Nader, K. (2001). Treatment methods for childhood trauma. In J. P. Wilson, M. Friedman, & J. Lindy (Eds.), *Treating psychological trauma and PTSD* (pp. 278–334). New York: Guilford Press.

Nader, K. (2003). *Assessing traumatic experiences in children and adolescents* Manuscript submitted for publication.

Nader, K. O., Blake, D. D., & Kriegler, J. A. (1994). *Instruction manual: Clinician Administered PTSD Scale, Child and Adolescent Version* (CAPS-C). White River Junction, VT: National Center for PTSD.

Nader, K., Dubrow, N., & Stamm, B. (Eds.). (1999). *Honoring differences: Cultural issues in the treatment of trauma and loss.* Philadelphia: Taylor & Francis.

Nader, K., & Fairbanks, L. (1994). The suppression of reexperiencing: Impulse control and somatic symptoms in children following traumatic exposure. *Anxiety, Stress and Coping: An International Journal, 7*, 229–239.

Nader, K. O., Kriegler, J. A., Blake, D. D., Pynoos, & R. S. (1994). *Clinician-Administered PTSD Scale, Child and Adolescent Version (CAPS-C).* White River Junction, VT: National Center for PTSD.

Nader, K. O., Kriegler, J. A., Blake, D. D., Pynoos, R. S., Newman, E., & Weathers, F. (1996). *Clinician-Administered PTSD Scale, Child and Adolescent Version (CAPS-C)*. White River Junction, VT: National Center for PTSD.

Nader, K., Newman, E., Weathers, F., Kaloupek, D., Kriegler, J., Blake, D., & Pynoos, R. (2004). *Clinician-Administered PTSD Scale for Children and Adolescents (CAPS-C)*. Los Angeles: Western Psychological Press.

Nader, K., Pynoos, R., Fairbanks, L., Al-Ajeel, M., & Al-Asfour, A. (1993). Acute post-traumatic stress reactions among Kuwait children following the Gulf Crisis. *British Journal of Clinical Psychology*, *32*, 407–416.

National Center for Study of Corporal Punishment and Alternatives in Schools. (1992). *My Worst Experience Survey*. Philadelphia, PA: Temple University.

Nesselroade, J. R. (1995). As the twig is bent, so grows the tree . . . sometimes. *Psychological Inquiry*, *6*(4), 343–348.

Newman, C. J. (1976). Children of disaster: Clinical observations at Buffalo Creek. *American Journal of Psychiatry*, *133*, 306–312.

Newman, E., Weathers, F., Nader, K., Kaloupek, D., Pynoos, R., Blake, D., & Kriegler, J. (1997). *Clinician-Administered PTSD Scale for Children and Adolescents manual* (CAPS-C manual). White River Junction, VT: National Center for PTSD.

Ollendick, T. H. (1983). Reliability and validity of the revised Fear Survey Schedule for Children (FSSC-R). *Behaviour Research and Therapy*, *21*, 685–692.

Pfefferbaum, B., Nixon, S. J., Tucker, P. M., Tivis, R. D., Moore, V. L., Gurwitch, R. H., et al. (1999). Posttraumatic stress responses in bereaved children after the Oklahoma City bombing. *Journal of the American Academy of Child and Adolescent Psychiatry*, *38*(11), 1372–1379.

Piaget, J. (1952). *The origins of intelligence in children*. New York: International Universities Press.

Piers, E. V., & Herzberg, D. S. (2002). *Piers–Harris Children's Self-Concept Scale manual* (2nd ed.). Los Angeles: Western Psychological Services.

Pinderhughes, E. (1998). Black genealogy revisited: Restorying an African American family. In M. McGoldrick (Ed.), *Re-visioning family therapy* (pp. 177–199). New York: Guilford Press.

Praver, F., Pelcovitz, D., & DiGiuseppe, R. (1994). *The Angie/Andy Child Rating Scales*. (Available from Dr. F. Praver, *drpraver@cs.com*; FAX: (516) 671-3269)

Praver, F., Pelcovitz, D., & DiGiuseppe, R. (1998). *The Angie/Andy Child Rating Scales*. Toronto, Ontario, Canada: Multi-Health Systems.

Putnam, F. W. (1993). Dissociative disorders in children: Behavioral profiles and problems. *Child Abuse and Neglect*, *17*, 39–45.

Putnam, F. W. (1998). Trauma models of the effects of childhood maltreatment. *Journal of Aggression, Maltreatment, and Trauma*, *2*, 51–66.

Pynoos, R., Frederick, C., Nader, K., Arroyo, W., Eth, S., Nunez, W., et al. (1987). Life threat and posttraumatic stress in school age children. *Archives of General Psychiatry*, *44*, 1057–1063.

Pynoos, R. S., & Nader, K. (1993). Issues in the treatment of posttraumatic stress disorder in children and adolescents. In J. Wilson & B. Raphael (Eds.), *The international handbook of traumatic stress syndromes* (pp. 535–539). New York: Plenum Press.

Pynoos, R. S., Rodriguez, N., Steinberg, A., Stuber, M., & Frederick, C. (1998). *UCLA PTSD Index for DSM-IV*. (Available from *Asteinberg@mednet.ucla.edu*)

Rabalais, A. E., Ruggiero, J. K., & Scotti, J. R. (2002). Multicultural issues in the response of children to disasters. In A. M. LaGreca, W. K. Silverman, E.. Vernberg, & M. C. Roberts (Eds.), *Helping children cope with disasters and terrorism* (pp. 73–89). Washington, DC: American Psychological Association Press.

Raphael, B., & Wilson, J. (Eds.). (2001). *Psychological debriefing: Theory, practice and evidence*. Cambridge, UK: Cambridge University Press.

Realmuto, G. M., Masten, A., Carole, L. F., Hubbard, J., Groteluschen, A., & Chun, B. (1992). Adolescent survivors of massive childhood trauma in Cambodia: Life events and current symptoms. *Journal of Traumatic Stress, 5*(4), 589–599.

Reich, W., & Earls, F. (1987). Rules for making psychiatric diagnoses in children on the basis of multiple sources of information: Preliminary strategies. *Journal of Abnormal Child Psychology, 15*(4), 601–616.

Reich, W., & Earls, F. (1990). Interviewing children by telephone: Preliminary results. *Comprehensive Psychiatry, 31*(3), 211–215.

Reich, W., & Kaplan, L. (1994). The effects of psychiatric and psychosocial interviews on children. *Comprehensive Psychiatry, 3*, 50–53.

Reich, W., Taibleson, C., & Shayka, J. J. (1992). Diagnostic Interview for Children and Adolescents (DICA), copyrighted, Washington University. Available from Washington University School of Medicine, Department of Psychiatry, 4940 Children's Place, St. Louis, MO, FAX: (314) 454-2330 Phone: (314) 454-2307

Reich, W., & Todd, R. D. (1997). *Missouri Assessment of Genetics Interview for Children*. St. Louis, MO: Washington University School of Medicine. (see Reich & Todd, 2002a).

Reich, W., & Todd, R. D. (2002a). *Missouri Assessment of Genetics Interview for Children*. St. Louis, MO: Washington University School of Medicine.

Reich, W., & Todd, R. D. (2002b). *Missouri Assessment of Genetics Interview for Children Specifications Manual*. St. Louis, MO: Washington University School of Medicine.

Reynolds, C. R. (1980). Concurrent validity of What I Think and Feel: The Revised Children's Manifest Anxiety Scale. *Journal of Consulting and Clinical Psychology, 48*, 774–775.

Reynolds, C. R., & Kamphaus, R. W. (1998). *Behavior Assessment System for Children manual*. Circle Pines, MN: American Guidance Service.

Reynolds, C. R., & Richmond, B. O. (1978). What I think and feel: A revised measure of children's manifest anxiety. *Journal of Abnormal Child Psychology, 6*(2), 271–280.

Richters, J. E., & Martinez, P. (1990). *Things I have seen and heard: A structured interview for assessing young children's violence exposure*. Unpublished measure, National Institute of Mental Health, Rockville, MD.

Richters, J. E., & Martinez, P. (1991). Community violence project: Children as victims or witnesses to violence. *Psychiatry, 56*, 7–21.

Roberts, B. W., & DelVecchio, W. F. (2000). The rank-order consistency of personality from childhood to old age: A quantitative review of longitudinal studies. *Psychological Bulletin, 126*, 3–25.

Rodriguez, N. (2001, December). *Youth PTSD assessment: Psychometric investigation of PTSD self-report instruments*. Paper presented at the International Society for Traumatic Stress Studies meeting, New Orleans, LA.

Rothbart, M. K., & Bates, J. E. (1998). Temperament. In W. Damon (Series Ed.) & N.

Eisenberg (Vol. Ed.), *Handbook of child psychology: Vol. 3. Social, emotional, and personality development* (5th ed., pp. 105–176). New York: Wiley.

Rutter, M., & Graham, P. (1967). A children's behavior questionnaire for completion by teachers: Preliminary findings. *Journal of Child Psychology and Psychiatry, 8*, 1–11.

Ruzek, J., & Watson, P. (2001). Early intervention to prevent PTSD and other trauma-related problems. *PTSD Research Quarterly, 12*(4), 1–7.

Scheeringa, M. S., Peebles, C. D., Cook, C. A., & Zeanah, C. H. (2001). Toward establishing procedural, criterion, and discriminant validity for PTSD in early childhood. *Journal of the American Academy of Child and Adolescent Psychiatry, 40*(1), 52–60.

Scheeringa, M. S., & Zeanah, C. H. (1995). Symptom expression and trauma variables in children under 48 months of age. *Infant Mental Health Journal, 16*, 259–270.

Shiang, J. (2000). Considering cultural beliefs and behaviors in the study of suicide. In R. Maris, S. Canetto, J. McIntosh, & M. Silverman (Eds.), *Review of suicidology* (pp. 226–241). New York: Guilford Press.

Silverman, W. K., & LaGreca, A. M. (2002). Children experiencing disasters: Definitions, reactions, and predictors of outcomes. In A. M. LaGreca, W. K. Silverman, E. M. Vernberg, & M. C. Roberts (Eds.), *Helping children cope with disasters and terrorism* (pp. 11–34). Washington, DC: American Psychological Association Press.

Singer, M. I., Anglen, T. M., Song, L. Y., & Lunghofer, L. (1995). Adolescents' exposure to violence and associated symptoms of psychological trauma. *Journal of American Medical Association, 273*(6), 477–482.

Stallard, P., Velleman, R., Langsford, J., & Baldwin, S. (2001). Coping and psychological distress in children involved in road traffic accidents. *British Journal of Clinical Psychology, 40*, 197–208.

Sternberg, K. J., Lamb, M. E., Greenbaum, C., Cicchetti, D., Dawud, S., Cortes, R. M., et al. (1993). Effects of domestic violence on children's behavior problems and depression. *Developmental Psychology, 29*(1), 44–52.

Swiss, S., & Giller, J. E. (1993). Rape as a crime of war: A medical perspective. *Journal of the American Medical Association, 270*(5), 612–615.

Terr, L. (1979). Children of Chowchilla: Study of psychic trauma. *Psychoanalytic Study of the Child, 34*, 547–623.

Terr, L. (1981). Psychic trauma in children: Observations following the Chowchilla school-bus kidnapping. *American Journal of Psychiatry, 138*(1), 14–19.

Terr, L. (1983). Chowchilla revisited: The effects of psychic trauma four years after a schoolbus kidnapping. *American Journal of Psychiatry, 140*, 1542–1550.

Terr, L. C. (1985). Remembered images and trauma: A psychology of the supernatural. *Psychoanalytic Study of the Child, 40*, 493–533.

Todd, R. D., Joyner, C. A., Heath, A. C., Neuman, R. J., & Reich, W. (2003). Reliability and stability of a semi-structured DSM-IV interview designed for family studies. *Journal of the American Academy of Child and Adolescent Psychiatry, 42*,(12), 1460–1468.

Tully, M. (1999). Lifting our voices: African American cultural responses to trauma and loss. In K. Nader, N. Dubrow, & B. Stamm (Eds.), *Honoring differences: Cultural issues in the treatment of trauma and loss* (pp. 23–48). Philadelphia: Taylor & Francis.

van der Kolk, B. A., Roth, S., Pelcovitz, D., & Mandel, F. S. (1992). *Disorders of extreme stress: Results from the DSM-IV field trials for PTSD*. Unpublished manuscript.

Vila, G., Porche, L., & Mouren-Simeoni, M. (1999). An 18-month longitudinal study of posttraumatic disorders in children who were taken hostage in their school. *Psychosomatic Medicine*, *61*, 746–754.

Webb, N. B. (Ed.). (2004). *Mass trauma and violence: Helping families and children cope*. New York: Guilford Press.

Weinstein, D., Staffelbach, D., & Biaggio, M. (2000). Attention-deficit hyperactivity disorder and posttraumatic stress disorder: Differential diagnosis in childhood sexual abuse. *Clinical Psychology Review*, *20*(3), 359–378.

Weissman, M., Wichkramaratne, P., Warner, V., John, K., Prusoff, B., Merikangas, K., & Gammon, D. (1987). Assessing psychiatric disorders in children. *Archives of General Psychiatry*, *44*, 747–753.

Wiedemann, J., & Greenwald, R. (2000, November). *Child trauma assessment with the CROPS and PROPS: Construct validity in a German translation*. Poster session presented at the annual meeting of the International Society for Traumatic Stress Studies, San Antonio, TX.

Wolfe, V. V., & Birt, J. H. (2002a). *The Children's Peritraumatic Experiences Questionnaire: A measure to assess DSM-IV PTSD criterion A2*. Manuscript submitted for publication.

Wolfe, V. V., & Birt, J. H. (2002b). *The Children's Impact of Traumatic Events Scale—Revised (CITES-R): Scale structure, internal consistency, discriminant validity, and PTSD diagnostic patterns*. Manuscript submitted for publication.

Wolfe, V. V., & Gentile, C. (2003). Children's Impact of Traumatic Events Scale (CITES-2). Available from Vicky Veitch Wolfe, PhD, Child & Adolescent Centre, 346 South Stree, London Health Sciences Centre, London, Ontario N6A 4G5 or *wolfev@lhsc.on.ca*

CHAPTER 19

Psychological Assessment of Child Abuse Effects in Adults

JOHN BRIERE

As a group, adults who were abused as children exhibit a wide range of psychological and interpersonal problems relative to those without an abuse history. Although a causal relationship between such difficulties and child abuse cannot easily be established, the extensive replication of findings, both cross-sectionally and prospectively, suggest that childhood maltreatment is a significant risk factor for later psychological disorder.

Probably due to the psychologically injurious aspects of child abuse, the rates of self-reported child maltreatment in clinical samples are considerably greater than in the general population. For example, the incidence of self-reported sexual abuse histories among women averages around 50% across outpatient, inpatient, and emergency room samples, as opposed to rates of about half that magnitude in general population samples (Briere, 1996; Briere & Elliott, 2003; Finkelhor, Hotaling, Lewis, & Smith, 1990; Wyatt, 1985).

This chapter reviews some of the assessment and measurement issues associated with evaluation of the long-term psychological effects of child maltreatment. Among the topics addressed are (1) how to systematically assess the specific details and context of the victimization experience, such as its type (i.e., sexual, physical, psychological), frequency, duration, and the victim's age at abuse onset and offset, because more severe and prolonged abuse appears to increase subsequent mental health impairment; and (2) how to accurately assess the specific nature and extent of any abuse-related symptomatology or dysfunction that might be present.

Because the study of child abuse and its impacts is still relatively new, there has been insufficient focus on the actual psychological evaluation of abuse-specific disturbance. As a result, until recently researchers and clinicians frequently have used nonstandardized measures of unknown or less than adequate psychometric properties or have applied more generic measurement strategies and instruments that were initially developed without reference to child abuse. Considerable development of standardized child abuse-relevant measures has occurred since the last edition of this volume, however.

Child abuse effects also may be difficult to measure adequately because of their complexity. Because child maltreatment may coexist with disrupted parent–child attachment (Alexander, 1992; Ogata, et al., 1990; Zlotnick, Zakriski, Shea, & Costello, 1996), interfere with normal psychological (and potentially neurophysiological) development (Cicchetti & Toth, 1995; Cole & Putnam, 1992), and motivate the development of avoidance strategies that are in and of themselves detrimental (Briere, 2002a), the direct and indirect effects of such trauma may be so diverse as to preclude their easy determination.

Among the known effects of child maltreatment are those seen in other forms of trauma, such as chronic posttraumatic stress (Elklit, 2002; Rowan, Foy, Rodriguez, & Ryan, 1994; Ullman & Brecklin, 2002) and dissociation (Chu & Dill, 1990; Simeon, Guralnik, Schmeidler, Sirof, & Knutelska, 2001). However, less trauma-specific symptoms and disorders may also be presented, such as helplessness, guilt, shame, and low self-esteem (Briere & Runtz, 1990; Feiring, Rosenthal, & Taska, 2000; Owens & Chard, 2001); easily triggered negative relational schema (Baldwin, Fehr, Keedian, Seidel, & Thompson, 1993; Briere, 2002a); anxiety, depression, and anger (Dutton, Starzomski, & Ryan, 1996; MacMillan, et al., 2001; Molnar, Buka, & Kessler, 2001); sexual dysfunction (Davis, Petretic-Jackson, & Ting, 2001; Wyatt, Newcomb, & Riederle, 1993); and somatization (Drossman, Li, Leserman, Toomey, & Hu, 1996; Katon, Sullivan, & Walker, 2001; Springs & Friedrich, 1992). Abuse survivors are also more likely to engage in drug and alcohol abuse (e.g., Briere, Woo, McRae, Foltz, & Sitzman, 1997; De Bellis, 2002; Molnar, Buka, & Kessler, 2001), as well as externalizing behaviors such as compulsive and indiscriminate sexual activity (Briere, Elliott, Harris, & Cotman, 1995; Davis, Combs-Lane, & Jackson, 2002), bingeing or chronic overeating (Connors & Morse, 1993; Waller, 1992; Webster & Palmer, 2000), antisocial behavior and aggression (Luntz & Widom,1994; Pollock et al., 1990), suicidal behavior (e.g., Molnar, Berkman, & Buka, 2001; Dube et al., 2001), and self-mutilation (Briere & Gil, 1998; van der Kolk, Perry, & Herman, 1991; Walsh & Rosen, 1988).

Given this complexity, psychological assessment can be incomplete if, for example, only a Minnesota Multiphasic Personality Inventory (MMPI-2; Butcher, Dahlstrom, Graham, Tellegen, & Kaemmer, 1989), a posttraumatic stress disorder (PTSD) measure, or a test of borderline traits is administered. Instead, a comprehensive assessment of abuse-related difficulties should involve multiple measures that encompass not only the usual tests of anxiety, depression, or PTSD but also, for example, dissociation, somatization, self-capacities, sexual issues, and cognitive distortions.

PSYCHOLOGICAL TESTS AND MEASURES USED IN ABUSE EFFECTS RESEARCH AND PRACTICE

As I have indicated, a wide variety of negative psychological states and traits are associated with a childhood history of abuse. In many cases, these have been tested with generic self-report instruments, such as the MMPI-2, the Millon Clinical Multiaxial Inventory—III (MCMI-III; Millon, 1994), and the Rorschach Inkblot Test (Rorschach, 1921/1981). All of these measures are examined in this chapter because of their frequent use in the assessment of child abuse survivors. In addition, a number of more directly trauma-relevant self-report measures are described as they relate to the evaluation of abuse survivors. Not included in this review, however, are structured clinical interviews (e.g., the Clinician-Administered PTSD Scale [CAPS; Blake, et al., 1995], the Structured Clinical Interview for DSM-IV Dissociative Disorders [SCID-D; Steinberg, 1994], and the Structured Interview for Disorders of Extreme Stress [SIDES; Pelcovitz et al., 1997]) that also are helpful in the assessment of abuse-related disturbance. The reader is referred to Weiss, Chapter 4, this volume, for detailed information on trauma-relevant clinical interviews.

Assessment Issues Relevant to Abuse Survivors

Before discussing specific assessment tools, I consider several issues relevant to the assessment of abuse survivors. Although less technical in nature than instrument psychometrics, these aspects of the testing process are critically important to effective evaluation.

Importance of Rapport and Sensitivity

Because most abuse survivors were, almost by definition, maltreated by authority figures, it is not uncommon for former victims to approach the psychological assessment process with some level of fear, distrust, or concerns about evaluation. As a result, the clinician must especially strive to provide a manifestly safe and nonjudgmental testing environment and to approach the issue of childhood maltreatment in a gradual and nonupsetting manner (Armstrong, 1995; Courtois, 1995). The psychological assessor with a brusque, dismissive, or intrusive manner runs the risk of motivating negativistic or avoidant responses in the client, as well as potentially increasing the survivor's scores on dysphoria and stress measures. This dynamic is more likely to occur if the evaluation includes a structured interview or projective (as opposed to objective) test, as the survivor must interact directly with the evaluator in order to produce test data.

The Role of Avoidance

As noted earlier, chronic child abuse promotes and reinforces the development of avoidance defenses. Unfortunately, this tendency to avoid or attenuate distress may decrease the survivor's response to psychological assessment, in some instances leading to a significant underpresentation of abuse history (Briere & Zaidi, 1989; Currier & Briere, 2000) and/or abuse effects (Courtois, 1988). Although unlikely to produce lasting harm, any assessment technique that intentionally or inadvertently requires the abuse survivor to recall or reexperience abuse-related events can activate upsetting thoughts or feelings and, and a result, may motivate denial or other cognitive avoidance responses.

On occasion, avoidance may present in its most extreme form, that of dissociative amnesia (Courtois, 1999), or, at lower levels, chronic suppression of negative thoughts or memories (Briere, 2002a). In such cases, the client may have insufficient narrative recall of abuse experiences as tapped by measures of childhood maltreatment history. Various studies suggest that some instances of childhood sexual and physical abuse may be relatively unavailable to conscious memory for extended periods of time, during which, presumably, the participants in these studies would deny or underestimate historical events that did, in fact, occur (see a review by Williams & Banyard, 1999). Although aspects of these studies have been criticized for their methodological shortcomings (e.g., Loftus, 1993), the repeated replication of reduced or absent memories of childhood abuse experiences suggests that individual self-reports of childhood maltreatment may be subject to a nontrivial rate of false negatives (Courtois, 1999).

Avoidance also can affect clients' reports of symptomatology on assessment instruments (Carlson, 1997; Epstein, 1993; Friedrich, 2002). Dissociative and cognitive avoidance of painful material are both prevalent in survivors of physical and sexual abuse, and both may suppress clients' scores on symptom measures. For example, Elliott and Briere (1994) report on a subsample of children for whom there was compelling evidence of sexual abuse but who, nonetheless, both denied that they had been abused and scored *lower* than control participants (children without sexual abuse histories) on the Trauma Symptom Checklist for Children (TSCC; Briere, 1996). As we noted, it is likely that these children were using denial and other cognitive avoidance strategies to keep from confronting both their abuse and its psychological impacts. In the absence of outside corroboration, these children probably would have been judged as nonabused (and, presumably, asymptomatic) on interview or by psychological evaluation.

Symptom underreporting, although potentially an important issue in the assessment of abuse survivors and other traumatized individuals, is obviously difficult to identify in any given individual. At present, the practitioner is limited to reliance on validity scales that, for example, index defensiveness or "fake good" responses (e.g., the L and K scales of the MMPI, the Positive Impression Management scale of the Personality Assessment Inventory [PAI], the Desirability scale of the MCMI, or the Response Level scale of the Trauma Symptom Inventory [TSI; Briere, 1995]). Unfortunately, although these validity indicators may point to more extreme examples of underreporting, it is likely that many other instances will go unidentified unless the clinician can somehow detect it during the evaluation interview (Shedler, Mayman, & Manis, 1993).

Overreporting, Confabulation, and Malingering

In addition to underreporting, some individuals misreport or falsely report abuse histories and/or abuse-related symptomatology. Occasionally, false reports of abuse may occur in psychosis or extreme personality disorders. On the other hand, the presence of either condition is not necessarily a risk factor for untruthfulness about abuse: Research suggests that borderline personality disorder may also *arise* from, among other things, severe sexual abuse (e.g., Briere & Zaidi, 1989; Herman, Perry, & van der Kolk, 1989; Ogata et al., 1990), and recent research implicates child abuse in at least some psychotic presentations (e.g., Read, 1997; Ross, Anderson, & Clark, 1994). In addition, I know of no data to suggest that more disturbed individuals have a lower probability of being abused than other people. As a result, the child abuse reports of psychotic or borderline individuals should not be discounted automatically but, instead, should be evaluated for their credibility in the same manner as any other historical data might be considered. Rather than excessive focus on the client's diagnosis to index response validity, consideration of issues such as current reality contact, memory function, or emotional stability may be more helpful in assessing whether a given protocol is credible.

It is also possible for individuals to confabulate abuse memories as a result of the demand characteristics associated with certain therapists and therapies. Specifically, overly directive therapists and the inappropriate use of hypnosis, "memory recovery" techniques, and other activities that especially capitalize on suggestion may reduce the accuracy of therapy-associated recollections of abuse (Courtois, 1999; Lindsay & Briere, 1997; Enns, McNeilly, Corkery, & Gilbert, 1995). Unfortunately, because not all therapy is good therapy, it may be necessary on occasion to query the client regarding the nature and impacts of previous therapeutic interventions—especially when the reported abuse appears especially unlikely.

Finally, it is not especially uncommon for some individuals who have suffered stigmatization and rejection (including child abuse) to amplify their subsequent complaints in an effort to draw attention to injuries that they believe would be overlooked otherwise. When this occurs on psychological tests, it is sometimes referred to as a "cry for help," typically involving a generic overendorsement of symptom items in order to call attention to one's distress. Unfortunately, as a result of such symptom amplification, the survivor's more accurate symptom reports may be overlooked or misinterpreted.

Although overreporting is likely to be considerably less frequent than underreporting in nonforensic clinical situations, it is obviously important to identify it when it occurs. Unfortunately, as per underreporting, it is not always easy to uncover cases of overreporting through the use of psychological tests. Overreporting or false reporting of symptomatology, for example, may be detected only in its most obvious instances through validity scale scores, such as elevations on the F or F_p scales of the MMPI, the Debasement scale of the MCMI, or the Negative Bias scale of the Detailed Assessment of Posttraumatic Stress (DAPS; Briere, 2001). Similarly, elevated psychosis scores on standardized instruments—if found to represent true psychotic disorder—may suggest instances in which the client is too cognitively disorganized or delusional to respond in valid ways to psychological tests of trauma. Finally, the client whose historical reports or symptom presentation appear especially unlikely (e.g., descriptions of alien abductions, technically impossible abuse scenarios, or especially bizarre symptomatology) obviously is likely to be misreporting or confabulating, although even such individuals may have experienced other, actual abuse events and may nevertheless report at least some events or symptoms accurately.

Moderating Phenomena

An additional issue in the assessment of abuse survivors is the role of "third variables" in participants' responses to psychological assessment. This issue arises because child abuse often occurs in the context of a wide variety of other potentially detrimental phenomena, including lower socioeconomic status (Finkelhor & Baron, 1986), early attachment difficulties (Alexander, 1992; Cicchetti & Toth, 1995), family disturbance (Briere & Elliott, 1993; Nash, Hulsey, Sexton, Harralson, & Lambert, 1993), parental substance abuse (Melchert, 2000), and other forms of coexisting child maltreatment (e.g., concomitant physical or psychological abuse in a sexual abuse victim; Briere & Runtz, 1990). These various factors may in and of themselves elevate symptom scales and thus confound what otherwise might be appear to be straightforward abuse effects.

A number of studies also indicate that childhood abuse is a significant risk factor for subsequent revictimization as an adult (Coid et al., 2001; Feerick, Haugaard, & Hien, 2002; Stermac, Reist, Addison, & Millar, 2002). As a result, what may appear to be the long-term effects of childhood abuse in a given individual may be, in fact, the effects of a more recent sexual or physical assault or the exacerbating interaction of child abuse and adult assault. In such an instance, the client's more recent trauma history must be taken into account before his or her symptoms can be attributed solely to childhood events.

Given these complexities, psychological assessment can rarely determine exactly which symptoms or difficulties in an adult survivor of abuse are, in fact, directly related to a given instance of abuse. Further, it will never be true that psychological testing alone can serve as an absolute litmus test for whether abuse has or has not occurred in a given individual. Instead, such data should be combined with all other available information (including the relevant child abuse literature) to provide hypotheses about what *may* be abuse effects in someone who has reported abuse. Other than in a court of law, however, the ultimate issue is less likely to be, Are these symptoms or dysfunctions directly due to a specific act of child abuse, devoid of all other potential mediating factors? but rather, What is the current symptom status of this individual for whom a child abuse history is known? Evaluation of the latter question best occurs when the client is administered not only generic psychological tests but also instruments that are more relevant to the specific difficulties of adults abused as children and thus more likely to tap symptoms or problems that otherwise might be overlooked or misinterpreted.

Commonly Used Abuse-Nonspecific Tests

There are several psychological tests that are widely applied to abuse survivors despite their lack of focus on abuse effects. In each case, the assessor must walk the delicate balance between (1) having access to data that, although not abuse specific, can be valid and useful and (2) running the risk of underassessing or distorting abuse effects though the use of generic measures. By becoming more aware of the strengths and weaknesses of these tests, the evaluator can maximize their helpfulness and lessen their problematic aspects.

MMPI

The MMPI and its successor, the MMPI-2, are very popular instruments and thus often have been applied to abuse survivors. The MMPI scores of sexual abuse survivors have been examined in a number of studies, wherein a profile characterized by elevations in scales 4 (Pd) and 8 (Sc) appears to be most prevalent, frequently followed by lesser elevations on 2 (D), 7 (Pt), and/or 6 (Pa; e.g., Belkin, Greene, Rodrigue, & Boggs, 1994; Engles, Moisan, & Harris, 1994; Hunter, 1991; Goldwater & Duffy, 1990; Lundberg-Love, Marmion, Ford, Geffner, & Peacock, 1992). The relationship between this two-point profile and a history of childhood sexual abuse has been documented for some time—for example, Caldwell and O'Hare (1975) noted almost three decades ago that women with elevated 4–8 profiles often report "a seductive and ambivalent father" and "a high frequency of incest" (p. 94).

Although a body of evidence suggests that sexual abuse survivors in therapy tend to present with a 4–8 profile (other profiles also are possible; see Carlin & Ward, 1992; Elhai, Klotz Flitter, Gold, & Sellers, 2001), it is not clear whether this configuration should be interpreted in the manner suggested by standard interpretive texts. In this regard, traditional approaches to MMPI interpretation may be misleading in the evaluation of abuse-related disturbance. For example, Lundberg-Love et al. (1992) note that

> Historically, clinically significant elevations on the Pd and Sc scales have been interpreted as evidence of sociopathy and schizophrenia, respectively. Indeed, Scott and Stone (1986) concluded that the results of their testing indicated that incest survivors possessed a general deviancy from societal standards and a tendency to act out in antisocial, immature, and egocentric ways. (p. 98)

Lundberg-Love et al. (1992) note that the sexual abuse survivors in their sample accomplished a 4–8 profile through the differential endorsement of certain Pd and Sc items (as measured by Harris & Lingoes, 1968, subscales) over others. Specifically, survivors' scale 4 elevations were due primarily to endorsement of familial discord and current feelings of alienation, rather than the authority and social imperturbability Pd items often endorsed by more antisocial individuals. Similarly, their sexual abuse sample scored highest on the social alienation and reduced ego mastery items of scale 8, as opposed to the clinical levels of endorsement of bizarre sensory experiences and emotional alienation often found in true schizophrenics. In another study, sexual abuse survivors' scale 8 elevations appeared to be due primarily to the dissociation and depression often associated with sexual abuse experiences (Elhai, Gold, Mateus, & Astaphan, 2001) rather than to psychotic symptoms. In fact, the tendency for scale 8 to index dissociative symptoms in abuse (and other trauma) survivors has been described in the assessment literature (e.g., Friedrich, 2002).

It is not only clinical scale interpretation of the MMPI that may suffer when applied to abuse survivors. Also potentially problematic is the F scale and other "fake bad" indices of this measure, which tend to be endorsed to a greater extent by former child abuse victims and other trauma survivors (Briere, in press; Carlson, 1997). Elliott (1993), for example, found that psychiatric inpatients with victimization histories had twice the likelihood of invalid MMPI profiles than their nonvictimized cohorts (30% vs. 15%). It is likely that, for some abused individuals, elevated F scores reflect the tendency for trauma-related dissociative and intrusive symptomatology to produce unusual experiences and chaotic, disorganized internal states. Under such conditions, an elevated F scale may not suggest a malingering response or invalid protocol so much as an accurate portrayal of extreme stress (Elliott, 1994).

A positive development with regard to the MMPI assessment of abuse-related disturbance is the inclusion of two PTSD scales in the MMPI-II: the PK (Keane, Malloy, & Fairbanks, 1984) and the PS (Schlenger & Kulka, 1989). The PK and PS scales, although of only moderate predictive validity with reference to true PTSD, are clearly more effective than other MMPI scales in assessing posttraumatic stress. Despite a paucity of data on the efficacy of these new scales in identifying child abuse trauma per se (although see Knisely, Barker, Ingersoll, & Dawson, 2000, and Zierhoffer, 1996), clinical experience suggests that they are helpful in pinpointing some of the symptoms associated with posttraumatic disturbance in victimized populations.

MCMI

The MCMI-II (Millon, 1987) and MCMI-III (Millon, 1994) are among the most popular of personality tests (Choca, Shanley, & Van Denburg, 1992; Piotrowski & Lubin, 1990). As such, they are widely applied in clinical situations, including in the assessment of abuse survivors. In several studies of the

MCMI and child abuse trauma (e.g., Allen, Coyne, & Huntoon, 1998; Bryer, Nelson, Miller, & Krol, 1987; Busby, Glenn, Steggell, & Adamson, 1993; Fisher, Winne, & Ley, 1993), physical and/or sexual abuse survivors score in the clinical range on a variety of MCMI-I and MCMI-II scales, most typically on the *Avoidant*, *Dependent*, *Passive-Aggressive*, and *Borderline* personality scales and the *Anxiety*, *Somatoform*, *Thought Disorder*, *Major Depression*, and *Delusional Disorder* syndrome scales. Also typically elevated on the MCMI-II is the *Self-Defeating* personality scale (e.g., Allen et al., 1998), although this unfortunately named scale is not present in the MCMI-III.

As with the MMPI, a potential problem associated with interpreting abuse survivors' responses to the MCMI is whether high scores on a given scale indicate that the survivor, in fact, "has" the relevant disorder or personality style. For example, clinical experience suggests that adults abused as children who have elevated scores on MCMI scales that involve psychosis (i.e., Thought Disorder and Delusional Disorder) do not necessarily show psychotic symptoms, nor do all of those with a clinical Borderline scale score necessarily have borderline personality disorder. Instead, the psychotic scales may tap the posttraumatic symptoms (especially reexperiencing and avoidance), dissociation, and chaotic internal experience of survivors of severe abuse, whereas the Borderline scale may be affected by the greater identity, affect regulation, and interpersonal difficulties of the severely abused (Briere, 2000a).

Reinforcing the potential for misidentification of abuse survivors on the MCMI, Choca et al. (1992) note that individuals with posttraumatic stress disorder (a common diagnosis among survivors of extreme childhood abuse, as noted earlier) often score in the clinical range on a variety of MCMI scales. They further note that these scale elevations "do not exclusively identify individuals with PTSD because there may be individuals with other diagnoses who also fit the same pattern of scale elevations" (p. 128). Stated in the reverse, individuals with PTSD are likely to appear to have other psychiatric disorders on the MCMI by virtue of the relevance of other scale items to posttraumatic symptomatology.

With the advent of the MCMI-III, some of these issues have been reduced to some extent, as this measure does have a PTSD (R) scale. The latter is loosely tied to DSM-IV criteria, although, like many trauma measures, the symptoms are not anchored to any specific traumatic event, and no time frame is specified for symptom duration. In addition, review of the items of this scale reveals a number of depressive items not directly associated with DSM-IV diagnostic criteria. Results of the MCMI-III validation studies indicate that the R scale is reliable (alpha = .89, test–retest = .94) and that it has reasonable specificity (.84) but poor sensitivity (.37) in the detection of participants diagnosed with PTSD (Millon, 1994). A second MCMI-III validity study (Millon, Davis, & Millon, 1997) suggested that the diagnostic utility of the MCMI-III vis-à-vis PTSD was better than previously reported, although some of that apparent improvement may have been due to methodological problems associated with both the 1994 and 1997 studies (Hsu, 2002). Clinical experience suggests that this scale does improve the interpretation of abuse survivors' MCMI scores by indicating the possible presence of posttraumatic stress. In such an instance, although other, less relevant, scales might also be elevated (e.g., Thought Disorder), the presence of a high PTSD score might alert the examiner to the possibility of alternate explanations for such elevations.

Personality Assessment Inventory

The Personality Assessment Inventory (PAI; Morey, 1991) is a 344-item inventory consisting of 4 validity scales and 18 nonoverlapping clinical scales, many of which have scorable subscales. Because of its relative recency, the PAI has not been well studied in terms of its association with child abuse trauma. However, it contains a PTSD subscale, evaluates both Axis I and Axis II disorders, and—as one of the latest generation of multitarget psychological tests—has superior psychometric characteristics.

The PTSD subscale (ARD-T) of the PAI is one of three components of the full *Anxiety-Related Disorders (ARD)* scale. Five items of *ARD-T* tap reexperiencing phenomena, and three are concerned with, respectively, guilt, loss of interest, and avoidance of memory-triggering stimuli. In the beta stage of test development, *ARD-T* had an alpha of .89 in 325 participants. In follow-up reliability studies, alphas ranged from .81 to .89 in community, college student, and clinical samples.

The few studies available on PAI scores among abuse survivors indicate that elevations on scales associated with Morey's (1991) *Cluster 2* (involving symptoms associated with trauma exposure and PTSD, including *ARD-T*) and "borderline" symptoms (i.e., the *BOR* subscales) are considerably more likely among child abuse survivors (Cherepon & Prinzhorn, 1994; Feder, 1996). More generally, this measure has wide content coverage (i.e., covering both Axis I and II disorders) and very good psychometric characteristics—qualities that should justify its frequent use in the assessment of those with childhood maltreatment histories.

Rorschach

In contrast to the MCMI or PAI, a number of studies have been done of child abuse survivors' Rorschach responses (e.g., Armstrong & Loewenstein, 1990; Meyers, 1988; Owens, 1984; Kamphuis, Kugeares, & Finn, 2000; Leavitt, 2000; Nash et al., 1993; Saunders, 1991). These studies document a number of response patterns especially common to clinical child abuse survivors, most of which parallel classic Rorschach indicators of borderline personality disorder or PTSD (Berg, 1983; Saunders, 1991; Sugarman, 1980; van der Kolk & Ducey, 1989). Those Rorschach indicators most frequently present in abuse survivor protocols appear to be higher color-dominated responses; more blood, anatomy, morbid, and sexual content; greater aggression; reduced texture; more active, passive, and atypical movement; greater bodily concerns; and more confabulation. The reader is referred to Luxenberg & Levin (Chapter 8, this volume) for a comprehensive review of indicators and issues associated with the Rorschach evaluation of traumatized individuals, much of which is relevant to child abuse survivors.

As is true of the other standard measures reviewed here, the Rorschach has both positive and negative qualities with regard to the assessment of former child abuse victims. On the one hand, the Rorschach provides an opportunity to avoid the constraints of objective testing, wherein the survivor typically is forced to respond to a specific test item and therefore to a specific minihypothesis regarding the structure of psychological disturbance. Instead, the Rorschach offers a set of relatively free-form stimuli, to which the client may respond in any manner he or she chooses. As a result, the productions of the client are less predetermined and therefore more free to reflect whatever abuse effects might be discoverable by such a method.

On the other hand, the interpretation approaches used to classify Rorschach responses (especially those other than Exner's [1986] system) are often theory driven and thus are subject to whatever level of sensitivity to (or distortion of) abuse effects the underlying interpretive model potentially entails. For example, the abuse-related indicators presented here are frequently viewed as reflective of a psychotic or near-psychotic process, yet the studies from which these abuse indicators were derived were not known to contain psychotic individuals. As well, although some PTSD sufferers revealed signs of thought disorder and/or impaired reality testing in van der Kolk and Ducey's (1989) Rorschach study of war veterans, these indicators "coexisted with an absence of psychotic thinking in clinical interviews, suggesting that the subjects possessed a basically intact reality orientation that was only overwhelmed by intrusive traumatic material in the context of unstructured tests" (Saunders, 1991, p. 50).

Abuse-Relevant Evaluation

Because adults abused as children present with a variety of relatively specific difficulties, their evaluation should include measures sensitive to such concerns and symptoms. For this reason, this section is devoted to those assessment issues most relevant to former child abuse victims. The subsequent section provides a more detailed analysis of those psychological tests that specifically tap abuse-relevant symptomatology. It should be reiterated, however, that being an abuse survivor does not, in some mysterious way, preclude one's being evaluated with generic psychological tests. Rather, it is likely that psychological assessment of the abuse survivor is most successful when it involves standard psychological measures such as the MMPI-2, PAI, or Rorschach, augmented with one or more abuse-specific measures.

Evaluating Abuse History

As noted by Norris and Hamblen (Chapter 3, this volume) in a broader context, detailed assessment of abuse-related difficulties must include evaluation of both the circumstances of the abuse and the psychological disturbance potentially arising from it. Unfortunately, most instruments that evaluate traumatic events in adulthood either overlook childhood abuse or merely include it as one of many traumas that the participant can endorse. There are, however, several scales that specifically examine childhood maltreatment history in adults. These instruments, briefly described next, vary considerably in terms of the number of forms of abuse or neglect they assess and the amount of abuse-specific detail they offer.

ASSESSING ENVIRONMENTS III, FORM SD

The Assessing Environments III, Form SD (AE III-Form SD; Rausch & Knutson, 1991), is a revision of the AE III, first introduced by Berger, Knutson, Mehm, and Perkins in 1988. This scale consists of 170 items forming the following scales: Physical Punishment Scale, Sibling Physical Punishment Scale, Perception of Discipline Scale, Sibling Perception of Punishment Scale, Deserving Punishment Scale, and Sibling Deserving Punishment Scale. The reliability of scales that make up the current (Form SD) version of the AE III was evaluated in a sample of 421 university students, yielding KR-20 coefficients ranging from .68 to .74 (Rausch & Knutson, 1991).

CHILDHOOD TRAUMA QUESTIONNAIRE

The Childhood Trauma Questionnaire (CTQ; Bernstein, et al., 1994) is a 70-item measure that assesses childhood trauma in six areas: physical, sexual, and emotional abuse, physical and emotional neglect, "and related areas of family dysfunction (e.g., substance abuse)" (Bernstein et al., 1994, p. 1133). Items in the CTQ begin with the phrase "When I was growing up" and are rated on 5-point Likert-type scales. Principal-components analysis of the CTQ in a sample of 286 substance-dependent patients yielded four factors that subsequently made up the scales of this measure: physical and emotional abuse, emotional neglect, sexual abuse, and physical neglect. Internal consistency of these factor subscales was moderately high (alphas range from .79 to .94) and, in a subsample of 40 patients, test–retest correlations ranged from .80 to .83 for an average intertest interval of 3.6 months (Bernstein et al., 1994). Later analyses suggest a 5-factor solution, wherein physical and emotional abuse form separate factors (Bernstein, Ahluvalia, Pogge, & Handelsman, 1997; Scher et al., 2001).

CHILD MALTREATMENT INTERVIEW SCHEDULE

The Child Maltreatment Interview Schedule (CMIS; Briere, 1992a) is a 46-item measure, with some items containing a large number of subquestions that yield greater detail on a given abuse or neglect experience. The CMIS evaluates the following areas of maltreatment, each limited to events that occurred before age 17: level of parental physical availability, parental disorder and substance abuse history, parental psychological availability, psychological abuse, physical abuse, emotional abuse, sexual abuse, and perception of physical and sexual abuse status. For each area, specific questions probe the age of onset, the relationship to the abuser, and the severity of the maltreatment. The Psychological Abuse component of the CMIS is a 7-item scale taken from Briere and Runtz (1988, 1990), which it has demonstrated moderate internal consistency (alphas ranging from .75 to .87). The CMIS is also available in a short form (CMIS-SF; Briere, 1992b).

CHILDHOOD MALTREATMENT QUESTIONNAIRE

The Childhood Maltreatment Questionnaire (CMQ; Demaré, 1993) focuses extensively on psychological abuse and neglect, although it includes scales for sexual and physical maltreatment. This questionnaire contains three components: the Psychological Maltreatment Questionnaire (PMQ), the Physical Abuse Questionnaire (PAQ), and the Sexual Abuse Questionnaire (SAQ). The PMQ has 12 scales, each tapping a form of child maltreatment identified as significant in the psychological abuse literature. These are: Rejecting, Degrading, Isolating, Corrupting, Denying Emotional Responsiveness, Exploiting (Nonsexual), Verbal Terrorism, Physical Terrorism, Witness to Violence, Unreliable and Inconsistent Care, Controlling and Stifling Independence, and Physical Neglect. Each CMQ item assesses the frequency of maltreatment behaviors on or before age 17. Validation trials, using large samples of university students, suggest that the scales of the CMQ are valid (alphas ranging from .76 to .95) and predictive of symptomatology (Demaré, 1993).

TRAUMATIC EVENTS SCALE

The Traumatic Events Scale (TES; Elliott, 1992) assesses a wide range of childhood and adult traumas. As with those scales reviewed by Norris and Hamblen (Chapter 3, this volume), the TES evaluates adult traumas in detail. Of the 30 specific traumas examined by the TES, however, 10 are devoted to childhood traumas, both interpersonal and environmental. Interpersonal traumas include physical abuse, psychological abuse, and sexual abuse, as well as witnessing spouse abuse. Considerable detail is obtained vis-à-vis characteristics of child abuse, including age at first and last incident, relationship to perpetrator, and level of distress about the abuse—both at the time it occurred and currently. Additional details are ascertained regarding sexual abuse in particular, such as whether the abuser used threats or force to gain sexual access and whether penetration occurred.

Abuse-Relevant Symptom Measures

Although a number of trauma-relevant measures are available to researchers, as described in other chapters of this volume, many of the older ones have insufficient normative or validity data to justify their regular use as clinical instruments. Two of these instruments are mentioned here, however, because of their great popularity and use in some clinical test batteries. Without norms, however, even these measures must be interpreted with care, and specific clinical conclusions should not be made on their basis alone.

Nonstandardized/Research Measures

IMPACT OF EVENT SCALE

The items and psychometric properties of the original and the relatively recently revised Impact of Event Scale (IES; Horowitz, Wilner, & Alvarez, 1979; IES-R; Weiss & Marmar, 1997) are described in other chapters of this volume (see Weiss, Chapter 7). As a result, only the association between IES scores and child abuse history is discussed here. This measure generates three scale scores (Intrusion, Avoidance, and Hyperarousal), as well as a total score. Adults abused as children appear to score higher on IES scales than nonabused individuals in a variety of nonclinical samples. Briere and Elliott (1998), for example, report that adults with sexual abuse histories in the general population score higher on both the Intrusion and Avoidance scales of the original IES.

DISSOCIATIVE EXPERIENCES SCALE

The Dissociative Experiences Scale (DES; Bernstein & Putnam, 1986) is the most popular measure of dissociation available (Carlson & Armstrong, 1994) and has been used to study many traumatized populations, including adults abused as children (e.g., Chu & Dill, 1990; DiTomasso & Routh, 1993; Draijer & Langeland, 1999; Swett & Halpern, 1993). A meta-analysis that included 26 studies of abuse survivor's DES scores found a moderate relationship between childhood physical or sexual abuse and DES scores, suggesting the potential utility of this measure in the assessment of abuse-related trauma (van IJzendoorn & Schuengel, 1996).

Because the DES has not been normed on the general population, however, it is difficult to interpret a given DES score clinically. A cutoff score (30 or higher) has been suggested for the probable presence of a dissociative disorder (Carlson et al., 1993); however, even those who use this value suggest interpretive caution (Armstrong, 1995). In addition to its use with the cutoff score, the DES may useful as a structured review of dissociative symptomatology, wherein any given item endorsement operates as qualitative information regarding a specific dissociative symptom.

Standardized Measures

As opposed to nonstandardized measures, a handful of psychological tests have been developed specifically to evaluate trauma-related disturbance in clinical settings. The majority of these have been normed on reasonably large and representative samples of the general population, or they have been shown to generate a DSM-IV diagnosis that agrees well with a "gold standard" diagnostic interview. In addition, standardized tests—trauma focused or otherwise—generally demonstrate good to very good reliability and evidence for psychometric validity. The instruments described in this section evaluate phenomena relevant to the presenting problems of child abuse survivors, including posttraumatic stress, dissociation, self-capacities, relational schema, and cognitive distortions.

TRAUMA SYMPTOM INVENTORY

The Trauma Symptom Inventory (TSI; Briere, 1995) is a 100-item instrument that evaluates acute and chronic posttraumatic symptomatology. It has 3 validity scales and 10 clinical scales, all of which yield normative *T*-scores. There are 12 critical items covering issues such as self-mutilation, suicidality, and potential violence against others. The validity scales of the TSI are Response Level, which measures a general underendorsement response style or a need to appear unusually symptom-free; Atypical Response, which evaluates psychosis or extreme distress, a general overendorsement response set, or an attempt to appear especially disturbed or dysfunctional; and Inconsistent Response, which measures unusually inconsistent responses to TSI item-pairs. The 10 clinical scales of the TSI are Anxious Arousal, Depression, Anger/Irritability, Intrusive Experiences, Defensive Avoidance, Dissociation, Sexual Concerns, Dysfunctional Sexual Behavior, Impaired Self-Reference, and Tension-Reduction Behavior. There is an alternate version (the TSI-A) that does not include Sexual Concerns or Dysfunctional Sexual Behavior items.

The TSI was standardized on a random sample of 828 adults from the general population and has been separately normed for military personnel based on a sample of 3,659 Navy recruits. Norms are available for four combinations of sex and age (males and females ages 18–54 and 55 or older). The clinical scales of the TSI are internally consistent (mean alphas ranging from .84 to .87 in general population, clinical, university, and military samples) and exhibit reasonable convergent, predictive, and incremental validity. Recent research suggests that the TSI is relatively sensitive to the lasting sequelae of childhood abuse (e.g., Briere & Elliott, 2003; Merrill, Thomsen, Sinclair, Gold, & Milner, 2001; Runtz & Roche, 1999).

POSTTRAUMATIC STRESS DIAGNOSTIC SCALE

In contrast to the TSI, the Posttraumatic Stress Diagnostic Scale (PDS; Foa, 1995) provides a DSM-IV diagnosis of PTSD. It examines four domains: exposure to potentially traumatic events, characteristics of the most traumatic event, the 17 symptoms listed in the DSM-IV for PTSD, and the extent of symptom interference in the individual's daily life. The frequency of each symptom is rated on a 4-point scale, ranging from 0 (*not at all or only one time* to 3 (*5 or more times a week/almost always*).

The PDS demonstrates positive psychometric characteristics, including high internal consistency (alpha = .92 for the 17 items), good test–retest reliability (kappa = .74), and reasonably good sensitivity and specificity with respect to PTSD diagnosis (.82 and .77, respectively). Although the PDS has not been normed on the general population, Foa (1995) reports PDS data for a group of 248 individuals sampled from treatment and research centers that have high numbers of PTSD sufferers. Because this instrument is criterion based (i.e., it evaluates whether a client meets or does not meet diagnostic criteria for PTSD), general population norms are not required for its central function. Instead of standardized *T*-scores, the PDS describes PTSD symptom severity as "mild," "moderate," "moderate to severe," or "severe."

Despite its psychometric qualities, the PDS does not consider childhood sexual abuse to be a potential trauma unless it involves bodily threat—in contrast to DSM-IV criteria that explicitly include sexual abuse without fear of death or injury as a codable criterion A event (American Psychiatric Association, 2000). As a result, the clinician should adapt the PDS for abuse survivors by informing them that childhood sexual victimization, regardless of whether there was physical harm or threat of harm, is a rateable trauma.

DETAILED ASSESSMENT OF POSTTRAUMATIC STRESS

The Detailed Assessment of Posttraumatic Stress (DAPS; Briere, 2001) is a 105-item standardized inventory that provides information on an adult client's history of various types of trauma exposure (Trauma Specification and Relative Trauma Exposure), as well as scales that tap his or her immediate cognitive, emotional, and dissociative reactions to the trauma (Peritraumatic Distress and Peritraumatic Dissociation), subsequent posttraumatic stress symptoms (Reexperiencing, Avoidance, and Hyperarousal), and level of experienced disability (Posttraumatic Impairment) in the context of a specific traumatic event. Like the PDS, the DAPS provides a tentative DSM-IV diagnosis of PTSD. This measure has two validity scales that evaluate under- and overreport of symptoms (Positive Bias and Negative Bias, respectively) and three scales that measure common trauma/PTSD-related comorbidities (Trauma-Specific Dissociation, Substance Abuse, and Suicidality). The DAPS was normed on 433 adults from the general population who had experienced at least one DSM-IV criterion A trauma. The scales of the DAPS are reliable and demonstrate various types of validity in clinical and nonclinical contexts. The DSM-IV PTSD diagnosis generated by the DAPS has good sensitivity (.88) and specificity (.86) with regard to the gold-standard CAPS diagnostic interview (Briere, 2001). The DAPS has coding options for childhood sexual abuse and childhood physical abuse, allowing clients to rate posttraumatic stress associated with their specific maltreatment histories.

MULTISCALE DISSOCIATION INVENTORY

The Multiscale Dissociation Inventory (MDI; Briere, 2002b) is a 30-item self-report test of dissociative symptomatology. It is normed on 444 trauma-exposed individuals from the general population and has subscales measuring six different types of dissociative responses: Disengagement, Depersonalization, Derealization, Emotional Constriction, Memory Disturbance, and Identity Dissociation. Scores on this measure can be converted to *T*-scores that allow for empirically based clinical interpretation of clients' actual level of dissociative disturbance. The MDI has been shown to be reliable and valid in a number of samples (e.g., Briere, 2002b; Dietrich, 2003), and a multisample factor analysis of over 1,300 participants' scores supports the factorial validity of the individual subscales (Briere, Weathers, & Runtz, in press). A raw Identity Dissociation scale score of 15 or higher has a specificity of .93 and a sensitivity of .92 with reference to an independent dissociative identity disorder (DID) diagnosis (Briere, 2002b).

TRAUMA AND ATTACHMENT BELIEF SCALE

The Trauma and Attachment Belief Scale (TABS; Pearlman, 2003) consists of 84 items that form 10 scales tapping schema about self and others on five dimensions: Safety, Trust, Esteem, Intimacy, and Control. There are norms from 1,743 individuals, age 17 and older, based primarily on a regression-method interpolation of scores from the previous version of the TABS, then known as the Traumatic Stress Institute Belief Scale, Revision L. The TABS has good internal consistency and test–retest reliability (e.g., median values across scales of .79 and .75, respectively, in a sample of 260 college students). Previous versions of the TABS have been employed as a measure of vicarious traumatization in therapists (e.g., Pearlman & Saakvitne, 1995) and as a measure of the effects of trauma (including those of childhood abuse) on college students, outpatients, battered women, and the homeless (Pearlman, 2003).

Although it is a newly published clinical instrument, research on earlier versions of this test and a review of the specific scales and items of the TABS suggest that it is an important addition to existing measures of child abuse–related disturbance. In contrast to more symptom-based tests, the TABS measures the self-reported needs and expectations of trauma survivors, especially as they predict self in relation to others. As a result, the TABS is likely to be helpful in understanding important assumptions that the client carries in his or her relationships to others, including the therapist, and in formulating more relational (i.e., not just symptom focused) treatment goals.

INVENTORY OF ALTERED SELF CAPACITIES

The Inventory of Altered Self Capacities (IASC; Briere, 2000a) is a standardized test that contains 63 items and seven scales measuring various types of "self-related" personality disturbance common to survivors of severe childhood abuse. Scales of the IASC are Interpersonal Conflicts, Idealization–Disillusionment, Abandonment Concerns, Identity Impairment (with two subscales: Self-Awareness and Diffusion), Susceptibility to Influence, Affect Dysregulation (with two subscales: Instability and Skills Deficits), and Tension Reduction Activities. Each symptom item is rated according to its frequency of occurrence over the prior 6 months, using a 4-point scale ranging from 1 (*never*) to 4 (*often*).

The IASC was normed on 620 participants from the general population and validated in community, clinical, and university samples. It is psychometrically reliable and demonstrates predictive validity in both normative and validation samples. The IASC scales have been shown to predict self-reported child abuse history, adult attachment style, "borderline" and "antisocial" personality features, relationship problems, suicidality, and substance abuse (Briere, 2000a). It also can be helpful in predicting—and thus, hopefully, forestalling—certain self–other issues (e.g., abandonment fears, idealization/devaluation, hypersusceptibility to interpretation) that can disrupt or derail the client–therapist relationship during treatment.

COGNITIVE DISTORTIONS SCALE

The Cognitive Distortions Scale (CDS; Briere, 2000b) is a 40-item test that measures five types of cognitive symptoms or distortions found among those who have experienced interpersonal victimization, including child abuse: Self-Criticism, Self-Blame, Helplessness, Hopelessness, and Preoccupation with Danger. Each item is rated according to its frequency of occurrence over the prior month, using a 5-point scale ranging from 1 (*never*) to 5 (*very often*). CDS scales are psychometrically reliable and have construct, predictive, and convergent validity in standardization and validity samples. Scales are normed separately for males and females and can be expressed as *T*-scores. In the standardization samples, individuals with psychological, sexual, and physical abuse histories had significantly elevated scores on the CDS.

DISCUSSION

This chapter has briefly reviewed some of the major issues associated with the assessment of abuse-related distress and dysfunction. In general, it appears that traditional measures of psychological symptoms and disorders are necessary but insufficient to provide a clear and detailed clinical picture of many abuse survivors' psychological functioning. Although such tests can provide important information regarding trauma-nonspecific conditions such as major depression or psychosis, they may overlook certain symptoms or misinterpret certain abuse effects as evidence of other, less relevant difficulties. When using generic measures, the clinician must be careful to consider the applicability of standard interpretation approaches to these measures. Especially important is the clinician's appreciation of the theory and underlying model of symptom development associated with any given test and the extent to which such theory is congruent with what is known about the breadth and form of abuse-related psychological dysfunction. Failure to take these issues into account may result in overpathologized assessments of abuse survivors or misspecification of abuse-specific responses as other disorders.

Partially because professional interest in the lasting effects of child abuse is a relatively new phenomenon, there are fewer abuse-relevant tests available to researchers than is true for other clinical phenomena. Further, clinicians are constrained by the absence of normative data for some of these measures—a minimal requirement for the valid interpretation of most psychological test results. As a result, until recently, the clinician was forced to choose between standardized but insensitive generic tests and specific but nonstandardized psychological measures in the evaluation of abuse effects. This situation has improved somewhat, although further test development is clearly indicated in the child abuse and general trauma fields. Given these limitations and the complexity of childhood maltreatment effects, the assessing practitioner must proceed with due caution. On the other hand, the evaluator who is well versed on the abuse effects literature, aware of the relative strengths and weaknesses of the tests he or she uses, and cognizant of new developments in the psychometrics of trauma response will find that abuse-relevant assessment strategies can provide valid and highly relevant data on the survivor's psychological functioning.

REFERENCES

Alexander, P. C. (1992). Application of attachment theory to the study of sexual abuse. *Journal of Consulting and Clinical Psychology*, *60*, 185–195.

Allen, J. G., Coyne, L., & Huntoon, J. (1998). Complex posttraumatic stress disorder in women from a psychometric perspective. *Journal of Personality Assessment*, *70*, 277–298.

American Psychiatric Association. (2000). *Diagnostic and statistical manual of mental disorders* (4th ed., text rev.). Washington, DC: Author.

Armstrong, J. (1995). Psychological assessment. In J. L. Spira (Ed.), *Treating dissociative identity disorder*. San Francisco: Jossey-Bass.

Armstrong, J. G., & Loewenstein, R. J. (1990). Characteristics of patients with multiple personality and dissociative disorders on psychological testing. *Journal of Nervous and Mental Disease*, *178*, 448–454.

Baldwin, M. W., Fehr, B., Keedian, E., Seidel, M., & Thompson, D. W. (1993). An exploration of the relational schemata underlying attachment styles: Self-report and lexical decision approaches. *Personality and Social Psychology Bulletin*, *19*, 746–754.

Belkin, D. S., Greene, A. F., Rodrigue, J. R., & Boggs, S. R. (1994). Psychopathology and history of sexual abuse. *Journal of Interpersonal Violence*, *9*, 535–547.

Berg, M. (1983). Borderline psychopathology as displayed on psychological tests. *Journal of Personality Assessment*, *47*, 120–133.

Berger, A. M., Knutson, J. F., Mehm, J. G., & Perkins, K. A. (1988). The self-report of punitive childhood experiences of young adults and adolescents. *Child Abuse and Neglect*, *12*, 251–262.

Bernstein, D. P., Ahluvalia, T., Pogge, D., & Handelsman, L. (1997). Validity of the Childhood Trauma Questionnaire in an adolescent psychiatric population. *Journal of the American Academy of Child and Adolescent Psychiatry*, *36*, 340–348.

Bernstein, D. P., Fink, L., Handelsman, L., Foote, J., Lovejoy, M., & Wenzel, K. (1994). Initial reliability and validity of a new retrospective measure of child abuse and neglect. *American Journal of Psychiatry*, *151*, 1132–1136.

Bernstein, E. M., & Putnam, F. W. (1986). Development, reliability, and validity of a dissociation scale. *Journal of Nervous and Mental Diseases*, *174*, 727–734.

Blake, D. D., Weathers, F. W., Nagy, L. M., Kaloupek, D. G., Gusman, F. D., Charney, D. S., & Keane, T. M. (1995). The development of a clinician-administered PTSD scale. *Journal of Traumatic Stress*, *8*, 75–90.

Briere, J. (1992a). *Child abuse trauma: Theory and treatment of the lasting effects.* Thousand Oaks, CA: Sage.

Briere, J. (1992b). *Child Maltreatment Interview Schedule, Short Form (CMIS-SF).* Retrieved February 11, 2004, from *http://www.JohnBriere.com/cmis.htm*

Briere, J. (1995). *Trauma Symptom Inventory*. Odessa, FL: Psychological Assessment Resources.

Briere, J. (1996). *Trauma Symptom Checklist for Children (TSCC)*. Odessa, FL: Psychological Assessment Resources.

Briere, J. (2000a). *Inventory of Altered Self Capacities (IASC)*. Odessa, FL: Psychological Assessment Resources.

Briere, J. (2000b). *Cognitive Distortions Scale (CDS)*. Odessa, FL: Psychological Assessment Resources.

Briere, J. (2001). *Detailed Assessment of Posttraumatic Stress (DAPS)*. Odessa, FL: Psychological Assessment Resources.

Briere, J. (2002a). Treating adult survivors of severe childhood abuse and neglect: Further development of an integrative model. In J. E. B. Myers, L. Berliner, J. Briere, C. T. Hendrix, T. Reid, & C. Jenny (Eds.), *The APSAC handbook on child maltreatment* (2nd ed., pp. 175–202). Thousand Oaks, CA: Sage.

Briere, J. (2002b). *Multiscale Dissociation Inventory*. Odessa. FL: Psychological Assessment Resources.

Briere, J. (in press). *Psychological assessment of adult posttraumatic states: Phenomenology, diagnosis, and measurement* (2nd ed.). Washington, DC: American Psychological Association.

Briere, J., & Elliott, D. M. (1993). Sexual abuse, family environment, and psychological symptoms: On the validity of statistical control. *Journal of Consulting and Clinical Psychology*, *61*, 284–288.

Briere, J., & Elliott, D. M. (1998). Clinical utility of the Impact of Event Scale: Psychometrics in the general population. *Assessment*, *5*, 135–144.

Briere, J., & Elliott, D. M. (2003). Prevalence and symptomatic sequelae of self-reported childhood physical and sexual abuse in a general population sample of men and women. *Child Abuse and Neglect*, *27*, 1205–1222.

Briere, J., Elliott, D. M., Harris, K., & Cotman, A. (1995). Trauma Symptom Inventory: Psychometrics and association with childhood and adult trauma in clinical samples. *Journal of Interpersonal Violence*, *10*, 387–401.

Briere, J., & Gil, E. (1998). Self-mutilation in clinical and general population samples:

Prevalence, correlates, and functions. *American Journal of Orthopsychiatry, 68*, 609–620.

Briere, J., & Runtz, M. (1988). Multivariate correlates of childhood psychological and physical maltreatment among university women. *Child Abuse and Neglect, 12*, 331–341.

Briere, J., & Runtz, M. (1990). Differential adult symptomatology associated with three types of child abuse histories. *Child Abuse and Neglect, 14*, 357–364.

Briere, J., Weathers, F. W., & Runtz, M. (in press). Is dissociation a multidimensional construct?: Data from the Multiscale Dissociation Inventory. *Journal of Traumatic Stress*.

Briere, J., Woo, R., McRae, B., Foltz, J., & Sitzman, R. (1997). Lifetime victimization history, demographics, and clinical status in female psychiatric emergency room patients. *Journal of Nervous and Mental Disease, 185*, 95–101.

Briere. J., & Zaidi, L. Y. (1989). Sexual abuse histories and sequelae in female psychiatric emergency room patients. *American Journal of Psychiatry, 146*, 1602–1606.

Bryer, J. B., Nelson, B. A., Miller, J. B., & Krol, P. A. (1987). Childhood sexual and physical abuse as factors in adult psychiatric illness. *American Journal of Psychiatry, 144*, 1426–1430.

Busby, D. M., Glenn, E., Steggell, G. L., & Adamson, D. W. (1993). Treatment issues for survivors of physical and sexual abuse. *Journal of Marital and Family Therapy, 19*, 377–391.

Butcher, J. N., Dahlstrom, W. G., Graham, J. R., Tellegen, A., & Kaemmer, B. (1989). *Minnesota Multiphasic Personality Inventory (MMPI-2): Manual for administration and scoring*. Minneapolis: University of Minnesota Press.

Caldwell, A. B., & O'Hare, C. (1975). *A handbook of MMPI personality types*. Santa Monica, CA: Clinical Psychological Services.

Carlin, A. S., & Ward, N. G. (1992). Subtypes of psychiatric inpatient women who have been sexually abused. *Journal of Nervous and Mental Disease, 180*, 392–397.

Carlson, E. B. (1997). *Trauma assessments: A clinician's guide*. New York: Guilford Press.

Carlson, E. B., & Armstrong, J. G. (1994). The diagnosis and assessment of dissociative disorders. In S. J. Lynn & J. W. Rhue (Ed.), *Dissociation: Clinical and theoretical perspectives* (pp. 159–174). New York: Guilford Press.

Carlson, E. B., Putnam, F. W., Ross, C. A., Torem, M. S., Coons, P. M., Dill, D. L., et al. (1993). Validity of the Dissociative Experiences Scale in screening for multiple personality disorder: A multicenter study. *American Journal of Psychiatry, 150*, 1030–1036.

Cherepon, J. A., & Prinzhorn, B. (1994). Personality Assessment Inventory (PAI) profiles of adult female abuse survivors. *Assessment, 1*, 393–399.

Choca, J. P., Shanley, L. A., & Van Denburg, E. (1992). *Interpretative guide to the Millon Clinical Multiaxial Inventory*. Washington, DC: American Psychological Association.

Chu, J. A., & Dill, D. L. (1990). Dissociative symptoms in relation to childhood physical and sexual abuse. *American Journal of Psychiatry, 147*, 887–892.

Cicchetti, D., & Toth, S. L. (1995). A developmental psychopathology perspective on child abuse and neglect. *Journal of the American Academy of Child and Adolescent Psychiatry, 34*, 541–565.

Coid, J., Petruckevitch, A., Feder, G., Chung, W., Richardson, J., & Moorey, S.

(2001). Relation between childhood sexual and physical abuse and risk of revictimisation in women: A cross-sectional survey. *Lancet, 358*, 450–454.
Cole, P. M., & Putnam, F. W. (1992). Effect of incest on self and social functioning: A developmental psychopathology perspective. *Journal of Consulting and Clinical Psychology, 60*, 174–184.
Connors, M. E., & Morse, W. (1993). Sexual abuse and eating disorders: A review. *International Journal of Eating Disorders, 13*, 1–11.
Courtois, C. A. (1988). *Healing the incest wound: Adult survivors in therapy*. New York: Norton.
Courtois, C. (1995). Assessment and diagnosis. In C. Classen (Ed.), *Treating women molested in childhood* (pp. 1–34). San Francisco: Jossey-Bass.
Courtois, C. (1999). *Recollections of sexual abuse: Treatment principles and guidelines*. New York: Norton.
Currier, G. W., & Briere, J. (2000). Trauma orientation and detection of violence histories in the psychiatric emergency service. *Journal of Nervous and Mental Disease, 188*, 622–624.
Davis, J. L., Combs-Lane, A. M., & Jackson, T. L. (2002). Risky behaviors associated with interpersonal victimization: Comparisons based on type, number, and characteristics of assault incidents. *Journal of Interpersonal Violence, 17*, 611–629.
Davis, J. L., Petretic-Jackson, P. A., & Ting, L. (2001). Intimacy dysfunction and trauma symptomatology: Long-term correlates of different types of child abuse. *Journal of Traumatic Stress, 14*, 63–79.
De Bellis, M. D. (2002). Developmental traumatology: A contributory mechanism for alcohol and substance use disorders. *Psychoneuroendocrinology, 27*, 155–170.
Demaré, D. (1993, August). *Childhood psychological maltreatment experiences as predictors of adulthood psychological symptomatology*. Paper presented at the annual meeting of the American Psychological Association, Toronto, Ontario, Canada.
Dietrich, A. M. (2003). Characteristics of child maltreatment, psychological dissociation, and somatoform dissociation of Canadian inmates. *Journal of Trauma and Dissociation, 4*, 81–100.
DiTomasso, M. J., & Routh, D. K. (1993). Recall of abuse in childhood and three measures of dissociation. *Child Abuse and Neglect, 17*, 477–485.
Draijer, N., & Langeland, W. (1999). Childhood trauma and perceived parental dysfunction in the etiology of dissociative symptoms in psychiatric inpatients. *American Journal of Psychiatry, 156*, 379–385.
Drossman, D. A., Li, Z., Leserman, J., Toomey, T. C., & Hu, Y. J. B. (1996). Health status by gastrointestinal diagnosis and abuse history. *Gastroenterology, 110*, 999–1007.
Dube, S. R., Anda, R. F., Felitti, V. J., Chapman, D. P., Williamson, D. F., & Giles, W. H. (2001). Childhood abuse, household dysfunction, and the risk of attempted suicide throughout the life span: Findings from the Adverse Childhood Experiences Study. *Journal of the American Medical Association, 286*, 3089–3096.
Dutton, D. G., Starzomski, A., & Ryan, L. (1996). Antecedents of abusive personality and abusive behavior in wife assaulters. *Journal of Family Violence, 11*, 113–132.
Elhai, J. D., Gold, S. N., Mateus, L. F., & Astaphan, T. A. (2001). Scale 8 elevations on the MMPI-2 among women survivors of childhood sexual abuse: Evaluating posttraumatic stress, depression, and dissociation as predictors. *Journal of Family Violence, 16*, 47–57.

Elhai, J. D., Klotz Flitter, J. M., Gold, S. N., & Sellers, A. H. (2001). Identifying subtypes of women survivors of childhood sexual abuse: An MMPI-2 cluster analysis. *Journal of Traumatic Stress, 14*, 157–175.

Elklit, A. (2002). Victimization and PTSD in a Danish national youth probability sample. *Journal of the American Academy of Child and Adolescent Psychiatry, 41*, 174–181.

Elliott, D. M. (1992). *Traumatic Events Survey*. Unpublished psychological test. Los Angeles: Harbor-UCLA Medical Center.

Elliott, D. M. (1993, November). *Assessing the psychological impact of recent violence in an inpatient setting*. Paper presented at the meeting of the International Society for Traumatic Stress Studies, San Antonio, TX.

Elliott, D. M. (1994). Assessing adult victims of interpersonal violence. In J. Briere (Ed.), *Assessing and treating victims of violence* (*New Directions for Mental Health Services*, MHS #64). San Francisco: Jossey-Bass.

Elliott, D. M., & Briere, J. (1994). Forensic sexual abuse evaluations of older children: Disclosures and symptomatology. *Behavioral Sciences and the Law, 12*, 261–277.

Engles, M. L., Moisan, D., & Harris, R. (1994). MMPI indices of childhood trauma among 110 female outpatients. *Journal of Personality Assessment, 63*, 135–147.

Enns, C. Z., McNeilly, C. L., Corkery, J. M., & Gilbert, M. S. (1995). The debate about delayed memories of child sexual abuse: A feminist perspective. *Counseling Psychologist, 23*, 181–279.

Epstein, R. S. (1993). Avoidant symptoms cloaking the diagnosis of PTSD in patients with severe accidental injury. *Journal of Traumatic Stress, 6*, 451–458.

Exner, J. E. (1986). *The Rorschach: A comprehensive system* (2nd ed.). New York: Wiley.

Feder, S. (1996). *Self-mutilation and childhood trauma*. Unpublished doctoral dissertation, Adelphi University, Institute of Advanced Psychological Studies.

Feerick, M. M., Haugaard, J. J., & Hien, D. A. (2002). Child maltreatment and adulthood violence: The contribution of attachment and drug abuse. *Child Maltreatment, 7*, 226–240.

Feiring, C., Rosenthal, S., & Taska, L. S. (2000). Stigmatization and the development of friendship and romantic relationships in adolescent victims of sexual abuse. *Child Maltreatment, 5*, 311–322.

Finkelhor, D., & Baron, L. (1986). High-risk children. In D. Finkelhor (Ed.), *A sourcebook on child sexual abuse* (pp. 60–88). Newbury Park, CA: Sage.

Finkelhor, D., Hotaling, G., Lewis, I. A., & Smith, C. (1990). Sexual abuse in a national survey of adult men and women: Prevalence, characteristics, and risk factors. *Child Abuse and Neglect, 14*, 19–28.

Fisher, P. M., Winne, P. H., & Ley, R. G. (1993). Group therapy for adult women survivors of child sexual abuse: Differentiation of completers versus dropouts. *Psychotherapy, 30*, 616–624.

Foa, E. B. (1995). *Posttraumatic Stress Diagnostic Scale*. Minneapolis, MN: National Computer Systems.

Friedrich, W. N. (2002). *Psychological assessment of sexually abused children and their families*. Thousand Oaks, CA: Sage.

Goldwater, L., & Duffy, J. F. (1990). Use of the MMPI to uncover histories of childhood abuse in adult female psychiatric patients. *Journal of Clinical Psychology, 46*, 392–398.

Harris, R., & Lingoes, J. (1968). *Subscales for the Minnesota Multiphasic Personality*

Inventory [Mimeographed materials]. Ann Arbor, MI: University of Michigan, Department of Psychology.

Herman, J. L., Perry, C., & van der Kolk, B. A. (1989). Childhood trauma in borderline personality disorder. *American Journal of Psychiatry, 146*, 490–494.

Horowitz, M. D., Wilner, N., & Alvarez, W. (1979). Impact of Event Scale: A measure of subjective stress. *Psychosomatic Medicine, 41*, 209–218.

Hsu, L. M. (2002). Diagnostic validity statistics and the MCMI-III. *Psychological Assessment, 14*, 410–422.

Hunter, J. A. (1991). A comparison of the psychosocial maladjustment of adult males and females sexually molested as children. *Journal of Interpersonal Violence, 6*, 205–217.

Kamphuis, J. H., Kugeares, S. L., & Finn, S. E. (2000). Rorschach correlates of sexual abuse: Trauma content and aggression indexes. *Journal of Personality Assessment, 75*, 212–224.

Katon, W. J., Sullivan, M., & Walker, E. A. (2001). Medical symptoms without identified pathology: Relationship to psychiatric disorders, childhood and adult trauma, and personality traits. *Annals of Internal Medicine, 134*, 917–925.

Keane, T. M., Malloy, P. F., & Fairbanks, J. A. (1984). Empirical development of an MMPI subscale for the assessment of combat-related posttraumatic stress disorder. *Journal of Consulting and Clinical Psychology, 52*, 888–891.

Knisely, J. S., Barker, S. B., Ingersoll, K. S., & Dawson, K. S. (2000). Psychopathology in substance-abusing women reporting childhood sexual abuse. *Journal of Addictive Diseases, 19*, 31–44.

Leavitt, F. (2000). Texture response patterns associated with sexual trauma of childhood and adult onset: Developmental and recovered memory implications. *Child Abuse and Neglect, 24*, 251–257.

Lindsay, D. S., & Briere, J. (1997). The controversy regarding recovered memories of childhood sexual abuse: Pitfalls, bridges, and future directions [Invited commentary]. *Journal of Interpersonal Violence, 12*, 631–647.

Loftus, E. F. (1993). The reality of repressed memories. *American Psychologist, 48*, 518–537.

Lundberg-Love, P. K., Marmion, S., Ford, K., Geffner, R., & Peacock, L. (1992). The long-term consequences of childhood incestuous victimization upon adult women's psychological symptomatology. *Journal of Child Sexual Abuse, 1*, 81–102.

Luntz, B. K., & Widom, C. S. (1994). Antisocial personality disorder in abused and neglected children grown up. *American Journal of Psychiatry, 151*, 670–674.

MacMillan, H. L., Fleming, J. E., Streiner, D. L., Lin, E., Boyle, M. H., Jamieson, E., et al. (2001). Childhood abuse and lifetime psychopathology in a community sample. *American Journal of Psychiatry, 158*, 1878–1883.

Melchert, T. P. (2000). Clarifying the effects of parental substance abuse, child sexual abuse, and parental caregiving on adult adjustment. *Professional Psychology: Research and Practice, 31*, 64–69.

Merrill, L. L., Thomsen, C. J., Sinclair, B. B., Gold, S., & Milner, J. (2001). Predicting the impact of child sexual abuse on women: The role of abuse severity, parental support, and coping strategies. *Journal of Consulting and Clinical Psychology, 69*, 992–1006.

Meyers, J. (1988). The Rorschach as a tool for understanding the dynamics of women with histories of incest. In H. D. Lerner & P. M. Lerner (Eds.), *Primitive mental states and the Rorschach* (pp. 203–228). Madison, CT: International Universities Press.

Millon, T. (1987). *Manual for the MCMI-II* (2nd ed.). Minneapolis, MN: National Computer Systems.

Millon, T. (1994). *Manual for the MCMI-III*. Minneapolis, MN: National Computer Systems.

Millon, T., Davis, R., & Millon, C. (1997). *MCMI-III manual* (2nd ed.). Minneapolis, MN: National Computer Systems.

Molnar, B. E., Berkman, L. F., & Buka, S. L. (2001). Psychopathology, childhood sexual abuse and other childhood adversities: Relative links to subsequent suicidal behaviour in the U.S. *Psychological Medicine*, *31*, 965–977.

Molnar, B. E., Buka, S. L., & Kessler, R. C. (2001). Child sexual abuse and subsequent psychopathology: Results from the National Comorbidity Survey. *American Journal of Public Health*, *91*, 753–760.

Morey, L. C. (1991). *Personality Assessment Inventory: Professional manual*. Odessa, FL: Psychological Assessment Resources.

Nash, M. R., Hulsey, T. L., Sexton, M. C., Harralson, T. L., & Lambert, W. (1993). Long-term sequelae of childhood sexual abuse: Perceived family environment, psychopathology, and dissociation. *Journal of Consulting and Clinical Psychology*, *61*, 276–283.

Ogata, S. N., Silk, K. R., Goodrich, S., Lohr, N. E., Westin, D., & Hill, E. M. (1990). Childhood sexual and physical abuse in adult patients with borderline personality disorder. *American Journal of Psychiatry*, *147*, 1008–1013.

Owens, G. P., & Chard, K. M. (2001). Cognitive distortions among women reporting childhood sexual abuse. *Journal of Interpersonal Violence*, *16*, 178–191.

Owens, T. H. (1984). Personality traits of female psychotherapy patients with a history of incest: A research note. *Journal of Personality Assessment*, *48*, 606–608.

Pearlman, L. A. (2003). *Trauma and Attachment Belief Scale (TABS) manual*. Los Angeles, CA: Western Psychological Services.

Pearlman, L. A., & Saakvitne, K. W. (1995). *Trauma and the therapist: Countertransference and vicarious traumatization in psychotherapy with incest survivors*. New York: Norton.

Pelcovitz, D., van der Kolk, B. A., Roth, S., Mandel, F., Kaplan, S., & Resick, P. (1997). Development of a criteria set and a structured interview for disorders of extreme stress (SIDES). *Journal of Traumatic Stress*, *10*, 3–16.

Piotrowsky, C., & Lubin, B. (1990). Assessment practices of health psychologists: Survey of APA Division 38 clinicians. *Professional Psychology: Research and Practice*, *21*, 99–106.

Pollock, V. E., Briere, J., Schneider, L., Knop, J., Mednick, S. A., & Goodwin, D. W. (1990). Childhood antecedents of antisocial behavior: Parental alcoholism and physical abusiveness. *American Journal of Psychiatry*, *147*, 1290–1293.

Rausch, K., & Knutson, J. F. (1991). The self-report of personal punitive childhood experiences and those of siblings. *Child Abuse and Neglect*, *15*, 29–36.

Read, J. (1997). Child abuse and psychosis: A literature review and implications for professional practice. *Professional Psychology: Research and Practice*, *28*, 448–456.

Rorschach, H. (1981). *Psychodiagnostics: A diagnostic test based upon perception* (P.

Lemkau & B. Kronemberg, Eds. & Trans., 9th ed.). New York: Grune & Stratton. (Original work published 1921)
Ross, C. A., Anderson, G., & Clark, P. (1994). Childhood abuse and the positive symptoms of schizophrenia. *Hospital and Community Psychiatry, 45*, 489–491.
Rowan, A. B., Foy, D. W., Rodriguez, N., & Ryan, S. (1994). Posttraumatic stress disorder in a clinical sample of adults sexually abused as children. *Child Abuse and Neglect, 18*, 51–61.
Runtz, M. G., & Roche, D. N. (1999). Validation of the Trauma Symptom Inventory in a Canadian sample of university women. *Child Maltreatment, 4*, 69–80.
Saunders, E. A. (1991). Rorschach indicators of chronic childhood sexual abuse in female borderline patients. *Bulletin of the Menninger Clinic, 55*, 48–71.
Scher, C. D., Stein, M. B., Asmundson, G. J. G., McCreary, D. R., & Forde, D. R. (2001). The Childhood Trauma Questionnaire in a community sample: Psychometric properties and normative data. *Journal of Traumatic Stress, 14*, 843–857.
Schlenger, W., & Kulka, R. A. (1989). *PTSD scale development for the MMPI-2*. Research Triangle Park, NC: Research Triangle Park Institute.
Scott, R. L., & Stone, D. A. (1986). MMPI measures of psychological disturbance in adolescent and adult victims of father–daughter incest. *Journal of Consulting and Clinical Psychology, 42*, 251–259.
Shedler, J., Mayman, M., & Manis, M. (1993). The illusion of mental health. *American Psychologist, 48*, 1117–1131.
Simeon, D., Guralnik, O., Schmeidler, J., Sirof, B., & Knutelska, M. (2001). The role of childhood interpersonal trauma in depersonalization disorder. *American Journal of Psychiatry, 158*, 1027–1033.
Springs, F. E., & Friedrich, W. N. (1992). Health risk behaviors and medical sequelae of childhood sexual abuse. *Mayo Clinic Proceedings, 67*, 527–532.
Steinberg, M. (1994). *Structured Clinical Interview for DSM-IV Dissociative Disorders—Revised (SCID-D-R)*. Washington, DC: American Psychiatric Press.
Stermac, L., Reist, D., Addison, M., & Millar, G. M. (2002). Childhood risk factors for women's sexual victimization. *Journal of Interpersonal Violence, 17*, 647–670.
Sugarman, A. (1980). The borderline personality organization as manifested on psychological tests. In J. S. Kwawer, H. D. Lerner, P. M. Lerner, & A. Sugarman (Eds.), *Borderline phenomena and the Rorschach* (pp. 39–57). New York: International Universities Press.
Swett, C., & Halpern, M. (1993). Reported history of physical and sexual abuse in relation to dissociation and other symptomatology in women psychiatric inpatients. *Journal of Interpersonal Violence, 8*, 545–555.
Ullman, S. E., & Brecklin, L. R. (2002). Sexual assault history, PTSD, and mental health service seeking in a national sample of women. *Journal of Community Psychology, 30*, 261–279.
van der Kolk, B. A., & Ducey, C. (1989). Clinical implications of the Rorschach in post-traumatic stress disorder. In B. A. van der Kolk (Ed.), *Post-traumatic stress disorder: Psychological and biological sequelae* (pp. 29–42). Washington, DC: American Psychiatric Press.
van der Kolk, B. A., Perry, J. C., & Herman, J. L. (1991). Childhood origins of self-destructive behavior. *American Journal of Psychiatry, 146*, 490–494.

van IJzendoorn, M. H., & Schuengel, C. (1996). The measurement of dissociation in normal and clinical populations: Meta-analytic validation of the Dissociative Experiences Scale (DES). *Clinical Psychology Review*, *16*, 365–382.

Waller, G. (1992). Sexual abuse and bulimic symptoms in eating disorders: Do family interaction and self-esteem explain the links? *International Journal of Eating Disorders*, *12*, 235–240.

Walsh, B. W., & Rosen, P. (1988). *Self-mutilation: Theory, research, and treatment*. New York: Guilford Press.

Webster, J. J., & Palmer, R. L. (2000). The childhood and family background of women with clinical eating disorders: A comparison with women with major depression and women without psychiatric disorder. *Psychological Medicine*, *30*, 53–60.

Weiss, D. S., & Marmar, C. R. (1997). The Impact of Event Scale—Revised. In J. P. Wilson & T. Keane (Eds.), *Assessing psychological trauma and PTSD* (pp. 399–411). New York: Guilford Press.

Williams, L. M., & Banyard, V. L. (Eds.). (1999). *Trauma and memory*. Thousand Oaks, CA: Sage.

Wyatt, G. E. (1985). The sexual abuse of Afro-American and white American women in childhood. *Child Abuse and Neglect*, *9*, 231–240.

Wyatt, G. E., Newcomb, M. D., & Riederle, M. H. (1993). *Sexual abuse and consensual sex: Women's developmental patterns and outcomes*. Newbury Park, CA: Sage.

Zierhoffer, D. M. (1996). *Validity of the PK and PS scales of the MMPI-2: PTSD and incest*. Unpublished dissertation, Indiana State University.

Zlotnick, C., Zakriski, A., Shea, T., & Costello, E. (1996). The long-term sequelae of sexual abuse: Support for a complex posttraumatic stress disorder. *Journal of Traumatic Stress*, *9*, 195–205.

CHAPTER 20

Gender Issues in the Assessment of PTSD

RACHEL KIMERLING
ANNABEL PRINS
DARRAH WESTRUP
TINA LEE

DEFINING THE ISSUES OF GENDER

The construct of posttraumatic stress disorder (PTSD) was derived largely from the stress reactions of two specific populations: "shell shock" observed among male combat veterans and "rape trauma syndrome" observed among female sexual assault survivors (Saigh & Bremner, 1999). As a result, our understanding of PTSD has been shaped by implicit judgments and assumptions about trauma and gender from its very inception. Gender has a substantial impact on the type of trauma exposure experienced by an individual, the social relationships that mediate the impact of exposure, and the subsequent systems of meaning into which the traumatic event is encoded. Despite the substantive role that gender plays in the experience of trauma, creating a framework to understand gender issues presents a significant challenge. However, an awareness and consideration of gender issues can only enhance our understanding of this disorder and our ability to help traumatized individuals.

A necessary first step in exploring gender issues in the assessment of PTSD is to identify sex differences observed between men and women. The reader is cautioned that these descriptive data do not lead to conclusions regarding the essential nature of men and women or how each sex responds to traumatic stress. Sex differences between men and women must be interpreted in context. Thus, when we refer to sex differences, we mean comparisons that are based only on the biological facts of male and female. When we refer to gender, we reference more broadly the social context and psychological experience of a male or female individual in a given culture. Gender issues can therefore be conceptualized as an interaction between biologically based sex differences and the individual's social context. This definition of gender differences accounts for intragender diversity, as well as differences between genders, by assuming that gender differences are context dependent. The focus of this chapter, therefore, is to examine components of psychological assessment and populations of patients in which the considerations of gender are relevant to an accurate understanding of an individual's trauma exposure and its sequelae.

In this chapter, we first provide a brief overview of gender differences in the prevalence of trauma exposure and PTSD. We then describe approaches to the assessment of PTSD that are sensitive to the gender issues of both men and women. These sections are followed by additional material addressing gender-sensitive assessment approaches to associated features of PTSD and cormorbid conditions. Suggestions regarding relevant domains of assessment, referral and collaboration among providers, and examples of effective psychometric instruments are provided. Conclusions include a summary of findings and suggestions for incorporating research on gender and PTSD into clinical assessments.

GENDER AND PREVALENCE OF TRAUMA AND PTSD

The essential paradox of gender and PTSD lies in the gender-based discrepancies in rates of trauma exposure and subsequent rates of PTSD. Research consistently finds that men are more likely to experience traumatic events, whereas women are more than twice as likely to develop PTSD. The attention drawn to this counterintuitive finding has led to much investigation of the different ways in which men and women respond to traumatic events. In this section, we briefly review the major studies that have established these prevalence estimates.

In a comprehensive analysis of this literature, Norris, Foster, and Weisshaar (2002) note that studies conducted in the United States and other countries, including Canada, Israel, New Zealand, Mexico, and China, consistently document elevated rates of trauma exposure among men when compared with women. Major studies in the United States indicate that approximately 61% of men and 51% of women report at least one lifetime traumatic event (Kessler, Sonnega, Bromet, Hughes, & Nelson, 1995). The majority of individuals exposed to trauma experience multiple events. Among individuals exposed to trauma, women report fewer events than do men, with men reporting an average of 5.3 events and women reporting 4.3 events (Breslau et al., 1998). However, the types of trauma men and women experience are not equivalent. Women are more likely to report sexual assault in childhood or adulthood, whereas men are more likely to report being shot or physically assaulted, or experiencing motor vehicle crashes and combat (Breslau et al., 1998; Norris, 1992). Although the cross-cultural research supporting gender differences in trauma exposure is compelling, we cannot yet rule out the possibility that the observed gender disparities in trauma exposure are confounded by the assessment process. Most epidemiological studies on trauma and PTSD have utilized interviews in which respondents are asked to indicate whether they have experienced a finite number of traumatic events, usually between 12 and 20. Despite findings that the use of trauma lists improves overall detection of trauma exposure by 10% (Franklin, Sheeran, & Zimmerman, 2002), the content validity and gender sensitivity of these trauma lists have not been systematically investigated and may result in the underreporting of traumatic events by women. For example, experiences such as a sudden miscarriage or stillbirth are not easily captured in these trauma lists, and references to "rape" or "sexual assault" are likely to miss early childhood experiences of sexual abuse by a close other, which are more common for women. Furthermore, the broad categorization of traumatic events—which equates experiences such as a single, brief, physical altercation with a stranger to those such as prolonged physical abuse by an intimate partner, all under the rubric of physical assault—may not be the most precise method for organizing exposure for the purpose of explaining gender differences in rates of PTSD.

General population studies consistently find that women are approximately twice as likely as males to meet criteria for PTSD at some point in their lives. Major studies that have used DSM-III-R criteria have documented prevalence rates of 10.4–11.3% in women and 5–6% in men (Breslau, Davis, Andreski, & Peterson, 1991; Kessler et al., 1995). The National Comorbidity Survey (NCS; Kessler et al., 1995) has documented that, among individuals exposed to trauma, 20.4% of women and 8.2% of men developed PTSD, suggesting that the gender difference associated with the conditional risk for PTSD is even stronger. The event with the highest conditional risk was rape for both men and women, although a higher proportion of women than men met criteria for PTSD for all nonrape trauma as well. On the basis of DSM-IV criteria, the conditional probability of lifetime PTSD is 13% in women and 6.2% in men (Breslau et al., 1998). These probabilities may be lower based on how the index event was identified. In the Breslau et al. (1998) study, estimates were made using a randomly selected event for those participants who endorsed multiple traumas. In the NCS, estimates were based on a self-identified "worst event," with resultant rates of 17.7% in women and 9.5% in men. PTSD is not only more frequent among women but also more chronic. PTSD becomes chronic, lasting several years, among about one-third of individuals ever diagnosed with the disorder (Kessler et al., 1995). Epidemiological data suggest that the median length of time from onset to remission is about 4 years for women, compared with only about 1 year for men (Breslau et al., 1998). Other research suggests that 22% of women will develop chronic PTSD, as compared with only 6% of men (Breslau & Davis, 1992).

In sum, women are twice as likely to suffer from PTSD than men. Women also experience more chronic forms of the disorder. Although earlier age at time of exposure and a high probability of sexual assault partially account for these gender differences, research has not yet been able to explain the disparities in these rates of PTSD. It is likely that characteristics of exposure (e.g., intensity, duration, physical injury) beyond the specific type of event and the age at which it occurs contribute to the observed gender differences in prevalence. Furthermore, factors beyond exposure, such as gender-related differences in cognitive processes (Tolin & Foa, 2002), or social roles and relationships, also play a role in explaining these gender differences.

ASSESSMENT METHODS AND APPROACHES

Cardinal Features of PTSD

Numerous psychometric measures and clinical interviews are used to assess the major symptom domains of PTSD. Gender issues are best addressed by selecting measures that are sensitive to the factors that distinguish the different characteristics of exposure and psychological sequelae experienced by men and women while retaining sufficient criterion-rated validity and generalizability to ensure adequate adherence to the PTSD construct and effective communication with other professionals. In this section, we review selected measures that are widely used with populations of men and women and comment on these issues of reliability and validity as they pertain to patient gender.

Trauma Exposure Measures

Three general factors affect the utility of trauma exposure measures to address gender issues: (1) the extent to which trauma exposure is queried in behaviorally specific language that is easily read and understood by respondents; (2) the extent to which specific characteristics of traumatic events are measured; and (3) the inclusiveness of events or experiences examined. The importance of wording trauma queries in behaviorally specific language became apparent in studies that found that women with sexual experiences that met the legal definition of rape did not label their experiences as such and, as a result, did not endorse questionnaire items such as "Have you ever been raped?" (Kilpatrick, Saunders, Amick-McMullan, & Best, 1989; Koss, 1985). Exposure measures that describe experiences in plain language are more sensitive to events that men and women experience. The Potential Stressful Events Interview (PSEI; Kilpatrick, Resnick, & Freedy, 1991) is an excellent example of an exposure measure that uses sensitive language. This structured interview was used in the DSM-IV field trials for PTSD and is appropriate for use with men and women. Queries for sexual assault include gender-specific items for both men and women, and the measure also obtains good detail for exposure characteristics, such as age at the time of the event, severity, and chronicity. The main consideration for use of this measure is that the PSEI takes approximately 60–90 minutes to complete.

Characteristics such as age at the time of the event, severity, and chronicity are especially important with respect to gender, as these characteristics define the parameters of exposure that appear to partially explain several gender differences in PTSD prevalence and comorbid symptoms. The Trauma History Questionnaire (THQ; Green, 1996) is a 23-item, self-report measure of exposure derived from the PSEI that uses behaviorally specific wording to query age, frequency, and chronicity. Measures such as these are able to differentiate multiple incidents of physical assault from repeated and chronic intimate partner violence or physical abuse. The measure has demonstrated good reliability and validity in samples of both men and women, and its brevity measure makes it appropriate for both clinical and research purposes.

Gender-sensitive measures include content relevant to the stressors and traumatic experiences of men and women. The Life Stressor Checklist (Wolfe & Kimerling, 1997) is an example of a measure specifically tailored to the trauma exposure and stressful life experiences of women. The current version of this instrument is the revised version (LSC-R). The LSC-R is a 30-item instrument that includes unique assessments for abortion, loss of a child, and domestic violence and that also differentiates sexual assault from rape. The LSC-R includes stressors relevant to the lives of women that do not usually meet criterion A for PTSD but that may be relevant to understanding the context of trauma exposure, such as prolonged and unwanted separation from children, caregiving for someone ill or disabled, and severe financial strain. The LSC-R uses behaviorally specific language and assesses age at the time of the event for the first occurrence (if there were multiple occurrences of the same event), chronicity, subjective distress, and DSM-IV criteria for life threat, intense fear, helplessness, and horror. Information regarding the respondent's relationship to the perpetrator is embedded in the item wording when relevant. The LSC and the LSC-R have demonstrated good criterion-rated validity for PTSD in diverse populations of women and in several languages (Brown, Stout, & Mueller, 1999; Gavrilovic, Lecic-Tosevski, Knezevic, & Priebe, 2002; Kimerling, Calhoun, et al., 1999). The content of the LSC-R makes it particularly useful for low-income and ethnic-minority samples, and it has been used in national studies of traumatic stress in these populations.

The Traumatic Life Events Questionnaire—3 (TLEQ; Kubany, Haynes, et al., 2000), like the LSC-R, is a self-report measure that uses behaviorally specific terms to describe 21 potentially traumatic events, including several gender-specific experiences (e.g., miscarriages, abortions), as well as one open-ended question that assesses exposure to "other" life-threatening or highly disturbing events. It includes information on the frequency of occurrence, as well as the presence of fear, helplessness, or horror at the time of the trauma. In a small sample of battered women, the temporal stability and discriminative validity of the TLEQ-3 was good to excellent. The interrater reliability was also good, and battered women scoring in the PTSD range on the Distressing Event Questionnaire (DEQ; see the next section) endorsed significantly more types of TLEQ events, higher total number of events, and more events that produced intense feelings of fear, helplessness, or horror than women whose DEQ scores did not suggest PTSD.

PTSD Measures

Many of the most widely used measures for PTSD are the result of research with combat trauma, in which participants are largely males, and of research with sexual assault trauma, in which participants are largely females. The measures that have emerged are quite similar and closely tied to DSM-IV criteria. As a result, the measures are commonly used with a variety of male and female PTSD populations. A gender-sensitive PTSD measure will allow for multiple traumatic events, as males tend to experience a greater number of events than women, and will limit the extent to which the respondent must tie symptoms to the event, as doing this is very difficult for individuals who were exposed to trauma in childhood (the majority of whom are women). Further confidence in the utility of measures for either gender is generated when psychometric properties of the measure are available for samples of both men and women.

The Clinician-Administered PTSD Scale (CAPS; Blake et al., 1995; Blake et al., 1990) is a good example of an interview that can be administered to individuals who have experienced multiple events and of one that does not require an individual to specifically link DSM-IV PTSD criteria C and D symptoms to a specific event. The CAPS also yields a dichotomous indicator of PTSD diagnostic status, as well as a continuous measure of PTSD severity. The CAPS was developed with male combat veterans but is widely used with samples of women. Studies of the instrument's reliability and validity with samples of women exclusively would make an important contribution to the literature; currently, most clinicians find that the CAPS has utility for female populations, and preliminary research suggests that the measure performs similarly to the PTSD Symptom Scale—Interview Version (PSS-I) in civilian populations (Foa & Tolin, 2000). The PSS-I differs from the CAPS in that it does not include follow-up prompts for symptom clarification and in that it combines frequency and intensity of symptoms into a single estimate of severity for each symptom. Furthermore, whereas the CAPS appears to have slightly higher specificity, the PSS-I shows a slightly higher sensitivity. Although the CAPS takes about 10 minutes longer to administer than the PSS-I, its inclusion of separate frequency and intensity ratings may make it more sensitive to the detection of change. We recommend excluding the section "associated and hypothesized features" when using the CAPS with samples of women because these features are more common to combat experience—for example, survivor guilt and disillusion with authority. We suggest that clinicians focus on the associated features of PTSD described later in this chapter.

The Composite International Diagnostic Interview (CIDI; McFarlane, 2001) and the Structured Clinical Interview for DSM-IV (SCID; First, Spitzer, Williams, & Gibbon, 2000) are also widely used clinical interviews in the assessment of PTSD DSM-IV criteria. The CIDI was developed by the World Health Organization and was validated using samples of men and women drawn from diverse cultures. It is available in a number of languages. Utility for diverse samples is a strength of the CIDI. The SCID is useful for its comparability with other studies because the SCID is so widely used as a diagnostic measure for Axis I disorders. Although both the CIDI and the SCID have established good psychometric properties in samples of men and samples of women, the instruments share several drawbacks. Neither interview is structured to account for multiple traumas, and both assess symptoms with respect to the "worst" event endorsed during a brief trauma probe. This method of assessment leads to the loss of valuable information and may result in underestimates of the rates of PTSD. The symptom queries of both instruments require respondents to link their symptoms to a specific traumatic event, which is difficult for survivors of early childhood trauma to do, especially when items ask the respondent to compare levels of functioning in specific domains before and after the event. When the SCID or the CIDI are used in assessments, we recommend the use of one of the trauma-exposure measures described previously to measure criterion A, as the trauma probes in these instruments are less sensitive.

Self-report formats are also useful in the assessment of PTSD in men and women. The Posttraumatic Stress Diagnostic Scale (PDS; Foa, Cashman, Jaycox, & Perry, 1997) assesses trauma exposure and DSM-IV criterion A and the 17 symptoms of criteria B, C, and D rated on a 4-point scale of frequency. The PDS also includes items that assess the impact of the trauma on social and occupational functioning, although respondents who were exposed to trauma in childhood may have difficulty determining the degree to which these experiences affect them as adults. A similar difficulty arises when respondents' premorbid level of social and occupational functioning was fairly low. The PDS is worded to refer to a single traumatic event. The measure yields a continuous measure of PTSD severity, as well as a dichotomous diagnostic score. The PDS was developed with both males and females and is appropriate for use with both genders, and the optimal cutoff score for a PTSD diagnosis does not appear to differ for men and women.

The Distressing Life Event Questionnaire (DEQ; Kubany, Leisen, Kaplan, & Kelly, 2000) matches the criteria of PTSD as specified in DSM-IV and assesses a few associated features such as guilt, anger, and unresolved grief. Like the PDS, it uses a 0–4 response format for frequency of symptoms, and symptoms are tied to a specific traumatic event. The DEQ was validated on both male Vietnam War veterans and a diverse group of abused women (i.e., women with childhood sexual abuse, women raped after the age of 12, battered women, and women with histories of prostitution). The DEQ has good psychometric properties, including excellent discriminative and convergent validity. The DEQ discriminated men and women with PTSD from those without PTSD. Importantly, the most accurate scoring algorithms for men and women were different. For example, the optimal cutoff scores for predicting PTSD for the abused women was 18 and for the male war veterans, 26. When the measure was scored according to DSM-IV criteria, a cutoff score of 2 was the optimal symptom scoring for men, whereas a symptom cutoff score of 1 resulted in the most accurate diagnoses for women. It is unclear whether this reflects a gender difference in response to trauma or whether the optimal scoring algorithm depends on the nature of the trauma. Analyses such as these should be considered with a variety of measures and populations and are important in determining the gender sensitivity of assessment instruments.

The PTSD Checklist (PCL; Blanchard, Jones-Alexander, Buckley, & Forneris, 1996; Weathers, Litz, Herman, Huska, & Keane, 1993) assesses the 17 items of the DSM-IV PTSD criteria B, C, and D. Unlike the PDS and DEQ, items on the PCL are rated on a 5-point scale for distress caused by the symptom in the past month, not frequency of the symptom. The PCL assesses PTSD with respect to a single event. The PCL was developed with research on both male and female veterans and is now widely used with various male and female trauma populations. Initial psychometric data indicate that the PCL has good internal consistency, test–retest reliability, and predictive validity for a PTSD diagnosis based on the SCID (Blanchard et al., 1996; Weathers et al., 1993). One advantage it has over the PDS is that the PCL is in the public domain and thus free to users.

The PCL can be scored using DSM-IV criteria or different cutoff scores. Scoring based on DSM-IV criteria requires symptom endorsement of 3 or greater on at least one reexperiencing symptom, three avoidance symptoms, and two arousal symptoms. Blanchard et al. (1996) argue against this approach and recommend using a total PCL score to increase diagnostic efficiency. The recommended cutoff score for detecting PTSD in male veterans is 50 (Weathers et al., 1993). Blanchard et al. (1996) found a slightly lower optimal cutoff score (44 vs. 50) in their sample of mostly female survivors of motor vehicle accidents. More recently, Walker, Newman, Dobie, Ciechanowski, and Katon (2002) reported an optimal cut score of 30 for a large sample of female HMO patients, and Dobie et al. (2002) found an optimal cutoff of 38 in a sample of female veterans (Dobie et al., 2002). Similar to the findings of Kubany, Leisen, et al. (2000), these results suggest that either gender differences or trauma type can influence cutoff scores. One disadvantage of the PDS, DEQ, and PCL is that they require a relatively high reading level. For example, the PCL has a Flesch grade level of 13.2 (Carlson, 2001).

The Screen for Posttraumatic Stress Symptoms (SPTSS) is a recent measure (Carlson, 2001) that offers several advantages over other self-report measures of PTSD. First, it does not require that symptoms be keyed to a single trauma. Second, it has a Flesch grade reading level of 7.5. Third, it utilizes a response format that obtains information on frequency of symptoms, although its response format (0–10 scale) lacks clear frequency anchors and assesses symptoms for the previous 2 weeks rather than the previous month. Fourth, the SPTSS was developed using both male and female psychiatric inpatients and has good internal consistency, concurrent validity with other PTSD and distress measures, and diagnostic sensitivity. Its specificity is weaker, and information pertaining to other populations is still needed.

Associated Features

In addition to the cardinal features of reexperiencing, avoidance, and hyperarousal, symptoms of impaired affect regulation, dissociation, and marked difficulties with interpersonal relationships co-occur in a significant portion of trauma-exposed individuals (Herman, 1992). Symptom presentations that include these domains are often referred to as "complex PTSD" or the proposed category of DESNOS (disorders of extreme stress not otherwise specified). Individuals who present with these features of PTSD may benefit from skills-based treatment targeting awareness and regulation of feeling states, distress tolerance, and the ability to maintain relationships and utilize social support prior to exposure-based treatment components (Cloitre, Koenen, Cohen, & Han, 2002). Attention to these symptom domains is therefore an important part of assessment and treatment planning.

Comprehensive semistructured interviews for these associated features have been developed. The Structured Interview for Disorders of Extreme Stress (SIDES; Pelcovitz et al., 1997) has received the most attention and empirical support. It was used in DSM-IV field trials for PTSD and requires clinicians to rate the severity of affect dysregulation (i.e., difficulty with affect modulation, unmodulated anger, self-destructivenes, suicidal behavior, unmodulated sexual involvement), as well as dissociation and somatization. Although they are conceptually and descriptively different, DSM-IV borderline personality disorder and complex PTSD display significant symptom overlap (Cloitre, Koenen, Gratz, & Jakupcak, 2002). A comprehensive interview frequently used for the assessment of borderline personality disorder that captures these similarities is the Diagnostic Interview for Borderline Personality Disorders—Revised (Zanarini, Gunderson, Frankenburg, & Chauncey, 1989). It contains a section on the experience of chronic negative mood (e.g. anger, depression, anxiety), unusual cognitive experiences (e.g., odd thinking, quasi-psychotic experiences), impaired impulse patterns (e.g., self-mutilation, substance abuse). and interpersonal relations (e.g., stormy relationships, devaluation). In addition to these comprehensive interviews, self-report measures of specific associated features are available and are reviewed later.

Affect Regulation

Affect regulation can be defined as the ongoing process of an individual's emotion patterns in response to moment-by-moment contextual demands (Cole, Michel, & Teti, 1994). Individuals with dysregulated affect experience low-threshold, high-intensity emotional reactions and slow return to baseline levels of arousal (Cloitre, Koenen, Cohen, & Han, 2002). These individuals often report that they get upset very easily, have trouble calming down, or feel overwhelmed by the experience of negative emotions.

Early experiences significantly influence the degree to which affect regulation processes are successfully developed (Cole et al., 1994). When exposure to trauma occurs in childhood, the process of learning to experience, identify, and talk about emotions, to observe how they function, and to develop strategies for modulating and utilizing emotions effectively is often disrupted (van der Kolk et al., 1996). This appears to be especially true for interpersonal violence and in cases in which the perpetrator is a family member or other intimate who would model or coach the child in emotional regulation strategies. As noted earlier, these forms of exposure are more common among women, and as a result symptoms of affective dysregulation may be seen more often among female patients. Gender differences may be magnified by the different ways in which men and women experience emotion. For example, women report more intense emotions and more negative and self-directed emotions, such as shame, sadness, and guilt (Kring & Gordon, 1998). Women are also more likely than men to utilize emotion-focused coping strategies in response to stress (Ptacek, Smith, & Dodge, 1994). It may be most effective for clinicians to use both female gender and childhood trauma as signals for the assessment of affect regulation symptoms.

Assessment of affect regulation should target emotional competence indices such as the ability to identify, articulate, and tolerate emotional states. The Toronto Alexithymia Scales (TAS; Taylor et al., 1988) and its revision (TAS-R; Bagby, Parker, & Taylor, 1994; Taylor, Bagby, & Parker, 1992) are reliable and well validated self-report measures that assess alexithymia. Alexithymia is often considered the hallmark of somatization, which is characterized by the inability to describe and differentiate the emotional valence of physiological states. Sifneos (1996) argued that these scales miss important features of alexithymia (e.g., paucity of fantasy life) and recommends a more comprehensive assessment that includes his Beth Israel Questionnaire (BIQ) and a nine-item rating scale to evaluate affective flattening. The General Expectancy for Negative Mood Regulation Scale (NMR; Cantanzaro & Mearns, 1990) is another brief (30–item) self-report measure that assesses the capacity to regulate negative mood. The NMR has good face validity, internal consistency, temporal stability, and discriminant validity from social desirability and locus of control. Interestingly, the NMR is not correlated with the experience of stressful life events, although it does add predictive validity to reports of depression following a stressful life event. Because problems with affect regulation are associated with maladaptive and often self-destructive attempts to manage overwhelming affect, especially anger (van der Kolk & Fisler, 1994), it is important for clinicians to assess for self-harm behaviors when assessing for affect regulation symptoms. The Self-Harm Inventory (Sansone, Wiederman, & Sansone, 1998) is a 22-item questionnaire that has been used as a diagnostic screen for borderline personality disorder. It has good diagnostic predictive validity with a cutoff score of 5, and it provides useful clinical information about both the number of times a client has engaged in self-harm behaviors and the recency of his or her self-harm behavior.

Dissociation

Dissociation is conceptually linked to affective regulation: Unsuccessful attempts at regulating emotional states can result in the processes of monitoring and avoiding emotionally arousing information (Thompson, 1994). Dissociation, which involves the internal redirection of attention, is an example of such a strategy and is likely to be used in situations in which escape or avoidance of emotionally arousing stimuli is impossible. Dissociative symptoms occur on a continuum, which ranges from common behaviors such as "tuning out" or daydreaming to depersonalization or derealization. These more severe forms of dissociation appear to be categorically distinct from the dissociative tendencies that characterize the general population (Waller, Putnam, & Carlson, 1996). These symptoms are not heritable, suggesting that trauma exposure plays the most significant role in their etiology (Waller & Ross, 1997). These more severe dissociative symptoms are most common among individuals who experience trauma during childhood, especially trauma perpetrated by family members, as well as more chronic forms of trauma (Dancu, Riggs, Hearst-Ikeda, Shoyer, & Foa, 1996; Gershuny & Thayer, 1999). Similar to affect regulation symptoms, dissociative symptoms are more closely linked to forms of exposure that are more common among women and may thus appear to have a higher prevalence among women. Dissociation at the time of the trauma predicts the development of PTSD among individuals who have experienced a variety of forms of exposure (Ehlers, Mayou, & Bryant, 1998; Tichenor, Marmar, Weiss, Metzler, & Ronfeldt, 1996). Recent research suggests that the relationship between peritraumatic dissociation and the development of PTSD may be stronger among women than men (Fullerton et al., 2001).

The assessment of dissociation can be particularly challenging. In our experience, the colloquial meaning of dissociation for patients is often similar to momentary distraction, daydreaming, or other problems with sustained attention that significantly differ from clinical dissociation. We suggest a careful interview, operationally defining the symptoms queried, as well as using standardized measures of dissociation. The most widely used and extensively researched screening instrument is the Dissociative Experiences Scale, or DES (Carlson et al., 1993). This measure has been shown to have strong test–retest and internal reliability and also good validity (Bernstein & Putnam, 1986; Carlson, 1994; Frischholz, Braun, Sachs, & Hopkins, 1990). It is also efficient, with 28 self-reported items that can be completed in about 10 minutes. Screening measures such as the DES work well in conjunction with a structured interview that provides more detailed information regarding the nature and extent of dissociative symptoms. The most widely used structured interview is the Structured Clinical Interview for DSM-IV Dissociative Disorders—Revised (SCID-D-R; Steinberg, Rounsville, & Cicchetti, 1990). The SCID-D-R is a highly refined measure that specifically yields DSM-IV dissociative diagnoses. In a recent review, the SCID-D-R was found have good-to-excellent reliability and validity, both in the United States and abroad (Steinberg, 2002).

Interpersonal Relationships

Individuals with PTSD may experience difficulties over a wide variety of domains, including impairment in interpersonal functioning in family and intimate relationships, problems accessing and receiving social support, and more generalized issues related to potential social stigma associated with the trauma. Careful assessment can yield important information regarding the symptoms experienced by the individual and the social resources available to cope with PTSD symptoms. Although pretrauma support is influential in determining subsequent social resources, factors such as gender and type of trauma can create additional obstacles for obtaining social support from the community and from intimate others.

For both men and women, the manifestations of PTSD often erode existing support systems and intimate relationships. Male veterans with PTSD report more problems with marital functioning and difficulties with intimacy, and they are more likely to separate or divorce than veterans without PTSD. All of these effects appear to stem from symptoms of emotional numbing (Riggs, Byrne, Weathers, & Litz, 1998). PTSD severity and hyperarousal symptoms in particular are also linked to the perpetration of intimate partner violence in these couples (Byrne & Riggs, 1996; Savarese, Suvak, King, & King, 2001). Female spouses of men with PTSD experience stress consistent with caregiver burden and decreased marital satisfaction (Beckham, Lytle, & Feldman, 1996; Calhoun, Beckham, & Bosworth, 2002). Children of male veterans with PTSD demonstrate poorer adjustment and more behavior problems than children of veterans without PTSD (Caselli & Motta, 1995).

Research with trauma-exposed women has not addressed PTSD to the same extent as it has with male veterans, and it has focused on exposure to child sexual abuse and adult sexual assault. Sexually abused or assaulted women are less likely to be married (Golding, Wilsnack, & Cooper, 2002) and more likely to be single mothers (Lipman, MacMillan, & Boyle, 2001). These women report less relationship satisfaction and more problems with trust and communication than nonabused women (DiLillo & Long, 1999), and they are more likely to be recipients of intimate partner violence (DiLillo, Giuffre, Tremblay, & Peterson, 2001). Similar to studies with males, partners of women sexually abused in childhood report poorer satisfaction with their relationships than do partners of nonabused women (Nelson & Wampler, 2000).

For both women and men, close interpersonal relationships are negatively affected by trauma exposure and PTSD. The research with males has primarily focused on combat veterans and has identified the role of emotional numbing as an obstacle to communication and partnership and of hyperarousal symptoms in the perpetration of relationship violence. The issues of trust, communication, and general difficulties in forming intimate relationships are consistent with numbing symptoms, as well as the interpersonal difficulties that are seen as the hallmark of prolonged trauma exposure during childhood (Cloitre, Scarvalone, & Difede, 1997).

Emotional validation of traumatic events and reactions may be more important components of intimate social support to women than to men. The positive effects of marital social support are more pronounced when partners of women accurately appraise the woman's stressor exposure (Ritter, Hobfoll, Lavin, Cameron, & Hulsizer, 2000). In contrast, women's accurate perceptions of their male partner's PTSD symptoms are not related to his satisfaction with spousal support (Taft, King, King, Leskin, & Riggs, 1999). These findings are consistent with findings that mutuality and relationship maintenance with close others may be more important to women than to men, the latter placing greater value on the ability to maintain independence (Josephs, Markus, & Tafarodi, 1992). Women's power relative to men's may also play a role in how symptoms of PTSD negatively affect close relationships. Whereas the hyperarousal cluster of symptoms for males is linked to risk of perpetration of intimate partner violence, research indicates that women's trauma-related anger and physical aggression are more often directed toward their children (DiLillo, Tremblay, & Peterson, 2000).

A promising tool for assessing interpersonal problems and distress associated with interpersonal problems is the Inventory of Interpersonal Problems (IIP; Horowitz, Rosenberg, Baer, Ureno, & Villasenor, 1988). The IIP is a 127-item self-report measure that was initially validated with a diverse psychiatric outpatient sample. It includes six subscales that assess difficulty with assertiveness, social interactions, intimacy, submissiveness, overcontrol, and excessive responsibility. The inventory has been shown to be sensitive to treatment effects, including treatment of child abuse–related PTSD (Cloitre, Koenen, Cohen, & Han, 2002). Although much of the attention paid by clinicians to social support focuses on intimate partners and the family, social resources from the survivor's community also play an important role in adjustment to trauma. Women's reports of general well-being (Acitelli & Antonucci, 1994) and marital satisfaction (Julien & Markman, 1991) are more strongly related to perceptions of social support in marriage than are men's reports. Thus the goal of increasing social support within an intimate relationship, as well as from the community, may be particularly important for women. These findings suggest that a comprehensive assessment of trauma and PTSD with women should include measures of social support. The Interpersonal Support Evaluation List (ISEL; Cohen & Hoberman, 1983) is a 48-item questionnaire that assesses the perceived availability of potential social resources. It assesses the availability of four separate functions of social support: (1) tangible support (i.e., availability of material aid); (2) belonging support (i.e., availability of people to do things with); (3) appraisal support (i.e., availability of a confidant); and (4) self-esteem support (i.e., perceived availability of positive comparisons to others). Although extensive psychometric information has not been obtained on the ISEL, it contains important conceptual distinctions that are relevant to gender and trauma. It also appears to be sensitive to treatments that directly target interpersonal functioning in trauma survivors (Cloitre, Koenen, Cohen, & Han, 2002).

Clinicians interested in a global assessment of social functioning may want to use the self-report Social Adjustment Scale (SAS-SR; Weissman & Bothwell, 1976). This measure has been used extensively and measures overall social adjustment for a 2-week period across several role areas (i.e., household, employment, family, marital, parental, financial, school, social/leisure). In treatment outcome studies with both borderline personality disorder and child abuse–related PTSD, this measure has shown pre- and posttreatment effects (Cloitre, Koenen, Cohen, & Han, 2002; Linehan, Tutek, Heard, & Armstrong, 1994). The Quality of Life Questionnaire (QLQ; Evans & Cope, 1989) is another measure that assesses the quality of life across 15 domains, including interpersonal relationships (i.e., marital, parent–child, extended family, and extramarital). The normative sample on which the QLQ is based was balanced for gender, and preliminary reports suggest that males with PTSD score on average 3 standard deviations below the normative sample (Freuh, Turner, Beidel, & Cahill, 2001).

Comorbidity

The prevalence of many psychiatric disorders differs among men and women. These different prevalence rates have been variously attributed to social and biological differences or to gender biases on the part of health care providers and the systems in which they work. The extent to which these gender differences show similar patterns in their comorbidity with PTSD is not fully understood. In the NCS, 59% of men and 43.6% of women had three or more additional diagnoses (Kessler et al., 1995). For men, the three most common comorbid conditions were alcohol abuse/dependence (52%), major depressive disorder (48%), and conduct disorder (43.3%). For women, the three most common comorbid conditions were major depressive disorder (48.5%), simple or social phobia (28–29%), and alcohol abuse/dependence (28%). Comorbidity has a substantial impact on the severity and course of PTSD and is an important domain of assessment for both men and women. In the following sections, we review the evidence for gender differences in disorders most often comorbid with PTSD in men and women and suggest adjunct methods for assessment.

Major Depression

Major depressive disorder (MDD) is an important assessment consideration in both women and men, as it is a common comorbid diagnosis with PTSD for both genders. As already noted, epidemiological surveys conducted in the United States that have included men and women have found similar rates of comorbid depression among both men and women. In veteran samples, however, women appear to be more likely than men to be assigned a diagnosis of comorbid MDD both within the previous 6 months (men = 16% and women = 23%) and over the course of their lifetimes (men = 26% and women = 42%; Kulka et al., 1990). The basis for the discrepancy in rates of comorbid depression in veteran samples as compared with community samples is unclear, but it may be partially due to the National Vietnam Veterans Readjustment Study's focus on combat-related trauma, which could result in underestimation of both PTSD symptoms and depression related to sexual assault and intimate partner violence among women.

The similarity of the rates of comorbid depression among the community sample of men and women with PTSD is striking given women's risk for depression in the absence of PTSD. Major life events, including trauma exposure, play an etiological role in depression and partly explain women's greater risk for the disorder (Nolen-Hoeksema & Girgus, 1994). The high rates of comorbid depression in men and women seems to indicate that PTSD (or trauma exposure of sufficient magnitude to lead to PTSD) may create a vulnerability toward depression in men that suppresses the protective effect of male gender.

Several researchers have, in fact, hypothesized that the high rates of overlap between PTSD and depression indicate two distinct, but functionally related, syndromes. This hypothesis stems from consistent findings that, among both women and men, trauma exposure demonstrates a graded increase in the risk for both PTSD and depression, with more severe exposure resulting in a greater likelihood of both disorders (McQuaid, Pedrelli, McCahill, & Stein, 2001). A history of depression also functions as a gender-specific risk factor for PTSD following trauma exposure and partially explains women's elevated risk for PTSD (Breslau, Davis, Andreski, & Peterson, 1997; Resnick, Kilpatrick, Best, & Kramer, 1992). A history of depression, as well as current symptoms, is therefore an important component in the assessment of posttraumatic stress, especially with women.

The overlap between current symptoms of depression and PTSD presents a notable assessment challenge. Three of the nine DSM-IV symptoms of major depression (i.e, diminished interest in activities, difficulty sleeping, and difficulty concentrating) are strikingly similar to those of PTSD. Expert clinicians have proposed several distinguishing features between the two disorders despite the apparent symptom overlap. For example, in PTSD, diminished interest in activities is circumscribed to cues of past trauma exposure; in major depression, inactivity and diminished interest are more generalized and are characterized by loss of energy and hopelessness (Keane, Taylor, & Penk, 1997). Sleep difficulties must be distinguished from trauma-relevant nightmares and hypervigilance that were not present before the traumatic exposure. Similarly, global difficulties in concentration must be distinguished from symptoms of dissociation and from intrusive trauma-relevant memories that were not present before traumatic exposure. Such discrimination may be more difficult among individuals with prolonged histories of childhood trauma, as the precise onset of traumatic stress symptoms may be difficult to pinpoint. Because such histories are more common among women (Breslau et al., 1997) and because the relationship between childhood maltreatment and adult psychopathology is stronger among women than men (MacMillan et al., 2001), gender may appear to be a confounding factor in discriminating PTSD from MDD.

Ruling out physical health disorders that could influence the presentation of depressive symptoms is another issue particularly relevant for assessment of depression among female PTSD patients (Orsillo, Raha, & Hammond, 2002). Thyroid disorders; adrenal, pituitary, and parathyroid disorders; seizure disorders; multiple sclerosis; and mitral valve prolapse can all produce symptoms that may be attributed to depression and/or anxiety. Many of these disorders, such as thyroid conditions and autoimmune conditions, are more common among women. The misdiagnosis of these physical disorders as psychiatric symptoms partially accounts for the overdiagnosis of depression in women (Klonoff, Landrine, & Lang, 1997).

Gender differences in the efficiency of detection and diagnosis of depression remain unclear, though research does suggest that practitioners may be more sensitive to depression in women and more specific when assessing depression among males. A recent study (Bertakis et al., 2001) found that women were 72% more likely than men to be identified as depressed by their primary care physicians, even after controlling for other variables such as severity of symptoms as reported by psychometric assessment, demographic variables (e.g., age, marital status), and utilization patterns.

A frequently used self-report measure of depression is the Beck Depression Inventory (BDI; Beck, Steer, & Garbin, 1988; Beck, Ward, Mendelson, Mock, & Erbaugh, 1961) and the revised version, the Beck Depression Inventory—II (BDI-II;Beck, Steer, & Brown, 1996). The BDI-II is a 21-item inventory that assesses many of the cardinal features of depression. Salokangas and colleagues (Salokangas, Vaahtera, Pacriev, Sohlman, & Lehtinen, 2002) recently proposed that gender differences observed using the BDI may not reflect true differences in degree of depression but rather gender bias in items. More specifically, they found that items such as loss of interest in sex and crying were reported more frequently by females than males. The authors argue that these items are psychologically, culturally, and/or biologically related to female gender and that their endorsement may be more a function of gender than depression. These findings also suggest that the extent to which gender differences in depressive symptoms are detected may be influenced by the specific assessment tool used.

Although more research with comorbid PTSD and MDD is needed, the literature concerning depression can serve to guide clinicians' efforts. In general, research suggests that practitioners are more likely to diagnose and treat depression among women (Badger et al., 1999). Given a diagnosis, women are more likely to seek mental health services than are men, despite their relative disadvantage in access to health insurance (Kessler et al., 1999). As a result, symptoms of depression are more likely to be detected and treated among women, though care should be taken not to overdiagnose and overpathologize women patients. Because male patients, on the other hand, are less likely to be diagnosed with depression, men with PTSD should be carefully assessed for comorbid depression given their comparable rates for this disorder with women.

Substance Use Disorders

The prevalence of substance use disorders (SUDs) among individuals with PTSD is high. Current population estimates for lifetime comorbidity indicate that approximately 30–50% of men and 25–30% of women with lifetime PTSD have a co-occurring SUD. Among the men with PTSD, rates are 52% for alcohol disorders and 35% for drug disorders. Among the women with PTSD, rates are 28% for alcohol disorders and 27% for drug disorders (Kessler et al., 1995). These estimates suggest that when clinicians encounter an individual with PTSD, a cormorbid diagnosis of a drug or alcohol use disorder is more likely if that patient is male. Screening for drug and alcohol disorders should be a part of any trauma assessment, though the issue may be particularly important in settings in which large numbers of male patients are seen.

If these comorbidity rates among men and women are considered in the context of base rates for SUDs in the general population, however, additional gender issues important for assessment become apparent. SUDs in the general population are higher among men, making it more likely that a male with PTSD will be diagnosed with a comorbid SUD because he is male, and not because of an association with PTSD. Though the rates of comorbidity are lower among women with PTSD than among men, the associations between PTSD and SUDs are actually stronger for women, especially with respect to drug disorders (Stewart, Ouimette, & Brown, 2002). This finding suggests that the functional relationship between PTSD and SUDs may differ among men and women.

Research suggests that the etiology of PTSD–SUD comorbidity may differ among men and women, and that men and women with PTSD appear to differ in the situations in which they use substances. For example, women are more likely than men to develop SUDs subsequent to trauma exposure and PTSD (Cottler, Nishith, & Compton, 2001; Kessler et al., 1995), with approximately 65–84% of women meeting criteria for PTSD before they develop substance use disorders. These findings are consistent with a "self-medication" hypothesis for PTSD–SUD comorbidity among women, in which women develop SUDs in an effort to cope with trauma-related symptoms. In males, however, the temporal pattern is more consistent with an increased risk for trauma exposure that is linked to behaviors surrounding substance use, which then results in PTSD.

These hypotheses regarding gender differences in the functional relations between PTSD and SUDs are further supported by data regarding the situational specificity of substance use in men and women. Both men and women with PTSD use substances more frequently than SUD-diagnosed individuals without PTSD, and they tend do so in negatively reinforcing situations, for example in response to negative emotions, interpersonal conflict, or physical discomfort (Sharkansky, Brief, Peirce, Meehan, & Mannix, 1999; Stewart, Conrod, Samoluk, Pihl, & Dongier, 2000). Male substance abusers, independent of PTSD status, are more likely than women with PTSD–SUD comorbidity to engage in substance-using behavior in situations that involve positive emotions, either alone or with others. It has been hypothesized (Stewart, Ouimette, & Brown, 2002) that positive emotions occur more rarely among women with PTSD–SUD comorbidity, due to more intensive emotional numbing. As a result, these cues less often trigger substance use. Although much research remains to be done in this area, existing data and hypotheses regarding gender-related differences in the functional relationship between PTSD and SUD can serve to inform clinicians' case formulations.

Given the high rates of comorbidity in both men and women, clinicians may want to consider routinely screening patients for SUDs. A number of brief measures are commonly used to detect high-risk individuals in treatment settings. For alcohol use disorders, among the most widely used is the AUDIT (Alcohol Use Disorder Identification Test), developed by the World Health Organization in order to detect International Classification of Diseases (ICD-10) criteria hazardous or harmful drinking (Babor, de la Fuente, Saunders, & Grant, 1992). The AUDIT was developed using a multinational sample and has demonstrated utility for ethnic minority populations in the United States. Using the standard cutoff of 8, it is less sensitive for women patients (Bradley, Boyd-Wickizer, Powell, & Burman, 1998) but appears to be effective using cut scores lower than 8. Another widely used screen is the CAGE (Mayfield, McLeod, & Hall, 1974), thus named for the four items that make up the measure (i.e., Cutdown, Annoyed, Guilty, and Eye-opener). The CAGE uses a cutoff of 2 to indicate high risk for problem drinking. It should be noted that the CAGE has been criticized for demonstrating less sensitivity in female populations (Volk, Cantor, Steinbauer, & Cass, 1997). A modified version of the CAGE, called the TWEAK (Tolerance, Worried, Eye-Opener, Amnesia, Cutdown), is a five-item screen developed for use with women patients that utilizes a cutoff of 1 or 2 (Russell et al., 1991). When these lower cutpoints are used, the TWEAK and AUDIT screens appear to be sensitive and effective in diverse samples of women patients (Bradley et al., 1998).

Sexual Functioning

Problems with sexual functioning are common among men and women exposed to both sexual and nonsexual trauma. Though patients may not list sexual concerns as a chief presenting problem at the onset of treatment, screening for sexual dysfunction or other intimacy issues is not only valuable for treatment planning and case formulation but also can serve to normalize problems in sexual functioning as being common sequelae of trauma exposure. Both men and women with PTSD report sexual dysfunction, as well as other alterations in sexual behavior, that appear to arise from trauma-related deficits in interpersonal functioning. Because a wide range of pharmacological agents, vascular conditions, and hormonal conditions can impair sexual functioning, both male and female patients should be referred to a physician as part of a comprehensive assessment of sexual function. It is important to remember that such exams may be retraumatizing for male and female patients who have survived sexual trauma. Clinicians should discuss the possibility with patients prior to referral and ensure good communication among the patient, physician, and therapist regarding the patient's needs and experiences.

Among male patients, sexual dysfunction has been observed in samples of combat veterans (Cosgrove et al., 2002) and civilians (Kotler et al., 2000) and in all phases of the sexual response cycle. Studies of treatment-seeking males with PTSD suggest that up to 80% of this population experiences clinically relevant sexual dysfunction, with the most common condition being male erectile dysfunction (Cosgrove et al., 2002; Letourneau, Schewe, & Frueh, 1997). When assessing sexual functioning in males, clinicians should be aware that many of the pharmacological treatments for PTSD, including certain serotonin reuptake inhibitors and beta-blockers, can impair male sexual functioning or exacerbate existing dysfunction. Studies of sexual dysfunction among women exposed to trauma have focused primarily on survivors of childhood sexual abuse, although research indicates that sexual dysfunction is common among female survivors of both sexual and nonsexual trauma (Letourneau, Resnick, Kilpatrick, & Saunders, 1996; Walker et al., 1999). Approximately 58% of these women report sexual dysfunction in all phases of the sexual response cycle.

Assessment can also address mechanistic processes: Fear of overwhelming affect may lead to hypervigilance for internal cues that signal emotional or physiological arousal (Barlow, 2002). Anxiety can alter cognitive and attentional processes during sexual activity, whereby the attentional shift serves to interfere with sexual responses and reception of sexually arousing stimuli (Rosen & Leiblum, 1995). For individuals exposed to sexual trauma, sexual dysfunction may be the result of cues to the traumatic memories, flashbacks, or dissociative experiences.

When assessing sexual functioning, clinicians should address interpersonal factors that affect intimacy and sexual negotiation, as well as screen for sexual dysfunction. These issues can be addressed via interview or psychometric assessment. The Golombok–Rust Inventory of Sexual Satisfaction (GRISS; Rust & Golombok, 1985) is a measure of sexual satisfaction. This instrument, composed of 28 items for women and 28 items for men, measures sexual functioning and relationship quality and can be completed in approximately 10 minutes. Domains assessed in women are anorgasmia, vaginismus, female avoidance, female nonsensuality, and female dissatisfaction. Domains assessed in men are impotence, premature ejaculation, male nonsensuality, male avoidance, and male dissatisfaction. Two domains, infrequency and noncommunication, are administered to both men and women. Frequency is assessed on a scale from 0 (*never*) to 4 (*always*), yielding a global sexual satisfaction, score as well as an individual profile of sexual functioning. Items pertaining to communication, as well as sexual functioning, make the GRISS useful for trauma populations, and it appears to be equally sensitive for both men and women. The GRISS is targeted toward heterosexual relationships and may not be appropriate for use with individuals with same-sex sexual partners.

Two other brief measures of sexual functioning are excellent examples of questionnaires that can be used with individuals with same-sex or opposite-sex sexual partners. The International Index of Erectile Function (IIEF; Rosen et al., 1997) is a brief 15-item measure for males that assesses domains of sexual activity, sexual intercourse, sexual stimulation, ejaculation and orgasm. It is sensitive to treatment-related changes in sexual functioning and is available in several languages. A brief five-item screen for sexual dysfunction has also been developed from this measure (Rosen, Cappelleri, Smith, Lipsky, & Pena, 1999). The Female Sexual Function Index (FSFI; Rosen et al., 2000) is a 19-item measure for women that assesses desire, arousal, lubrication, orgasm, satisfaction, and pain. The measure can discriminate between women diagnosed with DSM-IV sexual dsyfunctions and a comparison group for each of the five domains. Both the IIEF and the FSFI use clear, behaviorally specific language and take approximately 10 minutes to complete.

Medical Comorbidity

Both men and women with PTSD experience a greater degree of functional impairment from their illness and evidence a poorer course of disease for a variety of medical conditions. Although research has not yet delineated the full extent of medical cormorbidity with PTSD, ample evidence supports the importance of assessing health status among individuals exposed to traumatic stress. Readers are referred to several excellent reviews for an overview of this literature (Friedman & Schnurr, 1995; Kimerling, Clum, McQuery, & Schnurr, 2002; Koss, Koss, & Woodruff, 1991; Resnick, Acierno, & Kilpatrick, 1997; Schnurr & Jankowski, 1999). To date, we are not aware of published data that have directly compared women and men for the extent or type of medical comorbidity attendant to a diagnosis of PTSD. However, several disorders appear to occur with significant frequency among men and women with PTSD. The studies cited here have controlled for potentially confounding factors in the relationship between PTSD and health status, such as age, smoking, body mass index (BMI), and alcohol use.

Cardiovascular Disorders

Studies of men suggest that PTSD may be associated with increased risks of cardiovascular disorders. PTSD symptoms are associated with a greater risk for several categories of physician-diagnosed medical problems common to older males: arterial disorders, gastrointestinal disorders, dermatological problems, and musculoskeletal disorders (Schnurr, Spiro, & Paris, 2000). These results are corroborated by laboratory studies in which chronic PTSD is associated with ECG abnormalities, atrioventricular defects, and infarctions (Boscarino & Chang, 1999) and with poorer performance on laboratory stress tests (Shalev, Bleich, & Ursano, 1990). At this time, most studies finding increased risk of cardiovascular disorders among individuals with PTSD have been conducted with male participants and veteran samples. However, researchers and clinicians should not mistake the lack of empirical data to mean that cardiovascular disorders are not also a risk for women with PTSD. Cardiovascular disease remains the leading cause of death among women in the United States (Centers for Disease Control and Prevention, 1999). Given the morbidity and mortality of cardiovascular disease and lack of gender data, our recommendation is that cardiovascular assessments be carried out in both men and women with PTSD.

Gastrointestinal Disorders

Increased rates of gastrointestinal disorders have been observed among male veterans with PTSD (Schnurr et al., 2000) and among women exposed to intimate partner violence (Campbell, 2002). Conversely, increased rates of trauma and PTSD have been observed among individuals with gastrointestinal disorders. A study of male and female patients diagnosed with irritable bowel syndrome (IBS) found that 36% met criteria for a PTSD diagnosis that preceded the onset of IBS (Irwin et al., 1996). Gender comparisons in such studies have found only minimal differences thus far: Women may be likely to suffer from IBS and dyspepsia, whereas men may be more likely to suffer more from heartburn (Talley, Fett, Zinsmeister, & Melton, 1994.).

Recent investigations have also indicated that assessment of hepatitis C and liver disease may be relevant for both men and women. It is estimated that approximately 46.2% of male veterans with PTSD test positive for hepatitis C (Muir et al., 1999). Liver disease is an important consideration given the high rates of comorbid alcohol use disorder in women and men with PTSD. Women are more susceptible to alcohol-induced liver disease (Maddrey, 2000). We recommend assessment in both men and women for liver disease, viral hepatitis A, B, & C, irritable bowel syndrome, and gastroesophageal reflux disease (GERD)—the current nomenclature that includes heartburn.

Pain Disorders

The majority of research linking pain disorders to PTSD was done with male veterans. In this population, it has been estimated that 20–80% of male veterans with PTSD will experience a chronic musculoskeletal pain condition (Beckham et al., 1997; White & Faustman, 1989). Other studies have examined PTSD among individuals with PTSD conditions. In a study of men and women seeking treatment for fibromyalgia, 56% met criteria for PTSD (Sherman, Turk, & Okifuji, 2000). Trauma-exposed individuals also report more severe pain symptoms and pain in a greater number of body sites when compared with nonexposed individuals (Fillingim, Wilkinson, & Powell, 1999). Based on these findings and consistent with our clinical experience, fibromyalgia, musculoskeletal pain, low back pain, and migraine headaches seem to be seen more frequently in populations with PTSD and should be considered for assessment in these individuals. When available, referral to specialized chronic pain clinics in which multidisciplinary, multimodal approaches to pain management are taken should be considered.

Sexually Transmitted Diseases

Several studies have established a history of interpersonal violence among men and women with sexually transmitted diseases (STDs), with a focus on HIV infections (Kimerling, Armistead, & Forehand, 1999; Kimerling, Calhoun, et al., 1999; Zierler et al., 1991). One study of HIV-infected women estimated the lifetime rate of sexual assault at 43% (Zierler, Witbeck, & Mayer, 1996). In a large national survey of male veterans, men diagnosed with both PTSD and substance abuse were approximately 12 times more likely to be infected with HIV than veterans without either diagnosis (Hoff, Beam-Goulet, & Rosenheck, 1997). PTSD may affect course of disease, as well as risk for infection, as the disease progresses more rapidly among women diagnosed with PTSD than in women without PTSD, as evidenced by rate of CD4/CD8 cell decline and number of opportunistic infections (Kimerling, Armistead, & Forehand, 1999).

Researchers have proposed plausible behavioral mechanisms in which trauma exposure serves as risk factor for infection with STD, specifically, HIV infection. Violence can be linked to HIV and STDs through several pathways. Most directly, sexual assault can result in STD for both men and women if the perpetrator is infected (Gostin et al., 1994; Holmes, 1999; Kobernick, Seifert, & Sanders, 1985). Other studies have noted that intimate partner violence may contribute to the likelihood of STDs and HIV. One study found that partners in violent relationships were less likely to use condoms and that abuse or threatened abuse resulted from initiating discussions about condom use (Wingood & DiClemente, 1997). Similarly, among a group of women demographically and geographically at high risk for HIV infection, 42% reported engaging in unwanted, unprotected sexual activity as a result of force or threat of force (Kalichman, Williams, Cherry, Belcher, & Nachimson, 1998). For men who have sex with men, childhood sexual abuse may be linked to unwanted and unprotected sexual activity and relationship violence (Paul, Catania, Pollack, & Stall, 2001).

These observations have led researchers to focus on shared causal pathways for interpersonal violence and HIV infections influenced by social inequalities related to gender, minority, ethnicity, economic status, and sexual orientation (Zierler & Krieger, 1997). The studies reviewed suggest that for women and for men who have sex with men, especially those with a history of interpersonal violence, assessment of STDs and HIV is an important consideration.

Reproductive and Gynecological Disorders

Studies have linked trauma exposure to adverse reproductive health among women. Exposure during childhood is associated with increased risk of gynecological disorders such as sexually transmitted diseases, excessive bleeding, vaginitis, cervical dysplasia, dysmenorrhea, and infertility (Fildes, Reed, Jones, Martin, & Barrett, 1992; Frye, 2001). Intimate partner violence during pregnancy is associated with low maternal weight gain, infections, anemia, preterm labor, and shorter intervals between pregnancies (Berenson, Wiemann, Wilkinson, Jones, & Anderson, 1994; Cokkinides, Coker, Sanderson, Addy, & Bethea, 1999; Parker, McFarlane, & Soeken, 1994). Recent data suggest that intimate partner violence during pregnancy may be one of the leading causes of morbidity and mortality among pregnant women (Fildes et al., 1992; Frye, 2001). Although there are yet no comprehesive data concerning the reproductive health of women with PTSD, these studies suggest that women with PTSD should be referred for gynecological care and that prenatal and obstetrical assessment is especially important for pregnant women with diagnoses of PTSD or histories of trauma. Individuals with history of sexual trauma may need psychological support and assistance in communicating with medical providers in order to overcome their resistance to seeking care and to obtain sensitive, appropriate care.

Because health care assessments can involve mammography, gastrointestinal procedures, and breast, pelvic, and rectal exams, individuals with history of sexual trauma may need psychological support to undergo these evaluations. They may need assistance communicating to medical practitioners the need for a third party to be present during breast, pelvic, and rectal exams and requesting that the medical provider ask permission before initiating touch. If the medical intervention is clinically urgent, a therapist can communicate these issues directly to the medical practitioner after obtaining consent from the client. Whenever possible, however, patients should be encouraged to assume responsibility for informing medical practitioners of their concerns. Patients who are better able to interact with providers and to take charge of their physical health can feel an enhanced sense of well-being.

CONCLUSIONS AND FUTURE DIRECTIONS

As stated in the introduction, explicating the influence of gender on the vulnerability and recovery from traumatic stress is a complex process. Our review of the literature has identified the following considerations:

1. *Women are more than twice as likely as are men to be diagnosed with PTSD at some point in their lives.* This finding is not accounted for by the likelihood of trauma exposure and is only partially accounted for by the likelihood of traumatic events with high conditional risk for PTSD, such as sexual assault. However, trauma exposure may still play an important role in explaining a variety of gender differences in PTSD, particularly with respect to prevalence rates. For example, high-risk events such as sexual assault are associated with equally high rates of PTSD for both women and men. Exposure to sexual assault partially accounts for gender differences in PTSD because the larger culture and social context create environmental conditions in which exposure to this event is significantly overrepresented among women. Attention needs to be directed toward the qualitative characteristics of trauma exposure that, although they may occur more frequently among women, are likely risk factors for PTSD among both women and men. With respect to interpersonal violence (both sexual and physical), characteristics such as perpetration by an intimate partner or family member, chronic and repeated forms of exposure, exposure in ostensibly safe places such as in the home, and exposure during developmental years are factors that suggest an increased risk for PTSD and that are observed far more often in the traumatic experiences of women. Exposure factors such as these should not be overlooked in the assessment process with women or men.

2. *Women are more likely to experience more chronic and elaborated forms of PTSD than are men.* Characteristics of exposure that occur more frequently among women are conceptually linked to increased risk for more chronic forms of PTSD with associated features, such as impaired affect regulation, dissociation, and relationship problems. Until research suggests otherwise, we propose that characteristics of exposure, rather than patient gender, are the best markers for the importance of the assessment of these domains. However, this issue is complex. Sex differences are generally more pronounced in interpersonal interactions. These sex differences may be especially apparent in symptoms associated with and cued by early interpersonal trauma

that disrupts or confounds the development of effective social skills and self-regulatory systems necessary for relating to others. However, attention tends to focus on individual and dispositional foundations for such observed differences, rather than the social contextual and interactional basis for these differences—perhaps because these symptom clusters often include behaviors that are consistent with negative stereotypes of the female gender role. The pejorative connotations surrounding the diagnosis of borderline personality disorder are an example. Thus it sometimes appears that PTSD manifests differently among women because of some specific biological, genetic, or psychological characteristic of women. Although these domains are appropriate for assessment and research inquiry, environmental and social contextual factors should be accounted for as well.

3. *The social and environmental conditions under which women and men are exposed to and recover from traumatic stress are essential areas of assessment.* It is important to understand how gender differences in the frequency and chronicity of PTSD are related to the context in which the trauma occurred, as well as the recovery environment. In general, most childhood abuse appears to occur in a context of other adverse conditions in the home, such as interparental violence, substance abuse, or familial mental illness (Felitti et al., 1998). Rates of childhood abuse escalate in the wake of major natural disasters (Curtis, Miller, & Berry, 2000). Sexual assault and harassment in the military occurs significantly more frequently during wartime and combat (Wolfe et al., 1998), and disproportionately so for women in nontraditional occupations. Traumatic stress among women is also contextualized by a number of chronic stressors and environmental conditions. Women are far more likely than men to live in poverty, which appears to negatively affect women but not men with PTSD (Kimerling, 2004). Women experience traumatic stress in the context of caregiving, for both young children and elderly or disabled family members. Women's relative lack of social and material resources to cope with trauma doubtless makes the impact of exposure more pronounced. Furthermore, self-care needs compete with other priorities, such as securing resources to meet the basic needs of families and children. As noted by Moos (Moos, 2002), social systems maintain and reinforce characteristics of the individual that are congruent with the dominant aspects of the system. Therefore, when women's recovery from trauma occurs within a greater social system that grants them less influence and resources relative to men and within an immediate social system of poverty and the demands of multiple roles, the social context serves to maintain current symptoms, as well as the incidence of future stressors and chronic strains. Women's chronic, elaborated PTSD and comorbid conditions are consistent with these environmental influences.

4. *Effective assessment of PTSD utilizes assessment procedures and instruments that are sensitive to gender issues.* In addition to recognizing the social and environmental context of trauma exposure and PTSD, the selection and use of specific assessment *instruments* should be done with consideration

to the validity of the instrument for both women and men. For example, the selection of a trauma exposure measure should include an active questioning of content validity (i.e., Does it capture traumatic experiences common to women as well as men?) and the selection of a PTSD measure should include an awareness of the original validation sample (i.e., Were women included?) as well as any gender differences in clinically significant cutoff scores. Assessment of associated features and role functioning should be done with knowledge that the diagnostic validity of PTSD was originally established using single-event, adult-onset traumas, with pretrauma functioning able to be compared with posttrauma functioning. For survivors of multiple childhood traumas, such comparisons make little sense and do not begin to capture their affective and interpersonal disturbances. Much will be gained by the development and use of standardized assessment instruments that capture these problem areas.

REFERENCES

Acitelli, L. K., & Antonucci, T. C. (1994). Gender differences in the link between marital support and satisfaction in older couples. *Journal of Personality and Social Psychology*, *67*(4), 688–698.

Babor, T. F., de la Fuente, J. R., Saunders, J., & Grant, M. (1992). *AUDIT: The Alcohol Use Disorders Identification Test. Guidelines for use in primary health care.* Geneva, Switzerland: World Health Organization.

Badger, L. W., Bergaum, M., Carney, P. A., Dietrich, A. J., Owen, M., & Stem, J. T. (1999). Physician–patient gender and the recognition and treatment of depression in primary care. *Journal of Social Service Research*, *25*(3), 21–39.

Bagby, R. M., Parker, J. D., & Taylor, G. J. (1994). The twenty-item Toronto Alexithymia scale: 1. Item selection and cross-validation of the factor structure. *Journal of Psychosomatic Research*, *38*, 23–32.

Barlow, D. H. (2002). *Anxiety and its disorders: The nature and treatment of anxiety and panic* (2nd ed.). New York: Guilford Press.

Beck, A. T., Steer, R. A., & Brown, G. K. (1996). *Manual for the Beck Depression Inventory, 2nd ed.* San Antonio, TX: Psychological Corporation.

Beck, A. T., Steer, R. A., & Garbin, M. G. (1988). Psychometric properties of the Beck Depression Inventory: Twenty-five years of evaluation. *Clinical Psychology Review*, *8*, 77–100.

Beck, A. T., Ward, C. H., Mendelson, M., Mock, J., & Erbaugh, J. (1961). An inventory for measuring depression. *Archives of General Psychiatry*, *4*, 561–571.

Beckham, J. C., Crawford, A. L., Feldman, M. E., Kirby, A. C., Hertzberg, M. A., Davidson, J. R., et al. (1997). Chronic posttraumatic stress disorder and chronic pain in Vietnam combat veterans. *Journal of Psychosomatic Research*, *43*(4), 379–389.

Beckham, J. C., Lytle, B. L., & Feldman, M. E. (1996). Caregiver burden in partners of Vietnam War veterans with posttraumatic stress disorder. *Journal of Consulting and Clinical Psychology*, *64*(5), 1068–1072.

Berenson, A. B., Wiemann, C. M., Wilkinson, G. S., Jones, W. A., & Anderson, G.

D. (1994). Perinatal morbidity associated with violence experienced by pregnant women. *American Journal of Obstetrics and Gynecology, 170*(6), 1760–1766.

Bernstein, E. M., & Putnam, F. W. (1986). Development, reliability, and validity of a dissociation scale. *Journal of Nervous and Mental Disease, 174*, 727–735.

Bertakis, K. D., Helms, L. J., Callahan, E. J., Azari, R., Leigh, P., & Robbins, J. A. (2001). Patient gender differences in the diagnosis of depression in primary care. *Journal of Women's Health and Gender based Medicine, 10*(7), 689–698.

Blake, D. D., Weathers, F. W., Nagy, L. M., Kaloupek, D. G., Gusman, F. D., Charney, D. S., et al. (1995). The development of a Clinician-Administered PTSD Scale. *Journal of Traumatic Stress, 8*, 75–90.

Blake, D. D., Weathers, F. W., Nagy, L. M., Kaloupek, D. G., Klauminzer, G., Charney, D. S., et al. (1990). A clinician rating scale for assessing current and lifetime PTSD: The CAPS-1. *Behavior Therapist, 13*, 187–188.

Blanchard, E. B., Jones-Alexander, J., Buckley, T. C., & Forneris, C. A. (1996). Psychometric properties of the PTSD Checklist (PCL). *Behavior Research and Therapy, 8*, 669–673.

Boscarino, J. A., & Chang, J. (1999). Electrocardiogram abnormalities among men with stress-related psychiatric disorders: Implications for coronary heart disease and clinical research. *Annals of Behavioral Medicine, 21*(3), 227–234.

Bradley, K. A., Boyd-Wickizer, J., Powell, S. H., & Burman, M. L. (1998). Alcohol screening questionnaires in women: A critical review. *Journal of the American Medical Association, 280*(2), 166.

Breslau, N., & Davis, G. C. (1992). Posttraumatic stress disorder in an urban population of young adults: Risk factors for chronicity. *American Journal of Psychiatry, 149*(5), 671–675.

Breslau, N., Davis, G. C., Andreski, P., & Peterson, E. (1991). Traumatic events and posttraumatic stress disorder in an urban population of young adults. *Archives of General Psychiatry, 48*(3), 216–222.

Breslau, N., Davis, G. C., Andreski, P., & Peterson, E. L. (1997). Sex differences in posttraumatic stress disorder. *Archives of General Psychiatry, 54*(11), 1044–1048.

Breslau, N., Kessler, R. C., Chilcoat, H. D., Schultz, L. R., Davis, G. C., & Andreski, P. (1998). Trauma and posttraumatic stress disorder in the community: The 1996 Detroit Area Survey of Trauma. *Archives of General Psychiatry, 55*(7), 626–632.

Brown, P. J., Stout, R. L., & Mueller, T. (1999). Substance use disorder and posttraumatic stress disorder comorbidity: Addiction and psychiatric treatment rates. *Psychology of Addictive Behaviors, 13*(2), 115–122.

Byrne, C. A., & Riggs, D. S. (1996). The cycle of trauma: Relationship aggression in male Vietnam veterans with symptoms of posttraumatic stress disorder. *Violence and Victims, 11*(3), 213–225.

Calhoun, P. S., Beckham, J. C., & Bosworth, H. B. (2002). Caregiver burden and psychological distress in partners of veterans with chronic posttraumatic stress disorder. *Journal of Traumatic Stress, 15*(3), 205–212.

Campbell, J. C. (2002). Health consequences of intimate partner violence. *Lancet, 359*(9314), 1331–1336.

Cantanzaro, S. J., & Mearns, J. (1990). Measuring generalized expectations for negative mood regulation: Initial scale development and implications. *Journal of Personality Assessment, 54*, 546–563.

Carlson, E. B. (1994). Studying the interaction between physical and psychological states with the Dissociative Experiences Scale. In D. Spiegel (Ed.), *Dissociation: Culture, mind, and body* (pp. 41–58). Washington, DC: American Psychiatric Press.

Carlson, E. (2001). Psychometric study of a brief screen for PTSD: Assessing the impact of multiple traumatic events. *Assessment*, *8*(4), 431–441.

Carlson, E. B., Putnam, F. W., Ross, C., Torem, M., Coons, P., Dill, D. L., et al. (1993). Validity of the Dissociative Experiences Scale in screening for multiple personality disorder: A multicenter study. *American Journal of Psychiatry*, *15*(7), 1030–1036.

Caselli, L. T., & Motta, R. W. (1995). The effect of PTSD and combat level on Vietnam veterans' perceptions of child behavior and marital adjustment. *Journal of Clinical Psychology*, *51*(1), 4–12.

Centers for Disease Control and Prevention. (1999). Mortality patterns—United States, 1997. *Morbidity and Mortality Weekly Report*, *48*(30), 664–668.

Cloitre, M., Koenen, K. C., Cohen, L. R., & Han, H. (2002). Skills training in affective and interpersonal regulation followed by exposure: A phase-based treatment for PTSD related to childhood abuse. *Journal of Consulting and Clinical Psychology*, *70*(5), 1067–1074.

Cloitre, M., Koenen, K. C., Gratz, K. L., & Jakupcak, M. (2002). Differential diagnosis of PTSD in women. In R. Kimerling, P. Ouimette, & J. Wolfe (Eds.), *Gender and PTSD* (pp. 117–149). New York: Guilford Press.

Cloitre, M., Scarvalone, P., & Difede, J. A. (1997). Posttraumatic stress disorder, self- and interpersonal dysfunction among sexually retraumatized women. *Journal of Traumatic Stress*, *10*(3), 437–452.

Cohen, S., & Hoberman, H. M. (1983). Positive events and social supports as buffers of life change stress. *Journal of Applied Social Psychology*, *13*, 99–125.

Cokkinides, V. E., Coker, A. L., Sanderson, M., Addy, C., & Bethea, L. (1999). Physical violence during pregnancy: Maternal complications and birth outcomes. *Obstetrics and Gynecology*, *93*(5, Pt. 1), 661–666.

Cole, P. M., Michel, M. K., & Teti, L. O. (1994). The development of emotion regulation and dysregulation. *Monographs of the Society for Research in Child Development*, *59*(2–3), 73–100.

Cosgrove, D. J., Gordon, Z., Bernie, J. E., Hami, S., Montoya, D., Stein, M. B., et al. (2002). Sexual dysfunction in combat veterans with posttraumatic stress disorder. *Urology*, *60*(5), 881–884.

Cottler, L. B., Nishith, P., & Compton, W. M., III. (2001). Gender differences in risk factors for trauma exposure and posttraumatic stress disorder among inner-city drug abusers in and out of treatment. *Comprehensive Psychiatry*, *42*(2), 111–117.

Curtis, T., Miller, B. C., & Berry, E. H. (2000). Changes in reports and incidence of child abuse following natural disasters. *Child Abuse and Neglect*, *24*(9), 1151–1162.

Dancu, C. V., Riggs, D. S., Hearst-Ikeda, D., Shoyer, B. G., & Foa, E. B. (1996). Dissociative experiences and posttraumatic stress disorder among female victims of criminal assault and rape. *Journal of Traumatic Stress*, *9*(2), 253–267.

DiLillo, D., Giuffre, D., Tremblay, G. C., & Peterson, L. (2001). A closer look at the nature of intimate partner violence reported by women with a history of child sexual abuse. *Journal of Interpersonal Violence*, *16*(2), 116–132.

DiLillo, D., & Long, P. J. (1999). Perceptions of couple functioning among female survivors of child sexual abuse. *Journal of Child Sexual Abuse*, *7*(4), 59–76.

DiLillo, D., Tremblay, G. C., & Peterson, L. (2000). Linking childhood sexual abuse and abusive parenting: The mediating role of maternal anger. *Child Abuse and Neglect*, *24*(6), 767–779.

Dobie, D. J., Kivlahan, D. R., Maynard, C., Bush, K. R., McFall, M., Epler, A. J., et al. (2002). Screening for posttraumatic disorder in female Veteran's Affairs patients: Validation of the PTSD Checklist. *General Hospital Psychiatry*, *24*, 367–374.

Ehlers, A., Mayou, R. A., & Bryant, B. (1998). Psychological predictors of chronic posttraumatic stress disorder after motor vehicle accidents. *Journal of Abnormal Psychology*, *107*(3), 508–519.

Evans, D. R., & Cope, W. E. (1989). *Quality of Life Questionnaire: Manual*. Toronto, Ontario: Multi-Health Systems, Inc.

Felitti, V. J., Anda, R. F., Nordenberg, D., Williamson, D. F., Spitz, A. M., Edwards, V., et al. (1998). Relationship of childhood abuse and household dysfunction to many of the leading causes of death in adults: The Adverse Childhood Experiences ACE Study [see Comments]. *American Journal of Preventive Medicine*, *14*(4), 245–258.

Fildes, J., Reed, L., Jones, N., Martin, M., & Barrett, J. (1992). Trauma: The leading cause of maternal death. *Journal of Trauma*, *32*(5), 643–645.

Fillingim, R. B., Wilkinson, C. S., & Powell, T. (1999). Self-reported abuse history and pain complaints among young adults. *Clinical Journal of Pain*, *15*(2), 85–91.

First, M., Spitzer, R., Williams, J., & Gibbon, M. (2000). Structured Clinical Interview for DSM-IV Axis I Disorders (SCID-I). In American Psychiatric Association, *Handbook of psychiatric measures* (pp. 49–53). Washington, DC: American Psychiatric Association.

Foa, E. B., Cashman, L., Jaycox, L., & Perry, K. (1997). The validation of a self-report measure of posttraumatic stress disorder: The Posttraumatic Diagnostic Scale. *Psychological Assessment*, *9*, 445–451.

Foa, E. B., & Tolin, D. F. (2000). Comparison of the PTSD Symptom Scale—Interview Version and the Clinician-Administered PTSD scale. *Journal of Traumatic Stress*, *13*(2), 181–191.

Franklin, C. L., Sheeran, T., & Zimmerman, M. (2002). Screening for trauma history, posttraumatic stress disorder (PTSD) and subthreshold PTSD in psychiatric outpatients. *Psychological Assessment*, *14*, 467–471.

Freuh, B. C., Turner, S. M., Beidel, D. C., & Cahill, S. P. (2001). Assessment of social functioning in combat veterans with PTSD. *Aggression and Violent Behavior*, *6*, 79–90.

Friedman, M. J., & Schnurr, P. P. (1995). The relationship between trauma, posttraumatic stress disorder, and physical health. In M. Friedman, D. Charney, & A. Deutch (Eds.), *Neurobiological and clinical consequences of stress: From normal adaptation to posttraumatic stress disorder* (pp. 507–524). Philadelphia: Lippincott-Raven.

Frischholz, E. J., Braun, B. G., Sachs, R. G., & Hopkins, L. (1990). The Dissociative Experiences Scale: Further replication and validation. *Dissociation: Progress in the Dissociative Disorders*, *3*(3), 151–153.

Frye, V. (2001). Examining homicide's contribution to pregnancy-associated deaths. *Journal of the American Medical Association*, *285*(11), 1510–1511.

Fullerton, C. S., Ursano, R. J., Epstein, R. S., Crowley, B., Vance, K., Kao, T. C., et al.

(2001). Gender differences in posttraumatic stress disorder after motor vehicle accidents. *American Journal of Psychiatry, 158*(9), 1486–1491.

Gavrilovic, J., Lecic-Tosevski, D., Knezevic, G., & Priebe, S. (2002). Predictors of posttraumatic stress in civilians 1 year after air attacks: A study of Yugoslavian students. *Journal of Nervous and Mental Disease, 190*(4), 257–262.

Gershuny, B. S., & Thayer, J. F. (1999). Relations among psychological trauma, dissociative phenomena, and trauma-related distress: A review and integration. *Clinical Psychology Review, 19*(5), 631–657.

Golding, J. M., Wilsnack, S. C., & Cooper, M. L. (2002). Sexual assault history and social support: Six general population studies. *Journal of Traumatic Stress, 15*(3), 187–197.

Gostin, L. O., Lazzarini, Z., Alexander, D., Brandt, A. M., Mayer, K. H., & Silverman, D. C. (1994). HIV testing, counseling, and prophylaxis after sexual assault. *Journal of the American Medical Association, 271*(18), 1436–1444.

Green, B. (1996). Trauma History Questionnaire. In E. M. Varra (Ed.), *Measurement of stress, trauma and adaptation* (pp. 366–368). Lutherville, MD: Sidran Press.

Herman, J. L. (1992). *Trauma and recovery.* New York: Basic Books.

Hoff, R. A., Beam-Goulet, J., & Rosenheck, R. A. (1997). Mental disorder as a risk factor for human immunodeficiency virus infection in a sample of veterans. *Journal of Nervous and Mental Disease, 185*(9), 556–560.

Holmes, M. (1999). Sexually transmitted infections in female rape victims [see Comments]. *AIDS Patient Care and STDS, 13*(12), 703–708.

Horowitz, L. M., Rosenberg, S. E., Baer, B. A., Ureno, G., & Villasenor, V. S. (1988). Inventory of Interpersonal Problems: Psychometric properties and clinical applications. *Journal of Consulting and Clinical Psychology, 56*, 885–892.

Irwin, C., Falsetti, S. A., Lydiard, R. B., Ballenger, J. C., Brock, C. D., & Brener, W. (1996). Comorbidity of posttraumatic stress disorder and irritable bowel syndrome. *Journal of Clinical Psychiatry, 57*(12), 576–578.

Josephs, R. A., Markus, H. R., & Tafarodi, R. W. (1992). Gender and self-esteem. *Journal of Personality and Social Psychology, 63*(3), 391–402.

Julien, D., & Markman, H. J. (1991). Social support and social networks as determinants of individual and marital outcomes. *Journal of Social and Personal Relationships, 8*, 549–568.

Kalichman, S. C., Williams, E. A., Cherry, C., Belcher, L., & Nachimson, D. (1998). Sexual coercion, domestic violence, and negotiating condom use among low-income African American women. *Journal of Women's Health, 7*(3), 371–378.

Keane, T. M., Taylor, K. L., & Penk, W. E. (1997). Differentiating posttraumatic stress disorder (PTSD) from major depression (MDD) and generalized anxiety disorder (GAD). *Journal of Anxiety Disorders, 11*(3), 317–328.

Kessler, R. C., Sonnega, A., Bromet, E., Hughes, M., & Nelson, C. B. (1995). Posttraumatic stress disorder in the National Comorbidity Survey. *Archives of General Psychiatry, 52*(12), 1048–1060.

Kessler, R. C., Zhao, S., Katz, S. J., Kouzis, A. C., Frank, R. G., Edlund, M., et al. (1999). Past-year use of outpatient services for psychiatric problems in the National Comorbidity Survey. *American Journal of Psychiatry, 156*(1), 115–123.

Kilpatrick, D., Resnick, H., & Freedy, J. R. (1991). *The Potential Stressful Events Interview.* Charleston, SC: Medical University of South Carolina, Department of Psychiatry, Crime Victims Research and Treatment Center.

Kilpatrick, D. G., Saunders, B. E., Amick-McMullan, A., & Best, C. L. (1989). Victim and crime factors associated with the development of crime-related posttraumatic stress disorder. *Behavior Therapy*, *20*(2), 199–214.

Kimerling, R. (2004). An investigation of sex differences in nonpsychiatric morbidity associated with posttraumatic stress disorder. *Journal of the American Medical Women's Association*, *59*(1), 43–47.

Kimerling, R., Armistead, L., & Forehand, R. (1999). Victimization experiences and HIV infection in women: Associations with serostatus, psychological symptoms, and health status. *Journal of Traumatic Stress*, *12*(1), 41–58.

Kimerling, R., Calhoun, K. S., Forehand, R., Armistead, L., Morse, E., Morse, P., et al. (1999). Traumatic stress in HIV-infected women. *AIDS Education and Prevention*, *11*(4), 321–330.

Kimerling, R., Clum, G., McQuery, J., & Schnurr, P. P. (2002). PTSD and medical comorbidity. In R. Kimerling, P. Ouimette, & J. Wolfe (Eds.), *Gender and PTSD* (pp. 271–302). New York: Guilford Press.

Klonoff, E. A., Landrine, H., & Lang, D. L. (1997). Introduction: The state of research on black women in health psychology and behavioral medicine. *Women's Health*, *3*(3–4), 165–181.

Kobernick, M. E., Seifert, S., & Sanders, A. B. (1985). Emergency department management of the sexual assault victim. *Journal of Emergency Medicine*, *2*(3), 205–214.

Koss, M. P. (1985). The hidden rape victim: Personality, attitudinal, and situational characteristics. *Psychology of Women Quarterly*, *9*, 193–212.

Koss, M. P., Koss, P. G., & Woodruff, W. J. (1991). Deleterious effects of criminal victimization on women's health and medical utilization. *Archives of Internal Medicine*, *151*(2), 342–347.

Kotler, M., Cohen, H., Aizenberg, D., Matar, M., Loewenthal, U., Kaplan, Z., et al. (2000). Sexual dysfunction in male posttraumatic stress disorder patients. *Psychotherapeutics and Psychosomatics*, *69*(6), 309–315.

Kring, A. M., & Gordon, A. H. (1998). Sex differences in emotion: Expression, experience, and physiology. *Journal of Personality and Social Psychology*, *74*, 686–703.

Kubany, E. S., Haynes, S. N., Leisen, M. B., Owens, J. A., Kaplan, A. S., Watson, S. B., et al. (2000). Development and preliminary validation of a brief broad-spectrum measure of trauma exposure: The Traumatic Life Events Questionnaire. *Psychological Assessment*, *12*(2), 210–224.

Kubany, E. S., Leisen, M. B., Kaplan, A. S., & Kelly, M. P. (2000). Validation of a brief measure of posttraumatic stress disorder: The Distressing Life Event Questionnaire. *Psychological Assessment*, *12*, 197–209.

Kulka, R. A., Schlenger, W. E., Fairbank, J. A., Hough, R. L., Jordan, B. K., Marmar, C. R., et al. (1990). *Trauma and the Vietnam War generation: Report of findings from the National Vietnam Veterans Readjustment Study*: Philadelphia: Brunner/Mazel.

Letourneau, E. J., Resnick, H. S., Kilpatrick, D. G., & Saunders, B. E. (1996). Comorbidity of sexual problems and posttraumatic stress disorder in female crime victims. *Behavior Therapy*, *27*(3), 321–336.

Letourneau, E. J., Schewe, P. A., & Frueh, B. C. (1997). Preliminary evaluation of sexual problems in combat veterans with PTSD. *Journal of Traumatic Stress*, *10*(1), 125–132.

Linehan, M. M., Tutek, D. A., Heard, H. L., & Armstrong, H. E. (1994). Interpersonal outcome of cognitive behavioral treatment for chronically suicidal borderline patients. *American Journal of Psychiatry*, *151*(12), 1771–1776.

Lipman, E. L., MacMillan, H. L., & Boyle, M. H. (2001, January). Childhood abuse and psychiatric disorders among single and married mothers. *American Journal of Psychiatry, 158*(1), 73–77.

MacMillan, H. L., Fleming, J. E., Streiner, D. L., Lin, E., Boyle, M. H., Jamieson, E., et al. (2001). Childhood abuse and lifetime psychopathology in a community sample. *American Journal of Psychiatry, 158*(11), 1878–1883.

Maddrey, W. C. (2000). Alcohol-induced liver disease. *Clinical Liver Disease, 4*(1), 115–131.

Mayfield, D., McLeod, G., & Hall, P. (1974). The CAGE questionnaire: Validation of a new alcoholism screening instrument. *American Journal of Psychiatry, 131*(10), 1121–1123.

McFarlane, A. C. (2001). Comparing CIDI and clinical assessment. *Australia and New Zealand Journal of Psychiatry, 35*(6), 858–859.

McQuaid, J. R., Pedrelli, P., McCahill, M. E., & Stein, M. B. (2001). Reported trauma, posttraumatic stress disorder and major depression among primary care patients. *Psychological Medicine, 31*(7), 1249–1257.

Moos, R. H. (2002). The mystery of human context and coping: An unraveling of clues. *American Journal of Community Psychology, 30*(1), 67–88.

Muir, A., Butterfield, M., Meador, K. G., Bosworth, H., Stechuchak, K., & Frothingham, R. (1999, November). *The prevalence of Hepatitis C in a sample of severely mentally ill veterans.* Paper presented at the annual meeting of the Veterans Administration Health Services Research and Development, Washington, DC.

Nelson, B. S., & Wampler, K. S. (2000). Systemic effects of trauma in clinic couples: An exploratory study of secondary trauma resulting from childhood abuse. *Journal of Marital and Family Therapy, 26*(2), 171–184.

Nolen-Hoeksema, S., & Girgus, J. S. (1994). The emergence of gender differences in depression during adolescence. *Psychological Bulletin, 115*(3), 424–443.

Norris, F. H. (1992). Epidemiology of trauma: Frequency and impact of different potentially traumatic events on different demographic groups. *Journal of Consulting and Clinical Psychology, 60*(3), 409–418.

Norris, F. H., Foster, J. D., & Weisshaar, D. L. (2002). The epidemiology of sex differences in PTSD across developmental, societal, and research contexts. In R. Kimerling, P. Ouimette, & J. Wolfe (Eds.), *Gender and PTSD* (pp. 3–42). New York: Guilford Press.

Orsillo, S. M., Raha, S., & Hammond, C. (2002). Gender issues in PTSD with comorbid mental health disorders. In R. Kimerling, P. Ouimette, & J. Wolfe (Eds.), *Gender and PTSD* (pp. 207–231). New York: Guilford Press.

Parker, B., McFarlane, J., & Soeken, K. (1994). Abuse during pregnancy: Effects on maternal complications and birth weight in adult and teenage women. *Obstetrics and Gynecology, 84*(3), 323–328.

Paul, J. P., Catania, J., Pollack, L., & Stall, R. (2001). Understanding childhood sexual abuse as a predictor of sexual risk-taking among men who have sex with men: The Urban Men's Health Study. *Child Abuse and Neglect, 25*(4), 557–584.

Pelcovitz, D., van der Kolk, B., Roth, S., Mandel, F., Kaplan, S., & Resnick, P. (1997). Development of a criteria set and a structured interview for disorders of extreme stress (SIDES). *Journal of Traumatic Stress, 10*(1), 3–16.

Ptacek, J. T., Smith, R. E., & Dodge, K. L. (1994). Gender differences in coping with stress: When stressor and appraisals do not differ. *Personality and Social Psychology Bulletin, 20*, 421–430.

Resnick, H. S., Acierno, R., & Kilpatrick, D. G. (1997). Health impact of interpersonal violence: II. Medical and mental health outcomes. *Behavioral Medicine, 23*(2), 65–78.

Resnick, H. S., Kilpatrick, D. G., Best, C. L., & Kramer, T. L. (1992). Vulnerability–stress factors in development of posttraumatic stress disorder. *Journal of Nervous and Mental Disease, 180*(7), 424–430.

Riggs, D. S., Byrne, C. A., Weathers, F. W., & Litz, B. T. (1998). The quality of the intimate relationships of male Vietnam veterans: Problems associated with posttraumatic stress disorder. *Journal of Traumatic Stress, 11*(1), 87–101.

Ritter, C., Hobfoll, S. E., Lavin, J., Cameron, R. P., & Hulsizer, M. R. (2000). Stress, psychosocial resources, and depressive symptomatology during pregnancy in low-income, inner-city women. *Health Psychology, 19*(6), 576–585.

Rosen, R., Brown, C., Heiman, J., Leiblum, S., Meston, C., Shabsigh, R., et al. (2000). The Female Sexual Function Index (FSFI): A multidimensional self-report instrument for the assessment of female sexual function. *Journal of Sex and Marital Therapy, 26*(2), 191–208.

Rosen, R. C., Cappelleri, J. C., Smith, M. D., Lipsky, J., & Pena, B. M. (1999). Development and evaluation of an abridged, 5-item version of the International Index of Erectile Function (IIEF-5) as a diagnostic tool for erectile dysfunction. *International Journal of Impotence Research, 11*(6), 319–326.

Rosen, R. C., & Leiblum, S. R. (1995). Treatment of sexual disorders in the 1990s: An integrated approach. *Journal of Consulting and Clinical Psychology, 63*(6), 877–890.

Rosen, R. C., Riley, A., Wagner, G., Osterloh, I. H., Kirkpatrick, J., & Mishra, A. (1997). The international index of erectile function (IIEF): A multidimensional scale for assessment of erectile dysfunction. *Urology, 49*(6), 822–830.

Russell, M., Martier, S. S., Sokol, R. J., Jacobson, S., Jacobson, J., & Bottoms, S. (1991). Screening for pregnancy risk drinking: TWEAKING the tests. *Alcoholism, Clinical and Experimental Research, 15*(2), 638.

Rust, J., & Golombok, S. (1985). The Golombok–Rust Inventory of Sexual Satisfaction (GRISS). *British Journal of Clinical Psychology, 24*(Pt. 1), 63–64.

Saigh, P. A., & Bremner, J. D. (1999). The history of posttraumatic stress disorder. In J. D. Bremner (Ed.), *Posttraumatic stress disorder: A comprehensive text* (pp. 1–17). Boston: Allyn & Bacon.

Salokangas, R. K. R., Vaahtera, K., Pacriev, S., Sohlman, B., & Lehtinen, V. (2002). Gender differences in depressive symptoms: An artifact caused by measurement instruments? *Journal of Affective Disorders, 68*, 215–220.

Sansone, R. A., Wiederman, M.W., & Sansone, L. (1998). The Self-Harm Inventory (SHI): Development of a scale for identifying self-destructive behaviors and borderline personality disorder. *Journal of Clinical Psychology, 54*, 973–983.

Savarese, V. W., Suvak, M. K., King, L. A., & King, D. W. (2001). Relationships among alcohol use, hyperarousal, and marital abuse and violence in Vietnam veterans. *Journal of Traumatic Stress, 14*(4), 717–732.

Schnurr, P. P., & Jankowski, M. K. (1999). Physical health and post-traumatic stress disorder: Review and synthesis. *Seminars in Clinical Neuropsychiatry, 4*(4), 295–304.

Schnurr, P. P., Spiro, A., III, & Paris, A. H. (2000). Physician-diagnosed medical disorders in relation to PTSD symptoms in older male military veterans. *Health Psychology, 19*(1), 91–97.

Shalev, A. Y., Bleich, A., & Ursano, R. J. (1990). Somatic comorbidity of the posttraumatic stress disorder. In J. E. Lundeberg, U. Otto, & B. Rybeck (Eds.), *Wartime Medical Services Second International Conference* (pp. 25–29). Stockholm, Sweden.

Sharkansky, E. J., Brief, D. J., Peirce, J. M., Meehan, J. C., & Mannix, L. M. (1999). Substance abuse patients with posttraumatic stress disorder (PTSD): Identifying specific triggers of substance use and their associations with PTSD symptoms. *Psychology of Addictive Behaviors, 13*(2), 89–97.

Sherman, J. J., Turk, D. C., & Okifuji, A. (2000). Prevalence and impact of posttraumatic stress disorder-like symptoms on patients with fibromyalgia syndrome. *Clinical Journal of Pain, 16*(2), 127–134.

Sifneos, P. E. (1996). Alexithymia: Past and present. *American Journal of Psychiatry, 153*(7), 137–142.

Steinberg, M. (2002). Advances in the clinical assessment of dissociation: The SCID-D-R. *Bulletin of the Menninger Clinic, 64*(2), 146–163.

Steinberg, M., Rounsville, B., & Cicchetti, D. V. (1990). The Structured Clinical Interview for DSM-III-R Dissociative Disorders: Preliminary report on a new diagnostic instrument. *American Journal of Psychiatry, 147*, 76–82.

Stewart, S. H., Conrod, P. J., Samoluk, S. B., Pihl, R. O., & Dongier, M. (2000). PTSD symptoms and situation-specific drinking in women substance abusers. *Alcoholism Treatment Quarterly, 18*(3), 31–48.

Stewart, S. H., Ouimette, P., & Brown, P. J. (2002). Gender and the comorbidity of PTSD with substance use disorders. In R. Kimerling, P. Ouimette, & J. Wolfe (Eds.), *Gender and PTSD* (pp. 232–270). New York: Guilford Press.

Taft, C. T., King, L. A., King, D. W., Leskin, G. A., & Riggs, D. S. (1999). Partners' ratings of combat veterans' PTSD symptomatology. *Journal of Traumatic Stress, 12*(2), 327–334.

Talley, N. J., Fett, S. L., Zinsmeister, A. R., & Melton, L. J., III. (1994). Gastrointestinal tract symptoms and self-reported abuse: A population-based study. *Gastroenterology, 107*(4), 1040–1049.

Taylor, G. J., Bagby, R. M., & Parker, J. D. (1992). The Revised Toronto Alexithymia Scale: Some reliability, validity and normative data. *Psychotherapy and Psychosomatics, 57*, 34–41.

Taylor, G. J., Bagby, R. M., Ryna, D. P., Parkder, J. D. A., Doody, K. F., & Deefe, P. (1988). Critierion validity of the Toronto Alexithymia Scale. *Psychosomatic Medicine, 50*, 500–509.

Thompson, R. A. (1994). Emotion regulation: A theme in search of definition. *Monographs of the Society for Research in Child Development, 59*(2–3), 25–52.

Tichenor, V., Marmar, C. R., Weiss, D. S., Metzler, T. J., & Ronfeldt, H. M. (1996). The relationship of peritraumatic dissociation and posttraumatic stress: Findings in female Vietnam theater veterans. *Journal of Consulting and Clinical Psychology, 64*(5), 1054–1059.

Tolin, D. F., & Foa, E. B. (2002). Gender and PTSD: A cognitive model. In R. Kimerling, P. Ouimette, & J. Wolfe (Eds.), *Gender and PTSD* (pp. 76–97). New York: Guilford Press.

van der Kolk, B. A., & Fisler, R. E. (1994). Childhood abuse and neglect and loss of self-regulation. *Bulletin of the Menninger Clinic, 58*(2), 145–168.

van der Kolk, B. A., Pelcovitz, D., Roth, S., Mandel, F. S., McFarlane, A., & Herman, J. L. (1996). Dissociation, somatization, and affect dysregulation: The complexity of adaptation to trauma. *American Journal of Psychiatry, 153*(7S)(Suppl.), 83–93.

Volk, R. J., Cantor, S. B., Steinbauer, J. R., & Cass, A. R. (1997). Item bias in the CAGE Screening Test for Alcohol Use Disorders. *Journal of General Internal Medicine, 12*(12), 763–769.

Walker, E. A., Gelfand, A., Katon, W. J., Koss, M. P., Von Korff, M., Bernstein, D., et al. (1999). Adult health status of women with histories of childhood abuse and neglect. *American Journal of Medicine, 107*(4), 332–339.

Walker, E. A., Newman, E., Dobie, D. J., Ciechanowski, P., & Katon, W. (2002). Validation of the PTSD Checklist in an HMO sample of women. *General Hospital Psychiatry, 24*, 375–380.

Waller, N., Putnam, F. W., & Carlson, E. B. (1996). Types of dissociation and dissociative types: A taxometric analysis of dissociative experiences. *Psychological Methods, 1*(3), 300–321.

Waller, N. G., & Ross, C. A. (1997). The prevalence and biometric structure of pathological dissociation in the general population: Taxometric and behavior genetic findings. *Journal of Abnormal Psychology, 106*, 499–510.

Weathers, F. W., Litz, B. T., Herman, D. S., Huska, J. A., & Keane, T. M. (1993, October). *The PTSD checklist: Reliability, validity, and diagnostic utility.* Paper presented at the meeting of the International Society for Traumatic Stress Studies, San Antonio, TX.

Weissman, M. M., & Bothwell, S. (1976). Assessment of social adjustment by patient self-report. *Archives of General Psychiatry, 33*, 1111–1115.

White, P., & Faustman, W. (1989). Coexisting physical conditions among inpatients with posttraumatic stress disorder. *Military Medicine, 154*(2), 66–71.

Wingood, G. M., & DiClemente, R. J. (1997). The effects of an abusive primary partner on the condom use and sexual negotiation practices of African-American women. *American Journal of Public Health, 87*(6), 1016–1019.

Wolfe, J., & Kimerling, R. (1997). Gender issues in the assessment of posttraumatic stress disorder. In J. P. Wilson & T. M. Keane (Eds.), *Assessing psychological trauma and PTSD* (pp. 192–238). New York: Guilford Press.

Wolfe, J., Sharkansky, E. J., Read, J. P., Dawson, R., Martin, J. A., & Ouimette, P. C. (1998). Sexual harassment and assault as predictors of PTSD symptomatology among U.S. female Persian Gulf War military personnel. *Journal of Interpersonal Violence, 13*(1), 40–57.

Zanarini, M. C., Gunderson, J. G., Frankenburg, F. R., & Chauncey, D. L. (1989). The revised Diagnostic Interview for Borderlines: Discriminating BPD from other Axis II disorders. *Journal of Personality Disorders, 3*(1), 10–18.

Zierler, S., Feingold, L., Laufer, D., Velentgas, P., Kantrowitz-Gordon, I., & Mayer, K. (1991). Adult survivors of childhood sexual abuse and subsequent risk of HIV infection. *American Journal of Public Health, 81*(5), 572–575.

Zierler, S., & Krieger, N. (1997). Reframing women's risk: Social inequalities and HIV infection. *Annual Review of Public Health, 18*, 401–436.

Zierler, S., Witbeck, B., & Mayer, K. (1996). Sexual violence against women living with or at risk for HIV infection. *American Journal of Preventive Medicine, 12*(5), 304–310.

PART VI

Assessing Traumatic Injury in Litigation

CHAPTER 21

Forensic/Clinical Assessment of Psychological Trauma and PTSD in Legal Settings

JOHN P. WILSON
THOMAS A. MORAN

The forensic assessment of posttraumatic stress disorder (PTSD) in legal settings has grown in importance and scope since the formal nosological classification of the psychiatric disorder in 1980 (DSM-III; American Psychiatric Association, 1980). During the past two decades, the interface between the law and issues pertaining to PTSD as a psychological injury, mental disorder, or disabling condition as the direct result of trauma has brought the necessity of forensic and clinical assessment to the crossroads of science and the law, to the need to understand the effects of traumatization and their application to a wide range of legal problems and considerations. The understanding and application of PTSD as a stress disorder that results from different forms of trauma has found its way into almost every sector and domain of civil and criminal law (Wilson, 2000; Simon, 2000).

The purpose of this chapter is to present a general and practical overview of the forensic assessment of PTSD in legal settings and to identify the methods and processes necessary to establish adequately: (1) differential diagnosis; (2) the links or "causal connections" between a traumatic experience and the onset, development, and progression of PTSD as a stress syndrome and a psychiatric disorder; (3) the proper application of PTSD to legal questions; (4) the difference between PTSD, malingering, and factitious PTSD; and (5) the working alliance between attorneys, judges, adjudicators, and others and designated expert witnesses. We do not review the specific assessment technologies and psychometric measures available to aid in the use of diagnosis, in establishing a clinical/forensic opinion, or in defining a scientific finding for use in litigation. The other chapters in this book address the many different aspects of PTSD diagnosis and assessment. However, for an overview of PTSD and its psychological dynamics, see Wilson, Chapter 1, this volume. Further, although it is intrinsically interesting and relevant, we do not review the history of the use of PTSD in litigation. Elsewhere, reviews have been done of this phenomenon (Wilson, 1989, 2000; Sparr, White, Friedman, & Wiles, 1994; Sparr & Boehlein, 1990; Applebaum, Jick, Grisso, Givelber, Silver, & Stedman, 1993; Pitman, Sparr, Saunders, & McFarlane, 1996).

THE NEED TO UNDERSTAND PTSD AS A PROLONGED STRESS RESPONSE SYNDROME

Attorneys, judges, adjudicators, and mental health experts need to understand PTSD in its depth and complexity when relevant in legal arenas. *PTSD is a multidimensional phenomenon whose manifestations can be discerned at all levels of psychological functioning*:

1. *Mental processes*. Awareness, cognition, judgment, reasoning, executive functions, memory, consciousness, reality orientation, concentration, and so forth.
2. *Affects*. Range, frequency, duration and severity of various emotions (e.g., anger, anxiety, fear, terror, horror, rage, grief, sadness, etc.).
3. *Trauma-related coping styles*. Avoidance tendencies, isolation, psychic numbing or loss of feelings and capacity to experience self and others, withdrawal, detachment, alienation, estrangement, and social distancing.
4. *Hyperarousal states*. Increased levels of posttraumatic physiological reactivity that include sleep disturbance, startle responses, impaired cognitive processes, irritability, "short fuses," repetitive states of agitation, and expressions of heightened nervous system arousal (e.g., sweating, flushing, muscle tension, hyperventilation, heart palpitations, urinary urgency, etc.).
5. *Self-reference alterations and disturbances*. Low self-esteem, changes in sense of well-being, feeling different than one was before the trauma, change in identity, alterations in body or self-images, loss of dignity and integrity, shame and guilt, and having a sense of being victimized.

Understanding the multidimensional nature of PTSD is critical to many areas of forensic assessments and their application to civil and criminal law issues, such as the insanity defense, diminished capacity, impulse control, parental competence, fitness for duty, mental disability status, capacity to form intent, levels of psychiatric impairment, present or future needs for treatment, temporary versus permanent disability status, and so forth. A careful and thorough assessment of PTSD, as a complex form of a stress-related psychiatric disorder, is essential in order to (1) establish a sound scientific and empirical basis for an expert opinion; (2) demonstrate a "good fit" between objective data and facts and their relevance to the pertinent legal issues in civil, criminal, and administrative domains; (3) avoid misdiagnosis and the failure to detect malingering or factitious PTSD; (4) facilitate a credible and impartial professional presentation of scientific data that is replicable, testable, and likely to be verified by other independent mental health examiners.

TRAUMA AND THE LAW: CIVIL TORTS AND CRIMINAL LITIGATION

In civil, criminal, and international courts of law, PTSD has been used in litigation in many different ways. The subjects of litigation are as diverse as the nature of the traumatic events that bring them to a court of jurisdiction and include disasters of natural and human origin (e.g., war atrocities, technological disasters, industrial accidents, motor vehicle accidents, rape, assault, domestic violence), as well as other events that result in personal injury. Litigation (in a plaintiff or a defense position) may involve other traumatic events, such as childhood sexual and physical abuse, kidnapping, airplane crashes, and mass disasters. Traumatic exposure with potential legal consequences also include victims of hostage taking, negligent exposure to life-threatening diseases, war-related stressors, duty-related traumatic exposure (e.g., for police officers, EMTs, firefighters, rescue workers, emergency room medical staff), and the witnessing of horrific injury to others in unexpected fatal accidents or by deliberate infliction of pain and suffering.

Wilson and Walker (1990), Sparr and Boehnlein (1990), Modlin (1983), Simon (2000), and Wilson (2000) have noted that posttraumatic reactions are of concern in the forensic endeavors in the United States legal system in five major areas:

1. In *criminal litigation*, in which PTSD has been used as a *complete* defense for a crime (not guilty by reason of insanity [NGRI]), as a *partial* defense to refute an element of a crime (diminished capacity), or as *mitigation*, a basis for reduced sentencing.
2. In *civil litigation*, wherein psychologically traumatized individuals seek compensation for personal injury.
3. In *disability or pension claims* made to private, local, state, and federal organizations (e.g., Social Security disability claims; Veterans Administration service-connected disability claims associated with military service; disability pension claims from police and firefigher funds; workers' compensation bureaus and similar agencies).
4. In *courts of common pleas*, involving such issues as child custody disputes and domestic violence.
5. In religious–spiritual matters, in which PTSD may be considered as a basis to retain good standing in the Catholic Church following a divorce or as mitigation, for example, in canonical matters before the tribunal of a diocese (Wilson & Moran, 1997).

In each of these five areas, there is a potential interaction between the science of PTSD and the considerations of law.

LEGAL MATTERS CONCERNED WITH PERSONAL INJURY, ABUSE, HARM, AND TRAUMA

PTSD is among the primary DSM-IV (American Psychiatric Association, 1994) diagnostic classifications (code 309.81) associated with litigation that involves the issues of (1) *victimization* by willful or negligent harm, (2) *personal injury* caused deliberately or accidentally, (3) *compensation* for traumatization for personal injury caused by service or work duties, and (4) *criminal responsibility, culpability, and mitigation* in regard to the psychiatric disorder of persons with the stress syndrome.

In criminal and civil litigation the core areas of PTSD span a broad range of legal and psychological issues that bring together mental health professionals, attorneys, expert witnesses, judges, and juries into a common arena of determination and decision making as to the validity and reliability of simple and complex claims associated with traumas and their consequences in the lives of ordinary people.

FORENSIC ASSESSMENT WITH THE MATRIX CONCEPT: DETERMINING THE CAUSE OF PTSD

In medical–legal contexts, assessing the linkage between a traumatic event, the development of PTSD, and the forensic issues is a critical task for lawyers and experts alike. The *matrix concept* of assessing PTSD enables experts to obtain information pertinent to the differential diagnosis of PTSD and its relevance to a particular legal case (Wilson & Zigelbaum, 1986). To determine this potential relationship, it is important to gather as much information as possible as to the client's psychosocial functioning before, during, and after the trauma. Table 21.1 presents a schematic representation of the matrix concept and indicates where data and documents can be obtained that shed light on how a traumatic event may have affected a person's level of psychosocial functioning.

In cases involving civil or criminal litigation, information can be examined from the following sources: (1) relevant legal documents such as medical records, arrest records, police investigations, forensic and laboratory tests, hospital records, photographs of the trauma source, and so forth; (2) psychiatric and psychological evaluations, including the results of biomedical and psychometric testing (e.g., MMPI-2 PTSD subscales, neurological assessments, specialized tests); (3) personal witness statements, affidavits, and statements made by significant others about changes in the individual's behavior *after* the trauma; and (4) records of life-course experiences (e.g.,

TABLE 21.1. The Matrix Concept: Assessing Posttraumatic Functioning in Medical–Legal Contexts

	Forensic Assessment of PTSD (trauma time-line chronology)	
Pretrauma psychosocial adaptation	Traumatic event: Peritraumatic experience	Posttraumatic functioning: Changes in baseline functioning across assessment areas
Areas of psychological sssessment	Traumatic event[a] assessment: Stressor assessment of specific exposure	PTSD symptoms assessment
Affective states(emotional control)	Specific stressors experienced: Assess reactive affects.	B, C, D[b]
Personality characteristics	Nature of traumatic event experienced: Assess personality impacts.	B, C, D
Cognitive and intellectual functioning	Assess cognitive processing of trauma experience.	B, C, D
Interpersonal relations	Assess impact on interpersonal and social relations.	C
Work and industrial capacity	Assess changes in work disposition.	B, C, D
Self-concept and sense of ego identity	Assess changes in self-structure and identity.	C
Motivational states	Assess motives and goal striving.	C
Stress-related symptoms	Assess peritraumatic reactions (acute or persistent stress responses).	B, C, D
Preexisting psychopathology	Assess impact on preexisting Axis I or Axis II disorders.	I[c]
Psychobiological functioning	Assess psychobiological alterations (brain MRIs, PET scans, neurohormonal changes).	B, D

[a] Adapted from A criteria.
[b] B, C, and D are the primary DSM-IV PTSD symptom criteria categories likely to be manifested posttrauma for a specific area of psychosocial functioning.
[c] Preexisting psychopathology may be intensified.

military records, educational and employment records, medical and hospital records, etc.).

The Matrix Concept and Issues of Differential Diagnosis

The matrix concept of assessment is a procedure that can yield important information relevant to differential diagnosis. A review of the appropriate and relevant data sources can be applied within the framework of the matrix concept of assessing PTSD in medical–legal contexts. As Table 21.1 shows, there are at least 10 areas of assessment relevant to a determination of how a traumatic event might influence psychosocial functioning as rated by the Global Assessment of Functioning (GAF) scale in DSM-IV (American Psychiatric Association, 1994) or as observable changes in posttraumatic levels of adaptive behavior. In DSM-IV, the GAF scale "is for reporting the clinician's judgment of the individual's overall level of functioning" (American Psychiatric Association, 1994, p. 30) and ranges from 1 (extremely impaired) to 100 (superior functioning). On the other hand, observable changes in levels of adaptive behavior can be assessed from multiple sources of information, such as psychometric testing, job performance data, interviews with collaterals, specialized medical–psychiatric testing, or laboratory results. Using either the GAF scale or other methods, the matrix approach can assist in pinpointing the specific areas of psychosocial behavior that may have changed due to the trauma.

How does PTSD relate to the central issue in a forensic case? In terms of the matrix concept, discernible changes in psychosocial behavior of the person can be evaluated in the following areas: affective states, personality characteristics, cognitive and intellectual functioning, interpersonal and social relations, work and industrial capacity, self-concept and sense of ego identity, motivational states, stress-related symptoms, preexisting psychopathology, and baseline states of psychobiological functioning. In most, if not all, medical–legal contexts, the central most important issue with PTSD is how much of the behavior in question (e.g., level of injury or action in a criminal matter) is caused by trauma-induced PTSD and how much of the behavior in question is attributable to other factors. Stated differently, this is the issue of behavioral, statistical, and psychological variance: *How much of the total variance in a hypothetical or an actual "pie-chart" representation of the legal issues is caused by PTSD as a* trauma-related *"slice of the pie" and how much of the remaining segments of variance are from other sources of causation?*

Pre- and Posttraumatic Changes in Psychological Functioning

By utilizing the matrix concept of assessment, it is possible to ascertain three fundamental forensic issues relevant to the role of PTSD in litigation or legal matters: first, to determine changes in psychosocial functioning, personality dynamics, and adaptive behavior in proximity to the time of the trauma; second, to determine whether changes in psychological functioning can be attributed to the trauma, especially if PTSD is present; and third, to determine the relationship, if any, between PTSD and the forensic issues of consideration in a legal case.

In forensic evaluations in medical–legal contexts, there are many critical issues that lawyers and experts must weigh in their evaluation of a PTSD claim. Simon (1995) has suggested that there are at least five standard questions that are germane to the assessment of PTSD claims. These five criteria are consistent with the matrix concept of assessing psychosocial functioning before, during, and after a trauma and are as follows: (1) Does the alleged PTSD claim actually meet specific clinical criteria for this disorder? (2) Is the traumatic stressor that is alleged to have caused the PTSD of sufficient severity to produce this disorder? (3) What is the preincident psychiatric history of the claimant? (4) Is the diagnosis of PTSD based solely on the subjective reporting of symptoms by the claimant? (5) What is the claimant's actual level of functional psychiatric impairment? (See Simon, 1995, p. 33, for discussion.) These five factors should also be considered, along with questions of malingering and factitious PTSD, within the context of the matrix approach to differential diagnosis and psychological assessment.

THE FORENSIC/CLINICAL ASSESSMENT PROCEDURE: MULTIPLE CLIENT INTERVIEWS AND PSYCHOLOGICAL ASSESSMENTS

Assessing PTSD in its simple and complex forms requires a determination of how the person's psychological functioning has changed from its pretrauma baseline in the relevant areas of psychosocial adaptation and coping. A pre- and posttraumatic analysis of functioning is a minimal requirement for determining the nature and extent of emotional injuries. In essence, the critical question is, How has the person been changed by the experience? Although this is a central question in determining posttraumatic injuries, it must be recognized that there is a continuum of posttraumatic effects that range from minimal to catastrophic. In forensic settings, this question relates directly to issues of *scientific causation* of the traumatic damage and *legal liability* under rules of law. The forensic/clinical assessment process of PTSD requires several procedures and components.

Whenever possible, it is useful to conduct multiple interviews within a relatively short period of time (e.g., 1 month to 1 year). Multiple interviews are important in order to record a complete trauma and psychosocial history. Clinical and forensic wisdom has shown that the reporting of the trauma history (i.e., "trauma story") takes time and may not be fully disclosed or revealed in just one interview (Wilson, Friedman, & Lindy, 2001). The trauma story unfolds over time and changes in complexity, clarity, and detail as the emotions and memories of the traumatic event are reexperienced and tolerated by the individual (Wilson & Lindy, 1994). Because PTSD as a disorder involves symptoms of impaired concentration, memory, denial, dissociation, avoidance, and amnesia, there may be "gaps" or missing pieces of information in the client's account and recollection of the trauma experience. For these and other reasons, multiple interviews are recommended in order to explore carefully and in a way that can be tolerated by the client the various components of the trauma experience and how it was encoded and processed.

Multiple Interviewers, Assessments, and Methods

It is useful to have multiple interviews conducted by different examiners who work collaboratively on a case. Collateral interviews by an allied, rather than adversarial, examiner serve several functions that are important when addressing PTSD assessment in litigation.

First, these interviews verify information and facts reported by the client. Second, they help establish and confirm PTSD symptoms and/or other psychiatric symptoms or disorders. Third, they help acquire additional information, observations, and insights about the client's functioning. Fourth, they can verify and supplement the details of the trauma and psychosocial history. Fifth, they help to assess inconsistencies in the trauma story or personal history that might suggest malingering, lying, incorrect data, fabrication, faking, distortions, fantasy, or improbable actions.

Multiple interviews using multiple assessments and methods and conducted by collaborative professional examiners establish a process that "triangulates" forensic data. This multimethod process obtains information and identifies consistencies or inconsistencies in the trauma history that can be analyzed as part of the larger forensic "jigsaw puzzle" of how the relevant data fits together when addressing the forensic questions of relevance to litigation or other legal issues. The use of collaborative multiple interviews also reduces the risk of errors, biases, and omissions and aids in the discovery of inconsistencies in the self-presentation of the client.

Psychological Testing and the Clinical/Forensic Assessment of PTSD in Litigation Settings

Stressor Assessment

PTSD is a prolonged form of stress response to traumatic events. In forensic settings, it is the determination of the *link* between the traumatic event(s) and the subsequent onset of the symptoms or disorder that is relevant to legal issues. It is important to establish the cause of PTSD and its associated clinical features, such as depression, generalized anxiety, substance abuse, phobias, and so forth. What, exactly, is the connection between exposure to specific types of stressors in the traumatic event and the development of PTSD? Did these anxiety, depressive or PTSD symptoms exist before the trauma? Were they caused by a preexisting mental condition or other factors, such as an earlier traumatic experience?

As part of the forensic assessment process, the examiner should ascertain the nature and degree of exposure to specific stressors in the traumatic event. Several measures are available to assess the type and nature of exposure to such stressors. For example, the Life Events Checklist (LEC) from the National Center for PTSD (NC-PTSD) contains 17 categories of stressful life events that clients can endorse, indicating whether they have experienced any of them directly or indirectly and at what age. Similarly, the Impact of Event

Scale—R (see Weiss, Chapter 7, this volume) is a 22-item PTSD scale that asks the client to self-report traumatic experiences and PTSD symptoms directly relevant to the stated traumatic event.

It is also important to note that PTSD is not typically caused by a single dimension of a traumatic experience. Wilson and Lindy (1994) establish a taxonomy of traumatic events that includes 10 separate categories (e.g., childhood abuse, war trauma, technological disaster, duty-related events, etc.). They note that traumatic stressors involve direct or indirect experiences of exposure to harm or injury in five areas: (1) self; (2) others; (3) personal, affiliative attachments and relationships; (4) biosphere and physical structures; and (5) physical integrity, bodily functions, and health. Thus the forensic/clinical assessment of PTSD should attempt to assess as precisely as possible the nature, extent, and impact of specific stressors that would potentially cause PTSD or that, alternatively, have a very low probability of doing so. *The forensic process requires that the link between exposure to traumatic stressors and PTSD symptoms be established scientifically, and not solely on the examiner's opinion.*

Case Example: Exxon Valdez Oil Spill Litigation

One of us (JPW) served as an expert witness in the *Exxon Valdez* oil spill litigation, in which hundreds of claims for PTSD were being made due to exposure to the massive oil spill that leaked 13.5 million gallons of crude oil into the beautiful and pristine Prince William Sound, Alaska. The claims for PTSD by persons living in various geographical areas of Alaska, ranging from the port city of Valdez in Prince William Sound to the remote western island of Kodiak and those beyond toward Russia, were particularly interesting for several reasons.

First, did the oil spill from the tanker ship *Exxon Valdez* constitute a trauma? At what point does such a maritime transport disaster become traumatic? For example, in the Exxon Valdez case, not a single person was killed or injured due to the oil spill. Nor were any parts of constructed physical structures significantly damaged or destroyed. Second, the nature and magnitude of exposure to the oil spill varied in dispersion, from a massive oil slick near Bly Reef outside the town of Valdez to minimal oil splatters on beachfront land and islands hundreds of miles away. *Is such exposure scientifically sufficient to cause a psychiatric disorder* (e.g., PTSD)? Third, if there was no scientific, empirical evidence of a "dose–response" exposure relationship between oil scatters and seeing its effects on persons and the environment (e.g., dead birds, dirty beaches, etc.), how could PTSD be *causally* related to such an event? Fourth, although many litigation claimants from a wide range of geographical areas reported PTSD symptoms, careful analysis of their psychological test data and surveys revealed the presence of other traumatic experiences in their lives, such as domestic violence, childhood sexual abuse, exposure to violent alcoholic parents and spouses, exposure to teen suicide, and rapes. Did the oil spill cause PTSD or aggravate or reawaken preexisting conditions?

In a litigation case of the unprecedented magnitude of the *Exxon Valdez* case, how does the examiner rule out malingering or deliberate fabrication or exaggeration of symptoms when the defendant being sued is one of the wealthiest corporations in the world? *Thus it can be seen that assessment of specific stressor exposure in a particular traumatic event is important in establishing the causal link between the trauma experience and the development of PTSD symptoms.*

A review of the available records in the *Exxon Valdez* litigation showed that, in hundreds of cases analyzed, only a handful of litigants reported the *cardinal* reexperiencing PTSD symptoms of distressing, intrusive recollections of the oil spill (i.e., the alleged traumatic event); nightmares with *specific content* related to the tanker disaster; or increased psychological or physiological distress at exposure to cues (sights, environmental changes) of the oil spill. On the other hand, the freely reported symptoms of childhood abuse, exposure to alcoholic spouses or parents, and interpersonal family violence were prevalent by history. These facts clearly highlight the important issue in forensic settings of determining the "chicken and egg" problem of which causal factor came first. In tort litigation, this also applies to the "cracked eggshell" theory as to whether or not a client was premorbidly vulnerable, fragile, or had a preexisting mental disorder or other mental/medical condition that rendered him or her unusually susceptible to traumatic exposure. In PTSD-related research, it is known that there are persons with a higher risk probability for developing PTSD (Friedman, 2000; Weisaeth, 1994). These factors include gender, age, prior traumatization, childhood adversity, prior psychiatric history, family instability, and genetic variables. In formulating a forensic opinion, the totality of factors has to be sifted through and carefully weighed as to their relevance.

PSYCHOLOGICAL ASSESSMENT TECHNIQUES: STRUCTURED CLINICAL PROTOCOLS

The forensic/clinical assessment process typically involves the use of standardized psychometric procedures. In terms of understanding PTSD and personality processes, it is recommended that a variety of psychological questionnaires and protocols be employed as part of the assessment process. It is important to use standardized, reliable, and valid measures of PTSD and its associated features. This volume contains chapters that describe the features of such instruments as the Impact of Event Scale—Revised (IES-R); the Trauma Symptom Inventory (TSI); the Penn Inventory for PTSD; the MMPI-2 PTSD scales (PK and PS); the MCMI-III PTSD scale; the Mississippi Scale for PTSD; and many others (see Norris & Hamblen, Chapter 3, this volume, for a review).

It is also recommended that a structured clinical protocol for the assessment of PTSD be administered (see Weiss, Chapter 4, this volume, on structured clinical interview techniques). The CAPS, for example, was developed by the National Center for PTSD (NC-PTSD). The Clinician-Administered

PTSD Scale (CAPS; Blake et al., 1990a, 1990b) has different versions that assess current, lifetime, and childhood forms of PTSD. The user of the CAPS follows a systematic, standard protocol procedure in which all of the diagnostic symptoms for PTSD and its associated features are probed by questions designed to evoke responses that may be indicative of PTSD symptomatology. The CAPS is structured to measure the frequency, validity, and intensity of symptoms. The CAPS also has the advantage of allowing the examiner to follow up on probes and questions that might generate additional information or insights about the client's self-presentation. Among the advantages of using the CAPS are that: (1) it has established cutoff scores for a positive PTSD diagnosis; (2) it is a "standardized yardstick" that is used by all properly trained examiners in the same manner, thereby enhancing the accuracy and reliability of symptom assessment and eliminating or reducing interviewer bias; (3) it can be used to assess current and lifetime prevalence of symptoms for single or multiple traumatic events and the stressors associated with them; (4) it is available for use in determining the levels of social and occupational impairment produced by the symptoms of the disorder as an entity (i.e., the DSM-IV-TR [American Psychiatric Association, 2000] criterion F for PTSD); and (5) the CAPS findings can be correlated with data obtained from other psychometric procedures to support a diagnosis or illuminate potentially inconsistent or discrepant results from other psychological measures of PTSD or psychopathology.

Psychometric Assessment of Psychopathology and PTSD

The forensic/clinical examiner has a wide range of psychometric measures that can be employed to aid in the process of making a differential diagnosis. We recommend that the following instruments be administered as part of the overall procedure to assist in making an Axis I or Axis II clinical diagnosis.

Minnesota Multiphasic Personality Inventory–2

The Minnesota Multiphasic Personality Inventory–2 (MMPI-2) contains 567 true/false items that measure psychopathology, personality processes (e.g., depression, schizophrenia, anxiety states, type A personality, etc.), and PTSD (PK and PS subscales). The MMPI-2 has 10 clinical scales of psychopathology that assess major psychiatric symptom clusters. It also contains validity indices that measure faking, malingering, response consistency and inconsistency, defensiveness, and lying. These scales reflect the test taker's attitudes during the administration of the questionnaire and generate information relevant to understanding the client's mental state while completing the questionnaire (e.g., confusion, inattention, psychotic states, cries for help, and lack of language or reading skills.) Several reference books are available to aid clinicians and attorneys in interpreting the test results (e.g., Graham, 1993; Green, 1988; Butcher, Dahlstrom, Graham, Tellegen, & Raemmer, 1989).

Millon Clinical Multiaxial Inventory–III

The MCMI-III (Millon, 1997) is a 175-item true/false self-report questionnaire that is designed to assess DSM-IV Axis I and Axis II mental disorders (American Psychiatric Association, 1994). It also has a specific PTSD subscale (16 items), as well as indices on validity, reliability, defensiveness, and response inconsistencies (known respectively as scales V, X, Y, Z). The computer-scored questionnaire generates suggested Axis I and II diagnoses, as well as critical item analysis.

Symptom Checklist 90—Revised

The Symptom Checklist 90—Revised (SCL-90-R) is a self-report, 90-item measure of nine psychiatric symptom clusters. The instrument is scaled on the basis of frequency of symptoms reported across the 90 items. The computer-scored questionnaire generates "suggested" diagnoses and determines whether or not the symptoms qualify to be considered as "psychiatric caseness." The SCL-90-R has also been subject to construct validity, and a 28-item version for PTSD has been derived by Saunders, Arata, and Kilpatrick (1990). Unlike the MMPI-2 and MCMI-III, the instrument does not contain indices of malingering, defensiveness, faking, or lying. However, it does identify pathognomonic signs that are especially useful as they earmark specific symptoms that may require further probing and inquiry. Additionally, the pathognomonic signs can be cross-indexed and/or validated by data obtained from critical item analysis produced by the MMPI-2, MCMI-III, and the CAPS protocol. In this manner, then, the data from multiple sources of assessment can be triangulated scientifically to provide a clear picture of consistency in symptoms reported during the interview process.

Trauma Symptom Inventory

The Trauma Symptom Inventory (TSI) is a 100-item self-report questionnaire that assesses symptoms of PTSD and its associated clinical features (e.g., dissociation, impaired self-reference, sexual dysfunction, etc.). It contains three validity scales for atypical responses, defensiveness, and response inconsistencies among PTSD subscales. The computer-generated profile analysis presents a graphic summary of the test results and indicates various profile elevations that can be compared against standardized normative data on different trauma populations (Briere, 1995).

Impact of Event Scale—Revised

The Impact of Event Scale—Revised (IES-R) is a 22-item self-report questionnaire. It measures symptoms in three DSM-IV PTSD diagnostic categories (B, C, D) in response to a designated traumatic event. It is quickly administered and scored and has a high correlation with other measures of PTSD (see Weiss, Chapter 7, this volume, for a review).

COMPREHENSIVE DOCUMENT AND RECORD REVIEW

As part of the forensic/clinical process, it is important for the examiner to review documents pertinent to the case. If such documents are not provided by legal counsel, the expert examiner should request any documents that would provide information that will assist in formulating diagnoses and reaching a set of opinions that bear on the legal issues being considered in litigation or an arena of adjudication. A thorough and detailed analysis of documents is important for several reasons:

1. They are independently generated sources of data, facts, and information.
2. They may provide objective information about the nature and severity of the traumatic experiences.
3. They may assist in establishing a pretrauma baseline of adaptive functioning in terms of work, school, relationships, cognitive functioning, interpersonal relationships, and physical (medical) functioning.
4. They may document consistencies or inconsistencies in reported symptoms, levels of impairment, or objective criteria about activities of daily living.
5. They note important areas of change or disruptions in interpersonal, intimate, social, or love relationships.
6. They may indicate the use of alcohol or substances that may be associated with PTSD symptoms (see Najavits, Chapter 16, this volume).
7. They may shed light on the relationship of PTSD to bereavement, traumatic bereavement, and loss of significant others (see Raphael, Martinek, & Wooding, Chapter 17, this volume).

PROFESSIONAL EDUCATION, TRAINING, AND EXPERIENCE OF THE EXPERT EXAMINER

Professional Education and Background

The expert witness who is preparing an evaluative assessment or who will appear in court as an expert witness should have more than elementary knowledge of PTSD as a diagnosis that exists in DSM-IV or other publications. Professional training should include specific courses in PTSD, human stress response, psychopathology, crisis intervention, lifespan development, stress management, psychological assessment, psychiatric diagnosis, and so forth, as well as continuing education and legal courses on the many facets of PTSD.

Board Certification

The evaluator should have certification as an expert in PTSD from such organizations as the American Academy of Experts in Traumatic Stress, with subspecialty designation (e.g., forensic traumatology, crisis response, etc.); the American College of Forensic Examiners, with specialization in trauma, abuse and PTSD; or the American Psychological Association Board of Professional Psychologists (ABPP); or certification as a traumatic stress specialist (CTS) from the Association of Traumatic Stress Specialists.

Professional Organization Membership

The expert's background should reflect active membership in professional organizations primarily dedicated to PTSD, trauma studies, or dissociative phenomena, such as the International Society for Traumatic Stress Studies (ISTSS), International Society for Study of Dissociative Disorders (ISSD), the International Institute of Psychotraumatology (IIP), the American College of Forensic Examiners, and so forth.

Knowledge of Assessment Techniques

The examiner or expert should have knowledge of psychological assessment procedures developed during the past 25 years to specifically measure acute stress disorder, PTSD, dissociative states, and their associated features with scientifically validated instruments.

Knowledge of Treatment Modalities

The expert should have knowledge of effective scientific, medical, and psychological treatments for PTSD (see Wilson et al., 2001; Foa, Keane, & Friedman, 2000; for reviews), as well as professional experience in working directly with trauma clients who have experienced a wide range of traumatic stressors.

Knowledge of Peer-Reviewed Scientific Literature and Website Databases

It is critical for the expert to have knowledge and familiarity with peer-reviewed scientific literature in professional journals (e.g., *Journal of Traumatic Stress*; *Journal of Trauma and Dissociation*; *Journal of Trauma, Abuse and Violence*; *International Journal of Emergency Mental Health*; *American Journal of Psychiatry*; *Journal of Consulting and Clinical Psychology; National Center for Clinical PTSD Quarterly*; *National Center for PTSD Research Quarterly; Journal of Trauma Practice*; etc.). The expert should be familiar with website databases on scientific peer-reviewed articles and other information on trauma, PTSD, dissociative disorders, and so forth (e.g., *www.ncptsd.org*; *ncptsd.org/publications/pilots* database; Psychological Abstracts [*apa.org*]; National Clearinghouse on Child Abuse and Neglect Information [*http://nccanch.acf.hhs.gov/*]; etc.).

Forensic Rules of Evidence

The expert witness should have knowledge of forensic rules of evidence, the *Daubert* standard, courtroom proceedings, and direct and cross-examinations by attorneys and judges. Knowledge of the courtroom procedures and processes is useful to preparation and testimony under the stresses of litigation.

TESTIMONY OF THE EXPERT WITNESS

Admissibility of Testimony

The expert witness plays many roles in the process of litigation or in the adjudication of claims for PTSD. As an expert witness in the courtroom, the professional serves as an impartial, neutral witness with specialized experience and expertise in the area of trauma and PTSD. The opinions of the expert should be grounded in clinical/forensic/academic expertise that reflects knowledge of the field and of peer-reviewed scientific research and competence in the use of diagnostic testing. The role of the expert is to render information that will enable a jury, judge, or adjudicating official to form an accurate opinion or conclusion about the psychological functioning of the client. In this sense, the expert witness serves in a "teaching" role during the trial or adjudication process. Once credentialed and certified as an expert witness, the professional witness presents facts that are admissible as evidence relevant to the issues before those who try the facts, the court or the adjudicating officials who render decisions.

Rules of Evidence Pertaining to Expert Witness Testimony

The Frye Rule

For most of the 20th century, the admissibility of expert testimony was based on the *Frye* rule. The *Frye* rule was one of "general acceptance." The expert's opinion had to be based on information, data, or conclusions that were "generally accepted" by the majority of those in the expert's field of specialization.

The Federal Rules of Evidence

In 1973 the United States Federal Rules of Evidence began to address admissibility rules of evidence with specific applications to the bases, nature, and quality of evidence presented by expert witnesses. Technically, the pertinent U.S. federal rules are Rules 401, 402, 702, and 703. These federal rules lay out the definitions of relevant evidence and their limitations in court proceedings. Federal rules 702 and 703, for example, specified the bases of opinions that could be considered in determining the scope of expert testimony. Generally speaking, these rules allowed the expert to opine on information gathered other than "firsthand," in the tradition of general acceptance by peers in the profession. The Federal Rules of Evidence posed questions as to the sufficiency of the *Frye* statute and sought to create more precise guidelines by which expert testimony could be rendered.

The Daubert Standard

In 1993, the Supreme Court rejected the criteria of "general acceptance" in *Daubert v. Dow Pharmaceuticals Inc.* (*Daubert v. Merrell Dow Pharmaceuticals Inc.*, 113 S. Ct. 2786, 1993). The consequence of this ruling was to create a new litmus test for the admissibility of expert scientific testimony. The *Daubert* decision rejected the legal standard of the *Frye* rule and replaced it with one that emphasized the quality and adequacy of methodology and the theoretical soundness on which the expert's opinion was based. In brief, the *Daubert* standard emphasized the following points:

- Whether a theory or technique has been or could be tested scientifically.
- Whether the theory or technique has been subject to peer review and publication in scientific journals.
- The known or potential rates of error in the methodology.
- The "general acceptance" of the theory.

Relative to expert testimony in cases involving PTSD, the general guidelines for psychologists can be considered to have four interrelated dimensions: (1) testimony based *solely* or *primarily* on clinical experiences will likely be ruled inadmissible; (2) clinical psychologists who testify will be expected to refer to scientifically tested theories, methodology, and research in formulating opinions; (3) the discretion to differentiate between diagnostic and nondiagnostic syndromes (that is, the courts will rely on generally accepted scientific and medical criteria of psychological syndromes and officially classified disorders or mental processes); and (4) the court has the discretion to determine admissibility. The style, preparation, or presentation of the expert witness could enhance or interfere with the admissibility of the expert's opinions and testimony.

THE CLINICAL–FORENSIC REPORT AND FORMULATION OF ANSWERS TO THE ASSESSMENT QUESTIONS

The clinical–forensic report is used for different purposes in litigation that involves PTSD and traumatic injury. In earlier publications, Wilson (1989), Wilson and Zigelbaum (1986), and Keane (1995) reviewed some of the precedent cases in which PTSD was used as an insanity defense or as mitigation in criminal cases involving Vietnam veterans in the United States. Simon (2000) cites more recent cases in which PTSD was used in civil litigation. Whether a clinical–forensic report is prepared for civil or criminal litigation or for plaintiffs or defendants, it is the document that details the results of the forensic evaluation and constitutes one of the primary bases on which the expert witness will be deposed or cross-examined in a court of law. Unlike confidential clinical reports, forensic psychological reports have no limits of confidentiality and are typically distributed to the parties in a lawsuit, including opposing legal counsel, juries, the court, insurance companies, and opposing expert witnesses. Although most clients are aware of how the legal process works, it is important that they understand the limits of confidentiality and how the forensic report might be used in the litigation process. Traumatized clients, in particular, may not appreciate, recognize, or know what effects litigation may have on their PTSD symptoms.

As Table 21.2 summarizes, the forensic evaluation report for PTSD contains information about the data sources relied on in generating the report, as well as a description of the assessment process, psychosocial and trauma histories, results of psychometric testing, and specific measures of PTSD. The forensic report specifically addresses the issues pertaining to the litigation, including diagnostic conclusions reached using the DSM-IV multiaxial coding system. The forensic formulation of the case addresses the assessment question under evaluation and spells out the conclusions reached by the examiner.

MALINGERING AND FACTITIOUS PTSD

To malinger means:

- To fake being sick or having an illness/disorder
- Pretend illness, dissimilation
- Hide the truth, to play act
- Counterfeit, feigning
- False disposition, impostor
- Exaggerate sickness, shamming

The pervasiveness of personal injury lawsuits, claims for worker's compensation, pension claims, Social Security psychiatric disability claims, mental health disability pension claims, lawsuits alleging psychological damage, especially PTSD, from childhood sexual abuse that was repressed or unavailable to conscious awareness, as well as many other relevant applications in civil and criminal law, suggests that the issue of malingered PTSD must be considered in forensic evaluations. Resnick (1995); Wilson and Walker (1990); Sparr and Boehnlein (1990); Atkinson, Henderson, Sparr, and Deale (1982); Sparr and

TABLE 21.2. General Guidelines for Preparation of Clinical–Forensic Evaluation Report for PTSD Litigation

1. Purpose of forensic assessment
   a. Statement of questions to be addressed in the report
2. Referral source and legal considerations
3. Qualifications of the examiner
4. Data sources: Documents reviewed in preparation of the report
5. Identifying data
6. Persons interviewed: Claimant and collaterals
7. Assessment process: Description of methodology
   a. Clinical interview or structured clinical protocol
   b. Psychometric testing for PTSD
   c. Psychosocial history in comprehensive form (e.g., educational history, medical history, family background, substance use history, etc.)
8. Specialized test results
9. Trauma history and details of stressors experienced
10. Report of posttraumatic sequelae and impact on psychosocial functioning
11. Diagnostic considerations
    a. Definition of DSM-IV diagnostic axes
    b. Diagnostic impressions/formulation
    c. DSM-IV multiaxial assessment (Axes I–V)
12. Forensic formulation and answers to assessment questions
13. Prognosis and recommendations

Note. Adapted from Wilson (1989) and Keane (1995).

Atkinson (1986); and Lynn and Belza (1984), among others, have written on the nature of malingered PTSD, especially among Vietnam War veterans seeking service-connected benefits. However, the issue of malingering in PTSD cases extends well beyond the scope of military veteran populations. Hypothetically, virtually any claim for personal injury could involve malingering because of the potential benefits to the claimant. Moreover, because the diagnostic criteria for PTSD are readily available in the public domain and relatively easy to understand as a syndrome, the potential for faking must be understood to exist.

In DSM-IV (American Psychiatric Association, 1994), malingering is defined as "the intentional production of false or grossly exaggerated physical or psychological symptoms, motivated by external incentives such as avoiding military duty, avoiding work, obtaining financial compensation, evading criminal prosecution, or obtaining drugs" (p. 683). DSM-IV lists four criteria that clinicians should consider in regards to diagnosing malingering: "(1) medical–legal context of presentation; (2) marked discrepancy between the person's claimed stress or disability and the objective findings; (3) lack of cooperation during the diagnostic evaluation and in complying with the prescribed treatment regimen; (4) the presence of antisocial personality disorder" (p. 683).

Resnick (1995) presents a threshold model of malingering PTSD that includes the presence of two or more of eight potential indicators: poor work record; prior "incapacitating" injuries; discrepant capacity for work and recreation; unvarying, repetitive dreams; antisocial personality traits; overidealized functioning before the trauma; evasiveness; and inconsistency in symptom presentation. At the core of these factors appear to be three distinct processes that include inconsistencies in behavioral and self-presentation, deliberate falsification and/or aggrandized positive self-concept manifestation, and a history of irresponsible, hostile, reckless, and self-serving behavior that includes manipulation of others for personal gain. In this regard, Resnick's (1995) threshold model appears to be similar to the validity scales of the MMPI-2, which assess response inconsistency (e.g., scales TRIN, VRIN), faking "bad" or "good" (scales F, Fb), defensiveness (scale K), incompleteness (? cannot say) and other psychometric indices of malingering and dissimulation (Graham, 1993). Thus, through clinical interview, psychometric assessment, and Resnick's (1995) threshold checklist, the examiner may be able to differentiate malingered from genuine cases of PTSD.

In DSM-IV, factitious disorders are considered as a somewhat similar diagnostic entity to malingering, with the primary difference being that the person assumes a role of being psychologically disordered in the absence of external incentives. In factitious PTSD, the person intentionally produces the characteristic symptoms of the syndrome (e.g., reports of flashbacks, nightmares of the trauma, hyperarousal, psychic numbing, accounts of trauma stories, etc.) but has not experienced life events that would establish a valid diagnosis of the anxiety disorder. The next section summarizes studies of malingering and factitious PTSD.

Malingered PTSD is not a new phenomenon, despite the relative youth of PTSD as a distinct psychiatric disorder (DSM-III, American Psychiatric Association, 1980). In his review of the history of traumatic neuroses, Trimble (1981) notes that the assessment and determination of legitimate psychological trauma extends far back in history and was of special concern during the Industrial Revolution in England. After industrial accidents and other traumatic events, such as railroad collisions, individuals often complained of experiencing a wide range of psychological symptoms, including those that would today be considered posttraumatic stress symptoms. Moreover, during the industrialization of Western countries, workers injured on the job sought compensation for physical and psychological distress. Thus the medical examiners of the era faced the task of ascertaining whether or not the emotional distress was valid or being malingered for purpose of financial gain or other external incentives.

Similar considerations also arose in the context of war trauma. After the Civil War in the United States, soldiers complained of a condition that came to be known as "soldier's heart," in which PTSD and depressive symptoms were evident (Friedman, 2000). In World War I the existence of "shell shock" was widely recognized by the medical personnel attached to military units. After the cessation of hostilities, many former soldiers continued to manifest psychological distress. However, the etiology of shell shock was debated. Soldiers in the field of battle who were acutely traumatized were sometimes thought to be "cowards" who malingered to avoid duty or, alternatively, were considered to have suffered minor cerebral injury due to the concussive impact of exploding shells near trenches and battle lines (Trimble, 1981). When shell-shock symptoms persisted after the war, the issue of compensation neurosis arose, and it was generally assumed by the medical–psychiatric community that symptoms should abate upon cessation of the war stressors (Wilson, 1994b). Hence, the issue of malingering or faking illness once again was an area of controversy. Since World War II, in a variety of assessment contexts—including determining service-connected disability for Vietnam War veterans in the United States and Australia and, more recently, in Croatia following the dissolution of the former Yugoslavia[1] in 1995—the question of validly determining cases of genuine PTSD from malingered or pseudo-PTSD cases for combat veterans remains an important consideration in medical–legal contexts (Scurfield & Wilson, 2003).

Although many authors have written on the relevance of diagnosing malingering, Resnick (1995) suggests that it is a multidimensional construct and that there are different forms of expression in behavior. Pure malingering is the feigning of disease when it does not exist at all. Partial malingering is the conscious expression of existing symptoms or the fraudulent allegation that prior genuine symptoms are still present. In addition, the term "false imputation" refers to ascribing actual symptoms to a cause consciously recognized as having no relationship to the symptoms. For example, authentic psychiatric symptoms due to clearly defined stresses at home may be falsely attributed to a traumatic event at work in order to gain compensation.

Empirical Research on Malingered PTSD

Approaches to the study of malingered PTSD have been divergent. These include psychometric assessments to discern genuine from fake PTSD; studies of pseudo-PTSD claims in personal injury cases; clinical case study analysis of factitious PTSD; detection of differences on psychometric questionnaires for positively diagnosed PTSD cases versus control participants without the disorder; and checklist approaches that identified behavior patterns highly indicative of malingering.

Based on a review of the studies presented in Table 21.3, several overall conclusions may be reached:

---

[1]More than 50,000 Australian military personnel served as allied forces to the U.S. during the Vietnam War (1962–1975). More than 150,000 military personnel fought in Croatia against Bosnian and Serbian forces between 1991 and 1995.

TABLE 21.3. Studies of Malingering

Author (year)	Forensic content area	Description of study	Synopsis of findings
Resnick (1995)	Malingering	Evaluation criteria for malingered PTSD.	Guidelines for evaluating the threshold model for diagnosing malingered PTSD; special emphasis on Vietnam veterans.
Frueh & Kinder (1994)	Malingering in Vietnam veterans	Study of 40 male undergraduates and 20 Vietnam veterans.	Differences were obtained between groups on MMPI-2 and Rorschach tests. Students were more dramatic and less constricted than veterans.
Lacoursiere (1993)	Factitious PTSD	Motives for presenting with fictitious PTSD in Vietnam veterans.	Clinical discussion of the psychodynamics of fictitious PTSD. Motives and goals vary.
Perr (1992)	PTSD and asbestos exposure	Presents 9 case studies of pulmonary pathology and PTSD as basis of litigation.	Challenges validity of PTSD diagnosis in asbestos exposure litigation.
Binder (1990)	Malingering neuropsychology	Describes evaluation of potential malingering in neuropsychological assessment.	Emphasizes cases in which potential financial gain are present; i.e., worker's compensation and personal injury.
Jordan, Nunley, & Cook (1992)	Malingering	Compared service-related PTSD in Vietnam veterans to matched controls not receiving pension.	MMPI F-scales were highly elevated in both groups. No F-scale differentiation was found between groups.
Lees-Haley (1992)	Spurious PTSD claims	Study of 119 personal-injury claimants vs. 65 pseudo-PTSD participants and 64 control participants.	MMPI-2 and MCMI-II administration yielded differences on validity and other scales.
Lees-Haley (1992)	Malingering	MMPI-2 study of ego strength in 26 personal-injury malingerers vs. 21 nonmalingerers.	*T*-score > 30 correctly classified 88% of malingerers.
Lees-Haley (1992)	Malingering	Study of malingering using MMPI-2 F-scale and combined F-K scales for personal-injury malingerers vs. nonmalingerers.	Results show MMPI-2 instrumental capacity to differentiate between groups using alternative validity scales utilized in this experiment.

(continued)

TABLE 21.3. *(continued)*

Author (year)	Forensic content area	Description of study	Synopsis of findings
Lees-Haley (1992)	Malingering	MMPI-2 study of malingering for participants simulating motor vehicle accident, industrial stress, and toxic exposure vs. personal-injury plaintiffs.	Cutoff scores correctly differentiated between malingerers and nonmalingerers.
Westin & Daldy (1991)	Factitious PTSD	Case study of factitious Vietnam veteran.	Patient suffered from personality disorder but had history of childhood trauma.
Lees-Haley (1990)	Malingering	52 college students fake toxic exposure and complete an Impact of Event Scale.	Scores on IES were similar to valid PTSD among students faking psychopathology.
Perconte & Goreczny (1990)	Fabricated PTSD symptoms	Replication of Fairbank & Keane's study with 39 Vietnam veterans and controls.	Failed to duplicate results of earlier study. Correctly identified 43.59% of participants.
Salloway, Southwick, & Sadowsky (1990)	Malingering PTSD	Case study of masking opiate withdrawal by false PTSD presentation.	Opiate withdrawal may parallel some PTSD symptoms.
Lees-Haley (1989a)	Malingering PTSD	College students fake toxic exposure and complete SCL-90-R.	Participants fake psychopathology in range comparable to psychiatric patients.
Lees-Haley (1989b)	Malingering PTSD	Study of participants simulating an accident, then taking the MMPI.	Using Keane's cutoff scores, 52% of participants were misclassified with PTSD.
Levit (1989c)	Malingering worker's compensation PTSD	Review of PTSD assessment procedures.	Recommends reliance on psychometric testing for PTSD assessment.
Yudofsky (1989)	Malingering	*Handbook of Psychiatry* article.	Overview of malingering in medicine and psychiatry; discusses clinical features of malingering; lists index of suspicion and detection; and cross-references other psychiatric symptoms.

(continued)

TABLE 21.3. *(continued)*

Author (year)	Forensic content area	Description of study	Synopsis of findings
Green (1988)	Malingering	Reviews the detection of malingering with the MMPI, CPI, M-test and 18 PF.	Table summary of item endorsement with cutting scores for MMPI.
Hyer et al. (1988)	Malingering	Review of compensation neurosis and PTSD.	Review discussion of secondary gain in a wide range of psychiatric disorders.
Resnick (1988)	Malingering	Detailed psychiatric discussion of malingered PTSD.	Clinical presentation of criteria for detection of malingered PTSD. Review of terms for PTSD.
Ashlock, Walker, Starkey, Harmand, & Michel (1987)	Factitious PTSD	MMPI study of factitious Vietnam veterans.	Factitious self-report scores were higher on MMPI-F, MF, SC, and health concerns.
Hyer, Fallon, Harrison, & Boudewyns (1987)	MMPI Overreporting	Examined PTSD profiles in Vietnam veteran populations.	PTSD veterans tended to overreport on MMPI. Caution in use of MMPI for PTSD advised.
Lees-Haley (1986)	Malingering pseudo-PTSD	Examined factors that may influence the diagnosis of PTSD in litigation.	Pharmacological side effects and other factors may mimic certain PTSD symptoms.
Lees-Haley (1986)	Malingering	Detection of malingering in the workplace.	Reviews procedures that could help employers detect malingering on psychological tests.
Fairbank, McCaffrey, & Keane (1985)	Fabricated PTSD symptoms	Study comparing MMPI scores for PTSD-diagnosed Vietnam veterans, non-PTSD veterans, and mental health professionals.	Bona fide PTSD veterans scored higher on the F-scale and PTSD subscale than did control group. Predictor variables correctly classified over 90% of participants.
Hamilton (1985)	Malingering pseudo-PTSD	Case history and analysis of malingered, factitious, and pseudo-PTSD in three Vietnam veterans.	Recommends verification of service records and other objective sources. Cautions against taking story at face value.

(continued)

TABLE 21.3. *(continued)*

Author (year)	Forensic content area	Description of study	Synopsis of findings
Sparr & Atkinson (1986)	PTSD forensic content	Reviews cases of Vietnam veterans in criminal matters that faked PTSD.	Discusses the complexity of PTSD as an insanity defense.
Lynn & Belza (1984)	Factitious PTSD	7 case reports of factitious PTSD in Vietnam veterans.	Suggests factitious PTSD is more prevalent than expected. Recommends careful verification of trauma history.
Resnick (1984)	Malingering	Detection of malingering in psychosis and PTSD.	Reviews concept of malingering and clinical detection methods. Presents clues to detect malingered psychosis and PTSD. Citation of empirical research.
Rogers (1984)	Malingering empirical models	Reviews 5 years of studies on dissimulation. Reviews MMPI and deception.	Summarizes research literature into an empirical model of possible predictions.
Ziskin (1984)	Malingering	Overview of research on malingering.	Discusses forensic concerns in detection of malingering. Reviews MMPI F-K scales on malingering.
Sparr & Pankratz (1983)	Factitious PTSD	Case histories of factitious PTSD in Vietnam veterans.	Discusses simulation of PTSD and DSM-III criteria.
Atkinson, Henderson, Sparr, & Deale (1982)	PTSD VA claims malingering	Illustrates pitfalls in PTSD diagnosis.	Lists 12 key points to evaluate in making a legitimate diagnosis of PTSD.
Braveman (1978)	Malingering	Reviews studies on malingering.	Identifies various types of malingering. Psychodynamic orientation to subject matter. Discusses psychotraumatic injury in industrial-injury cases.
Lipman (1962)	Malingering Personal injury Litigation	Examines malingering in PI cases by frequency, motivation, causation, detection, differential diagnosis, and courtroom-related issues.	Review of various types of malingering. Discussion of legal aspects of malingering in litigation. Cites posttraumatic overevaluation in personal-injury cases.

1. The various psychometric studies yield equivocal results as to their specificity in detecting genuine from exaggerated or faked PTSD. For example, Fairbank, McCaffrey, and Keane (1985) were able to correctly identify over 90% of Vietnam veterans with PTSD from a control group. However, in a replication study, Hyer, Fallon, Harrison, and Boudewyns (1987) failed to achieve similar results, as did Perconte and Goreczny (1990). On the other hand, Frueh and Kinder (1994) were able to differentiate successfully PTSD positive symptoms that were not present in college control participants without PTSD, as would be expected. Jordan, Nunley, and Cook (1992) found no differences on the MMPI F-scale for Vietnam veterans with PTSD who either had a pension or did not receive one from the Veterans Administration. Thus the variation in results may reflect differences in sample characteristics, methodology, or research setting. Green (1988) found that, using a multimethod testing procedure, it was possible to establish cutting scores that identify parameters of true malingering.

2. In a series of studies between 1989 and 1992, Lees-Haley (1989a, 1989b, 1989c, 1990, 1992) has employed psychometric assessment to see whether commonly used PTSD measures (e.g., MMPI-2; SCL-90; IES, etc.) could be faked by instructing students to assume a test-taking attitude of having had a traumatic experience of varying types. In general, the results indicate that, when prompted by the induction of an *attitude set* (i.e., imagining one has had the traumatic experience), the students *sometimes* generated test results similar to those for known trauma victims with PTSD. However, in a less contrived study, Lees-Haley (1992) found significant differences in a study of 119 actual personal injury claimants versus controls using the MMPI-2 and the MCMI-III questionnaires. This finding seems congruent with Green's (1988) suggestion that psychometric discrimination is quite possible but that further studies are needed.

3. The studies on factitious PTSD are much clearer in their outcome than some of the psychometric experiments.

The "Red Flag": Critical Indices of Malingering PTSD

Forensic and clinical examiners have attempted to establish a core set of critical indicators or "red flags," for malingered PTSD (see Resnick, 1995; Rogers, 1997; Gorman, 1982; Wilson, 2000). In an overly simplified way, we can distinguish between malingering and genuine PTSD.

What Is Malingering?

Malingering is *not* a mental disorder. Malingering *is* the "intentional production of false or grossly exaggerated incentives" (American Psychiatric Association, 1994, p. 683). Malingering *is* faking illness when it does not exist. Malingering may be the conscious exaggeration of existing symptoms. Malingering invariably involves *inconsistencies* between reported symptoms, actual behaviors, and the report of the nature of stressors in the trauma experience.

What Are the Critical Clues to Malingering?

There are many clues to malingered PTSD, which could make up a long list. The 10 critical indices that we have developed follow.

- Noncooperation with psychological and medical assessment requests and procedures (e.g., psychological testing, medical evaluations, etc.).
- Evasiveness, vagueness and inability to produce details about the trauma.
- Incorrect details of the stressors or providing improbable or implausible information about the trauma experience.
- Manifestation of behaviors inconsistent with known scientific/medical/clinical patterns of PTSD.
- A general tendency to focus blame for all problems on symptoms of the trauma.
- Falsification or alteration of documents, certificates, reports, or other forms of "evidence" (e.g., DD214 military discharge papers).
- An overemphasis on PTSD-related "flashback" experiences relative to other PTSD symptom clusters.
- Psychometric testing shows a pattern of inconsistency, defensiveness, malingering (faking, bad or good), or lying but *does not* indicate probable PTSD (e.g., low scores on measures of PTSD on MMPI, TSI, IES-R, etc.).
- A history of antisocial personality or behaviors or previous claims for compensation or lawsuits (i.e., litigation proneness) that preceded the traumatic event.

Studies of Factitious PTSD

The following characterize factitious PTSD (trauma-like (traumatoid) psychiatric states):

- Artificially created, mythological
- False colors, simulated
- Illusory, make-believe
- Imagined, ungrounded

The review of the available data on factitious PTSD uses a different methodology from the psychometric approaches. To discern factitious PTSD, clinicians carefully review records regarding the patient's life history and claims of suffering from PTSD. Detailed analysis of the pertinent documents typically reveal major discrepancies between the patient's account of his or her trauma story and the actual records. Further, among the intriguing aspects of factitious PTSD (i.e., what could be termed "traumatoid states"), especially among Vietnam-era veterans, is that their clinical presentations are often quite convincing to mental health professionals in terms of the details of their traumatic events, affective demeanor, and purported patterns of adjustment and psychosocial functioning. For this reason, many investigators have suggested procedures to avoid a misdiagnosis of PTSD (e.g., Hamilton, 1985; Atkinson et al., 1982; Sparr & Pankratz, 1983; Westin & Daldy, 1991; Lynn & Belza, 1984; Lacoursiere, 1993).

Among the central issues of importance is to obtain *objective* evidence that the claimant was exposed to a traumatic event that would cause PTSD and that documents verify the potential psychological impact to the person. Perr (1992), for example, challenges the validity of the diagnosis of PTSD in cases in which personal injury claims were filed for asbestos exposure, because it was difficult to discern whether mere exposure alone met the prime criterion for the diagnosis of PTSD. Although Perr does not minimize the aspects of pulmonary pathology, the issue of posttraumatic psychological symptomatology associated with knowledge of the disease was challenged. Clearly, similar arguments could be applied to other traumatized persons or populations.

The issue of factitious PTSD is perhaps more interesting from a psychodynamic point of view than from a purely forensic science analysis. The central question for the practitioner is to understand why the patient assumes the role of being a traumatized individual. Lacoursiere (1993) notes that the motives and goals of assuming a factitious PTSD role vary widely, and, indeed, some individuals who show factitious presentations—for example, of being a combat veteran of the Vietnam War—have had a prior history of victimization. And, unlike malingering, in which there are clearly discernible external incentives, factitious PTSD is an enigma because the person often seems to relish portraying him- or herself as suffering from the stress disorder. As noted by Hyler, Reider, Spitzer, and Williams (1982), secondary gain is always an important consideration in such cases. On the other hand, the question could be studied as to whether factitious PTSD is a façade for trauma from a life event that is *hidden beneath the image of self-deception*. Stated differently, does a posture of trauma, in reality, mask trauma that may be obscure, hidden, and dormant in expression?

Psychometric Indications of Malingered (Faked) PTSD

Table 21.4 presents a capsule summary of some commonly used psychometric indices of malingered PTSD on the MMPI-2, MCMI-III, TSI, IES-R, and Rorschach questionnaires. The MMPI contains at least 10 validity scales, which assist in detecting malingered PTSD. For example, on the MMPI-2, inconsistency in responding to test items (scales F, Fb); failure to answer more than 30 items out of 567; inconsistency in answering paired items (scales VRIN, TRIN); low scores on the PTSD subscales (PK, PS); and the absence of critical

TABLE 21.4. Common Psychometric Indications of Malingered PTSD

Instrument	Scales	Malingering indications
MMPI-2		
Infrequency	F	$T > 100$
Lie	L	$T > 65$
Variable Response Inconsistency	VRIN	$T > 80$
True Response Inconsistency	TRIN	$T > 80$
Posttraumatic Stress Disorder (Keene)	PK	$T < 65$
Posttraumatic Stress Disorder (Schlenger)	PS	$T < 65$
Critical Item Analysis	Critical Item	Absence of PTSD symptoms
Cannot Say (No Answer)	?	30 items or more unanswered
Infrequency Back Part	Fb	$T > 100$
Defensiveness	K	$T > 71$ or $T < 40$
MCMI-III		
Validity	V	One or more items
Disclosure	X	BR < 34 or BR > 178
Desirability	Y	BR > 75
Debasement	Z	BR > 75
PTSD	R	BR < 75
Trauma Symptom Inventory		
Inconsistent Response	INC	$T > 75$
Response Level	RL	$T > 75$
Atypical Response	ATR	$T > 90$
PTSD Scale (A_1)		$T < 65$
Impact of Event Scale—Revised		
Intrusion Subscale (I)		All responses extreme or minimal
Avoidance Subscale (Av)		
Hyperarousal Subscale (Hyper)		
Rorschach Inkblot		Excessive P (popular) responses; minimal total responses; many deliberate unusual responses

test items that correspond to PTSD diagnostic symptom criteria would constitute a basis for suspecting malingering. Similarly, on the Trauma Symptom Inventory (TSI), high levels of response inconsistency (scale INC); high "no" response level (scale RL; i.e., answering "zero" or no symptoms reported), and atypical responses (scale ATR) inconsistent with PTSD are suggestive of malingering. On the MCMI-III, malingering should be considered when the validity index (scale V) is high on one or more of three highly improbable events or situations (i.e., "I flew across the Atlantic 30 times last year; I have not seen a car in the last 10 years") and the indices of defensiveness and the motive to appear socially desirable are elevated. On the Rorschach Inkblot Test, malingering should be suspected when there are very few total responses, a large number of P (popular) responses, or many deliberate unusual responses.

LITIGATION AND SYMPTOM SEVERITY

The course of litigation itself must be taken into consideration when conducting a forensic evaluation for PTSD. Individuals suffering from PTSD find relatively little reduction of symptoms during the course of litigation. It is likely that PTSD symptoms will increase until the litigation ends, for reasons that include: (1) reliving the trauma by having to retell the story and history of trauma-related events, (2) psychiatric/psychological examination by experts, (3) stressful depositions, (4) the need for the client to review documents regarding traumatic injury, and (5) the prospect or actual requirement of testifying in court before a judge and jury. These factors have a strong potential to reactivate and amplify current thoughts and emotions about the traumatic experiences. Simon (1995) notes that, although there is no substantial evidence that litigation causes PTSD or PTSD symptoms, cases of pseudo-PTSD and factitious PTSD do exist (Lynn & Belza, 1984). Further, empirical studies of disaster and the litigation process show that after court settlements, PTSD symptoms diminish in severity but do not necessarily resolve completely (Gleser, Green, & Winget, 1981; Green et al., 1993). For example, in a follow-up study of the 1974 Buffalo Creek Dam Disaster in Logan County, West Virginia, a $13.5 million settlement was reached for the plaintiffs. Gleser et al. (1981) observed a postsettlement rebound effect to PTSD symptoms and that "one-third continue to suffer symptoms as severe as when seen initially" (p. 136).

Whether the rebound phenomenon of PTSD symptoms occurs in all litigation with PTSD is a matter for further study. However, what is patently clear is that the psychological task of resolving and integrating PTSD begins when the stress of litigation ends.

LEXIS AND WESTLAW: NOT JUST FOR LAWYERS, BARRISTERS, AND SOLICITORS

The interaction between the psychological sciences and the law has been the subject of debate and controversy for a long time (Trimble, 1981). As the complexities of the psychological sciences have grown, the knowledge available in the scientific literature, especially in the area of traumatic stress syndromes, has increasing relevance and application to legal issues. As noted in the beginning of this chapter, the four principal areas in which PTSD and the law meet in common ground are: (1) in criminal litigation (e.g., insanity defense); (2) civil litigation (e.g., personal injury); (3) disability claims (e.g., duty-related pension compensations); and (4) in courts of common pleas (e.g., claims of domestic violence, sexual harassment, etc.).

It was one of the goals of this chapter to attempt to develop an organizational framework that examines the relation of PTSD to forensic issues. As part of this process, our research has uncovered more information in the databases (e.g., Medline, PsycINFO, PILOTS, Lexis, Westlaw, etc.) than could be reviewed or incorporated in this chapter. However, given the importance of these data to those concerned with trauma and the law in forensic settings throughout the world and of Internet resources, it would be beneficial to the field of traumatic stress studies to have a larger database systematically organized and catalogued so that the information could be used for research, as well as litigation purposes.

CONCLUSION

Traumatic events have the potential to inflict psychological injury in the form of PTSD, as well as other psychiatric conditions. Since the classification of PTSD as a distinct psychiatric disorder in DSM-III (American Psychiatric Association, 1980), the sheer number of published articles has grown quite rapidly.[2] As the database has expanded, so has the application of findings in many areas, including medical–legal contexts. As indicated in this chapter, the research studying the link between PTSD and legal issues has many different connections in the areas of criminal law, disability claims, worker's compensation, personal injury (tort law), and other areas.

The future will see not only more applications of the diagnosis of PTSD to medical–legal settings but also a much greater degree of sophistication and accuracy in diagnosis, assessment, and treatment. As the field advances, we will have a greater ability to apply the concept of PTSD within forensic settings. Clearly, victims of trauma deserve special attention and, when appropriate, financial compensation and just settlements.

In the area of justice, the effects of trauma and PTSD will be evaluated in terms of human compassion and a recognition of the conditions that led to victimization in the first place. However, a legal ruling, no matter how salutary, cannot alter the scars of trauma to the human psyche. Just and equitable outcomes serve to validate the pain and suffering of the trauma survivor. Healing from traumatic injury is a psychological task that transcends the meaning of a financial settlement or beneficial court rulings. The victims of trauma ultimately must search for meaning on their own and, as individuals, place the tragedy of the trauma into their life stories. In that regard, justice through the courts becomes elusive and ephemeral. The search for ultimate justice is that of the human search for meaning of trauma in the individual's life.

---

[2]The National Center for PTSD in White River Junction, Vermont, maintains the PILOTS database, with more than 22,000 published articles as of April 2003.

REFERENCES

American Psychiatric Association. (1980). *Diagnostic and statistical manual of mental disorders* (3rd ed.). Washington, DC: Author.

American Psychiatric Association. (1994). *Diagnostic and statistical manual of mental disorders* (4th ed.). Washington, DC: Author.

American Psychiatric Association. (2000). *Diagnostic and statistical manual of mental disorders* (text rev.). Washington, DC: Author.

Apostle, D. T. (1980). The unconscious defense as applied to posttraumatic stress disorder in a Vietnam veteran. *Bulletin of the American Academy of Psychiatry and the Law*, *8*, 426–430.

Applebaum, P. S., Jick, R. Z., Grisso, T., Givelber, D., Silver, E., & Steadman, H. J. (1993). Use of posttraumatic stress disorder to support an insanity defense. *American Journal of Psychiatry*, *150*, 229–234.

Ashlock, L. E., Walker, J., Starkey, T. W., Harmand, J., & Michel, D. (1987). Psychometric characteristics of factitious PTSD. *VA Practitioner*, *4*(2), 37–41.

Atkinson, R. M., Henderson, R. G., Sparr, L. F., & Deale, S. (1982). Assessment of Vietnam veterans for PTSD in VA disability claims. *American Journal of Psychiatry*, *139*, 1118–1121.

Binder, M. (1990). Malingering following mild head trauma. *Clinical Neuropsychology*, *4*, 25–46.

Blake, D. D., Weathers, F. W., Nagy, N., Kaloupek, D. G., Klauminzer, G., Charney, D. S., & Keane, T. M. (1990a). A clinician rating scale for assessing current and lifetime PTSD: The CAPS-1. *Behavior Therapist*, *18*, 187–188.

Blake, D., Weathers, F., Nagy, L., Kaloupek, D., Klauminzer, G., Charney, D., & Keane, T. M. (1990b). *Clinician-Administered PTSD Scale*. Boston, MA: National Center for PTSD, Behavioral Sciences Division; West Haven, CT: Neurosciences Division.

Braverman, M. (1978). Post injury malingering is a seldom calculated ploy. *Occupational Health and Safety*, *47*, 36–48.

Briere, J. (1995). *Trauma Symptom Inventory*. Odessa, FL: Psychological Assessment Resources.

Butcher, J. N., Dahlstrom, W. G., Graham, J. R., Tellegen, A., & Raemmer, B. (1989). *Minnesota Multiphasic Personality Inventory—2 (MMPI-2): Manual for administration and scoring*. Minneapolis: University of Minnesota Press.

Fairbank, J. A., McCaffrey, R. J., & Keane, T. M. (1985). Psychometric detection of fabricated symptoms of posttraumatic stress disorder. *American Journal of Psychiatry*, *142*(4), 501–503.

Foa, E., Keane, T. M., & Friedman, M. J. (2000). *Effective treatments for PTSD*. New York: Guilford Press.

Friedman, M. J. (2000). *Posttraumatic stress disorder: The latest assessment and treatment strategies*. Kansas City: Compact Clinicals.

Frueh, B. C., & Kinder, B. N. (1994). The susceptibility of the Rorschach Inkblot Test to malingering of combat-related PTSD. *Journal of Personality Assessment*, *62*(2), 280–298.

Gleser, G. C., Green, B. L., & Winget, C. N. (1981). *Prolonged psychosocial effects of disaster: A study of Buffalo Creek*. New York: Academic Press.

Gorman, W. F. (1982). Defining malingering. *Journal of Forensic Sciences*, *27*(2), 401–407.

Graham, J. R. (1993). *MMPI-2: Assessing personality and psychopathology*. New York: Oxford University Press.

Green, B. L., Grace, M. C., Vary, M. G., Kramer, T. L., Gleser, G. C., & Leonard, A. C. (1993). Children of disaster in the second decade: A 17-year follow-up of Buffalo Creek survivors. *Journal of the American Academy of Child and Adolescent Psychiatry*, *33*, 71–79.

Green, R. (1988). *The MMPI*. Boston: Allyn & Bacon.

Hamilton, J. D. (1985). Pseudo-posttraumatic stress disorder. *Military Medicine*, *150*(7), 353–356.

Hyer, L. A., Boudewyns, P. A., Harrison, W. R., O'Leary, W. C., Bruno, R. D., Saucer, R. T., & Blount, J. B. (1988). Vietnam veterans: Overreporting versus acceptable reporting of symptoms. *Journal of Personality Assessment*, *52*(3), 475–486.

Hyer, L. A., Fallon, J. H., Harrison, W. R., & Boudewyns, P. A. (1987). MMPI overreporting by Vietnam combat veterans. *Journal of Clinical Psychology*, *43*(1), 79–83.

Hyler, S., Rieder, R., Spitzer, R., & Williams, J. (1982). *The Personality Diagnostic Questionnaire (PDQ)*. New York: New York State Psychiatric Institute.

Jordan, R. G., Nunley, T. V., & Cook, R. R. (1992). Symptom exaggeration in a PTSD inpatient population: Response set of claim for compensation. *Journal of Traumatic Stress*, *5*(4), 633–642.

Keane, T. M. (1995). Guidelines for the forensic psychological assessment of PTSD claimants. In R. I. Simon (Ed.), *PTSD in litigation* (pp. 99–117). Washington, DC: American Psychiatric Press.

Lacoursiere, R. B. (1993). Diverse motives for fictitious post-traumatic stress disorder. *Journal of Traumatic Stress*, *6*(1), 141–149.

Lees-Haley, P. R. (1986). Pseudo-posttraumatic stress disorder. *Trial Diplomacy Journal*, *9*(4), 17–20.

Lees-Haley, P. R. (1989a). Malingering emotional distress on the SCL-90-R: Toxic exposure and cancerphobia. *Psychological Reports*, *65*(3), 1203–1208.

Lees-Haley, P. R. (1989b). Malingering posttraumatic stress disorder on the MMPI. *Forensic Reports*, *2*, 89–91.

Lees-Haley, P. R. (1989c). Malingering traumatic mental disorder on the Beck Depression Inventory: Cancerphobia and toxic exposure. *Psychological Reports*, *65*(2), 623–626.

Lees-Haley, P. R. (1990). Malingering mental disorder on the Impact of Event (IES) Scale: Toxic exposure and cancerphobia. *Journal of Traumatic Stress*, *3*, 315–321.

Lees-Haley, P. R. (1992). Efficacy of MMPI-2 validity scales and MCMI-III modifier scales for detecting spurious PTSD claims: F, F-K, Fake Bad Scale, Ego Strength, Subtle-Obvious Subscales, DIS, and DEB. *Journal of Clinical Psychology*, *48*(5), 681–689.

Levit, H. I. (1989). Posttraumatic stress disorder in workers' compensation cases. *American Journal of Forensic Psychology*, *7*(1), 75–80.

Lipman, F. D. (1962). Malingering in personal injury cases. *Temple Law Quarterly*, *35*, 141–162.

Lynn, E. J., & Belza, M. (1984). Factitious posttraumatic stress disorder: The veteran who never got to Vietnam. *Hospital and Community Psychiatry*, *35*(7), 697–701.

Modlin, H. C. (1983). Traumatic neurosis and other injuries. *Psychiatric Clinics of North America*, *6*, 661–682.

Perconte, S. T., & Goreczny, A. J. (1990). Failure to detect fabricated posttraumatic stress disorder with the use of the MMPI in a clinical population. *American Journal of Psychiatry, 147*, 1057–1060.

Perr, I. N. (1992). Asbestos exposure and psychic injury: A review of 48 claims. *Bulletin of the American Academy of Psychiatry and the Law, 20*(4), 383–393.

Pitman, R. K., Sparr, L. F., Saunders, L. S., & McFarlane, A. C. (1996). Legal issues in PTSD. In B. van der Kolk, A. C. McFarlane, & L. Weisaeth (Eds.), *Traumatic stress: The effects of overwhelming experience on mind, body, and society*. New York: Guilford Press.

Resnick, P. J. (1984). The detection of malingered mental illness. *Behavioral Sciences and the Law, 2*(1), 21–38.

Resnick, P. (1988). Detection of malingering. In R. Rogers (Ed.), *Malingering and deception in clinical practice*. New York: Guilford Press.

Resnick, P. J. (1995). Guidelines for the evaluation of malingering in posttraumatic stress disorder. In R. I. Simon (Ed.), *Posttraumatic stress disorder in litigation: Guidelines for forensic assessment* (pp. 117–134). Washington, DC: American Psychiatric Press.

Rogers, R. (1984). Towards an empirical model of malingering and deception. *Behavioral Sciences and the Law, 2*(1), 93–111.

Rogers, R. (1997). *Clinical assessment of malingering and deception*. New York: Guilford Press.

Salloway, S., Southwick, S. M., & Sadowsky, M. (1990). Opiate withdrawal presenting as posttraumatic stress disorder. *Hospital and Community Psychiatry, 41*(6), 666–667.

Saunders, B., Arata, C., & Kilpatrick, D. (1990). Development of a crime-related posttraumatic stress disorder scale for women with the Symptom Checklist—90 Revised. *Journal of Traumatic Stress, 3*, 439–448.

Scurfield, R. M., & Wilson, J. P. (2003). Ask not for whom the bell tolls. *Journal of Trauma, Abuse and Violence, 4*(2), 112–127.

Simon, R. I. (1995). *Posttraumatic stress disorder in litigation*. Washington, DC: American Psychiatric Press.

Simon, R. I. (2000). *Posttraumatic stress disorder in litigation* (2nd ed.). Washington, DC: American Psychiatric Press.

Sparr, L. F., & Atkinson, R. M. (1986). Posttraumatic stress disorder as an insanity defense: Medicolegal quicksand. *American Journal of Psychiatry, 143*, 608–613.

Sparr, L. F., & Boehnlein, J. K. (1990). Posttraumatic stress disorder in tort actions: Forensic minefield. *Bulletin of the American Academy of Psychiatry and the Law, 18*, 283–302.

Sparr, L. F., & Pankratz, L. D. (1983). Factitious posttraumatic stress disorder. *American Journal of Psychiatry, 140,* 1016–1019.

Sparr, L. F., White, R., Friedman, M. J., & Wiles, D. B. (1994). Veterans psychiatric benefits: Enter courts and attorneys. *Bulletin of the American Academy of Psychiatry and the Law, 22*, 205–222.

Trimble, M. (1981). *The traumatic neuroses*. New York: Wiley.

Weisaeth, L. (1994). Psychological and psychiatric aspects of technological disasters. In R. J. Ursano, B. McCaughey, & C. S. Fullerson (Eds.), *Individual and community response to disaster: The structure of human chaos*. New York: Cambridge University Press.

Westin, J., & Daldy, T. M. (1991). Factitious PTSD masquerading childhood sexual abuse. *Journal of Clinical Psychiatry, 53,* 315–318.

Wilson, J. P. (Ed.). (1989). *Trauma transformation and healing*. New York: Brunner/Mazel.

Wilson, J. P. (1994a). The historical evolution of PTSD diagnostic criteria: From Freud to DSM-IV. *Journal of Traumatic Stress*, *7*, 681–689.

Wilson, J. P. (1994b). The need for an integrative theory of posttraumatic stress disorder. In M. B. Williams (Eds.), *Handbook of PTSD therapy* (pp. 11–29). New York: Greenwood.

Wilson, J. P. (2000). Trauma and the law: Traumatic symptoms and PTSD from a legal perspective. In Z. Solomon (Ed.), *Mental/psychological disability: Medical research, social and legal rehabilitation agreements*. Tel Aviv: Ministry of Defense Publication.

Wilson, J. P., Friedman, M. J., & Lindy, J. D. (2001). *Treating psychological trauma and PTSD*. New York: Guilford Press.

Wilson, J. P., Harel, Z., & Kahana, B. (1988). *Human adaptation to extreme stress: From Holocaust to Vietnam*. New York: Plenum Press.

Wilson, J. P., & Lindy, J. (1994). *Countertransference in the treatment of PTSD*. New York: Guilford Press.

Wilson, J. P., & Moran, T. (1997). Psychological trauma: PTSD and spirituality. *Journal of Psychology and Theology*, *26*(2), 168–178.

Wilson, J. P., Smith, W. K., & Johnson, S. K. (1985). A comparative analysis among various survivor groups. In C. R. Figley (Ed.), *Trauma and its wake: The study and treatment of posttraumatic stress disorder*. New York: Brunner/Mazel.

Wilson, J. P., & Walker, A. J. (1990). Toward an MMPI trauma profile. *Journal of Traumatic Stress*, *3*, 151–168.

Wilson, J. P., & Zigelbaum, S. D. (1986). PTSD and the disposition to criminal behavior. In C. R. Figley (Ed.), *Trauma and its wake* (Vol. II, pp. 305–321). New York: Brunner/Mazel.

Yudofsky, S. (1989). Malingering. *Handbook of psychiatry*. New York: Sanders.

Ziskin, J. (1984). Malingering of psychological disorders. *Behavioral Sciences and the Law, 2*(1).

Author Index

B

C

D

E

F

G

H

I

J

K

L

N

O

P

Q

R

S

T

U

V

X

Y

Z

Subject Index

E

Q

R

T